Essential
CLINICAL ANATOMY

THIRD EDITION

Essential
CLINICAL ANATOMY

THIRD EDITION

Keith L. Moore, PhD, FIAC, FRSM

Professor Emeritus, Division of Anatomy,
Department of Surgery
Former Chair of Anatomy and Associate Dean for Basic Medical Sciences
Faculty of Medicine, University of Toronto
Toronto, Ontario, Canada

Anne M. R. Agur, BSc (OT), MSc, PhD

Associate Professor, Division of Anatomy, Department of Surgery
Department of Physical Therapy and Department of Occupational Therapy
Division of Biomedical Communications, Institute of Communications and Culture
Institute of Medical Science, Graduate Department of Rehabilitation Science
University of Toronto
Toronto, Ontario, Canada

In collaboration with, and with content provided by,

Arthur F. Dalley II, PhD

Director, Medical Gross Anatomy and Anatomical Donations Program
Department of Cell and Developmental Biology
Vanderbilt University School of Medicine
Nashville, Tennessee, USA

With the expertise of,

Valerie Oxorn, BA, MA, MSc, BMC

Medical Illustrator
and

Marion E. Moore, BA

Developmental Assistant

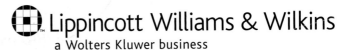

Philadelphia · Baltimore · New York · London
Buenos Aires · Hong Kong · Sydney · Tokyo

Acquisitions Editor: Crystal Taylor
Developmental Editor: Kathleen H. Scogna
Editorial Assistant: Ariel Winter
Marketing Manager: Valerie Shannahan
Production Editor: Paula C. Williams
Art Director: Doug Smock
Cover design by Valerie Oxorn and Doug Smock
Compositor: Maryland Composition, Inc.
Printer: R. R. Donnelley & Sons - Willard

351 West Camden Street
Baltimore, MD 21201

530 Walnut Street
Philadelphia, PA 19106

The publisher is not responsible (as a matter of product liability, negligence, or otherwise) for any injury resulting from any material contained herein. This publication contains information relating to general principles of medical care that should not be construed as specific instructions for individual patients. Manufacturers' product information and package inserts should be reviewed for current information, including contraindications, dosages, and precautions.

Printed in the United States of America

First Edition, 1995
Second Edition, 2002

Library of Congress Cataloging-in-Publication Data

Moore, Keith L.
  Essential clinical anatomy / Keith L. Moore, Anne M. R. Agur ; in collaboration with, and with content provided by, Arthur F. Dalley II ; with the expertise of medical illustrator Valerie Oxorn and the developmental assistance of Marion E. Moore. — 3rd ed.
      p. ; cm.
  Includes bibliographical references and index.
  ISBN 0-7817-6274-X (alk. paper)
  1. Human anatomy. 2. Human anatomy--Atlases.   I. Agur, A. M. R. II. Title.
  [DNLM: 1. Anatomy--Handbooks.   QS 39 M822e 2007]
  QM23.2.M673 2007
  611—dc22

                                                              2006003452

The publishers have made every effort to trace the copyright holders for borrowed material. If they have inadvertently overlooked any, they will be pleased to make the necessary arrangements at the first opportunity.

To purchase additional copies of this book, call our customer service department at **(800) 638-3030** or fax orders to **(301) 223-2320.** International customers should call **(301) 223-2300.**

Visit Lippincott Williams & Wilkins on the Internet: http://www.LWW.com. Lippincott Williams & Wilkins customer service representatives are available from 8:30 am to 6:00 pm, EST.

06 07 08 09 10
1 2 3 4 5 6 7 8 9 10

Preface

More than a decade has passed since the first edition of Essential Clinical Anatomy was published. As in the previous two editions, the main aim of the third edition is to provide a compact yet thorough textbook of clinical anatomy for students and practitioners in the health care professions and related disciplines. The presentations are concise and

- Provide a basic text of human anatomy for use in current health sciences curricula.
- Present an appropriate amount of clinically relevant anatomical material in a readable and interesting form.
- Place emphasis on clinical anatomy that is important for practice.
- Provide a concise clinically oriented anatomical reference for clinical courses in subsequent years.
- Serve as a rapid review when preparing for examinations, particularly those prepared by the National Board of Medical Examiners.
- Offer enough information for those wishing to refresh their knowledge of anatomy.

This edition has been thoroughly revised, keeping in mind the many invaluable comments received from students, colleagues, and reviewers. The larger trim size of the book has resulted in a new design that has larger figures, easier readability, and more white space to prevent crowding. The key features include the following:

- The revised text has a stronger clinical orientation.
- A significant number of new illustrations have been created, and many existing illustrations have been revised, recolored and resized. Most illustrations are in full color and are designed to highlight important facts and show their relationship to clinical medicine and surgery.
- More illustrated clinical correlations, known as "blue boxes," have been included to help with the understanding of the practical value of anatomy.
- New color photographs have been added in the surface anatomy sections to demonstrate the relationship between anatomy and physical examination, diagnosis and clinical procedures.
- New medical images (via radiography, computed tomography, magnetic resonance imaging, positron emission tomography, and ultrasonography) have been included, often with correclative illustrations. Current diagnostic imaging techniques demonstrate anatomy as it is often viewed clinically.
- Interactive case studies are included on the accompanying web site, providing further clinical integration of anatomy.

The terminology conforms with the Terminologica Anatomica (1998) approved by the International Federation of Anatomists (IFAA). The official English-equivalent terms are used throughout the present edition. When new terms are introduced, however, the Latin forms as used in Europe, Asia, and other parts of the world appear in parentheses. The roots and derivation of terms are included to help students understand the meaning of the terminology. Eponyms, although not endorsed by the IFAA, appear in parentheses to assist students during their clinical studies—for example, rectouterine pouch (pouch of Douglas).

The parent of this book, Clinically Oriented Anatomy (COA), is recommended as a resource for more detailed descriptions of human anatomy and its relationship and importance to medicine and surgery. Resources for instructors, including images exportable for PowerPoint presentations, are available—both specific to Essential Clinical Anatomy and through the institutional version of Dynamic Human Anatomy, which includes resources from the Lippincott Williams & Wilkins (LWW) portfolio of anatomy products.

We again welcome your comments and suggestions for improvements in future editions.

Keith L. Moore
Anne M. R. Agur
University of Toronto
Faculty of Medicine

Acknowledgments

We wish to thank the following colleagues who were invited by the publisher to assist with the development of this third edition.

- James H. Baker, PhD, Chairman, Department of Anatomy, Howard University, College of Medicine, Washington, D.C.
- Mary Lou Bareither, Clinical Assistant Professor, Department of Movement Sciences University of Illinois at Chicago, Chicago, Illinois
- Anne M. Burrows, PhD, Assistant Professor, Department of Physical Therapy Duquesne University, Pittsburgh, Pennsylvania
- Osvaldo Bustos, MD, Adjunct Associate Professor, Department of Anatomy and Cell Biology George Washington University School of Medicine and Health Sciences, Washington, D.C.
- Thomas J. Collins, PhD, Associate Professor, Department of Neuroscience and Cell Biology University of Texas Medical Branch, Galveston, Texas
- Patrick M. Coughlin, PhD, Professor, Department of Anatomy, Philadelphia College of Osteopathic Medicine, Philadelphia, Pennsylvania
- Frank J. Daly, PhD, Associate Professor, Department of Biological Sciences, University of New England, Biddeford, Maine
- Richard L. Doolittle, PhD, Professor and Head, Department of Medical Sciences, Rochester Institute of Technology, Rochester, New York
- Sherry A. Downie, PhD, Assistant Professor, Department of Anatomy and Structural Biology, Albert Einstein College of Medicine, Bronx, New York
- Kathleen L. Ehrhardt, MMS, PA-C, Academic Coordinator, Physician Assistant Department, DeSales University, Center Valley, Pennsylvania
- Mark L. Gabriele, PhD, Assistant Professor, Department of Biology, James Madison University, Harrisonburg, Virginia
- Stephen M. Gatesy, PhD, Associate Professor of Biology, Department of Ecology and Evolutionary Biology, Brown University, Providence, Rhode Island
- Peter Haase, Ph.D., Professor, Department of Anatomy and Cell Biology, University of Western Ontario, London, Ontario, Canada
- June A. Harris, MD, Associate Professor of Anatomy, Department of Basic Medical Sciences, Memorial University of Newfoundland, St. John's, Newfoundland, Canada
- Susan K. Hillman, MS, MA, ATC, PT, Associate Professor, Department of Human Anatomy A. T. Still University, Mesa, Arizona
- Alan W. Hrycyshyn, PhD, Professor, Division of Clinical Anatomy Department of Anatomy and Cell Biology, Schulick School of Medicine and Dentistry, University of Western Ontario, London, Ontario, Canada
- Adam Michael Jensen, BS, Third-year medical student, Arizona College of Osteopathic Medicine, Midwestern University, Glendale, Arizona
- Marjorie Johnson, PhD, Assistant Professor, Department of Anatomy and Cell Biology, Division of Clinical Anatomy, University of Western Ontario, London, Ontario, Canada
- Kathleen M. Klueber, PhD, Associate Professor, Department of Anatomical Sciences and Neurobiology, University of Louisville, Louisville, Kentucky
- Elisa M. Konieczko, PhD, Associate Professor, Department of Biology, Gannon University, Erie, Pennsylvania
- Randy J. Kulesza Jr., PhD, Assistant Professor of Anatomy, Department of Anatomy, Lake Erie College of Osteopathic Medicine, Erie, Pennsylvania
- Phil McClure PhD, PT, Associate Professor, Department of Physical Therapy, Arcadia University, Glenside, Pennsylvania
- Arezou Minooee, MS, Medical student, University of Vermont College of Medicine, Burlington, Vermont
- George W. Mulheron, PhD, Assistant Professor, Department of Neuroscience and Cell Biology, UMDNJ-Robert Wood Johnson Medical School, Piscataway, New Jersey
- Matthew B. R. Nessetti, PhD, MD, ABMP, Associate Professor, Department of Medicine International, University of the Health Sciences, Lincoln, Nebraska
- Bruce W. Newton, PhD, Associate Professor, Department of Neurobiology and Developmental Sciences, University of Arkansas for Medical Sciences, Little Rock, Arkansas
- Gary L. Nieder, PhD, Professor, Department of Neuroscience, Cell Biology and Physiology, Wright State University School of Medicine, Dayton, Ohio

- Akef Obeidat, MD PhD, Assistant Professor, Department of Cellular and Molecular Medicine, University of Ottawa, Ottawa, Ontario, Canada
- Larry J. Petterborg, PhD, Professor, School of Physical Therapy, Texas Woman's University, Dallas, Texas
- Kameelah Phillips, MSIV, Medical student, Keck School of Medicine at the University of Southern California, Los Angeles, California
- Dale Ritter, PhD, Morphology Course Coordinator, Department of Ecology and Evolutionary Biology, Brown University, Providence, Rhode Island
- Myra Bluestein Rufo, PhD, Senior Lecturer, Department of Anatomy and Cellular Biology, Tufts University School of Medicine, Boston, Massachusetts
- Tanyka Sam, Medical Student, SUNY at Buffalo—School of Medicine and Biomedical Sciences, Buffalo, New York
- David Seiden, PhD, Professor and Associate Dean, Department of Neuroscience and Cell Biology, UMDNJ-Robert Wood Johnson Medical School, Piscataway, New Jersey
- Shinil K. Shah, BS, Medical student, University of Medicine and Dentistry of New Jersey—School of Osteopathic Medicine, Stratford, New Jersey
- Lex C. Towns, PhD, Professor and Chairman, Department of Anatomy, Kirksville College of Osteopathic Medicine, Kirksville, Missouri
- R. Shane Tubbs, MS, PA-C, PhD, Assistant Professor, Department of Cell Biology, University of Alabama at Birmingham, Birmingham, Alabama
- Omair Vicaruddin, BSc, Medical student, University of Alberta Medical School, Edmonton, Alberta, Canada,
- Arthur Washburn, PhD, Assistant Professor, Department of Anatomy and Cell Biology, Temple University School of Medicine, Philadelphia, Pennsylvania

We would also like to acknowledge members of the Lippincott Williams & Wilkins Anatomy Advisory Board who provided feedback and suggestions for this edition.

In addition to reviewers, many people, some of them unknowingly, helped us by discussing parts of the manuscript and/or providing constructive criticisms of the text and illustrations in the present and previous editions:

- Dr. Peter Abrahams, Consultant Clinical Anatomist, University of Cambridge and examiner to the Royal College of Surgeons of Edinburgh.
- Dr. Robert D. Acland, Professor of Surgery/Microsurgery, Division of Plastic and Reconstructive Surgery, University of Louisville.
- Dr. Julian J. Baumel, Professor Emeritus of Biomedical Sciences, Creighton University School of Medicine.
- Dr. Edna Becker, Associate Professor of Medical Imaging, University of Toronto, Faculty of Medicine.
- Dr. Gerald D. Buckberg, Professor of Cardiac Surgery, David Geffen School of Medicine, University of California at Los Angeles.
- Dr. Donald R. Cahill, Professor of Anatomy (retired; formerly Chair), Mayo Medical School; former Editor-In-Chief of Clinical Anatomy.
- Dr. Joan Campbell, Assistant Professor of Medical Imaging, University of Toronto, Faculty of Medicine.
- Dr. Stephen W. Carmichael, Professor and Chair Emeritus of Anatomy, Mayo Medical School, Editor-In-Chief of Clinical Anatomy.
- Dr. Carmine D. Clemente, Professor of Anatomy and Orthopedic Surgery, University of California, Los Angeles School of Medicine.
- Dr. James D. Collins, Professor of Radiological Sciences, University of California, Los Angeles School of Medicine/Center for Health Sciences.
- Dr. Raymond F. Gasser, Professor of Anatomy, Louisiana State University School of Medicine.
- Dr. Ralph Ger, Professor of Anatomy and Structural Biology, Albert Einstein College of Medicine; Professor of Surgery, State University of New York at Stony Brook; Associate Chairman, Department of Surgery, Nassau County Medical Center.
- Dr. Douglas J. Gould, Associate Professor, University of Kentucky.
- Dr. Daniel O. Graney, Professor of Biological Structure, University of Washington School of Medicine.
- Dr. David G. Greathouse, Professor and Chair, Belmont University School of Physical Therapy.
- Dr. Masoom Haider, Assistant Professor of Medical Imaging, University of Toronto, Faculty of Medicine.
- Dr. John S. Halle, Professor, Belmont University School of Physical Therapy.
- Dr. Jennifer L. Halpern, Resident in Orthopedic Surgery and Rehabilitation, Vanderbilt University School of Medicine.
- Dr. Walter Kuchareczyk, Professor and Chair of Medical Imaging, University of Toronto Faculty of Medicine.
- Dr. Nirusha Lachman, Program Chair, Anatomy, Durban Institute of Technology.
- Dr. H. Wayne Lambert, Instructor, Cell and Developmental Biology and Cancer Biology, Vanderbilt University School of Medicine.
- Dr. Michael von Lüdinghausen, University Professor, Anatomy Institute, University of Würtzburg.
- Dr. Shirley McCarthy, Director of MRI, Department of Diagnostic Radiology, Yale University School of Medicine.
- Dr. Lillian Nanney, Professor of Plastic Surgery, Vanderbilt University School of Medicine.
- Dr. Todd R. Olson, Professor of Anatomy and Structural Biology, Albert Einstein College of Medicine.

- Dr. David Peck, Associate Professor of Anatomy and Neurobiology (retired), University of Kentucky School of Medicine.
- Dr. Wojciech Pawlina, Professor and Chair, Department of Anatomy, Mayo Medical School.
- Dr. T. V. N. Persaud, Professor of Human Anatomy and Cell Science, Faculties of Medicine & Dentistry, University of Manitoba.
- Dr. Thomas H. Quinn, Professor of Biomedical Sciences, Creighton University School of Medicine.
- Dr. George E. Salter, Professor of Anatomy, Department of Cell Biology, University of Alabama at Birmingham.
- Dr. Tatsuo Sato, Professor and Head (retired), Second Department of Anatomy, Tokyo Medical and Dental University Faculty of Medicine.
- Dr. Andreas H. Weiglein, Associate Professor, Institut fur Anatomie, Medical University Graz.
- Professor Colin P. Wendell-Smith, Department of Anatomy and Physiology, University of Tasmania.
- Dr. David G. Whitlock, Professor of Anatomy, University of Colorado Medical School.

We wish to acknowledge the dedication and effort of Kathleen Scogna, Senior Developmental Editor, in bringing this book to publication. Her suggestions, encouragement and advocacy helped lay a solid foundation for this edition.

All the new illustrations and changes to the existing artwork were done by Valerie Oxorn, a talented medical illustrator. We extend our sincere appreciation to her, not only for her illustrations but also for her design and creation of the cover of the book. Her meticulous work and insight into anatomy is invaluable. We also thank Kam Yu, who prepared the illustrations for the first edition. Other illustrations from the fifth edition of Clinically Oriented Anatomy and the eleventh edition of Grant's Atlas were prepared by Angela Cluer, Nina Kilpatrick, Stephen Mader, David Mazierski, Sari O'Sullivan, Bart Vallecoccia, J/B Woolsey Associates, and Rob Duckwall of Dragonfly Media Group. E. Anne Raynor, Senior Photographer, Vanderbilt Medical Art Group, did an excellent job photographing the surface anatomy models, working in conjunction with Dr. Arthur F. Dalley II and with the co-author (Anne M. Agur).

Our appreciation and thanks are extended to the editorial and production team at Lippincott Williams & Wilkins: Betty Sun, Executive Editor; Crystal Taylor, Acquisitions Editor; Ariel Winter, Editorial Assistant; Valerie Shannahan, Marketing Manager; Paula Williams, Production Editor; and Doug Smock, Art Director.

Keith L. Moore
Anne M. R. Agur

Contents

8 Neck / 583

9 Review of Cranial Nerves / 633

Clinical Correlation Blue Boxes

Introduction to Clinical Anatomy

Chapter Outline

Essential Clinical Anatomy relates the structure and function of the body to what is commonly required in the general practice of medicine, dentistry, and the allied health sciences. Because the number of details in anatomy overwhelms many beginning students, *Essential Clinical Anatomy* simplifies, correlates, and integrates the information so that it is easier to understand. The *clinical correlation boxes* (blue boxes) and *clinical case studies* (accompanying web site) illustrate the clinical applications of anatomy. The *surface anatomy boxes* (orange boxes) provide an understanding of what lies under the skin and the *medical imaging techniques* (green boxes) included throughout and at the end of each chapter) illustrate how anatomy is visualized clinically.

Approaches to Studying Anatomy

There are three main approaches to studying human gross anatomy: regional, systemic, and clinical (applied). In this introductory chapter, the systemic approach is used; in subsequent chapters, the clinical and regional approaches are used.

Regional anatomy is based on the organization of the body into parts: the head, neck, trunk (further subdivided into thorax, abdomen, pelvis/perineum, back) and paired upper and lower limbs. Emphasis is placed on the relationships of various systemic structures (e.g., muscles, nerves, and arteries) within the region (Fig. I.1). Each region is not an isolated part and must be put into the context of adjacent regions and of the body as a whole. Surface anatomy is an essential part of the regional approach, providing a knowledge of what structures are visible and/or palpable (perceptible to touch) in the living body at rest and in action. The physical examination of patients is the clinical extension of surface anatomy. In people with stab wounds, for example, the healthcare worker must be able to visualize the deep structures that might be injured.

Systemic anatomy is an approach to anatomical study organized by *organ systems* that work together to carry out complex functions. None of the organ systems functions in isolation. For example, much of the skeletal, articular, and muscular systems constitute the *locomotor system*. And although the structures directly responsible for locomotion are the muscles, bones, joints, and ligaments, other sys-

tems are involved as well. The arteries and veins of the circulatory system supply oxygen to them and remove waste from them, and the nerves of the nervous system stimulate them to act. Brief descriptions of the systems of the body and their fields of study (in parentheses) follow:

- The *integumentary system* (dermatology) consists of the skin (integument) and its appendages such as the hair and nails. The skin, an extensive sensory organ, forms a protective covering for the body.
- The *skeletal system* (osteology) consists of bones and cartilage. It provides support for the body and protects vital organs. The muscular system acts on the skeletal system to produce movements.
- The *articular system* (arthrology) consists of joints and their associated ligaments. It connects the bony parts of the skeletal system and provides the sites at which movements occur.
- The *muscular system* (myology) is composed of muscles that act (contract) to move or position parts of the body (e.g., the bones that articulate at joints).
- The *nervous system* (neurology) consists of the *central nervous system* (brain and spinal cord) and the *peripheral nervous system* (nerves and ganglia, together with their motor and sensory endings). The nervous system controls and coordinates the functions of the organ systems.
- The *circulatory system* (angiology) consists of the cardiovascular and lymphatic systems, which function in parallel to distribute fluids within the body.
  - The *cardiovascular system* (cardiology) consists of the heart and blood vessels that propel and conduct blood through the body.
  - The *lymphatic system* is a network of lymphatic vessels that withdraws excess tissue fluid (lymph) from the body's interstitial (intercellular) fluid compartment, filters it through lymph nodes, and returns it to the bloodstream.
- The *digestive* or *alimentary system* (gastroenterology) consists of the organs and glands associated with the ingestion, mastication (chewing), deglutition (swallowing), digestion, and absorption of food and the elimination of feces (solid wastes) after the nutrients have been absorbed.
- The *respiratory system* (pulmonology) consists of the air passages and lungs that supply oxygen and eliminate carbon dioxide. The control of air flow through the system produces tone, which is further modified into speech.
- The *urinary system* (urology) consists of the kidneys, ureters, urinary bladder, and urethra, which filter blood and subsequently produce, transport, store, and intermittently excrete liquid waste (urine).
- The *reproductive system* (gynecology for females; andrology for males) consists of the gonads (ovaries and testes) that produce oocytes (eggs) and sperms and the other genital organs concerned with reproduction.

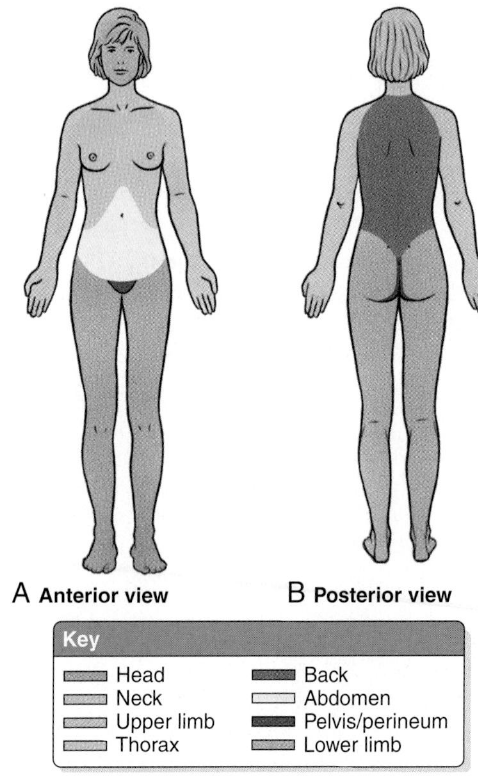

A Anterior view   **B** Posterior view

Key	
Head	Back
Neck	Abdomen
Upper limb	Pelvis/perineum
Thorax	Lower limb

Figure I.1. Anatomical position and regions of body.

- The *endocrine system* (endocrinology) consists of discrete ductless glands, (e.g., thyroid gland) as well as cells of the intestine and blood vessel walls and specialized nerve endings that secrete hormones. Hormones are distributed by the cardiovascular system to reach receptor organs in all parts of the body. These glands influence metabolism and coordinate and regulate other processes (e.g., the menstrual cycle).

Clinical (applied) anatomy emphasizes aspects of the structure and function of the body important in the practice of medicine, dentistry, and the allied health sciences. It encompasses both the regional and the systemic approaches to studying anatomy and stresses clinical application.

Anatomicomedical Terminology

Anatomy has an international vocabulary that is the foundation of medical terminology. This nomenclature enables precise communication among health professionals worldwide as well as among scholars in basic and applied health sciences. Although *eponyms* (names of structures derived from the names of people) are not used in official anatomical terminology, those commonly used by clinicians appear in parentheses throughout this book to reduce ambiguity and misunderstanding. Similarly, formerly used terms appear in parentheses on first mention—for example, internal thoracic artery (internal mammary artery). The terminology in this book conforms with the *Terminologia Anatomica: International Anatomical Terminology* (Federative Committee on Anatomical Terminology, 1998).

Anatomical Position

All anatomical descriptions are expressed in relation to the anatomical position (Fig. I.1) to ensure that the descriptions are not ambiguous. The anatomical position refers to people—regardless of the actual position they may be in—as if they were standing erect, with their:

- Head, eyes (gaze), and toes directed anteriorly (forward).
- Upper limbs by the sides with the palms facing anteriorly.
- Lower limbs close together with the feet parallel and the toes directed anteriorly.

Anatomical Planes

Anatomical descriptions are based on four imaginary planes that intersect the body in the anatomical position (Fig. I.2). There are many sagittal, frontal, and transverse planes, but there is only one median plane.

- **Median (median sagittal) plane** is the vertical plane passing longitudinally through the center of the body, dividing it into right and left halves.

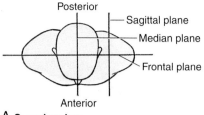

A Superior view

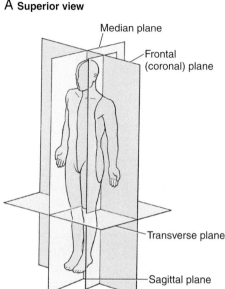

B Anterolateral view

Figure I.2. Planes of body.

- **Sagittal planes** are vertical planes passing through the body *parallel to the median plane*. It is helpful to give a point of reference to indicate the position of a specific plane—for example, a sagittal plane through the midpoint of the clavicle. A plane parallel and near the median plane may be referred to as a *paramedian plane*.
- **Frontal (coronal) planes** are vertical planes passing through the body *at right angles to the median plane*, dividing it into anterior (front) and posterior (back) portions—for example, a frontal plane through the heads of the mandible.
- **Transverse planes** are planes passing through the body *at right angles to the median and frontal planes*. A transverse plane divides the body into superior (upper) and inferior (lower) parts—for example, a transverse plane through the umbilicus. Radiologists refer to transverse planes as *transaxial planes* or simply *axial planes*.

Terms of Relationship and Comparison

Various adjectives, arranged as pairs of opposites, describe the relationship of parts of the body in the anatomical position and compare the position of two structures relative to each other. These pairs of adjectives are explained and illustrated in Table I.1 For example, the eyes are superior to the nose, whereas the nose is inferior to the eyes.

Table I.1 Commonly Used Terms of Relationship and Comparison

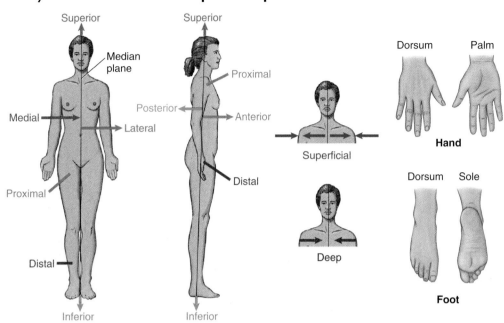

Term	Meaning	Usage
Superior (cranial)	Nearer to head	Heart is superior to stomach
Inferior (caudal)	Nearer to feet	Stomach is inferior to heart
Anterior (ventral)	Nearer to front	Sternum is anterior to heart
Posterior (dorsal)	Nearer to back	Kidneys are posterior to intestine
Medial	Nearer to median plane	Fifth digit (little finger) is on medial side of hand
Lateral	Farther from median plane	First digit (thumb) is on lateral side of hand
Proximal	Nearer to trunk or point of origin (e.g., of a limb)	Elbow is proximal to wrist; proximal part of artery is its beginning
Distal	Farther from trunk or point of origin (e.g., of a limb)	Wrist is distal to elbow; distal part of lower limb is foot
Superficial	Nearer to or on surface	Muscles of arm are superficial to its bone (humerus)
Deep	Farther from surface	Humerus is deep to arm muscles
Dorsum	Dorsal surface of hand or foot	Veins are visible in dorsum of hand
Palm	Palmar surface of hand	Skin creases are visible on palm
Sole	Plantar surface of foot	Skin is thick on sole of foot

Combined terms describe intermediate positional arrangements:

- **Inferomedial** means nearer to the feet and closer to the median plane—for example, the anterior parts of the ribs run inferomedially.
- **Superolateral** means nearer to the head and farther from the median plane.

Proximal and **distal** are directional terms used when describing positions—for example, whether structures are nearer to the trunk or point of origin (i.e., proximal). **Dorsum** refers to the superior or dorsal (back) surface of any part that protrudes anteriorly from the body, such as

the *dorsum of the foot, hand, penis, or tongue.* It is easier to understand why these surfaces are considered dorsal if one thinks of a quadripedal plantigrade animal that walks on its soles, such as a dog. The **sole** indicates the inferior aspect or bottom of the foot, much of which is in contact with the ground when standing barefoot. The **palm** refers to the flat of the hand, excluding the five digits, and is the opposite of the dorsum of the hand.

Terms of Laterality

Paired structures having right and left members (e.g., the kidneys) are **bilateral**, whereas those occurring on one side only (e.g., the spleen) are **unilateral. Ipsilateral** means occurring on the same side of the body; the right thumb and right great toe are ipsilateral, for example. **Contralateral** means occurring on the opposite side of the body; the right hand is contralateral to the left hand.

Terms of Movement

Various terms describe movements of the limbs and other parts of the body (Table I.21). Although most movements take place at joints where two or more bones or cartilages articulate with one another, several non-skeletal structures exhibit movement (e.g., tongue, lips, and eyelids). Movements taking place at joints are described relative to the axes around which the part of the body moves and the plane in which the movement takes place—for example, flexion and extension of the shoulder take place in the sagittal plane around a frontal (coronal) axis.

Anatomical Variations

Although anatomy books describe the structure of the body observed in most people (i.e., the most common pattern), the structure of individuals varies considerably in the details. Students are often frustrated because the bodies they are examining or dissecting do not conform to the atlas or textbook they are using. Students should expect anatomical variations when dissecting or studying prosected specimens. The bones of the skeleton vary among themselves not only in their basic shape but also in the details of surface structure. There is also a wide variation in the size, shape, and form of the attachment of muscles. Similarly, there is variation in the method of division of vessels and nerves, and the greatest variation occurs in veins. Apart from racial and sexual differences, humans exhibit considerable genetic variation. Approximately 3% of newborns show one or more significant congenital anomalies (Moore and Persaud, 2003).

Integumentary System

The skin, the largest organ of the body, is readily accessible, and is one of the best indicators of general health (Swartz, 2001) *The skin provides*

- *Protection* for the body from environmental effects, such as abrasions and harmful substances.
- *Containment* of the tissues, organs, and vital substances of the body, preventing dehydration.
- *Heat regulation* through sweat glands, blood vessels, and fat deposits.
- *Sensation* (e.g., pain) by way of superficial nerves and their sensory endings.
- *Synthesis and storage* of vitamin D.

The skin consists of a superficial cellular layer, the epidermis, which creates a tough protective outer surface, and a basal (deep) regenerative and pigmented connective tissue layer, the dermis (Fig. I.3).

The **epidermis** is a keratinized stratified (layered) epithelium with a tough outer surface composed of keratin (a fibrous protein). The outer layer of the epidermis is continuously "shed" or rubbed away with replacement of new cells from the basal layer. This process renews the epidermis of the entire body every 25–45 days. The epidermis is avascular (no blood vessels or lymphatics) and is nourished by the vessels in the underlying dermis. The skin is supplied by afferent nerve endings that are sensitive to touch, irritation (pain), and temperature. Most nerve terminals are in the dermis, but a few penetrate the epidermis.

The **dermis** is formed by a dense layer of interlacing *collagen and elastic fibers*. These fibers provide skin tone and account for the strength and toughness of the skin. The pattern of collagen fibers in a particular region determines the characteristic tension lines (cleavage lines) and wrinkle lines in the skin. The deep layer of the dermis contains hair follicles, with their associated smooth arrector (L. *arrector pili*) muscles and sebaceous glands. Contraction of the **arrector muscles** erects the hairs (causing goose bumps), thereby compressing the sebaceous glands and helping them secrete their oily product onto the skin. Other integumentary structures include the hair, nails, mammary glands, and the enamel of teeth.

The **subcutaneous tissue** (superficial fascia) is composed of loose connective tissue and fat. Located between the dermis and underlying deep fascia, the subcutaneous tissue contains the deepest parts of the sweat glands, the blood and lymphatic vessels, and cutaneous nerves that are distributed to the skin. The subcutaneous tissue provides for most of the body's fat storage, so its thickness varies greatly, depending on nutritional state. **Skin ligaments** (L. *retinacula cutis*), consisting of numerous small fibrous bands, extend through the subcutaneous tissue and attach the deep surface of the dermis to the underlying deep fascia. The length and density of these ligaments determine the mobility of the skin over deep structures.

The **deep fascia** is a dense, organized connective tissue layer, devoid of fat, that envelopes most of the body deep to the skin and subcutaneous tissue. Extensions from its internal surface:

- Invest deeper structures, such as individual muscles and neurovascular bundles (**investing fascia**).
- Divide muscles into groups or compartments (**intermuscular septa**).
- Lie between the musculoskeletal walls and the serous membranes lining body cavities (**subserous fascia**).

The deep fascia also forms **retinacula**, which hold tendons in place during joint movement, and **bursae** (closed

Table I.2 Terms of Movement

Flexion means bending of a part or decreasing the angle between body parts. **Extension** means straightening a part or increasing the angle between body parts. Except for the thumb, flexion and extension movements are in the sagittal plane.

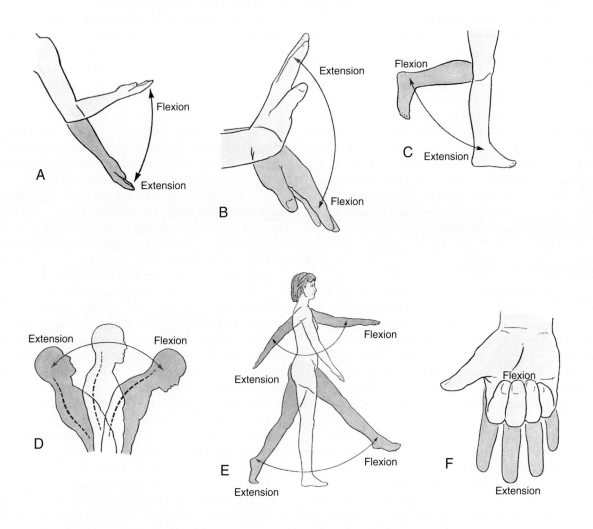

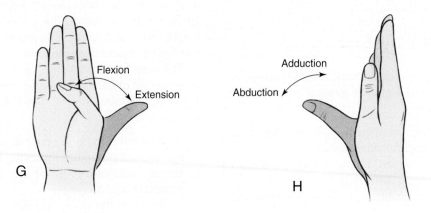

Table I.2 Terms of Movement (*continued*)

Abduction means moving away from the median plane of the body in the frontal plane. **Adduction** means moving toward the median plane of the body in the frontal (coronal) plane. When referring to the digits (fingers and toes), abduction means spreading them, and adduction means drawing them together. **Rotation** means moving a part of the body around its long axis. *Medial rotation* turns the anterior surface medially, and *lateral rotation* turns this surface laterally. **Circumduction** is the circular movement of the limbs, or parts of them, combining in sequence the movements of flexion, extension, abduction, and adduction. **Pronation** is a medial rotation of the forearm and hand so that the palm faces posteriorly. **Supination** is a lateral rotation of the forearm and hand so that the palm faces anteriorly, as in the anatomical position. **Eversion** means turning the sole of foot outward. **Inversion** means turning the sole of foot inward. **Protrusion** (protraction) means to move the jaw anteriorly. **Retrusion** (retraction) means to move the jaw posteriorly. **Elevation** raises or moves a part superiorly. **Depression** lowers or moves a part inferiorly.

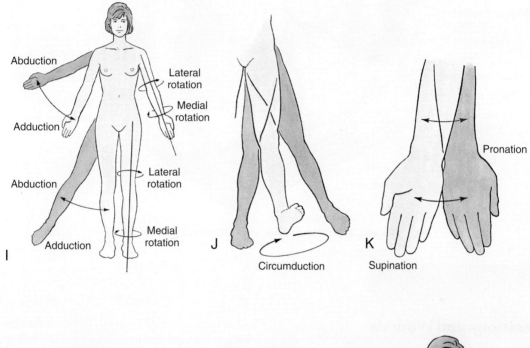

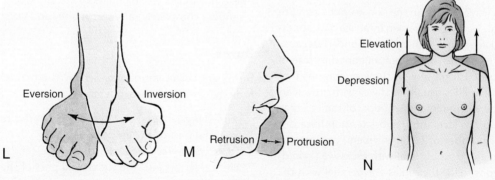

sacs containing fluid), which prevent friction and enable structures to move freely over another.

In living people, **fascial planes** (interfascial and intrafascial) are potential spaces between adjacent fascias or fascia-lined structures. During operations, surgeons take advantage of these planes, separating structures to create actual spaces that allow access to deeply placed structures. These planes are often fused in the embalmed cadaver.

Skeletal System

The skeleton of the body is composed of bones and cartilages and has two main parts (Fig. I.4):

- The **axial skeleton** consists of the bones of the head (cranium), neck (cervical vertebrae), and trunk (ribs, sternum, vertebrae, and sacrum).

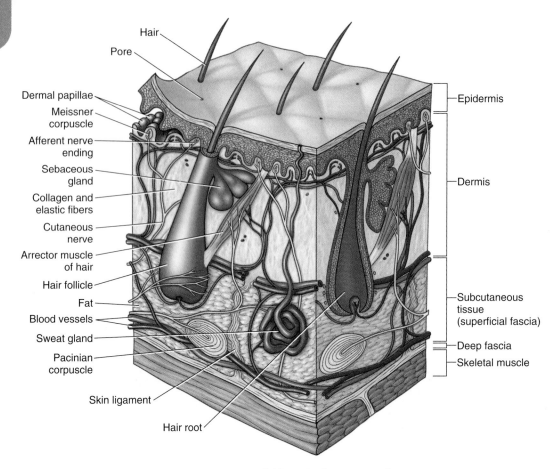

Hair

Pore

Dermal papillae

Meissner corpuscle

Afferent nerve ending

Sebaceous gland

Collagen and elastic fibers

Cutaneous nerve

Arrector muscle of hair

Hair follicle

Fat

Blood vessels

Sweat gland

Pacinian corpuscle

Skin ligament

Hair root

Epidermis

Dermis

Subcutaneous tissue (superficial fascia)

Deep fascia

Skeletal muscle

Figure I.3. **Structure of skin and subcutaneous tissue.**

Skin Incisions and Wounds

Tension lines (cleavage lines) in the skin keep the skin under tension. Stab wounds in the skin by an ice pick, for example, are usually slitlike rather than rounded because the pick splits the dermis in the predominant direction of the collagen fibers. Lacerations or surgical incisions that parallel the tension lines usually heal well with little scarring because there is minimal disruption of the collagen fibers. An incision or laceration across tension lines disrupts a greater number of collagen fibers, causing the wound to gape and possibly heal with excessive (keloid) scarring. Surgeons make their incisions parallel with the tension lines when other considerations (e.g., adequate exposure, avoiding nerves) are not of greater importance.

Stretch Marks in Skin

The collagen and elastic fibers in the dermis form a tough, flexible meshwork of tissue. The skin can distend considerably when the abdomen enlarges, as during pregnancy, for example. However, if stretched too far, it can result in damage to the collagen fibers in the dermis. Bands of thin wrinkled skin, initially red, become purple and later white. Stretch marks appear on the abdomen, buttocks, thighs, and breasts during pregnancy. These marks also form in obese individuals. Stretch marks generally fade (but never disappear completely) after pregnancy and weight loss.

Burns

Burns are tissue injuries caused by thermal, electrical, radioactive, or chemical agents.

- In *first-degree burns,* the damage is limited to the superficial part of the epidermis.
- In *second-degree burns,* the damage extends through the epidermis into the superficial part of the dermis. However, except for their most superficial parts, the sweat glands and hair follicles are not damaged and can provide the source of replacement cells for the basal layer of the epidermis.
- In *third-degree burns,* the entire epidermis, dermis, and perhaps underlying muscle are damaged. A minor degree of healing may occur at the edges, but the open ulcerated portions require skin grafting.

The extent of the burn (percent of total body surface affected) is generally more significant than the degree (severity of depth) in estimating its effect on the victim.

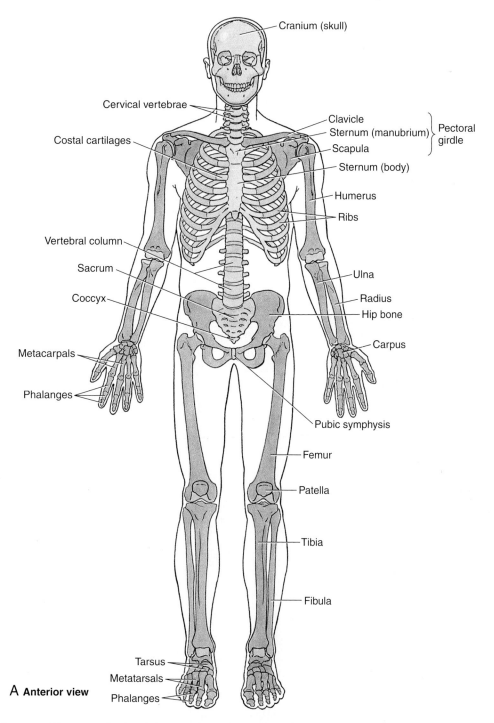

Cranium (skull)

Cervical vertebrae

Costal cartilages

Clavicle
Sternum (manubrium) ⎫ Pectoral
Scapula   ⎬ girdle
Sternum (body)

Humerus

Ribs

Vertebral column

Sacrum

Coccyx

Ulna

Radius

Hip bone

Carpus

Metacarpals

Phalanges

Pubic symphysis

Femur

Patella

Tibia

Fibula

Tarsus

Metatarsals

Phalanges

A **Anterior view**

Figure I.4. Skeletal system. The appendicular skeleton is shown in *purple* to distinguish it from the axial skeleton (*yellow*). Cartilages are colored *blue*.

• The **appendicular skeleton** consists of the bones of the limbs, including those forming the pectoral (shoulder) and pelvic girdles.

Bone, a living tissue, is a highly specialized, hard form of connective tissue that makes up most of the skeleton and is the chief supporting tissue of the body. *Bones provide*

• Protection for vital structures.
• Support for the body.
• The mechanical basis for movement.

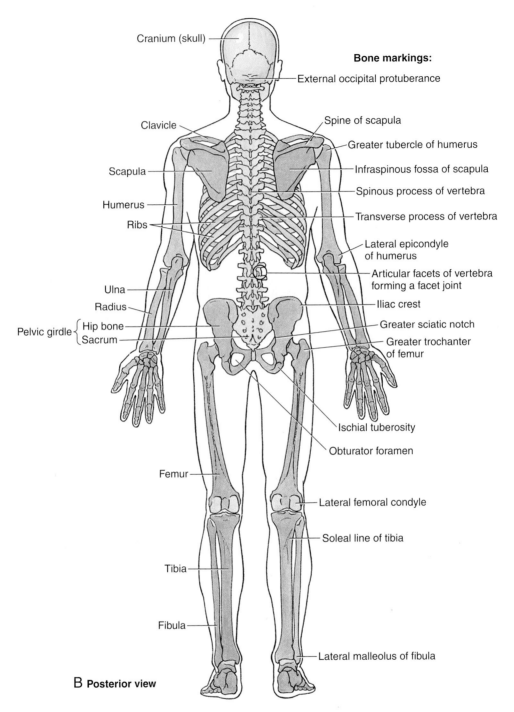

Bone markings:

Cranium (skull)

External occipital protuberance

Clavicle

Spine of scapula

Greater tubercle of humerus

Scapula

Infraspinous fossa of scapula

Spinous process of vertebra

Humerus

Ribs

Transverse process of vertebra

Lateral epicondyle of humerus

Articular facets of vertebra forming a facet joint

Ulna

Radius

Iliac crest

Pelvic girdle { Hip bone Sacrum

Greater sciatic notch

Greater trochanter of femur

Ischial tuberosity

Obturator foramen

Femur

Lateral femoral condyle

Soleal line of tibia

Tibia

Fibula

Lateral malleolus of fibula

B Posterior view

Figure I.4. Skeletal system. *(continued)*

- Storage for salts (e.g., calcium).
- A continuous supply of new blood cells (produced by the marrow within many bones).

Cartilage is a resilient, semirigid, avascular form of connective tissue that forms parts of the skeleton where more flexibility is necessary (e.g., the costal cartilages that attach the ribs to the sternum). The articulating surfaces of bones participating in a synovial joint are capped with **articular cartilage**, which provides smooth, low-friction gliding surfaces for free movement of the articulating bones (e.g., blue areas of the humerus in Fig. I.4A). Cartilage is avascular and is, therefore, nourished by diffusion. The proportion of bone and cartilage in the skeleton changes as the body grows; the younger a person is, the greater the contribution of cartilage. The bones of a newborn infant are soft and flexible because they are mostly composed of cartilage.

The fibrous connective tissue covering that surrounds bone is **periosteum**; that surrounding cartilage elements, excluding articular cartilage, is **perichondrium** (Fig. I.7). The periosteum and perichondrium help nourish the tissue, are capable of laying down more cartilage or bone (particularly during fracture healing), and provide an interface for attachment of tendons and ligaments.

Bones

There are two types of bone: **compact** and **spongy** (trabecular or cancellous). The differences between these types of bone depend on the relative amount of solid matter and the number and size of the spaces they contain (Fig. I.5). All bones have a superficial thin layer of compact bone around a central mass of spongy bone, except where the latter is replaced by a **medullary (marrow) cavity**. Within this cavity of adult bones, and between the spicules of spongy bone, blood cells and platelets are formed. The architecture of spongy and compact bone varies according to function.

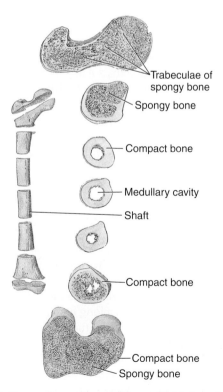

Trabeculae of spongy bone

Spongy bone

Compact bone

Medullary cavity

Shaft

Compact bone

Compact bone

Spongy bone

Figure I.5. Transverse sections of femur (thigh bone). Observe the trabeculae (tension and pressure lines) related to the weight-bearing function of this bone.

Compact bone provides strength for weight bearing. In long bones, designed for rigidity and attachment of muscles and ligaments, the amount of compact bone is greatest near the middle of the shaft (body) of the bone, where it is liable to buckle. Living bones have some elasticity (flexibility) and great rigidity (hardness).

CLASSIFICATION OF BONES

Bones are classified according to their shape (Fig. I.4).

- **Long bones** are tubular structures (e.g., humerus in the arm; phalanges in the fingers).
- **Short bones** are cuboidal and are found only in the ankle (tarsus) and wrist (carpus).
- **Flat bones** usually serve protective functions (e.g., those of the cranium protect the brain).
- **Irregular bones,** such as those in the face, have various shapes other than long, short, or flat.
- **Sesamoid bones** (e.g., patella, or kneecap) develop in certain tendons. These bones protect the tendons from excessive wear and often change the angle of the tendons as they pass to their attachments.

BONE MARKINGS

Bone markings appear wherever tendons, ligaments, and fascia are attached or where arteries lie adjacent to or enter bones. Other formations occur in relation to the passage of a tendon (often to direct the tendon or improve its leverage) or to control the type of movement occurring at a joint. *Some markings and features of bones are as follows* (Fig. I.4B):

- **Condyle:** rounded articular area (e.g., condyles of the femur).
- **Crest:** ridge of bone (e.g., iliac crest).
- **Epicondyle:** eminence superior to a condyle (e.g., epicondyles of the humerus).

Heterotopic Bones

Bones sometimes form in soft tissues where they are not normally present. Horse riders often develop heterotopic bones in their thighs or buttocks (*rider's bones*), probably because of chronic muscle strain resulting in small hemorrhagic (bloody) areas that undergo calcification and eventual ossification.

- **Facet:** smooth flat area, usually covered with cartilage, where a bone articulates with another bone (e.g., articular facets of a vertebra).
- **Foramen:** passage through a bone (e.g., obturator foramen).
- **Fossa:** hollow or depressed area (e.g., infraspinous fossa of the scapula).
- **Line:** linear elevation (e.g., soleal line of the tibia).
- **Malleolus:** rounded prominence (e.g., lateral malleolus of the fibula).
- **Notch:** indentation at the edge of a bone (e.g., greater sciatic notch in the posterior border of the hip bone).
- **Process:** projecting spine-like part (e.g., spinous process of a vertebra).
- **Protuberance:** projection of bone (e.g., external occipital protuberance of the cranium).
- **Spine:** thorn-like process (e.g., spine of the scapula).
- **Trochanter:** large blunt elevation (e.g., greater trochanter of the femur).

Trauma to Bone and Bone Changes

Bones are living organs that hurt when injured, bleed when fractured, remodel in relationship to stress placed on them, and change with age. Like other organs, bones have blood vessels, lymphatic vessels, and nerves, and they may become diseased. Unused bones, such as in a paralyzed or immobilized limb, *atrophy* (decrease in size). Bone may be absorbed, which occurs in the mandible after teeth are extracted. Bones *hypertrophy* (enlarge) when they have increased weight to support for a long period.

Trauma to a bone may *fracture* (break) it. For a fracture to heal properly, the broken ends must be brought together approximating their normal position (*reduction of fracture*). During bone healing, the surrounding *fibroblasts* (connective tissue cells) proliferate and secrete collagen that forms a *collar of callus* to hold the bones together. Remodeling of bone occurs in the fracture area, and the callus calcifies. Eventually, the callus is resorbed and replaced by bone.

Osteoporosis

As people age, both the organic and the inorganic components of bone decrease, often resulting in *osteoporosis,* a reduction in the quantity of bone, or atrophy of skeletal tissue. The bones become brittle, lose their elasticity, and fracture easily.

- **Tubercle:** small raised eminence (e.g., greater tubercle of the humerus).
- **Tuberosity:** large rounded elevation (e.g., ischial tuberosity).

BONE DEVELOPMENT

All bones are derived from **mesenchyme** (embryonic connective tissue) by one of two different processes: intramembranous ossification (directly from mesenchyme) and endochondral ossification (from cartilage derived from mesenchyme). The histology of a bone is the same either way.

- In **intramembranous ossification** (membranous bone formation), mesenchymal models of bone form during the embryonic period, and direct ossification of the mesenchyme begins in the fetal period.
- In **endochondral ossification** (cartilaginous bone formation), cartilage models of bones form from mesenchyme during the fetal period, and bone subsequently replaces most of the cartilage.

The following brief description of endochondral ossification explains how long bones grow. The mesenchymal cells condense and differentiate into *chondroblasts,* dividing cells in growing cartilage tissue, thereby forming a *cartilaginous bone model* (Fig. I.6A). In the midregion of the bone model, the cartilage *calcifies* (becomes impregnated with calcium salts), and *periosteal capillaries* (capillaries from the fibrous sheath surrounding the model) grow into the calcified cartilage of the bone model and supply its interior. These blood vessels, together with associated *osteogenic* (bone-forming) cells, form a **periosteal bud.** The capillaries initiate the **primary ossification center,** so named because the bone tissue it forms replaces most of the cartilage in the shaft (body) of the bone model. The shaft of a bone ossified from a primary ossification center is the **diaphysis,** which grows as the bone develops.

Most **secondary ossification centers** appear in other parts of the developing bone after birth; the parts of a bone ossified from these centers are **epiphyses.** Epiphysial arteries grow into the developing cavities with associated osteogenic cells. The flared part of the diaphysis nearest the epiphysis is the **metaphysis** (Fig. I.6B). For growth to continue, the bone formed from the primary center in the diaphysis does not fuse with that formed from the secondary centers in the epiphyses until the bone reaches its adult size. Thus, during growth of a long bone, cartilaginous **epiphysial plates** intervene between the diaphysis and the epiphyses. These growth plates are eventually replaced by bone at each of its two sides, diaphysial and epiphysial. When this occurs, bone growth ceases, and the diaphysis fuses with the epiphyses. The seam formed during this process (*synostosis*) is dense and appears in radiographs as an **epiphysial line** (Fig. I.7). The epiphysial fusion of bones occurs progressively from puberty to maturity.

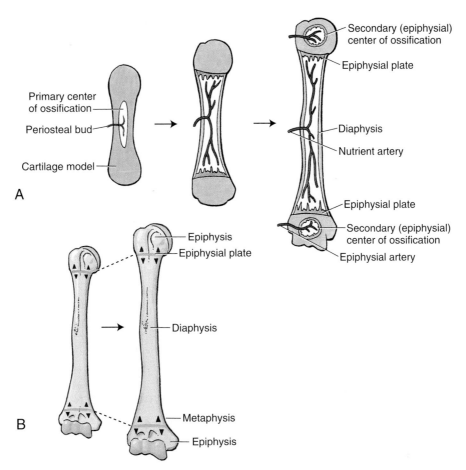

Figure I.6. Growth of long bone. A. The formation of primary and secondary centers of ossification is shown. **B.** Growth in the length of the bone occurs on both sides of the epiphysial plates (*arrowheads*).

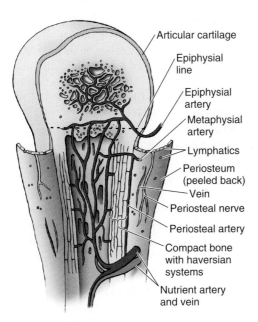

Figure I.7. Vasculature and innervation of long bone. The bulk of compact bone is composed of haversian systems (osteons). The haversian canal in the system houses one or two small blood vessels for nourishing the osteocytes (bone cells).

VASCULATURE AND INNERVATION OF BONES

Bones are richly supplied with blood vessels (Fig. I.7). The arterial supply is from:

- **Nutrient arteries** (one or more per bone) that arise outside the periosteum, pass through the shaft of a long bone via *nutrient foramina,* and split in the medullary cavity into longitudinal branches. These vessels supply the bone marrow, spongy bone, and deeper portions of the compact bone.
- Small branches from the **periosteal arteries** of the periosteum supply most of the compact bone. Consequently, if the periosteum is removed, the bone will die.
- **Metaphysial** and **epiphysial arteries** supply the ends of the bones. These vessels arise mainly from the arteries that supply the joints.

Veins accompany arteries through the *nutrient foramina.* Many large veins leave through foramina near the articular ends of the bones. **Lymphatic vessels** are abundant in the periosteum.

Accessory Bones

Accessory (supernumerary) bones develop when additional ossification centers appear and form extra bones. Many bones develop from several centers of ossification, and the separate parts normally fuse. Sometimes one of these centers fails to fuse with the main bone, giving the appearance of an extra bone; however, careful study shows that the apparent extra bone is a missing part of the main bone. Circumscribed areas of bone called *sutural (wormian) bones* are often seen along the sutures of the cranium where the flat bones come together. It is important to know that accessory bones are common in the foot to avoid mistaking them for bone fragments in medical images (e.g., radiographs).

Assessment of Bone Age

Knowledge of the sites where ossification centers occur, the times of their appearance, the rate at which they grow, and the times of fusion (*synostosis*) of the sites is used to determine the age of a person in clinical medicine, forensic science, and anthropology. The main criteria for determining bone age are (1) the appearance of calcified material in the diaphysis and/or epiphyses and (2) the disappearance of the dark line representing the epiphysial plate (absence of this line indicates epiphysial fusion has occurred; fusion occurs at specific times for each epiphysis). The fusion of epiphyses with the diaphysis occurs 1–2 years earlier in girls than in boys. Determination of bone age can be helpful in predicting adult height in early- or late-maturing adolescents and in establishing the approximate age of human skeletal remains in medicolegal cases.

Nerves accompany the blood vessels supplying bones. The **periosteum** is richly supplied with sensory nerves—**periosteal nerves**—that carry pain fibers. The periosteum is especially sensitive to tearing or tension, which explains the acute pain from bone fractures. Bone itself is relatively sparsely supplied with sensory endings. Within bones, *vasomotor nerves* cause constriction or dilation of blood vessels, regulating blood flow through the bone marrow.

Avascular Necrosis

Loss of blood supply to an epiphysis or other parts of a bone results in death of bone tissue, or *avascular necrosis* (G. *nekrosis,* deadness). After every fracture, small areas of adjacent bone undergo necrosis. In some fractures, avascular necrosis of a large fragment of bone may occur.

Joints

A joint is an articulation, or the place of union or junction between two or more rigid components (bones, cartilages, or even parts of the same bone). Joints exhibit a variety of forms and functions. Some joints have no movement; others allow only slight movement, and some are freely movable, such as the glenohumeral (shoulder) joint.

CLASSIFICATION OF JOINTS

The three types of joints (fibrous, cartilaginous, and synovial) are classified according to the manner or type of material by which the articulating bones are united (Table I.3):

- The articulating bones of **fibrous joints** are united by fibrous tissue. The amount of movement occurring at a fibrous joint depends in most cases on the length of the fibers uniting the articular bones. A **syndesmosis** type of fibrous joint unites the bones with a sheet of fibrous tissue, either a ligament or fibrous membrane. Consequently, this type of joint is partially movable. A **gomphosis** (*dentoalveolar syndesmosis*) is a type of fibrous joint in which a peg-like fibrous process stabilizes a tooth and provides proprioceptive information (e.g., about how hard we are chewing or clenching our teeth).

- The articulating structures of **cartilaginous joints** are united by hyaline cartilage or fibrocartilage. *Primary cartilaginous joints (synchondroses)* are united by hyaline cartilage. These joints permit growth of the length of the bone and allow slight bending during early life, until the epiphysial plate converts to bone and the epiphyses fuse with the diaphysis. *Secondary cartilaginous joints (symphyses)* are strong, slightly mobile joints, united by fibrocartilage.

- The articular cavity of **synovial joints** is a potential space that contains a small amount of synovial fluid. Synovial fluid serves the dual function of nourishing the articular cartilage and lubricating the joint surfaces. The distinguishing features of a synovial joint are illustrated and

Table I.3 Types of Joints

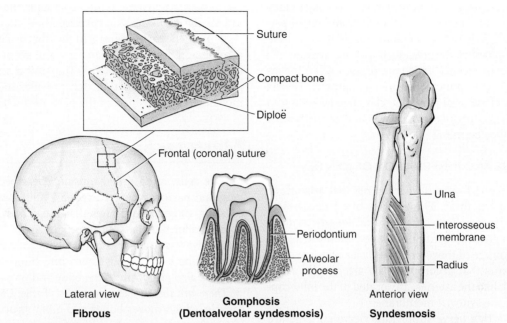

Fibrous
Lateral view

Gomphosis
(Dentoalveolar syndesmosis)

Syndesmosis
Anterior view

In **fibrous joints,** articulating bones are joined by fibrous tissue. Sutures of the cranium are fibrous joints in which bones are close together and united by fibrous tissue, often interlocking along a wavy line. Flat bones consist of two plates of compact bone separated by spongy bone and marrow (diploë). In a **syndesmosis joint,** the bones are joined by a sheet of fibrous tissue (e.g., the interosseous membrane joining the forearm bones). In a **gomphosis joint,** a peg-like process fits into a socket (e.g., the articulation between the root of the tooth and the alveolar process). Fibrous tissue, the periodontium, anchors the tooth in the socket.

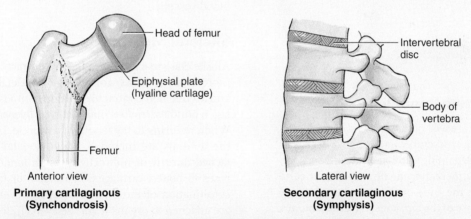

Primary cartilaginous
(Synchondrosis)
Anterior view

Secondary cartilaginous
(Symphysis)
Lateral view

In **cartilaginous joints,** articulating bones are united by fibrocartilage or hyaline cartilage. In a **synchondrosis,** such as that in a developing long bone, the bony epiphysis and body are joined by an epiphysial plate (hyaline cartilage). In a **symphysis,** the binding tissue is a fibrocartilaginous disc (e.g., between two vertebrae).

In a **synovial joint** (articulation), the two bones are separated by the characteristic joint cavity (containing synovial fluid) but are joined by an articular capsule (fibrous capsule lined with synovial membrane). The bearing surfaces of the bones are covered with articular cartilage. Synovial joints are functionally the most common and important type of joint. They provide free movement between the bones they join and are typical of nearly all joints of the limbs.

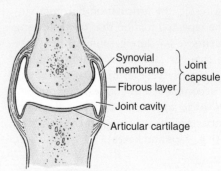

Synovial joint

described in Table I.3. Synovial joints, the most common type of joint, are usually reinforced by accessory ligaments that are either separate (extrinsic) or are a thickened part of the joint capsule (intrinsic). Some synovial joints have other distinguishing features, such as fibrocartilaginous *articular discs* or *menisci*, which are present when the articulating surfaces of the bones are incongruous. The six major types of synovial joints are classified according to the shape of the articulating surfaces and/or the type of movement they permit (Table I.4).

VASCULATURE AND INNERVATION OF JOINTS

Joints receive blood from *articular arteries* that arise from vessels around the joint. The arteries often *anastomose* (communicate) to form networks (*periarticular arterial anastomoses*), which ensure a continuous blood supply to a joint throughout its range of movement. *Articular veins* are communicating veins that accompany the arteries (L. *venae comitantes*) and, like the arteries, are located in the joint capsule, mostly in the synovial membrane.

Joints have a rich nerve supply; the nerve endings are numerous in the joint capsule. In the distal parts of limbs, the *articular nerves* are branches of the cutaneous nerves supplying the overlying skin. Otherwise, most articular nerves are branches of nerves that supply the muscles that cross and therefore move the joint. Hilton's Law states that the nerves supplying a joint also supply the muscles moving the joint and the skin covering their attachments.

Pain fibers are numerous in the fibrous layer of the joint capsule and associated ligaments; the synovial membrane is relatively insensitive. Joints transmit a sensation called *proprioception*, information that provides an awareness of movement and position of the parts of the body.

Muscular System

Muscle cells, often called muscle fibers because they are long and narrow when relaxed, are specialized contractile cells, organized into tissues that move body parts or temporarily alter the shape of internal organs. The associated connective tissue conveys nerve fibers and capillaries to the muscle fibers as it binds them into bundles or fascicles. Muscles also give form to the body and provide heat.

There are three types of muscles (Table I.5): (1) **skeletal muscle**, which moves bones and other structures (e.g., the eyes); (2) **cardiac muscle**, which forms most of the walls of the heart and adjacent parts of the great vessels; and (3) **smooth muscle**, which forms part of the walls of most vessels and hollow organs, moves substances through viscera such as the intestine, and controls movement through blood vessels.

Skeletal Muscle

All skeletal muscles have a fleshy contractile portion (one or more *heads* or *bellies*) composed of skeletal striated muscle and a white non-contractile portion composed mainly of collagen bundles: *tendons* (*rounded*) and *aponeuroses* (*flat sheets*). When referring to the length of a muscle, both the belly and the tendons are included. Most skeletal muscles are attached directly or indirectly through tendons and aponeuroses to bones, cartilages, ligaments, or fascia or to some combination of these structures; however, some muscles are attached to organs (e.g., the eyeball), to skin (e.g., facial muscles), and to mucous membranes (intrinsic tongue muscles). Muscles are organs of movement but they also provide static support and give form to the body and provide heat. Figure I.8 identifies some of the superficial muscles; the deep muscles are identified when each region is studied.

Most muscles are named on the basis of their function or the bones to which they are attached. The abductor digiti minimi, for example, abducts the little finger. The sternocleidomastoid (L. *kleidos,* bolt) attaches inferiorly to the sternum and clavicle and superiorly to the mastoid process of the temporal bone of the cranium. Other muscles are named on the basis of their shape (G. *deltoid*, triangle), position (medial, lateral, anterior, or posterior), length (brevis, short; longus, long), size (maximus, minimus), or number

Degenerative Joint Disease

Synovial joints are well designed to withstand wear, but heavy use over several years can cause degenerative changes. Beginning early in adult life and progressing slowly thereafter, aging of articular cartilage occurs on the ends of the articulating bones, particularly those of the hip, knee, vertebral column, and hands. These irreversible degenerative changes in joints result in the articular cartilage becoming less effective as a shock absorber and a lubricated surface. As a result, the articulation becomes vulnerable to the repeated friction that occurs during joint movements (e.g., during running). In some people these changes cause considerable pain. *Degenerative joint disease*, osteoarthritis (osteoarthrosis), is often accompanied by stiffness, discomfort, and pain. *Osteoarthritis* is common in older people and usually affects joints that support the weight of their bodies (e.g., hips and knees).

Table I.4 Types of Synovial Joints

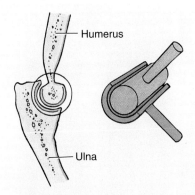

Hinge joints (uniaxial) permit flexion and extension only (e.g., the elbow joint).

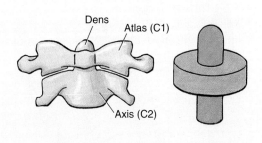

Pivot joints (uniaxial) allow rotation. A round process of bone fits into a bony ligamentous socket (e.g., the atlantoaxial joint between the atlas [C1] and axis [C2]).

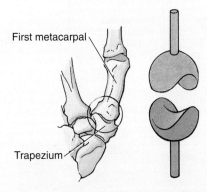

Saddle joints (biaxial) are shaped like a saddle—that is, they are concave and convex where the bones articulate (e.g., the joint between the metacarpal and the trapezium).

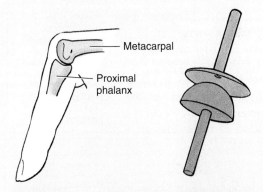

Condyloid joints (biaxial) permit flexion and extension, abduction and adduction, and circumduction (e.g., the metacarpophalangeal [knuckle] joints of fingers).

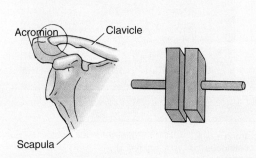

Plane joints permit gliding or sliding movements (e.g., the acromioclavicular joint).

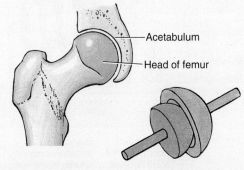

Ball and socket joints (multiaxial) permit movement in several axes (e.g., flexion-extension, abduction-adduction, medial and lateral rotation, and circumduction). A rounded head fits into a concavity (e.g., the hip joint).

Table I.5 Types of Muscles

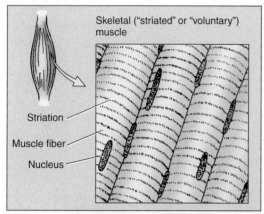

Skeletal ("striated" or "voluntary") muscle

Striation

Muscle fiber

Nucleus

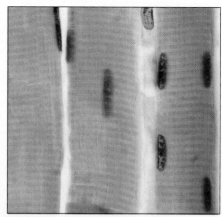

Location	Appearance	Type of Activity	Stimulation
Composes gross named muscles (e.g., the biceps of the arm) attached to the skeleton and/or fascia of limbs, body wall, and head/neck	Large, long, unbranched, cylindrical fibers with transverse striations (stripes) arranged in parallel bundles; multiple, peripherally located nuclei	Strong, quick intermittent (phasic) contraction above a baseline tonus; acts primarily to produce movement or resist gravity	Voluntary (or reflexive) by the somatic nervous system (SNS, p.34)

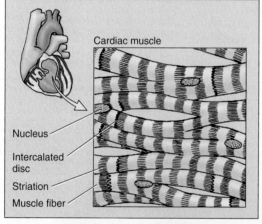

Cardiac muscle

Nucleus

Intercalated disc

Striation

Muscle fiber

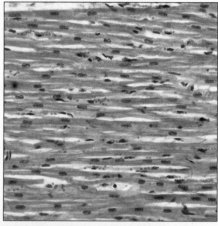

Location	Appearance	Type of Activity	Stimulation
Muscle of heart (myocardium) and adjacent portions of the great vessels (aorta, vena cava)	Branching and anastomosing shorter fibers with transverse striations (stripes) running parallel and connected end-to-end by complex junctions (intercalated discs); single, central nucleus	Strong, quick, continuous rhythmic contraction; acts to pump blood from heart	Involuntary; intrinsically (myogenically) stimulated and propagated; rate and strength of contraction modified by autonomic nervous system (ANS, p. 34)

Table I.5 Types of Muscles *(continued)*

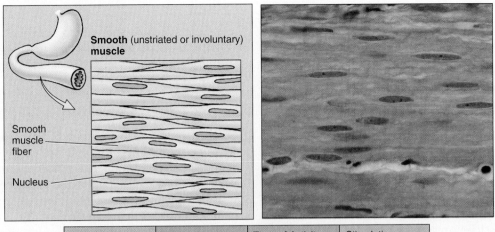

Location	Appearance	Type of Activity	Stimulation
Walls of hollow viscera and blood vessels, iris, and ciliary body of eye; attached to hair follicles of skin (arrector muscle of hair)	Single or agglomerated small, spindle-shaped fibers without striations; single, central nucleus	Weak, slow, rhythmic, or sustained tonic contraction; acts mainly to propel substances (peristalsis) and to restrict flow (vasoconstriction and sphincteric activity)	Involuntary by autonomic nervous system (ANS)

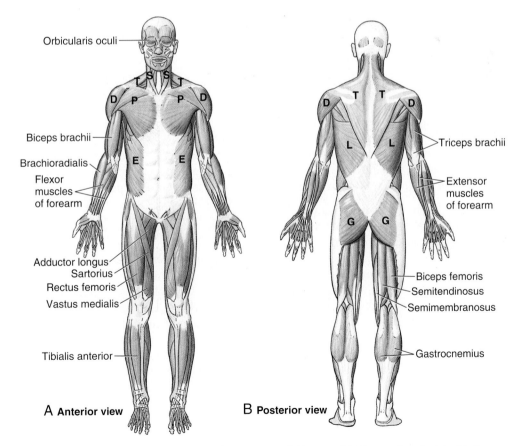

Figure I.8. Skeletal muscles. Some larger muscles are labeled. *S,* sternocleidomastoid; *T,* trapezius; *D,* deltoid; *P,* pectoralis major; *E,* external oblique; *L,* latissimus dorsi; *G,* gluteus maximus.

of attachments (biceps, triceps). Muscles may be described according to their shape and architecture (Fig. I.9). For example:

- **Pennate** muscles are feather-like in the arrangement of their fascicles (fiber bundles): unipennate, bipennate, or multipennate (L. *pennatus,* feather).
- **Fusiform** muscles are spindle shaped (round, thick belly, and tapered ends).
- In **parallel** muscles, the fascicles lie parallel to the long axis of the muscle; flat muscles with parallel fibers often have aponeuroses.
- **Convergent muscles** have a broad attachment from which the fascicles converge to a single tendon.
- **Circular muscle** surrounds a body opening or orifice constricting it when contracted

CONTRACTION OF MUSCLES

When muscles contract, the fibers shorten to about 70% of their resting length. Muscles with a long parallel fascicle arrangement shorten the most, providing considerable range of movement at a joint, but are not powerful. Muscle power increases as the total number of muscle cells increases. Therefore, the shorter, wide pennate muscles that "pack in" the most fiber bundles, shorten less but are most powerful.

When a muscle contracts and shortens, one of its attachments usually remains fixed and the other one moves. Attachments of muscles are commonly described as the origin and insertion; the *origin* is usually the proximal end of the muscle, which remains fixed during muscular contraction, and the *insertion* is usually the distal end of the muscle, which is movable. However, some muscles can act in both directions under different circumstances. Therefore, the terms *proximal* and *distal* or *medial* and *lateral* are used in this book when describing most muscle attachments.

Skeletal muscle can undergo contraction in three ways:

1. **Reflexive contraction** is automatic and not voluntarily controlled—for example, respiratory movements of the diaphragm. Muscle stretch is produced by tapping a tendon with a reflex hammer.
2. **Tonic contraction** is a slight contraction (**muscle tone**) that does not produce movement or active resistance but gives the muscle firmness, assisting the stability of joints and the maintenance of posture.
3. There are two principal types of **phasic contraction.** In **isometric contractions**, the muscle length remains the same—no movement occurs but muscle tension is increased above tonic levels (e.g., the deltoid holds the arm in abduction). In **isotonic contractions**, the muscle changes length to produce movement. There are two forms of isotonic contraction: **concentric contraction**, in which movement occurs owing to muscle shortening (e.g., the deltoid shortens to raise the arm into abduction), and **eccentric contraction**, in which the contracting muscle lengthens (e.g., the deltoid lengthens to lower arm in adduction).

The structural unit of a muscle is a **muscle fiber** (Fig. I.10). Connective tissue covering individual muscle fibers is called **endomysium**, a group of fibers (fiber bundles) is invested by **perimysium**, and the entire muscle is surrounded by **epimysium.** The functional unit of a muscle, consisting of a motor neuron and the muscle fibers it controls, is a **motor unit.** When a motor neuron in the spinal cord is stimulated, it initiates an impulse that causes all the muscle fibers supplied by that motor unit to contract simultaneously. The number of muscle fibers in a motor unit varies from one to several hundred, according to the size and function of the muscle. Large motor units, in which one neuron supplies several hundred muscle fibers, are found in the large trunk and thigh muscles. In the small eye and hand muscles, where precision movements are required, the motor units contain only a few muscle fibers.

Muscles serve specific functions in moving and positioning the body. The same muscle may act as a prime mover, antagonist, synergist, or fixator under specific conditions. The functions include:

- A **prime mover** or **agonist** is the main muscle responsible for producing a specific movement of the body (e.g., concentric contraction).
- **Fixators** steady the proximal parts of a limb while movements are occurring in distal parts.
- A **synergist** complements the action of prime movers—for example, by preventing movement of the intervening joint when a prime mover passes over more than one joint.
- An **antagonist** is a muscle that opposes the action of a prime mover. As a prime mover contracts, the antagonist progressively relaxes, producing a smooth movement.

Cardiac Muscle

Cardiac muscle forms the muscular wall of the heart—the **myocardium** (Table I.5). Some cardiac muscle is also present in the walls of the aorta, pulmonary vein, and superior vena cava (Fig. I.11). Cardiac muscle contractions are not under voluntary control. Heart rate is regulated intrinsically by a *pacemaker,* composed of special cardiac muscle fibers that are influenced by the autonomic nervous system (discussed later in this chapter).

Smooth Muscle

Smooth muscle, named for the absence of microscopic striations, forms a large part of the middle coat or layer

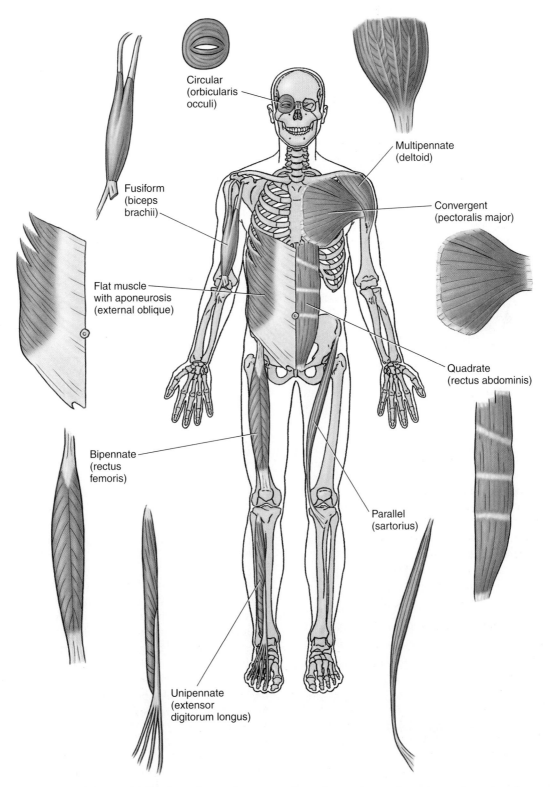

Circular
(orbicularis
occuli)

Fusiform
(biceps
brachii)

Multipennate
(deltoid)

Convergent
(pectoralis major)

Flat muscle
with aponeurosis
(external oblique)

Quadrate
(rectus abdominis)

Bipennate
(rectus
femoris)

Parallel
(sartorius)

Unipennate
(extensor
digitorum longus)

Figure I.9. Architecture and shape of skeletal muscles. Various types of muscles are shown whose shapes depend on the arrangement of fibers.

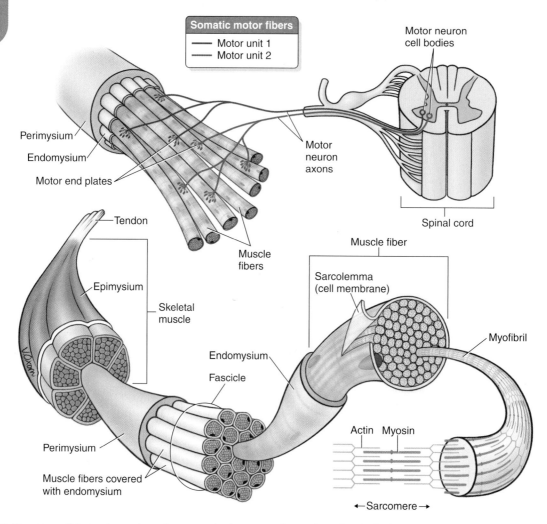

Figure I.10. Structure of skeletal muscle and motor unit. A motor unit consists of a single motor neuron and all the muscle fibers innervated by it. Actin (thin) and myosin (thick) filaments are contractile elements in the muscle fibers.

Muscle Testing

Muscle testing helps an examiner diagnose nerve injuries. This technique enables the examiner to gauge the power of the person's movement. Usually muscles are tested in bilateral pairs for comparison. There are two common testing methods:

1. The person performs movements that resist those produced by the examiner. For example, the person keeps the forearm flexed while the examiner attempts to extend it.
2. The examiner performs movements against resistance produced by the person. When testing flexion of the forearm, the examiner asks the person to flex his or her forearm, while the examiner resists the effort.

Electromyography

The electrical stimulation of muscles through electromyography (EMG) is another method for testing muscle action. The examiner places surface electrodes over a muscle and asks the person to perform certain movements. The examiner then amplifies and records the differences in electrical action potentials of the muscles. A normal resting muscle shows only a baseline activity (tonus), which disappears only during sleep, paralysis, and when under anesthesia. Contracting muscles demonstrate variable peaks of phasic activity. EMG makes it possible to analyze the activity of an individual muscle during different movements. EMG may also be part of the treatment program for restoring the action of muscles.

Muscular Atrophy

Wasting of the muscular tissue (atrophy) of a limb, for example, may result from a primary disorder of the muscle or from a lesion of a motor unit. Muscle atrophy may also be caused by immobilization of a limb, such as with a cast.

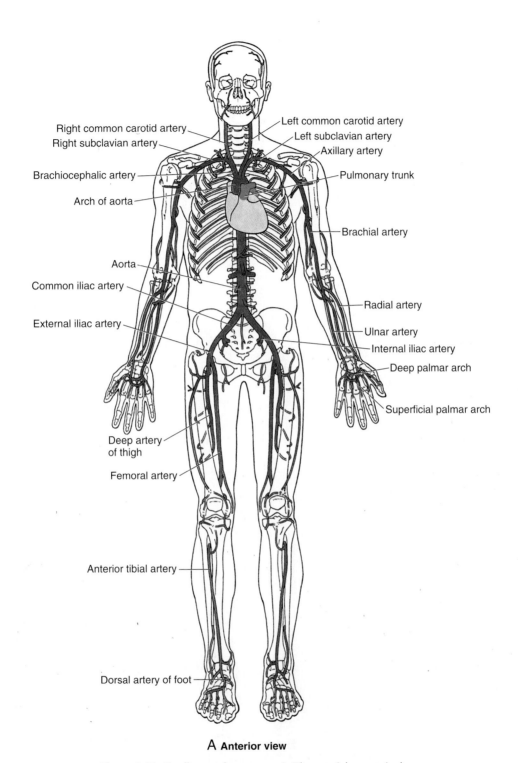

Right common carotid artery
Right subclavian artery
Brachiocephalic artery
Arch of aorta
Aorta
Common iliac artery
External iliac artery
Deep artery of thigh
Femoral artery
Anterior tibial artery
Dorsal artery of foot

Left common carotid artery
Left subclavian artery
Axillary artery
Pulmonary trunk
Brachial artery
Radial artery
Ulnar artery
Internal iliac artery
Deep palmar arch
Superficial palmar arch

A Anterior view

Figure I.11. Cardiovascular system. A. The arterial system is shown.

(tunica media) of the walls of most blood vessels and the muscular part of the wall of the digestive tract and ducts (Fig. I.12A; Table I.5). Smooth muscle is also found in skin (*arrector muscles* associated with hair follicles [Fig. I.3]) and in the eyeball (to controls lens thickness and pupil size). Like cardiac muscle, smooth muscle is innervated by the autonomic nervous system (Table I.5); hence it is

involuntary muscle that can undergo partial contraction for long periods. This is important in regulating the size of the lumen of tubular structures; in the walls of the digestive tract, uterine tubes, and ureters, the smooth muscle cells undergo rhythmic contractions (peristaltic waves). This process (**peristalsis**) propels the contents along these tubular structures.

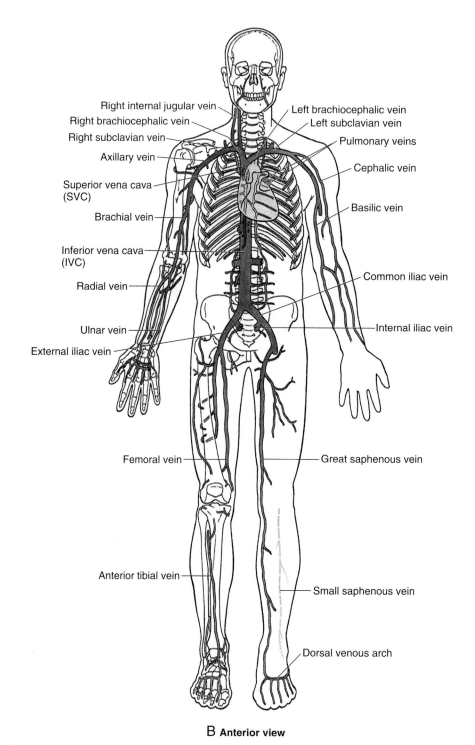

Right internal jugular vein

Right brachiocephalic vein

Right subclavian vein

Axillary vein

Superior vena cava (SVC)

Brachial vein

Inferior vena cava (IVC)

Radial vein

Ulnar vein

External iliac vein

Femoral vein

Anterior tibial vein

Left brachiocephalic vein

Left subclavian vein

Pulmonary veins

Cephalic vein

Basilic vein

Common iliac vein

Internal iliac vein

Great saphenous vein

Small saphenous vein

Dorsal venous arch

B Anterior view

Figure I.11. Cardiovascular system. *(continued)* **B.** The superficial veins are shown in the left limbs, and the deep veins are shown in the right limbs. Most arteries carry oxygenated blood away from the heart, and most veins carry deoxygenated blood to the heart; however, the pulmonary arteries arising from the pulmonary trunk carry deoxygenated blood (*blue*) to the lungs, and the pulmonary veins carry oxygenated blood (*red*) from the lungs to the heart.

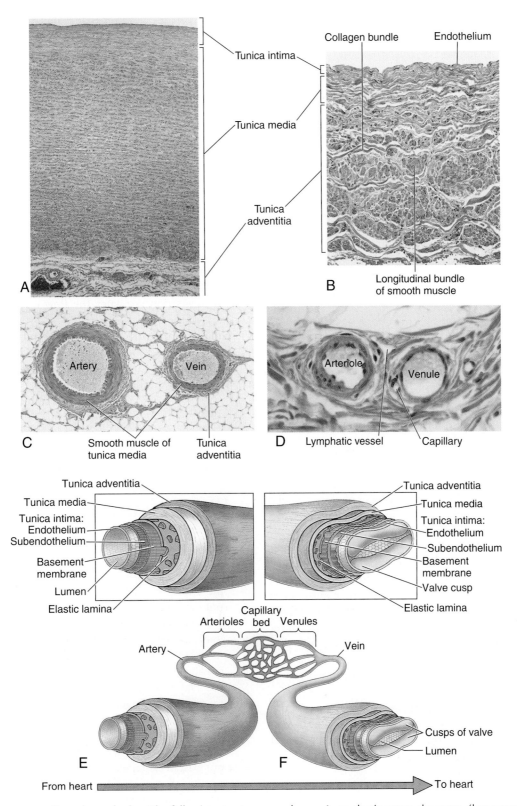

Figure I.12. Structures of arteries and veins. The following structures are shown: **A,** an elastic artery, the aorta, (low power); **B,** the inferior vena cava (low power); **C,** a muscular artery and vein (low power); and **D,** an arteriole and venule (high power). **E.** The structure of blood vessels is shown.

Hypertrophy

In *compensatory hypertrophy*, the myocardium responds to increasing demands by increasing the size of its fibers (cells). When cardiac muscle fibers are damaged during a heart attack, the tissue becomes necrotic (dies) and fibrous scar tissue that develops forms a *myocardial infarct* (MI), an area of *myocardial necrosis* (death of myocardial tissue). Smooth muscle cells also undergo compensatory hypertrophy in response to increased demands. During pregnancy, the smooth muscle cells in the wall of the uterus increase not only in size (*hypertrophy*) but also in number (*hyperplasia*).

Cardiovascular System

The **circulatory system** transports fluids throughout the body; it consists of the cardiovascular and lymphatic systems. The heart and blood vessels form the blood transportation network, the **cardiovascular system** (Fig. I.11). The heart pumps blood through the body's vast system of vessels. The blood carries nutrients, oxygen, and waste products to and from cells. There are three types of blood vessels: **arteries**, **veins**, and **capillaries**. Blood under high pressure leaves the heart and is distributed to the body by a branching system of thick-walled arteries. The final distributing vessels, **arterioles**, deliver oxygenated blood to capillaries. **Capillaries** form a capillary bed, where the interchange of oxygen, nutrients, waste products, and other substances with the extracellular fluid occurs (Fig. I.12*E*). Blood from the capillary bed passes into thin-walled venules, which resemble wide capillaries. **Venules** drain into small veins that open into larger veins. The largest veins, the superior vena cava (SVC) and inferior vena cava (IVC), return poorly oxygenated blood to the heart.

Most vessels of the circulatory system have three tunics or coats: **tunica intima**, the thin endothelial lining of vessels; **tunica media**, the middle smooth muscle layer; and **tunica adventitia**, the outer connective tissue coat.

Arteries

Arteries carry blood away from the heart and distribute it to the body (Fig. I.11*A*). Blood passes from the heart through arteries of ever decreasing caliber. The different types of arteries are distinguished from each other on the basis of overall size, relative amounts of elastic tissue or muscle in the tunica media, and the thickness of the wall relative to the lumen (Fig. I.12). Artery size and type is a continuum—that is, there is a gradual change in morphological characteristics from one type to another. There are three types of arteries:

- **Large elastic arteries** (conducting arteries) have many elastic layers in their walls; examples are the aorta and its branches from the arch of the aorta (Fig.I.12*A*). The maintenance of blood pressure in the arterial system between contractions of the heart results from the elasticity of these arteries. This quality allows them to expand when the heart contracts and to return to normal between cardiac contractions.
- **Medium muscular arteries** (distributing arteries) have walls that consist mainly of smooth muscle, circularly arranged; one example is the femoral artery (Fig. I.12*C*). The ability of these arteries to decrease their diameter (vasoconstrict) regulates the flow of blood to different parts of the body as required.
- **Small arteries and arterioles** have relatively narrow lumina and thick muscular walls (Fig. I.12*D*). The degree of arterial pressure within the vascular system is mainly regulated by the degree of tonus (firmness) in the smooth

Anastomoses, Collateral Circulation, and Terminal (End) Arteries

Anastomoses (communications) between the multiple branches of an artery provide numerous potential detours for blood flow in case the usual pathway is obstructed by compression, the position of a joint, pathology, or surgical ligation. If a main cannel is occluded, the smaller alternate channels can usually increase in size, providing a *collateral circulation* that ensures the blood supply to structures distal to the blockage. However, collateral pathways require time to develop; they are usually insufficient to compensate for sudden occlusion or ligation. There are areas where collateral circulation does not exist or is inadequate to replace the main vessel. Arteries that do not anastomose with adjacent arteries are true *terminal* (end) *arteries*. Occlusion of a terminal artery disrupts the blood supply to the structure or segment of an organ it supplies. For example, occlusion of the terminal arteries of the retina will result in blindness. Although not true terminal arteries, *functional terminal arteries* (arteries with ineffectual anastomoses) supply segments of the brain, liver, kidney, spleen, and intestines.

Arteriosclerosis: Ischemia and Infarction

The most common acquired disease of arteries is *arteriosclerosis* (hardening of arteries), a group of diseases characterized by thickening and loss of elasticity of arterial walls. *Atherosclerosis,* a common form of arteriosclerosis, is associated with the buildup of fat (mainly cholesterol) in the arterial walls. Calcium deposits then form an *atheromatous plaque,* resulting in arterial narrowing and irregularity. This may result in thrombosis (local clotting), which may occlude the artery or be flushed into the bloodstream, resulting in ischemia (reduction of blood supply to an organ or region) and infarction (local death of an organ or tissue). Among the consequences of a thrombus are myocardial infarction (heart attack), stroke, and gangrene (necrosis in parts of the limbs) (Fig BI.1).

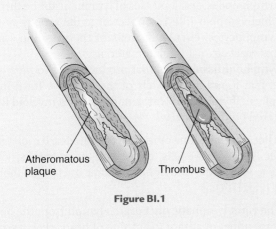

Atheromatous plaque

Thrombus

Figure BI.1

muscle of the arteriolar walls. If the tonus of muscle in the anterior wall is above normal, *hypertension* (high blood pressure) results.

Veins

Veins return poorly oxygenated blood to the heart from the capillary beds. The large pulmonary veins are atypical in that they carry well-oxygenated blood from the lungs to the heart (Fig. I.11*A*). Because of the lower blood pressure in the venous system the walls of veins are thinner than those of their companion arteries (Fig. I.12). The smallest veins, **venules,** unite to form larger veins that usually form *venous plexuses,* such as the **dorsal venous arch** of the foot (Fig. I.11). *Medium veins* in the limbs and other locations where the flow of blood is opposed by the pull of gravity have **valves** that permit blood to flow toward the heart but not in the reverse direction (Figs. I.12 and I.13*A*). **Large veins,** such as the SVC and IVC, are characterized by wide bundles of longitudinal smooth muscle and a well-developed tunica adventitia (Fig. I.12*B*). Systemic veins are more variable than the arteries and more frequently form anastomoses.

Although often depicted as single vessels, veins tend to be double or multiple. The veins that accompany deep arteries (accompanying veins) surround them in a branching network (Fig.I.13*B*) and occupy a relatively unyielding *vascular sheath* with the artery they accompany. As a result, they are stretched and flattened as the artery expands during contraction of the heart, which assists in driving the venous blood toward the heart. The outward expansion of the bellies of contracting skeletal muscles in the legs, for example, compresses the veins, "milking" the blood superiorly toward the heart; this is known as the *musculovenous pump* (Fig. I.13*A*).

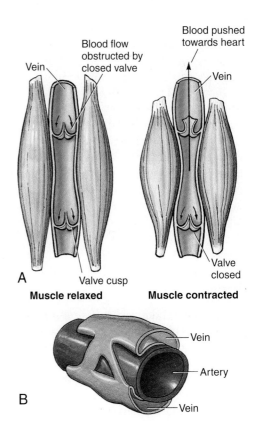

Blood flow obstructed by closed valve

Blood pushed towards heart

Vein

Vein

Vein

A   Valve cusp

Valve closed

Muscle relaxed   **Muscle contracted**

Vein

Artery

B   Vein

Figure I.13. Veins. A. The musculovenous pump is shown. The *arrows* indicate the direction of blood flow. **B.** Accompanying veins are shown (L. *venae comitantes*).

Varicose Veins

When the walls of veins lose their elasticity, they become weak and dilate under the pressure of supporting a column of blood against gravity. This results in *varicose veins*, abnormally swollen, twisted veins, most often seen in the legs (Fig BI.2).

Varicose veins have a caliber greater than normal and their valve cusps do not meet or have been destroyed by inflammation. These veins have *incompetent valves;* thus the column of blood ascending toward the heart is unbroken, placing increased pressure on the weakened walls of the veins and exacerbating their varicosities.

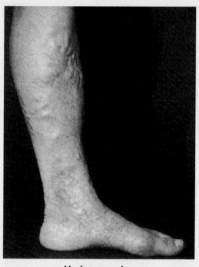

Varicose veins

Figure BI.2

Capillaries

Capillaries are simple endothelial tubes connecting the arterial and venous sides of the circulation. They are generally arranged in networks (**capillary beds**) between the arterioles and venules (Fig. I.12*E*). The blood flowing through the capillaries is brought to them by arterioles and carried away from them by venules. As the hydrostatic pressure in the arterioles forces blood through the capillary bed, oxygen, nutrients, and other cellular materials are exchanged with the surrounding tissue. In some regions, such as in the fingers, there are direct connections between the small arteries and veins proximal to the capillary beds they supply and drain. The sites of

such communications—**arteriovenous anastomoses (AV shunts)**—permit blood to pass directly from the arterial to the venous side of the circulation without passing through capillaries. AV shunts are numerous in the skin, where they have an important role in conserving body heat.

Lymphatic System

The lymphatic system provides for the drainage of surplus tissue fluid and leaked plasma proteins to the bloodstream and for the removal of cellular debris and infection (Fig. I.14). This system collects surplus extracellular tissue fluid as **lymph**. Lymph is usually clear and watery and is similar in composition to blood plasma. The lymphatic system consists of:

- **Lymphatic plexuses**, networks of small lymphatic vessels, **lymphatic capillaries**, that originate in the extracellular spaces of most tissues.
- **Lymphatic vessels (lymphatics)**, a nearly bodywide network of thin-walled vessels with abundant *valves*, originating from lymphatic plexuses along which lymph nodes are located. Lymphatic vessels occur almost everywhere blood capillaries are found, except, for example, teeth, bone, bone marrow, and the entire central nervous system (excess fluid here drains into the cerebrospinal fluid).
- **Lymph nodes**, small masses of lymphatic tissue through which lymph is filtered on its way to the venous system.
- **Lymphocytes**, circulating cells of the immune system that react against foreign materials.
- **Lymphoid tissue**, sites that produce lymphocytes, such as that found in the walls of the digestive tract; in the **spleen, thymus**, and lymph nodes; and in **myeloid tissue** in red bone marrow.

After traversing one or more lymph nodes, lymph enters larger lymphatic vessels, called lymphatic trunks, which unite to form either the right lymphatic duct or the thoracic duct (Fig. I.14).

- The **right lymphatic duct** drains lymph from the body's right upper quadrant (right side of head, neck, and thorax and the entire right upper limb). The duct ends in the right subclavian vein at its angle of junction with the right internal jugular vein, called *the right venous angle.*
- The **thoracic duct** drains lymph from the remainder of the body. This duct begins in the abdomen as a sac, the **chyle cistern** (L. *cisterna chyli*), and ascends through the thorax and enters the junction of the left internal jugular and left subclavian veins, called *the left venous angle.*

Superficial lymphatic vessels in the skin and subcutaneous tissue eventually drain into *deep lymphatic vessels* in the deep fascia between the muscles and the subcutaneous tissue; the deep vessels accompany the major blood vessels.

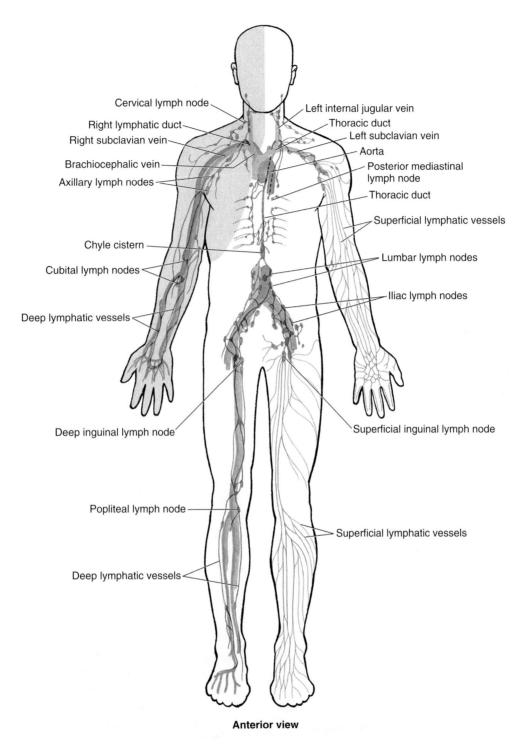

Anterior view

Figure I.14. Lymphatic system. The right lymphatic duct drains lymph from the right side of the head and neck and the right upper limb (*shaded*). The thoracic duct drains the remainder of the body. Deep lymphatic vessels are shown on the right, and superficial lymphatic vessels are shown on the left.

Additional functions of the lymphatic system include:

- *Absorption and transport of dietary fat,* in which special lymphatic capillaries (lacteals) receive all absorbed fat (chyle) from the intestine and convey it through the thoracic duct to the venous system.

- *Formation of a defense mechanism for the body.* When foreign protein drains from an infected area, antibodies specific to the protein are produced by immunologically competent cells and/or lymphocytes and dispatched to the infected area.

Lymphangitis, Lymphadenitis, and Lymphedema

The terms *lymphangitis* and *lymphadenitis* refer to the secondary inflammation of lymphatic vessels and lymph nodes, respectively. These pathological processes may occur when the lymphatic system is involved in the *metastasis* (spread) of cancer—the lymphogenous dissemination of cancer cells. *Lymphedema* (the accumulation of interstitial fluid) occurs when lymph is not drained from an area of the body. For instance, if *cancerous lymph nodes* are surgically removed from the axilla (armpit), lymphedema of the upper limb may result.

Nervous System

The nervous system enables the body to react to continuous changes in its external and internal environments. It controls and integrates various activities of the body, such as

circulation and respiration. For descriptive purposes, the human nervous system is divided as follows:

- Structurally into the *central nervous system* (CNS), made up of the brain and spinal cord, and the *peripheral nervous system* (PNS), consisting of nerve fibers and cell bodies outside the CNS that conduct impulses to or away from the CNS.
- Functionally into the *somatic nervous system* (SNS), the voluntary nervous system, which carries sensation (e.g., pain) from the skin and joints (e.g., position sense) and supplies skeletal muscle, and the *autonomic nervous system* (ANS), the involuntary/visceral nervous system, which supplies smooth muscle (e.g., in the wall of blood vessels), glands (e.g., sweat glands) and viscera (internal organs) in the body cavities (e.g., heart, stomach, and bladder).

Nervous tissue consists of two main cell types: neurons (nerve cells) and neuroglia (non-neuronal, non-excitable glial cells).

- **Neurons** are the structural and functional units of the nervous system specialized for rapid communication (Fig. I.15). A neuron is composed of a **cell body** with processes (extensions) called **dendrites** and an **axon**, which carry impulses to and away from the cell body, respectively. **Myelin**, layers of lipid and protein substances,

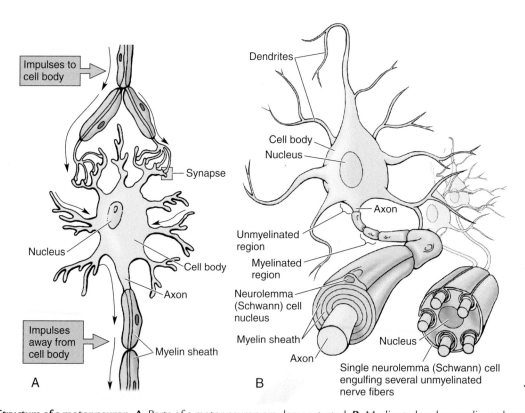

Figure I.15. Structure of a motor neuron. A. Parts of a motor neuron are demonstrated. **B.** Myelinated and unmyelinated nerves are shown.

forms a **myelin sheath** around some axons, greatly increasing the velocity of impulse conduction. Neurons communicate with each other at **synapses**, points of contact between neurons. The communication occurs by means of *neurotransmitters,* chemical agents released or secreted by one neuron, which may excite or inhibit another neuron, continuing or terminating the relay of impulses or the response to them.

- **Neuroglia** (glial cells or glia) are approximately five times as abundant as neurons, are non-neuronal, non-excitable cells that form a major component (scaffolding) of nervous tissue. Neuroglia support, insulate, and nourish the neurons.

Central Nervous System

The **central nervous system** consists of the **brain** and **spinal cord** (Fig. I.16). The principal roles of the CNS are to integrate and coordinate incoming and outgoing neural signals and to carry out higher mental functions, such as thinking and learning.

A collection of nerve cell bodies in the CNS is a **nucleus** (Fig. I.16*B*). A bundle of nerve fibers (axons) connecting neighboring or distant nuclei of the CNS is a **tract.** The nerve cell bodies lie within and constitute the **gray matter;** the interconnecting fiber tract systems form the **white matter** (Fig. I.17). In transverse sections of the spinal cord, the gray matter appears roughly as an H-shaped area embedded in a matrix of white matter. The struts (supports) of the H are **horns**; therefore, there are right and left **posterior (dorsal)** and **anterior (ventral) gray horns.**

Three membranous layers—pia mater, arachnoid mater, and dura mater—collectively constitute the **meninges** (Fig. I.17). The meninges and the **cerebrospinal fluid (CSF)** surround and protect the CNS. The brain and spinal cord are intimately covered on their outer surface by the innermost meningeal layer, a delicate, transparent covering, the **pia mater (pia).** The CSF is located between the pia and the **arachnoid mater (arachnoid),** in the subarachnoid space. External to the pia and arachnoid is the thick, tough **dura mater (dura),** which is intimately related to the internal aspect of the bone of the surrounding neurocranium (braincase). The dura of the spinal cord is separated from the vertebral column by a fat-filled space, the epidural space.

Peripheral Nervous System

The **peripheral nervous system** is made up of *nerve fibers* and *nerve cell bodies* that connect the CNS with peripheral structures (Fig. I.16). **Peripheral nerves** consist of bundles of nerve fibers, their connective tissue coverings, and blood vessels (vasa vasorum). A *peripheral nerve fiber* consists of an **axon,** the single process of a neuron; its **neurolemma,** the neurolemma (Schwann) cells that immedi-

Damage to CNS

When the CNS is damaged, the injured axons do not recover in most circumstances. Their proximal stumps begin to regenerate, sending sprouts into the area of the lesion; however, growth is blocked by astrocyte (a type of glial cell) proliferation at the site of injury. As a result, permanent disability follows destruction of a tract in the CNS.

ately surround the axon separating it from other axons; and its **endoneurium,** a connective tissue sheath. In the PNS, the neurolemma may take two forms, creating two classes of nerve fibers (Fig. I.18):

1. The neurolemma of **myelinated nerve fibers** have a neurolemmal (myelin) sheath that consists of a continuous series of neurolemma (Schwann) cells enwrapping an *individual axon,* forming myelin.
2. The neurolemma of **unmyelinated nerve fibers** consist of *multiple axons* separately embedded within the cytoplasm of each neurolemma (Schwann) cell. These neurolemma cells do not produce myelin. Most fibers in cutaneous nerves (nerves that supply sensation to the skin) are unmyelinated.

Peripheral nerves are fairly strong and resilient because the nerve fibers are supported and protected by three connective tissue coverings (Fig. I.18):

1. **Endoneurium,** a delicate connective tissue sheath that surrounds the neurolemma cells and axons.
2. **Perineurium,** a layer of dense connective tissue that encloses a fascicle (bundle) of peripheral nerve fibers, providing an effective barrier against penetration of the nerve fibers by foreign substances.
3. **Epineurium,** a thick connective tissue sheath that surrounds and encloses a bundle of fascicles, forming the outermost covering of the nerve; it includes fatty tissues, blood vessels, and lymphatics.

A peripheral nerve is much like a telephone cable: The axons are the individual wires insulated by the neurolemma and endoneurium, the insulated wires are bundled by the perineurium, and the bundles are surrounded in turn by the epineurium forming the outer wrapping of the "cable."

A collection of nerve cell bodies outside the CNS is a **ganglion.** There are both motor (autonomic) and sensory ganglia.

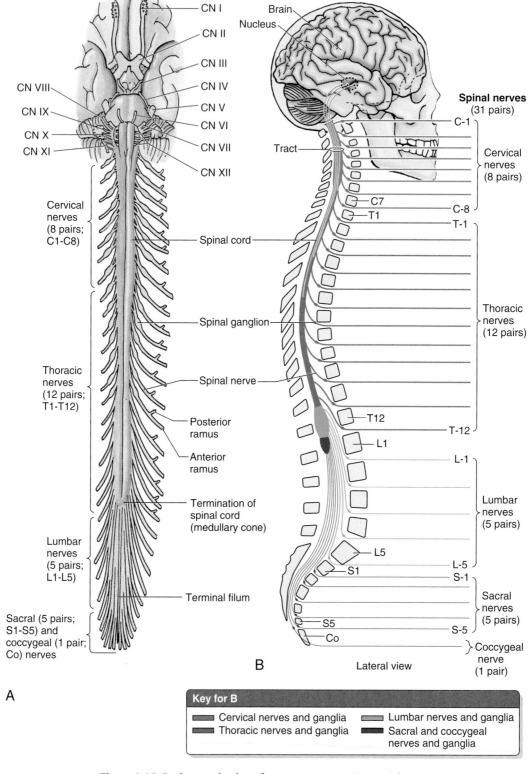

CN I
CN II
CN III
CN IV
CN V
CN VI
CN VII
CN XII

CN VIII
CN IX
CN X
CN XI

Cervical nerves (8 pairs; C1-C8)

Thoracic nerves (12 pairs; T1-T12)

Lumbar nerves (5 pairs; L1-L5)

Sacral (5 pairs; S1-S5) and coccygeal (1 pair; Co) nerves

Spinal cord

Spinal ganglion

Spinal nerve

Posterior ramus

Anterior ramus

Termination of spinal cord (medullary cone)

Terminal filum

A

Brain
Nucleus

Tract

Spinal nerves (31 pairs)

C-1
C7
T1
T12
L1
L5
S1
S5
Co

C-8
T-1
T-12
L-1
L-5
S-1
S-5

Cervical nerves (8 pairs)

Thoracic nerves (12 pairs)

Lumbar nerves (5 pairs)

Sacral nerves (5 pairs)

Coccygeal nerve (1 pair)

B   Lateral view

Key for B

Cervical nerves and ganglia
Thoracic nerves and ganglia

Lumbar nerves and ganglia
Sacral and coccygeal nerves and ganglia

Figure I.16. Basic organization of nervous system. *CN,* cranial nerve.

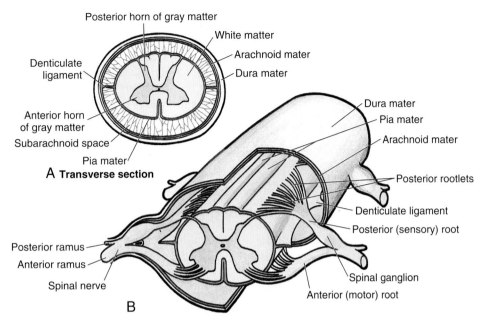

A **Transverse section**

B

Figure I.17. **Spinal cord and meninges.**

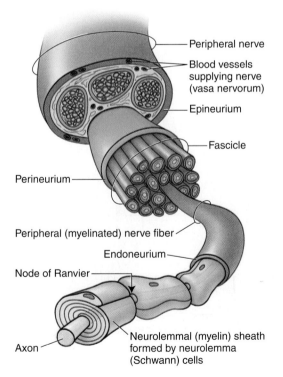

Figure I.18. **Arrangement and ensheathment of peripheral nerve fibers.** The nodes of Ranvier are intervals in the myelin sheath, i.e., where short lengths of axon are not covered by myelin.

Peripheral Nerve Degeneration

When peripheral nerves are crushed or severed, their axons degenerate distal to the lesion because they depend on their cell bodies for survival. A *crushing nerve injury* damages or kills the axons distal to the injury site; however, the nerve cell bodies usually survive and the connective tissue coverings of the nerve are intact. No surgical repair is needed for this type of nerve injury because the intact connective tissue sheaths guide the growing axons to their destinations. Surgical intervention is necessary if the nerve is cut because the regeneration of axons requires apposition of the cut ends by sutures through the epineurium. The individual fascicles (bundles of nerve fibers) are realigned as accurately as possible. Compromising a nerve's blood supply for a long period, produces *ischemia* by compression of the vasa nervorum (Fig. I.18), which can also cause nerve degeneration. Prolonged ischemia of a nerve may result in damage no less severe than that produced by crushing or even cutting the nerve.

Peripheral nerves are either cranial or spinal nerves. Of the 12 pairs of **cranial nerves (CN)**, only 11 arise from the brain; the 12th pair (CN XII) arises mostly from the superior part of the spinal cord. All cranial nerves exit the cranial cavity through foramina in the cranium (G. *kranion,* skull). All 31 pairs of **spinal nerves**—8 cervical (C), 12 thoracic (T), 5 lumbar (L), 5 sacral (S), and 1 coccygeal (Co)—arise from the spinal cord and exit through intervertebral foramina in the vertebral column (Fig I.16*B*).

Somatic Nervous System

The **somatic nervous system,** or voluntary nervous system, composed of somatic parts of the CNS and PNS, provides general sensory and motor innervation to all parts of the body (G. *soma*), except the viscera in the body cavities, smooth muscle, and glands (Fig. I.19). The *somatic (general) sensory fibers* transmit sensations of touch, pain, temperature, and position from sensory receptors. The *somatic motor fibers* permit voluntary and reflexive movement by causing contraction of skeletal muscles, such as occurs when one touches a candle flame.

Autonomic Nervous System

The visceral efferent (motor) fibers of the **autonomic nervous system** are accompanied by visceral afferent (sensory) fibers (L. *viscera,* internal organs). The **visceral efferent (motor) fibers** innervate involuntary (smooth) muscle, in the walls of organs and blood vessels, modified cardiac muscle (the intrinsic stimulating and conducting tissue of the heart; see Chapter 1), and glands. In their role as the afferent component of autonomic reflexes and in conducting visceral pain impulses, **visceral afferent (sensory) fibers** also regulate visceral function (Fig. I.20).

VISCERAL AFFERENT SENSATION

Visceral afferent fibers have important relationships to the ANS, both anatomically and functionally. We are usually unaware of the sensory input of these fibers, which provides information about the condition of the body's internal environment. This information is integrated in the CNS, often triggering visceral or somatic reflexes or both. Visceral reflexes regulate blood pressure and chemistry by altering such functions as heart and respiratory rates and vascular resis-

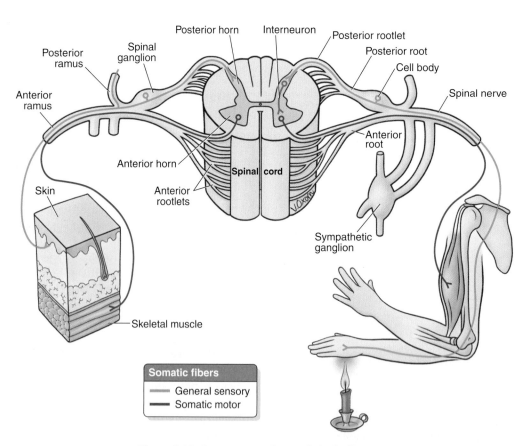

Figure I.19. Components of somatic (spinal) nerves.

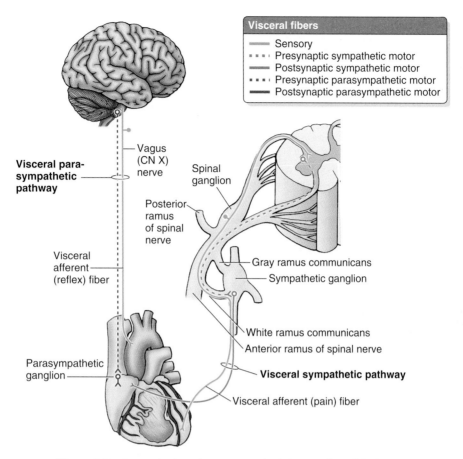

Visceral fibers
- — Sensory
- · · · · Presynaptic sympathetic motor
- — Postsynaptic sympathetic motor
- ▪ ▪ ▪ Presynaptic parasympathetic motor
- — Postsynaptic parasympathetic motor

Vagus (CN X) nerve

Visceral para-sympathetic pathway

Spinal ganglion

Posterior ramus of spinal nerve

Visceral afferent (reflex) fiber

Gray ramus communicans

Sympathetic ganglion

White ramus communicans

Anterior ramus of spinal nerve

Visceral sympathetic pathway

Parasympathetic ganglion

Visceral afferent (pain) fiber

Figure I.20. Sympathetic and parasympathetic innervation of the heart.

tance. Visceral sensation that reaches a conscious level is generally categorized as pain that is usually poorly localized and may be perceived as hunger or nausea. However, adequate stimulation, such as the following, may elicit true pain: sudden distention, spasms or strong contractions, chemical irritants, mechanical stimulation (especially when the organ is active), and pathological conditions (especially *ischemia*—inadequate blood supply) that lower the normal thresholds of stimulation. Normal activity usually produces no sensation but may do so when there is ischemia. Most visceral reflex (unconscious) sensation and some pain travel in visceral afferent fibers that accompany the parasympathetic fibers retrograde. Most visceral pain impulses (from the heart and most organs of the peritoneal cavity) travel centrally along visceral afferent fibers accompanying sympathetic fibers.

VISCERAL MOTOR INNERVATION

The efferent nerve fibers and ganglia of the ANS are organized into two systems or divisions:

1. **Sympathetic (thoracolumbar) division.** In general, the effects of sympathetic stimulation are *catabolic* (preparing the body to "flight or fight").

2. **Parasympathetic (craniosacral) division.** In general, the effects of parasympathetic stimulation are *anabolic* (promoting normal function and conserving energy).

Although both sympathetic and parasympathetic systems innervate the same structures, they have different (usually contrasting) but coordinated effects (Table 1.6).

Conduction of impulses from the CNS to the effector organ involves a series of two neurons in both sympathetic and parasympathetic systems. The cell body of the **presynaptic (preganglionic) neuron** (*first neuron*) is located in the gray matter of the CNS. Its fiber (axon) synapses on the cell body of a **postsynaptic (postganglionic) neuron**, the *second neuron* in the series (Fig. I.20). The cell bodies of such second neurons are located in autonomic ganglia outside the CNS, and the postsynaptic fibers terminate on the effector organ (smooth muscle, modified cardiac muscle, or glands). A functional distinction of pharmacological importance in medical practice is that the postsynaptic neurons of the two systems generally liberate different neurotransmitter substances: *norepinephrine by the sympathetic division* (except in the case of sweat glands) and *acetylcholine by the parasympathetic division*. The anatomical distinction between the sympathetic and the parasympa-

Table I.6 Functions of Autonomic Nervous System

Organ, Tract, or System		Effect of Sympathetic Stimulation[a]	Effect of Parasympathetic Stimulation[b]
Eyes	Pupil	Dilates pupil (admits more light for increased acuity at a distance)	Constricts pupil (protects pupil from excessively bright light)
	Ciliary body		Contracts ciliary muscle, allowing lens to thicken for near vision (accommodation)
Skin	Arrector muscle of hair	Causes hairs to stand on end (gooseflesh or goose bumps)	No effect (does not reach)[c]
	Peripheral blood vessels	Vasoconstricts (blanching of skin and lips; turning fingertips blue)	No effect (does not reach)[c]
	Sweat glands	Promotes sweating[d]	No effect (does not reach)[c]
Other glands	Lacrimal glands	Slightly decreases secretion[e]	Promotes secretion
	Salivary glands	Secretion decreases, becomes thicker, more viscous[e]	Promotes abundant, watery secretion
Heart		Increases rate and strength of contraction; inhibits effect of parasympathetic system on coronary vessels, allowing them to dilate[e]	Decreases rate and strength of contraction (conserving energy); constricts coronary vessels in relation to reduced demand
Lungs		Inhibits effect of parasympathetic system, resulting in bronchodilation and reduced secretion, allowing for maximum air exchange	Constricts bronchi (conserving energy) and promotes bronchial secretion
Digestive tract		Inhibits peristalsis and constricts blood vessels to digestive tract so blood is available to skeletal muscle; contracts internal anal sphincter to aid fecal continence	Stimulates peristalsis and secretion of digestive juices; contracts rectum and inhibits internal anal sphincter to cause defecation
Liver and gallbladder		Promotes breakdown of glycogen to glucose (for increased energy)	Promotes building/conservation of glycogen; increases secretion of bile
Urinary tract		Vasoconstriction of renal vessels slows urine formation; internal sphincter of bladder contracted to maintain urinary continence	Inhibits contraction of internal sphincter of bladder, contracts detrusor muscle of bladder wall, causing urination
Genital system		Causes ejaculation and vasoconstriction, resulting in remission of erection	Produces engorgement (erection) of erectile tissues of external genitals
Suprarenal medulla		Release of adrenaline into blood	No effect (does not innervate)

Underlying general principles:

[a] In general, the effects of sympathetic stimulation are catabolic, preparing body for the flight-or-fight response.

[b] In general, the effects of parasympathetic stimulation are anabolic, promoting normal function and conserving energy.

[c] The parasympathetic system is restricted in its distribution to the head, neck, and body cavities (except for erectile tissues of genitalia); otherwise, parasympathetic fibers are never found in the body wall and limbs. Sympathetic fibers, by comparison, are distributed to all vascularized portions of the body.

[d] With the exception of the sweat glands, glandular secretion is parasympathetically stimulated.

[e] With the exception of the coronary arteries, vasoconstriction is sympathetically stimulated; the effects of sympathetic stimulation on glands (other than sweat glands) are the indirect effects of vasoconstriction.

thetic motor divisions of the ANS is based primarily on (1) the location of the presynaptic cell bodies and (2) which nerves conduct the presynaptic fibers from the CNS. These differences are discussed in more detail later in this chapter.

Structure and Components of a Typical Spinal Nerve

A typical spinal nerve arises from the spinal cord by **nerve rootlets,** which converge to form two nerve roots (Fig. I.19): the **anterior (ventral) root** consists of motor (efferent) fibers passing from nerve cell bodies in the anterior horn of the spinal cord gray matter to effector organs located peripherally. The **posterior (dorsal) root** consists of sensory (afferent) fibers that convey neural impulses to the CNS from sense organs (e.g., the eyes) and from sensory receptors in various parts of the body (e.g., in the skin). The posterior root carries general sensory fibers to the posterior horn of the spinal cord. The anterior and posterior roots unite at the intervertebral foramen to form a **spinal nerve,** which immediately divides into two rami (branches): a posterior ramus and an anterior ramus. As branches of a mixed spinal nerve, the anterior and posterior rami also carry both motor and sensory nerves, as do all their branches.

- The **posterior rami** supply nerve fibers to synovial joints of the vertebral column, deep muscles of the back, and the overlying skin.
- The **anterior rami** supply nerve fibers to the much larger remaining area, consisting of anterior and lateral regions of the trunk and the upper and lower limbs arising from them.

The components of a typical spinal nerve include

- **Somatic sensory fibers and motor fibers.**
  - *General sensory (general somatic afferent) fibers* transmit sensations from the body to the CNS; they may be *exteroceptive sensations* (pain, temperature, touch, and pressure) from the skin or pain and *proprioceptive sensations* from muscles, tendons, and joints. Proprioceptive sensations are subconscious sensations that convey information on joint position and the tension of tendons and muscles, providing information on how the body and limbs are oriented in space, independent of visual input. The unilateral area of skin innervated by the general sensory fibers of a single spinal nerve is called a **dermatome.** From clinical studies of lesions of the posterior roots or spinal nerves, *dermatome maps* have been devised that indicate the typical pattern of innervation of the skin by specific spinal nerves (Fig. I.21). However, a lesion of a single posterior root or spinal nerve would rarely result in numbness over the area demarcated for that

nerve in these maps because the general sensory fibers conveyed by adjacent spinal nerves overlap almost completely as they are distributed to the skin, providing a type of double coverage. Clinicians need to understand the dermatomal innervation of the skin so they can determine, using sensory testing (e.g., with a pin) whether a particular spinal nerve/spinal cord segment is functioning normally.
  - *Somatic motor (general somatic efferent)* fibers transmit impulses to skeletal (voluntary) muscles (Fig. I.19). The unilateral muscle mass receiving innervation from the somatic motor fibers conveyed by a single spinal nerve is a **myotome** (Fig. I.21). Each skeletal muscle is usually innervated by the somatic motor fibers of several spinal nerves; therefore, the muscle myotome will consist of several segments. The muscle myotomes have been grouped by joint movement to facilitate clinical testing—for example, muscles that flex the glenohumeral (shoulder) joint are innervated primarily by the C5 spinal nerve, and muscles that extend the knee joint are innervated by the L3 and L4 spinal nerves.
- **Visceral sensory fibers and motor fibers** of the sympathetic and parasympathetic nervous systems.
  - *Visceral sensory (general visceral afferent)* fibers transmit pain or subconscious visceral reflex sensations from hollow organs, glands, and blood vessels to the CNS. Both types of sensory fiber—visceral sensory and general sensory—have their cell bodies in spinal ganglia or sensory ganglia of cranial nerves.
  - *Visceral motor (general visceral efferent) fibers* transmit impulses to involuntary (smooth and cardiac) muscle and glandular tissues. The two varieties of fibers (*presynaptic* and *postsynaptic*) work together to conduct impulses from the CNS to smooth muscle or glands (Fig. I.20).
- **Connective tissue coverings** (Fig. I.18).
- **Vasa nervorum,** the blood vessels supplying the nerves.

Sympathetic Visceral Motor Innervation

The cell bodies of *presynaptic* neurons of the sympathetic division of the ANS are located in the **intermediolateral cell columns** (IMLs) or nuclei of the spinal cord (Fig. I.22). The paired (right and left) IMLs are a part of the gray matter, extending between the first thoracic (T1) and the second or third lumbar (L2 or L3) segments of the spinal cord. In horizontal sections of this part of the spinal cord, the IMLs appear as small **lateral horns** of the H-shaped gray matter, looking somewhat like an extension of the cross-bar of the H between the posterior and the anterior horns of matter. The cell bodies of *postsynaptic* neurons of the sympathetic nervous system occur in two

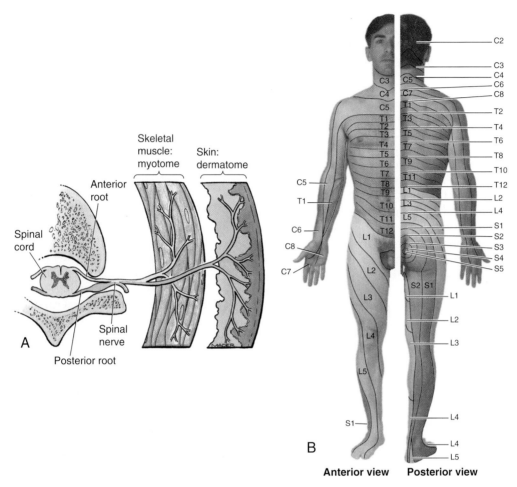

Figure I.21. Dermatomes and myotomes. A. A dermatome and myotome are shown. **B.** An example of a dermatome map is shown.

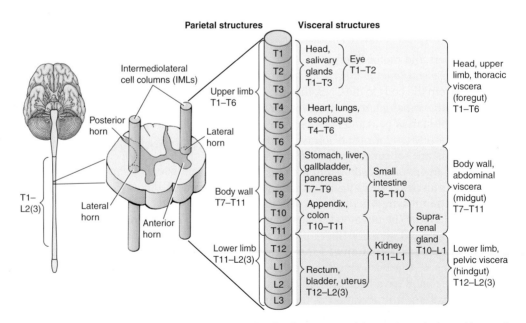

Figure I.22. Intermediolateral cell columns. The paired intermediolateral cell columns or nuclei constitute the lateral horn of gray matter, seen in the section of spinal cord segments T1 through L2 or L3, and consist of the cell bodies of presynaptic neurons of the sympathetic nervous system. Distribution of the postsynaptic fibers is also shown.

locations, the paravertebral and prevertebral ganglia (Fig. I.23):

- **Paravertebral ganglia** are linked to form right and left *sympathetic trunks* (*chains*) on each side of the vertebral column that extend essentially the length of this column. The superior paravertebral ganglion—the **superior cervical ganglion** of each sympathetic trunk— lies at the base of the cranium. The **ganglion impar** forms inferiorly, where the two trunks unite at the level of the coccyx.
- **Prevertebral ganglia** are in the plexuses that surround the origins of the main branches of the abdominal aorta (for which they are named), such as the large **celiac ganglia** that surround the origin of the celiac trunk (a major vessel arising from the aorta).

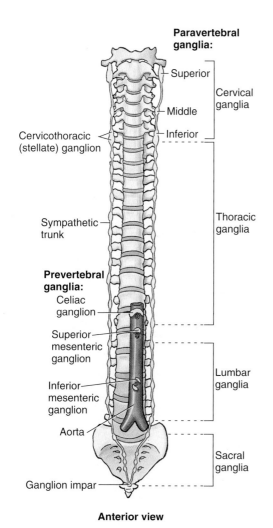

Paravertebral ganglia:

Superior
Middle
Inferior
} Cervical ganglia

Cervicothoracic (stellate) ganglion

Sympathetic trunk

Prevertebral ganglia:
Celiac ganglion

Superior mesenteric ganglion

Inferior mesenteric ganglion

Aorta

Thoracic ganglia

Lumbar ganglia

Sacral ganglia

Ganglion impar

Anterior view

Figure I.23. Sympathetic ganglia. *Paravertebral ganglia* are associated with all spinal nerves, although at the cervical level, eight spinal nerves share three ganglia. *Prevertebral (preaortic) ganglia* occur in the plexuses that surround the origins of the main branches of the abdominal aorta, such as the celiac artery.

Because they are motor fibers, the axons of presynaptic neurons leave the spinal cord through anterior roots and enter the anterior rami of spinal nerves T1 through L2 or L3 (Fig. I.22). Almost immediately after entering the rami, all the presynaptic sympathetic fibers leave the anterior rami of these spinal nerves and pass to the *sympathetic trunks* through **white rami communicantes.** Within the sympathetic trunks, presynaptic fibers follow one of four possible courses: (1) ascend or (2) descend in the sympathetic trunk to synapse with a postsynaptic neuron of a higher or lower paravertebral ganglion; or (3) enter and synapse immediately with a postsynaptic neuron of the paravertebral ganglion a that level; or (4) pass through the sympathetic trunk without synapsing, continuing on through an abdominopelvic splanchnic nerve (innervates abdominopelvic viscera) to reach the prevertebral ganglia (Fig. I.24).

Presynaptic sympathetic fibers that provide autonomic innervation within the head, neck, body wall, limbs, and thoracic cavity follow one of the first three courses, synapsing within the paravertebral ganglia. Presynaptic sympathetic fibers innervating viscera within the abdominopelvic cavity follow the fourth course.

Postsynaptic sympathetic fibers greatly outnumber the presynaptic fibers; they are destined for distribution within the neck, body wall, and limbs, passing from the paravertebral ganglia of the sympathetic trunks to adjacent anterior rami of spinal nerves through **gray rami communicantes.** By this means, they enter all branches of all 31 pairs of spinal nerves, including the posterior rami, to stimulate contraction of blood vessels (*vasomotion*) and the arrector muscles of hair (*pilomotion,* resulting in goose bumps) and to cause sweating (*sudomotion*). Postsynaptic sympathetic fibers that perform these functions in the head (plus innervation of the dilator muscle of the iris) all have their cell bodies in the **superior cervical ganglion** at the superior end of the sympathetic trunk. They pass from the ganglion by means of a **cephalic arterial branch** to form **periarterial plexuses** of nerves (Fig. I.24), which follow branches of the carotid arteries, or they may pass directly to nearby cranial nerves to reach their destination in the head.

Splanchnic nerves convey visceral efferent (autonomic) and afferent fibers to and from viscera of the body cavities (Figs. I.24 and I.25). Postsynaptic sympathetic fibers destined for viscera of the thoracic cavity (e.g., heart, lungs, and esophagus) pass through *cardiopulmonary splanchnic nerves* to enter the cardiac, pulmonary, and esophageal plexuses. The presynaptic sympathetic fibers involved in innervation of viscera of the abdominopelvic cavity (e.g., the stomach and intestines) pass to the prevertebral ganglia through *abdominopelvic splanchnic nerves* (the greater, lesser, least, and lumbar splanchnic nerves). All presynaptic sympathetic

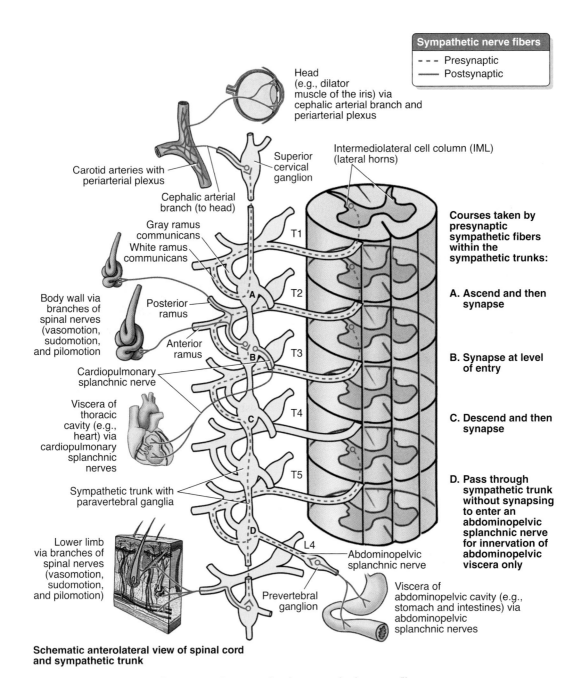

Sympathetic nerve fibers	
- - -	Presynaptic
———	Postsynaptic

Head
(e.g., dilator
muscle of the iris) via
cephalic arterial branch and
periarterial plexus

Superior
cervical
ganglion

Intermediolateral cell column (IML)
(lateral horns)

Carotid arteries with
periarterial plexus

Cephalic arterial
branch (to head)

Gray ramus
communicans
White ramus
communicans

T1

Courses taken by
presynaptic
sympathetic fibers
within the
sympathetic trunks:

Body wall via
branches of
spinal nerves
(vasomotion,
sudomotion,
and pilomotion)

Posterior
ramus

T2

A. Ascend and then
synapse

Anterior
ramus

T3

Cardiopulmonary
splanchnic nerve

B. Synapse at level
of entry

Viscera of
thoracic
cavity (e.g.,
heart) via
cardiopulmonary
splanchnic
nerves

T4

C. Descend and then
synapse

T5

Sympathetic trunk with
paravertebral ganglia

D. Pass through
sympathetic trunk
without synapsing
to enter an
abdominopelvic
splanchnic nerve
for innervation of
abdominopelvic
viscera only

Lower limb
via branches of
spinal nerves
(vasomotion,
sudomotion,
and pilomotion)

L4

Abdominopelvic
splanchnic nerve

Prevertebral
ganglion

Viscera of
abdominopelvic cavity (e.g.,
stomach and intestines) via
abdominopelvic
splanchnic nerves

Schematic anterolateral view of spinal cord
and sympathetic trunk

Figure I.24. Courses taken by sympathetic motor fibers.

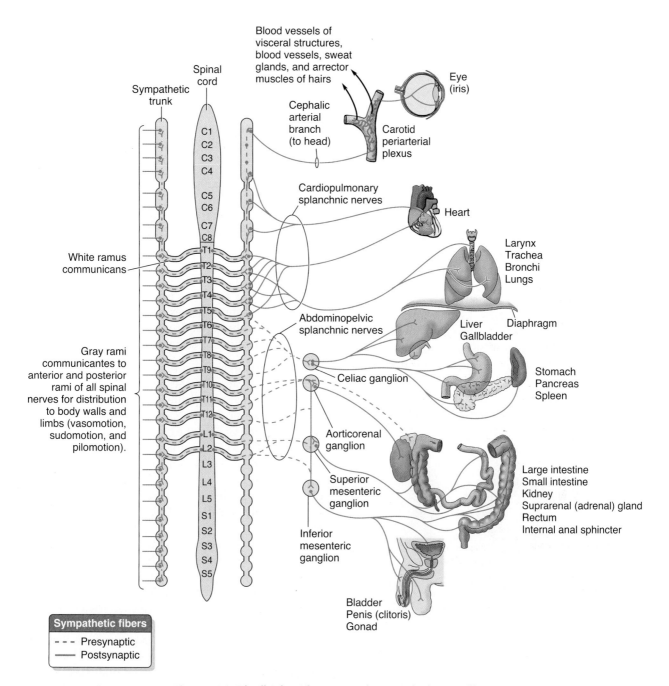

Figure I.25. Distribution of postsynaptic sympathetic nerve fibers.

fibers of the abdominopelvic splanchnic nerves, except those involved in innervating the suprarenal (adrenal) glands, synapse in the prevertebral ganglia. The postsynaptic fibers from the prevertebral ganglia form periarterial plexuses, which follow branches of the abdominal aorta to reach their destination.

Some presynaptic sympathetic fibers that pass through the prevertebral (celiac) ganglia without synapsing terminate directly on cells in the medulla of the **suprarenal gland** (Fig. I.26). The suprarenal medullary cells function as a special type of postsynaptic neuron that, instead of releasing their neurotransmitter substance onto the cells of a specific effector organ, release it into the bloodstream to circulate throughout the body, producing a widespread sympathetic response. Thus the sympathetic innervation of this gland is exceptional.

As described earlier, postsynaptic sympathetic fibers are components of virtually all branches of all spinal nerves. By this means and via periarterial plexuses, they extend to and innervate all the body's blood vessels (the sympathetic system's primary function) as well as sweat glands, arrector muscles of hairs, and visceral structures. Thus the sympathetic nervous system reaches virtually all parts of the body, with the rare exception of avascular tissues, such as cartilage and nails. The presynaptic fibers are relatively short,

whereas the postsynaptic fibers are relatively long, having to extend to all parts of the body.

Parasympathetic Visceral Motor Innervation

Presynaptic parasympathetic neuron cell bodies are located in two sites within the CNS (craniosacral); their fibers exit by two routes (Fig. I.27). This accounts for the alternate name of the parasympathetic (craniosacral) division of the ANS.

- In the gray matter of the brainstem, the fibers exit the CNS within CN III, CN VII, CN IX, and CN X; these fibers constitute the **cranial parasympathetic outflow.**
- In the gray matter of the sacral segments of the spinal cord (S2–S4), the fibers exit the CNS through the anterior roots of spinal nerves S2–S4 and the pelvic splanchnic nerves that arise from their anterior rami; these fibers constitute the **sacral parasympathetic outflow.**

Not surprisingly, the cranial outflow provides parasympathetic innervation of the head, and the sacral outflow provides the parasympathetic innervation of the pelvic viscera. However, in terms of the innervation of thoracic and abdominal viscera, the cranial outflow through the vagus nerve (CN X) is dominant. It provides innervation to all the thoracic viscera and most of the gastrointestinal (GI) tract from the esophagus through most of the large intestine (to its left colic flexure). The sacral outflow supplies only the descending and sigmoid colon and rectum.

Regardless of the extensive influence of its cranial outflow, the parasympathetic system is much more restricted than is the sympathetic system in its distribution. The parasympathetic system distributes only to the head, visceral cavities of the trunk, and erectile tissues of the external genitalia. With the exception of the latter, it does not reach the body wall or limbs, and except for initial parts of the anterior rami of spinal nerves S2–S4, its fibers are not components of spinal nerves or their branches.

Four discrete pairs of parasympathetic ganglia occur in the head (see Chapters 7 and 9). Elsewhere, presynaptic parasympathetic fibers synapse with postsynaptic cell bodies, which occur singly in or on the wall of the target organ (*intrinsic* or *enteric ganglia*). Most presynaptic parasympathetic fibers are long, extending from the CNS to the effector organ, whereas the postsynaptic fibers are short, running from a ganglion located near or embedded in the effector organ.

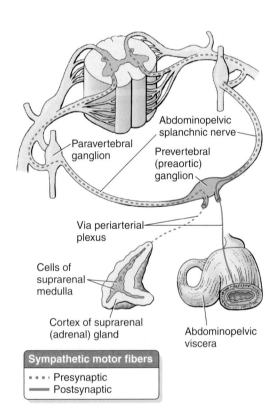

Sympathetic motor fibers
- ···· Presynaptic
- —— Postsynaptic

Figure I.26. Sympathetic supply to medulla of suprarenal gland.

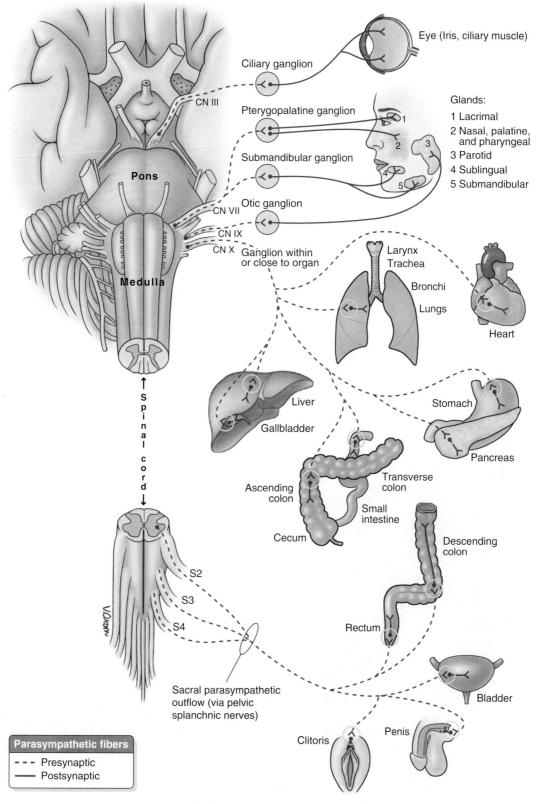

Figure I.27. Distribution of parasympathetic nerve fibers.

Imaging of Body Systems

Familiarity with imaging techniques commonly used in clinical settings enables one to recognize abnormalities such as congenital anomalies, tumors, and fractures. The introduction of contrast media allows the study of various luminal or vascular organs and potential or actual spaces, such as the digestive or alimentary system, blood vessels, kidneys, synovial cavities, and subarachnoid space. This section consists of short descriptions of the principles of some of the commonly used diagnostic imaging techniques:

- Conventional radiography (ordinary X-ray images).
- Computerized tomography (CT).
- Ultrasonography (US).
- Magnetic resonance imaging (MRI).
- Positron emission tomography (PET).

Conventional Radiography

The essence of a radiological examination is that a highly penetrating beam of X-rays transilluminates the patient, showing tissues of differing densities of mass within the body as images of differing densities of light and dark on the X-ray film (Fig. I.28). A tissue or organ

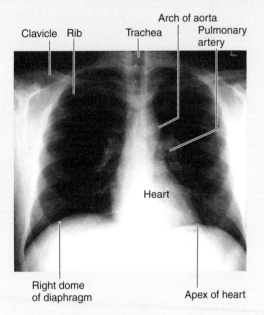

Posteroanterior (PA) projection

Figure I.28. Radiograph of thorax (chest). (Courtesy of Dr. E. L. Landsdown, Professor of Medical Imaging, University of Toronto, Toronto, Ontario, Canada.)

Table I.7 Basic Principles of X-Ray Image Formation

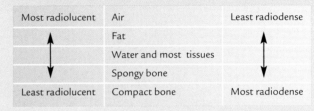

Most radiolucent	Air	Least radiodense
↑	Fat	↑
↕	Water and most tissues	↕
↓	Spongy bone	↓
Least radiolucent	Compact bone	Most radiodense

that is relatively dense in mass, such as compact bone in a rib, absorbs more X-rays than does a less dense tissue, such as spongy (cancellous) bone (Table I.7). Consequently, a dense tissue or organ produces a relatively transparent area on the X-ray film because relatively fewer X-rays reach the emulsion in the film. Therefore, relatively fewer grains of silver are developed at this area when the film is processed. A very dense substance is *radiopaque*, whereas a substance of less density is *radiolucent*.

Computerized Tomography

Computerized tomography (CT) shows images of the body that resemble transverse anatomical sections (Fig. I.29). A beam of X-rays is passed through the body as the X-ray tube and detector rotate around the axis of the body. The amount of radiation absorbed by each different type of tissue of the chosen body plane varies with the amount of fat, bone, and water in each element. A computer compiles and generates images as two-dimensional (2D) slices and total three-dimensional (3D) reconstructions.

Ultrasonography

Ultrasonography is a technique that allows visualization of superficial or deep structures in the body by recording pulses of ultrasonic waves reflecting off the tissues (Fig. I.30). The images can be viewed in real time to demonstrate the motion of structures and flow within blood vessels (Doppler US) and then recorded as single images or as a movie. Because ultrasonography is non-invasive and does not use radiation it is the standard method of evaluating the growth and development of the embryo and fetus.

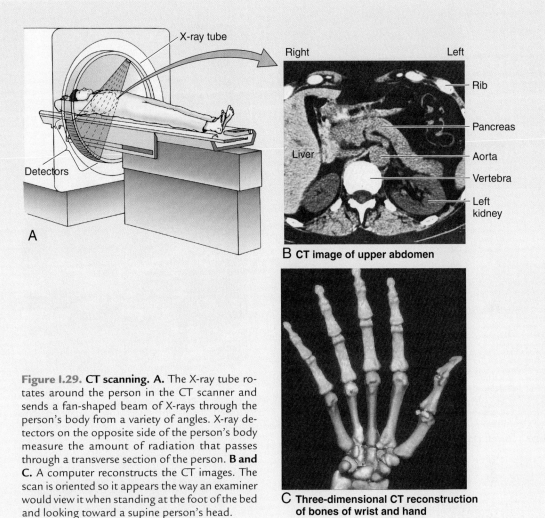

Figure I.29. CT scanning. A. The X-ray tube rotates around the person in the CT scanner and sends a fan-shaped beam of X-rays through the person's body from a variety of angles. X-ray detectors on the opposite side of the person's body measure the amount of radiation that passes through a transverse section of the person. **B and C.** A computer reconstructs the CT images. The scan is oriented so it appears the way an examiner would view it when standing at the foot of the bed and looking toward a supine person's head.

B **CT image of upper abdomen**

C **Three-dimensional CT reconstruction of bones of wrist and hand**

Magnetic Resonance Imaging

Magnetic resonance imaging (MRI) shows images of the body similar to those produced by CT, but they are better for tissue differentiation (Fig. I.31). Using MRI, the clinician is able to reconstruct the tissues in *any plane,* even arbitrary oblique planes. The person is placed in a scanner with a strong magnetic field, and the body is pulsed with radio waves. Signals subsequently emitted from the patient's tissues are stored in a computer and may be reconstructed in 2D or 3D images. The appearance of tissues on the generated images can be varied by controlling how radiofrequency pulses are sent and received. Scanners can be gated or paced to visualize moving structures, such as the heart and blood flow, in real time.

Positron Emission Tomography

Positron emission tomography (PET) scanning uses cyclotron-produced isotopes of extremely short half-life that emit positrons. PET scanning is used to evaluate the physiological functions of organs such as the brain on a dynamic basis. Areas of increased brain activity will show selective uptake of the injected isotope (Fig. I.32).●

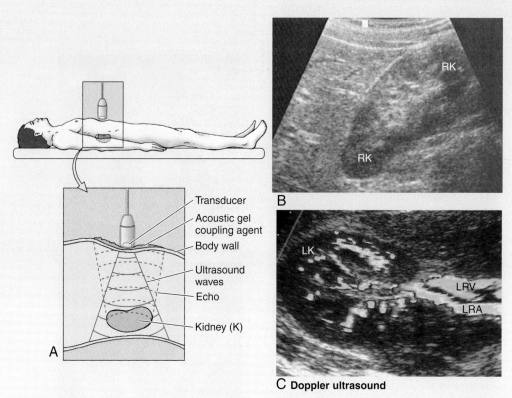

Figure I.30. Ultrasonography. A. The image results from the echo of ultrasound waves from structures of different densities. **B.** The image of a right kidney (*RK*) is displayed. **C.** Doppler US shows blood flow to and away from the kidney. *LRV*, left renal vein; *LRA*, left renal artery; *LK*, left kidney.

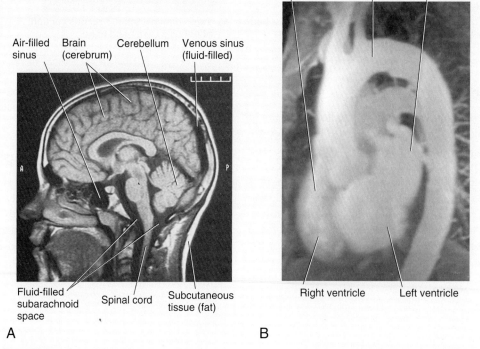

Figure I.31. MRI studies. A. A sagittal MRI study of the head and upper neck is shown. **B.** In this MR angiogram, the heart and great vessels are visualized.

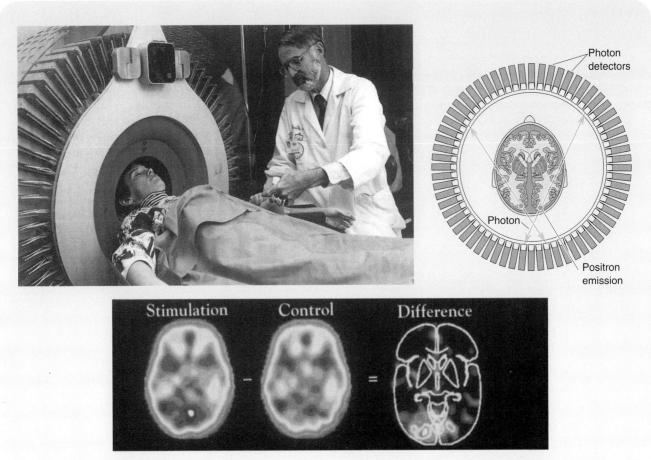

Photon
detectors

Photon

Positron
emission

Stimulation   Control   Difference

Figure I.32. PET scan. Observe the differences in brain activity associated with the planning and execution of a specific task in contrast to a control brain.

1

Thorax

Chapter Outline

The thorax (chest) is the superior part of the trunk between the neck and abdomen. The **thoracic cavity,** surrounded by the **thoracic wall,** contains the heart, lungs, thymus, distal part of the trachea, and most of the esophagus. To perform a physical examination of the thorax, a working knowledge of its structure and vital organs is required.

Thoracic Wall

The thoracic wall consists of skin, fascia, nerves, vessels, muscles, and bones. The functions of the thoracic wall include protecting of the thoracic and abdominal internal organs; resisting the negative internal pressures generated by the elastic recoil of the lungs and inspiratory movements; providing attachment for and supporting the weight of the upper limbs; and providing attachment for many of the muscles of the upper limbs, neck, abdomen and back, and the muscles of respiration. The mammary glands of the breasts are in the subcutaneous tissue overlying the pectoral muscles covering the anterolateral thoracic wall.

Skeleton of Thoracic Wall

The **thoracic skeleton** forms the osteocartilaginous *thoracic cage* (Fig. 1.1). The thoracic skeleton (bony thorax) includes 12 pairs of ribs and costal cartilages, 12 thoracic vertebrae and intervertebral (IV) discs, and the sternum. Costal cartilages form the anterior continuation of the ribs, providing a flexible attachment at their articulation with the sternum (Fig. 1.1*A*). Ribs and their cartilages are separated by **intercostal spaces**, which are occupied by intercostal muscles, vessels, and nerves.

RIBS AND COSTAL CARTILAGES

The ribs are curved, flat bones that form most of the thoracic cage (Fig. 1.1). They are remarkably light in weight yet highly resilient. Each rib has a spongy interior containing bone marrow, which forms blood cells (hematopoietic tissue). There are three types of ribs:

- **True (vertebrocostal) ribs** (1st–7th ribs) attach directly to the sternum through their own costal cartilages.
- **False (vertebrochondral) ribs** (8th–10th ribs) have cartilages that are joined to the cartilage of the rib just superior to them; thus their connection with the sternum is indirect.
- **Floating (free) ribs** (11th–12th ribs and sometimes the 10th rib) have rudimentary cartilages that do not connect even indirectly with the sternum; instead, they end in the posterior abdominal musculature.

Typical ribs (3rd–9th) have a:

- **Head** that is wedge-shaped and two facets that are separated by the **crest of the head** (Fig. 1.2*A*). One facet is for articulation with the numerically corresponding vertebra, and one facet is for the vertebra superior to it.
- **Neck** that connects the head with the body at the level of the tubercle.

- **Tubercle** at the junction of the neck and body. The tubercle has a smooth *articular part* for articulating with the corresponding transverse process of the vertebra and a rough *non-articular part* for the attachment of the costotransverse ligament.
- **Body** (shaft) that is thin, flat, and curved, most markedly at the **angle** where the rib turns anterolaterally. The concave internal surface has a **costal groove** that protects the intercostal nerve and vessels (Fig. 1.2*B*).

Atypical ribs (1st, 2nd, and 10th–12th) are dissimilar (Figs. 1.1 and 1.3):

- The **1st rib** is the broadest (i.e., its body is widest and is nearly horizontal), shortest, and most sharply curved of the seven true ribs; it has two grooves crossing its superior surface for the subclavian vessels; the grooves are separated by a **scalene tubercle** and ridge.
- The **2nd rib** is thinner, less curved, and much longer than the 1st rib; it has two facets on its head for articulation with the bodies of the T1 and T2 vertebrae.
- The **10th–12th ribs**, like the 1st rib, have only one facet on their heads.
- The **11th and 12th ribs** are short and have no necks or tubercles.

Costal cartilages prolong the ribs anteriorly and contribute to the elasticity of the thoracic wall. *Intercostal spaces* separate the ribs and their costal cartilages from one another. The spaces and neurovascular structures are named according to the rib forming the superior border of the space—that is, there are 11 intercostal spaces and 11 intercostal nerves. The *subcostal space* is below the 12th rib and the anterior ramus of spinal nerve T12 is the subcostal nerve.

THORACIC VERTEBRAE

Thoracic vertebrae are typical vertebrae in that they are independent and have bodies, vertebral arches, and seven processes for muscular and articular connections (see Chapter 5). Characteristic features of thoracic vertebrae include

- Bilateral costal facets (demifacets) on their bodies for articulation with the heads of ribs (Fig. 1.4); atypical thoracic vertebrae have one whole costal facet in place of the demifacets.
- Costal facets on their transverse processes for articulation with the tubercles of ribs, except for the inferior two or three thoracic vertebrae.
- Long inferiorly slanting spinous processes.

STERNUM

The sternum is the flat, vertically elongated bone that forms the middle of the anterior part of the thoracic cage. The

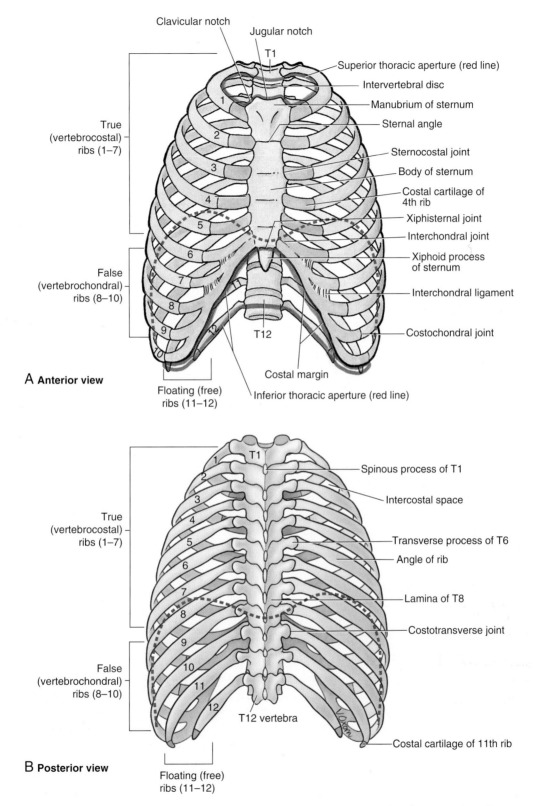

Clavicular notch
Jugular notch
T1
Superior thoracic aperture (red line)
Intervertebral disc
Manubrium of sternum
Sternal angle
Sternocostal joint
Body of sternum
Costal cartilage of 4th rib
Xiphisternal joint
Interchondral joint
Xiphoid process of sternum
Interchondral ligament
Costochondral joint

True (vertebrocostal) ribs (1–7)

False (vertebrochondral) ribs (8–10)

T12

Costal margin

Inferior thoracic aperture (red line)

Floating (free) ribs (11–12)

A Anterior view

True (vertebrocostal) ribs (1–7)

False (vertebrochondral) ribs (8–10)

T1

Spinous process of T1
Intercostal space
Transverse process of T6
Angle of rib
Lamina of T8
Costotransverse joint

T12 vertebra

Costal cartilage of 11th rib

Floating (free) ribs (11–12)

B Posterior view

Figure 1.1. Thoracic skeleton. The superior and inferior thoracic apertures are outlined in *pink*. Ribs are numbered *1–12*. *T1,* body of 1st thoracic vertebra; *T12,* body of 12th thoracic vertebra. The dotted lines indicate the position of the diaphragm, which separates the thoracic and abdominal cavities.

Role of Costal Cartilages

Costal cartilages prolong the ribs anteriorly and contribute to the elasticity of the thoracic wall, preventing many blows from fracturing the sternum and/or ribs. In elderly people, the costal cartilages undergo calcification, making them less resiliant and radiopaque.

Rib Excision

Rib excision is performed by surgeons who need access to the thoracic cavity. An incision is made through the periosteum along the curve of the rib and a piece of rib is removed. After the operation, the rib regenerates from the osteogenic layer of the preserved periosteum.

Rib Fractures

The weakest part of a rib is just anterior to its angle. Rib fractures commonly result from direct blows or indirectly from crushing injuries. The middle ribs are most commonly fractured. Direct violence may fracture a rib anywhere, and its broken ends may injure internal organs such as a lung and/or the spleen.

Flail Chest

Flail chest occurs when a sizable segment of the anterior and/or lateral thoracic wall moves freely because of *multiple rib fractures.* This condition allows the loose segment of the wall to move paradoxically (inward on inspiration and outward on expiration). Flail chest is an extremely painful injury and impairs ventilation, thereby affecting oxygenation of the blood. During treatment, the loose segment is often fixed by hooks and/or wires so that it cannot move.

Supernumerary Ribs

People usually have 12 ribs on each side, but the number may be increased by the presence of cervical and/or lumbar ribs or decreased by failure of the 12th pair to form. **Cervical ribs** (present in up to 1% of people) articulate with the C7 vertebra and are clinically significant because they may compress spinal nerves C8 and T1 or the inferior trunk of the brachial plexus supplying the upper limb. Tingling and numbness may occur along the medial border of the forearm. They may also compress the subclavian artery, resulting in *ischemic muscle pain* (caused by poor blood supply) in the upper limb. **Lumbar ribs** are less common than cervical ribs but have clinical significance in that they may confuse the identification of vertebral levels in diagnostic images.

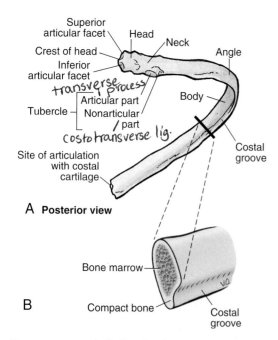

Figure 1.2. Typical rib. The features (**A**) and midbody cross section (**B**) of a typical rib are demonstrated.

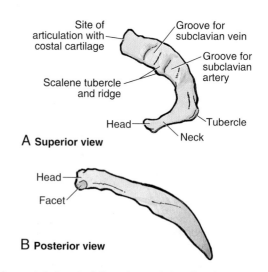

Figure 1.3. Atypical ribs. The 1st (**A**) and 12th (**B**) ribs are shown.

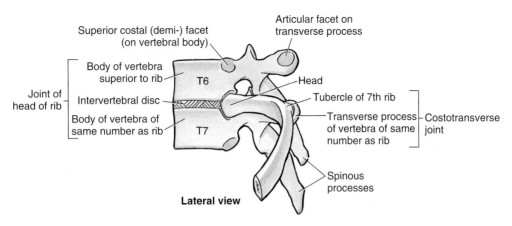

Figure 1.4. **Costovertebral joints.** The elements of the joint of the head of the rib and the costotransverse joint are identified.

sternum consists of three parts: manubrium, body, and xiphoid process (Figs. 1.1*A* and 1.5).

The **manubrium,** the superior part of the sternum, is a roughly trapezoidal bone that lies at the level of the bodies of the T3 and T4 vertebrae. Its thick superior border is indented by the **jugular notch** (suprasternal notch). On each side of this notch, a **clavicular notch** articulates with the sternal (medial) end of the clavicle. Just inferior to this notch, the costal cartilage of the 1st rib fuses with the lateral border of the manubrium. The manubrium and body of the sternum lie in slightly different planes; hence, forms a projecting **sternal angle** (of Louis). This readily palpable clinical landmark is located opposite the 2nd pair of costal cartilages at the level of the IV disc between the T4 and T5 vertebrae (Fig. 1.5*B*).

The **body** of the sternum (T5–T9 vertebral level) is longer, narrower, and thinner than the manubrium. Its width varies because of the scalloping of its lateral borders by the **costal notches** for articulation with the costal cartilages.

The **xiphoid process** (T10 vertebral level) is the smallest and most variable part of the sternum. It is relatively thin and elongated but varies considerably in form. The process is cartilaginous in young people but more or less ossified in adults older than 40 years. In elderly people, the xiphoid process may fuse with the sternal body. It is a midline marker for the superior level of the liver, the central tendon of the diaphragm, and the inferior border of the heart.

Sternal Fractures

Sternal fractures are not common, but crush injuries can occur during traumatic compression of the thoracic wall (e.g., in automobile accidents when the driver's chest is driven into the steering column). When the body of the sternum is fractured, it is usually a *comminuted fracture* (broken into several pieces). The most common site of sternal fracture occurs at the sternal angle, resulting in dislocation of the manubriosternal joint. In sternal injuries the concern is for the likelihood of heart and pulmonary injury.

Median Sternotomy

To gain access to the thoracic cavity for surgical operations—on the heart and great vessels, for example—the sternum is divided ("split") in the median plane and retracted (spread apart). After surgery, the halves of the sternum are reunited and held together with wire sutures.

Sternal Biopsies

The sternal body is often used for *bone marrow needle biopsy* because of its breadth and subcutaneous position. The needle pierces the thin cortic bone and enters the vascular trabecular (spongy) bone. Sternal biopsy is commonly used to obtain specimens of bone marrow for transplantation and for detection of metastatic cancer.

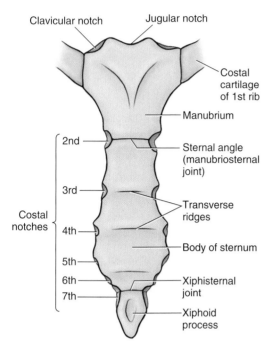

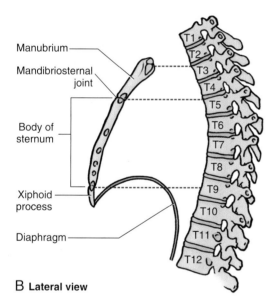

Figure 1.5. Sternum. A. The features of the sternum are shown. **B.** The relationship of the sternum to the vertebral column is demonstrated.

Thoracic Apertures

The thoracic cavity communicates with the neck and upper limb through the **superior thoracic aperture**, the anatomical *thoracic inlet* (Fig. 1.1*A*). Structures entering and leaving the thoracic cavity through this aperture include the trachea, esophagus, vessels, and nerves. The adult superior thoracic aperture measures approximately

6.5 cm anteroposteriorly and 11 cm transversely. Because of the obliquity of the 1st pair of ribs, the superior thoracic aperture slopes anteroinferiorly. The superior thoracic aperture is bounded:

- Posteriorly by the T1 vertebra.
- Laterally by the 1st pair of ribs and their costal cartilages.
- Anteriorly by the superior border of manubrium.

The thoracic cavity communicates with the abdomen through the **inferior thoracic aperture**, the anatomical *thoracic outlet* (Fig. 1.1*A*). In closing the inferior thoracic aperture, the diaphragm separates the thoracic and abdominal cavities almost completely. The inferior thoracic aperture is more spacious than the superior thoracic aperture. Structures passing to or from the thorax to the abdomen pass through openings in the diaphragm (e.g., the inferior vena cava and esophagus) or posterior to it (e.g., aorta).

The inferior thoracic aperture is bounded:

- Posteriorly, by the T12 vertebra.
- Posterolaterally, by the 11th and 12th pairs of ribs.
- Anterolaterally, by the joined costal cartilages of ribs 7–10, forming the costal margin.
- Anteriorly, by the xiphisternal joint.

Joints of Thoracic Wall

Although movements of the joints of the thoracic wall are frequent e.g., during respiration, the range of movement at the individual joints is small. Any disturbance that reduces the mobility of these joints interferes with respiration. *Joints of the thoracic wall* occur between the (Table 1.1):

- Vertebrae (intervertebral joints).
- Ribs and vertebrae (costovertebral joints: joints of the heads of ribs and the costotransverse joints).

Thoracic Outlet Syndrome

When clinicians refer to the superior thoracic aperture as the thoracic "outlet," they are emphasizing the important nerves and arteries that pass through this aperture into the lower neck and upper limb. Hence various types of thoracic outlet syndromes exist, such as the ***costoclavicular syndrome***—pallor and coldness of the skin of the upper limb and diminished radial pulse—resulting from compression of the subclavian artery between the clavicle and the 1st rib, particularly when the angle between the neck and the shoulder is increased.

Table 1.1 Joints of Thoracic Wall

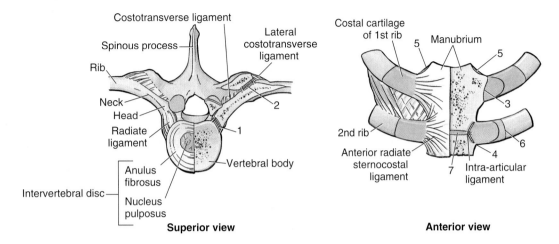

Superior view   **Anterior view**

Joint[a]	Type	Articulations	Ligaments	Comments
Intervertebral	Symphysis (secondary cartilaginous joint)	Adjacent vertebral bodies bound together by IV disc	Anterior and posterior longitudinal	
Costovertebral joints of head of ribs (**1**)	Synovial plane of joint	Head of each rib with superior demifacet or costal facet of corresponding vertebral body and inferior demifacet or costal facet of vertebral body superior to it	Radiate and intra-articular ligaments of head of rib	Heads of 1st, 11th, and 12th ribs (sometimes 10th) articulate only with corresponding vertebral body
Costotransverse (**2**)		Articulation of tubercle of rib with transverse process of corresponding vertebra	Lateral and superior costotransverse	11th and 12th ribs do not articulate with transverse process of corresponding vertebrae
Sternocostal (**3, 4**)	1st: primary cartilaginous joint	Articulation of 1st costal cartilages with manubrium of sternum		
	2nd–7th: synovial plane joints	Articulation of 2nd–7th pairs of costal cartilages with sternum	Anterior and posterior radiate sternocostal	
Sternoclavicular (**5**)	Saddle type of synovial joint	Sternal end of clavicle with manubrium and 1st costal cartilage	Anterior and posterior sternoclavicular ligaments; costoclavicular ligament	Joint is divided into two compartments by articular disc
Costochondral (**6**)	Primary cartilaginous joint	Articulation of lateral end of costal cartilage with sternal end of rib	Cartilage and bone; bound together by periosteum	Normally, no movement occurs
Interchondral (Fig. 1.1**A**)	Synovial plane joint	Articulation between costal cartilages of 6th-7th, 7th-8th, and 8th-9th ribs	Interchondral ligaments	Articulation between costal cartilages of 9th-10th ribs is fibrous
Manubriosternal (7)	Secondary cartilaginous joint (symphysis)	Articulation between manubrium and body of sternum		Often fuse and become synostosis in older people
Xiphisternal (Fig. 1.1**A**)	Primary cartilaginous joint (synchondrosis)	Articulation between xiphoid process and body of sternum		

[a]Numbers in parentheses refer to the figures.
IV, intervertebral disc.

Dislocation of Ribs

A rib dislocation (**slipping rib syndrome**) or **dislocation of a sternocostal joint** is the displacement of a costal cartilage from the sternum. This causes severe pain, particularly during deep respiratory movements. The injury produces a lump-like deformity at the dislocation site. Rib dislocations are common in body contact sports, and possible complications are pressure on or damage to nearby nerves, vessels, and muscles.

Separation of Ribs

A rib separation **refers to dislocation of a costochondral junction** between the rib and its costal cartilage. In separations of the 3rd–10th ribs, tearing of the perichondrium and periosteum usually occurs. As a result, the rib may move superiorly, overriding the rib above, causing pain.

- Sternum and costal cartilages (sternocostal joints).
- Sternum and clavicle (sternoclavicular joints).
- Ribs and costal cartilages (costochondral joints).
- Costal cartilages (interchondral joints).
- Parts of the sternum (manubriosternal and xiphisternal joints) in young people; usually the manubriosternal joint and sometimes the xiphisternal joint are fused in the elderly.

The *intervertebral joints* between the bodies of adjacent vertebrae are joined together by longitudinal ligaments and *intervertebral discs*. These joints are discussed with the back (see Chapter 4).

Movements of Thoracic Wall

Movements of the thoracic wall and diaphragm during inspiration increase the intrathoracic volume and diameters of the thorax. Consequent pressure changes result in air being drawn into the lungs (inspiration) through the nose, mouth, larynx, and trachea. During passive expiration, the diaphragm, intercostal muscles, and other muscles relax, decreasing *intrathoracic volume* and increasing *intrathoracic pressure*, expelling air from the lungs (expiration) through the same passages. The stretched elastic tissue of the lungs recoils, expelling most of the air. Concurrently, *intra-abdominal pressure decreases* and the abdominal viscera are decompressed.

The *vertical dimension* (height) of the central part of the thoracic cavity increases during inspiration as the contracting diaphragm descends, compressing the abdominal viscera (Fig. 1.6A & B). During expiration (Fig. 1.6A & C), the vertical diameter returns to the neutral position as the elastic recoil of the lungs produces subatmospheric pressure in the pleural cavities, between the lungs and the thoracic wall. As a result of this and the absence of resistance to the previously compressed viscera, the domes of the diaphragm ascend, diminishing the vertical dimension. The *anteroposterior* (AP) *dimension* of the thorax increases considerably when the intercostal muscles contract (Fig. 1.6D & E). Movement of the upper ribs at the costovertebral joints, about an axis passing through the neck of the ribs, causes the anterior ends of the ribs to rise like pump handles—the "pump-handle movement" (Fig. 1.6E). Because the ribs slope inferiorly, their elevation also results in anterior–posterior movement of the sternum, especially its inferior end, with slight movement occurring at the manubriosternal joint in young people (in whom the joint has not yet fused). In addition, the *transverse dimension* of the thorax increases slightly when the intercostal muscles contract, raising the middle i.e., lateralmost parts of the ribs, especially the most inferior ones. This is known as the "bucket-handle movement" (Fig. 1.6B & D).

Breasts

Both males and females have breasts (L. *mammae*); normally, the mammary glands are well developed only in women. **Mammary glands** in women are accessory to reproduction, but in men they are functionless, consisting of only a few small ducts or cords. The mammary glands are modified sweat glands and therefore have no special capsule or sheath. The contour and volume of the breasts are produced by subcutaneous fat, except during pregnancy when the mammary glands enlarge and new glandular tissue forms. During puberty (8–15 years of age), the female breasts normally grow because of glandular development and increased fat deposition. Breast size and shape result from genetic, racial, and dietary factors.

The roughly circular base of the female breast extends transversely from the lateral border of the sternum to the midaxillary line and vertically from the 2nd–6th ribs. A small part of the breast may extend along the inferolateral edge of the pectoralis major muscle toward the axillary fossa, forming an **axillary process** or **tail** (of Spence). Two thirds of the breast rests on the **pectoral fascia** covering the pectoralis major; the other third rests on the fascia covering the serratus anterior muscle (Figs. 1.7 and 1.8A). Between the breast and the deep pectoral fascia is a loose connective tissue plane or potential space—the **retromammary space** (bursa). This plane, containing a small amount of fat, allows the breast some degree of movement on the deep

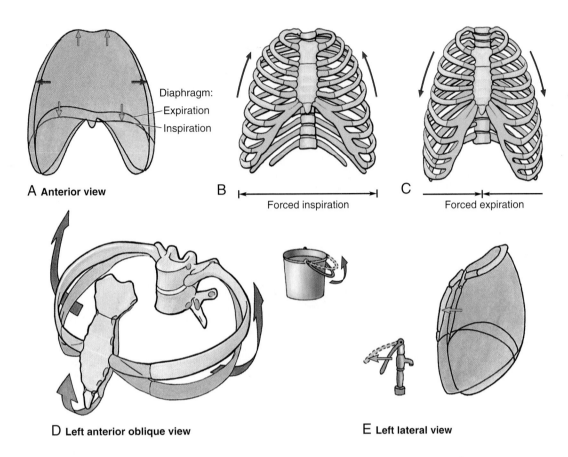

Diaphragm:
Expiration
Inspiration

A **Anterior view**

B Forced inspiration

C Forced expiration

D **Left anterior oblique view**

E **Left lateral view**

Figure 1.6. Movements of thoracic wall during respiration. A. Note the increased vertical (*green arrows*) and transverse (*red arrows*) diameters during inspiration. **B.** The thoracic cage widens during forced inspiration as the ribs are elevated (*arrows*). **C.** The thoracic cage narrows during expiration as the ribs are depressed (*arrows*). **D.** Observe the increased AP (*blue arrow*) and transverse (*red arrows*) diameters. The middle parts of the lower ribs move laterally when they are elevated (bucket-handle movement). **E.** The AP diameter of the thorax is increased (pump-handle movement); a greater excursion (increase) occurs inferiorly.

Paralysis of Diaphragm

One can detect paralysis of the diaphragm radiographically by noting its paradoxical movement. Paralysis of half of the diaphragm because of *injury to its motor supply from the phrenic nerve* does not affect the other half because each dome has a separate nerve supply. Instead of descending on inspiration, the paralyzed dome is pushed superiorly by the abdominal viscera that are being compressed by the active side. The paralyzed dome descends during expiration as it is pushed down by the positive pressure in the lungs (Fig. B1.1).

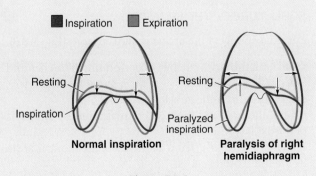

■ Inspiration   ■ Expiration

Resting
Inspiration

Normal inspiration

Resting
Paralyzed inspiration

Paralysis of right hemidiaphragm

Figure B1.1.

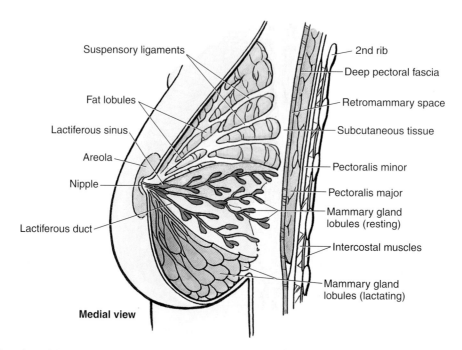

Figure 1.7. Sagittal section of female breast. The *upper part* of the figure shows the fat lobules and suspensory ligaments. The *middle part* shows the appearance of glandular tissue in the non-lactating (resting) breast. The *lower part* shows the appearance of glandular tissue in the lactating breast.

pectoral fascia. The mammary gland is firmly attached to the dermis of the overlying skin by the **suspensory ligaments** (of Cooper). These ligaments, particularly well developed in the superior part of the gland (Fig. 1.7), help support the **mammary gland lobules.**

At the greatest prominence of the breast is the **nipple**, surrounded by a circular pigmented area (the **areola**). The breast contains 15–20 **lobules** of glandular tissue, which constitute the parenchyma of the mammary gland. Each lobule is drained by a **lactiferous duct**, which opens independently on the nipple. Just deep to the areola, each duct has a dilated portion, the **lactiferous sinus** (Fig. 1.7).

VASCULATURE OF THE BREAST

The arterial supply of the breast is derived from (Fig. 1.8B):

- **Medial mammary branches of perforating branches** and *anterior intercostal branches of the internal thoracic artery*, originating from the subclavian artery.
- **Lateral thoracic** and **thoracoacromial arteries**, branches of the axillary artery.
- *Posterior intercostal arteries*, branches of the thoracic aorta in the intercostal spaces.

The **venous drainage of the breast** (Fig. 1.8C) is mainly to the **axillary vein**, but there is some drainage to the *internal thoracic vein*.

The **lymphatic drainage of the breast** is important because of its role in the metastasis (spread) of cancer cells. Lymph passes from the nipple, areola, and lobules of the gland to the **subareolar lymphatic plexus** (Fig. 1.8A), and from it:

- Most lymph (> 75%), especially from the lateral quadrants of the breasts, drains to the **axillary lymph nodes** (pectoral, humeral, subscapular, central, and apical), initially for the most part to the *pectoral (anterior) nodes*. However, some lymph may drain directly to other axillary nodes, or to interpectoral, deltopectoral, supraclavicular, or inferior deep cervical nodes.
- Most of the remaining lymph, particularly from the medial breast quadrants, drains to the **parasternal lymph nodes** or to the opposite breast. Lymph from the inferior breast quadrants may pass deeply to **abdominal lymph nodes** (inferior phrenic nodes).

Lymph from the axillary nodes drains to infraclavicular and supraclavicular nodes and from them to the **subclavian lymphatic trunk**. Lymph from the parasternal nodes enters the **bronchomediastinal trunks**, which ultimately drain into the thoracic or right lymphatic duct.

NERVES OF THE BREAST

The nerves of the breasts derive from the anterior and lateral cutaneous branches of the **4th–6th intercostal nerves** (Fig. 1.9). These branches of the intercostal nerves pass

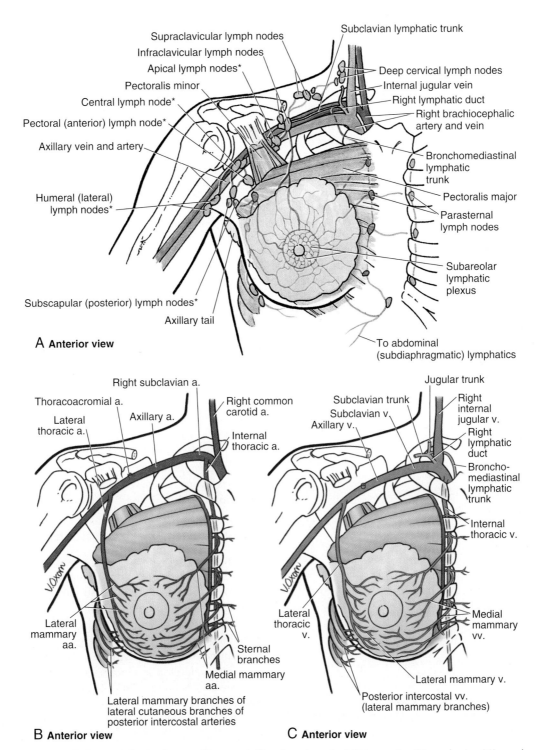

Supraclavicular lymph nodes
Infraclavicular lymph nodes
Apical lymph nodes*
Pectoralis minor
Central lymph node*
Pectoral (anterior) lymph node*
Axillary vein and artery
Humeral (lateral) lymph nodes*
Subscapular (posterior) lymph nodes*
Axillary tail

A Anterior view

Subclavian lymphatic trunk
Deep cervical lymph nodes
Internal jugular vein
Right lymphatic duct
Right brachiocephalic artery and vein
Bronchomediastinal lymphatic trunk
Pectoralis major
Parasternal lymph nodes
Subareolar lymphatic plexus
To abdominal (subdiaphragmatic) lymphatics

Thoracoacromial a.
Lateral thoracic a.
Axillary a.
Right subclavian a.
Right common carotid a.
Internal thoracic a.
Lateral mammary aa.
Medial mammary aa.
Sternal branches
Lateral mammary branches of lateral cutaneous branches of posterior intercostal arteries

B Anterior view

Jugular trunk
Subclavian trunk
Subclavian v.
Axillary v.
Right internal jugular v.
Right lymphatic duct
Broncho-mediastinal lymphatic trunk
Internal thoracic v.
Lateral thoracic v.
Medial mammary vv.
Lateral mammary v.
Posterior intercostal vv. (lateral mammary branches)

C Anterior view

Figure 1.8. Lymphatic drainage and vasculature of breast. Axillary lymph nodes* (**A**), arteries (**B**), and veins (**C**) are demonstrated.

Breast Quadrants

For the anatomical location and description of pathology (e.g., cysts and tumors), the breast is divided into four quadrants. The *axillary tail* is an extension of the mammary gland of the upper outer quadrant (Fig. B1.2).

Breast Cancer

Understanding the lymphatic drainage of the breasts is of practical importance in predicting the *metastasis* (spread) of breast cancer. Interference with the lymphatic drainage by cancer may cause lymphedema (edema, excess fluid in the subcutaneous tissue), which in turn may result in deviation of the nipple and a leathery, thickened appearance of the breast skin (Fig. B1.3). Prominent (puffy) skin between dimpled pores may develop, which gives the skin an orange-peel appearance (*peau d'orange sign*). Often the skin is dimpled because of cancerous invasion of the suspensory ligaments. Although breast cancer is uncommon in men, the consequences are serious because the tumor is often undetected until extensive metastases have occurred.

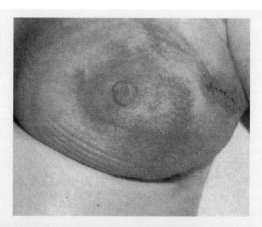

Figure B1.3. Inflamed carcinoma (cancer) of breast.

Mastectomy (breast excision) is not as common as it once was as a treatment for breast cancer. In *simple mastectomy,* the breast is removed down to the retromammary space. *Radical mastectomy,* a more extensive surgical procedure, involves removal of the breast, pectoral muscles, fat, fascia, and as many lymph nodes as possible in the axilla and pectoral region. In current practice, often only the tumor and surrounding tissues are removed—a *lumpectomy* or *quadrantectomy* (breast-conserving surgery using a wide local excision)—followed by radiation therapy.

Supernumerary Breasts and Nipples

Supernumerary (exceeding two) *breasts* (*polymastia*) or nipples (*polythelia*) may occur superior or inferior to the normal breasts. Usually supernumerary breasts consist of only a rudimentary nipple and areola. A supernumerary breast may appear anywhere along a line extending from the axilla to the groin, the location of the embryonic mammary ridge (milk line) from which the breasts develop in mammals with multiple breasts (Moore and Persaud, 2003). In either sex, there may be no breast development (amastia).

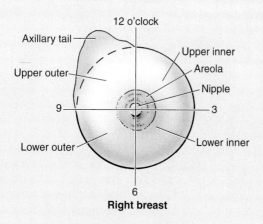

Figure B1.2. Breast quadrants.

through the deep pectoral fascia covering the pectoralis major to reach the skin. The branches thus convey sensory fibers to the skin of the breast and sympathetic fibers to the blood vessels in the breasts and smooth muscle in the overlying skin and nipple.

Muscles of Thoracic Wall

Several upper limb (axioappendicular) muscles attach to the thoracic cage: pectoralis major, pectoralis minor, serratus anterior anteriorly, and latissimus dorsi posteriorly (Fig.

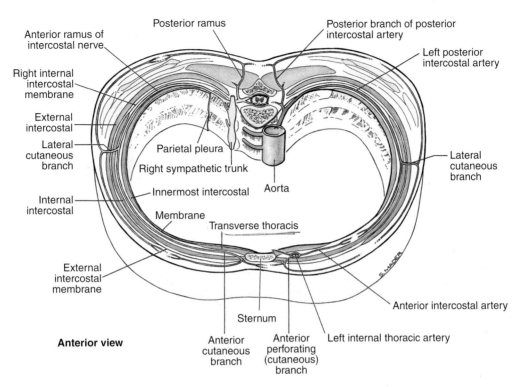

Posterior ramus

Posterior branch of posterior
intercostal artery

Anterior ramus of
intercostal nerve

Left posterior
intercostal artery

Right internal
intercostal
membrane

External
intercostal

Parietal pleura

Lateral
cutaneous
branch

Right sympathetic trunk

Lateral
cutaneous
branch

Innermost intercostal   Aorta

Internal
intercostal

Membrane

Transverse thoracis

External
intercostal
membrane

Anterior intercostal artery

Anterior view

Sternum

Anterior
cutaneous
branch

Anterior
perforating
(cutaneous)
branch

Left internal thoracic artery

Figure 1.9. Transverse section of thorax. Observe the contents of an intercostal space. The nerves are shown on the right and arteries on the left.

1.8A). In addition, the anterolateral abdominal muscles and some neck and back muscles attach to the thoracic cage. The pectoralis major, pectoralis minor, and the inferior part of serratus anterior may also function as accessory muscles of respiration, helping expand the thoracic cavity when inspiration is deep and forceful. The scalene muscles, passing from the neck to the 1st and 2nd ribs (see Chapter 8), also function as accessory respiratory muscles by fixing these ribs and enabling the muscles connecting the ribs below to be more effective in elevating the lower ribs during forced

inspiration. The intercostal, transverse thoracic (continuous with the transverse abdominal), subcostal (slips vary in size and number), levatores costarum, and serratus posterior are muscles of the thoracic wall (Table 1.2).

Typical intercostal spaces contain three layers of intercostal muscles (Figs. 1.9 and 1.10). The superficial layer is formed by the **external intercostal muscles** (fiber bundles oriented inferoanteriorly), the middle layer is formed by the **internal intercostal muscles** (fiber bundles oriented inferoposteriorly), and the deepest layer is formed by the **innermost intercostal muscles** (similar to internal intercostals). Anteriorly, the fleshy external intercostal muscles are replaced by **external intercostal membranes**; and posteriorly, the fleshy internal intercostal muscles are replaced by **internal intercostal membranes**. The innermost intercostal muscles are found only at the lateralmost parts of the intercostal spaces.

Nerves of Thoracic Wall

The thoracic wall has 12 pairs of thoracic spinal nerves. As they leave the IV foramina, they divide into anterior and posterior rami (Fig. 1.9). The anterior rami of T1–T11 comprise the **intercostal nerves** that run along the extent of the intercostal spaces. The anterior rami of the T12 nerves, inferior to the 12th ribs, form the **subcostal nerves** (see Chapter 3). The posterior rami of the thoracic spinal nerves pass posteriorly immediately lateral to the articular processes of

Dyspnea—Difficult Breathing

When people with respiratory problems such as *asthma*, emphysema, or with *heart failure* struggle to breathe, they use their accessory respiratory muscles to assist the expansion of their thoracic cavities. They typically lean on a table or their thighs to fix their pectoral girdles (clavicles and scapulae) so the muscles are able to act on their rib attachments and expand the thorax.

Table 1.2 Muscles of the Thoracic Wall

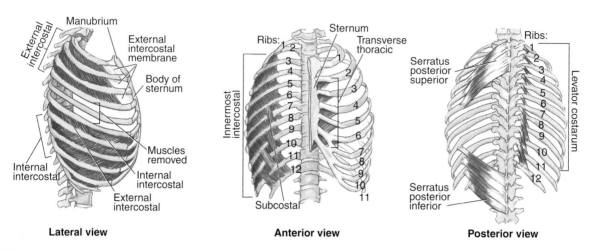

Lateral view   Anterior view   Posterior view

Muscles	Superior Attachment	Inferior Attachment	Innervation	Main Action[a]
External intercostal				During forced inspiration: elevate ribs
Internal intercostal	Inferior border of ribs	Superior border of ribs below		During forced inspiration: interosseous part depresses ribs; interchondral part elevates ribs
Innermost intercostal			Intercostal nerve	
Transverse thoracic	Posterior surface of lower sternum	Internal surface of costal cartilages 2–6		Weakly depresses ribs
Subcostal	Internal surface of lower ribs near their angles	Superior borders of 2nd or 3rd ribs below		Probably act in same manner as internal intercostal muscles
Levator costarum	Transverse processes of T7–T11	Subjacent ribs between tubercle and angle	Posterior rami of C8–T11 nerves	Elevate ribs
Serratus posterior superior	Nuchal ligament, spinous processes of C7–T3 vertebrae	Superior borders of 2nd–4th ribs	2nd–5th intercostal nerves	Elevate ribs[b]
Serratus posterior inferior	Spinous processes of T11–L2 vertebrae	Inferior borders of 8th–12th ribs near their angles	9th–11th intercostal nerves subcostal (T12) nerve	Depress ribs[b]

[a]All intercostal muscles keep the intercostal spaces rigid, thereby preventing them from bulging out during expiration and from being drawn in during inspiration. The role of individual intercostal muscles and accessory muscles of respiration in moving the ribs is difficult to interpret, despite many electromyographic studies.
[b]Action traditionally assigned based on attachments; these muscles appear to be largely proprioceptive in function.

the vertebrae, to supply the bones, joints, deep back muscles, and skin of the back in the thoracic region.

Typical intercostal nerves (3rd–6th) run initially along the posterior aspects of the intercostal spaces, between the parietal pleura (serous lining of the thoracic cavity) and the internal intercostal membrane. At first they run across the internal surface of the internal intercostal membrane and muscle near the middle of the intercostal space. Near the angles of the ribs, the nerves pass between the internal in-

tercostal and innermost intercostal muscles (Fig. 1.10). Here the nerves pass to and then continue to course within the **costal grooves**, lying just inferior to the intercostal arteries (which in turn lie inferior to the intercostals veins) (Fig. 1.11). Collateral branches of these nerves arise near the angles of the ribs and run along the superior border of the rib below. The nerves continue anteriorly between the internal and the innermost intercostal muscles, giving branches to these and other muscles and giving rise to

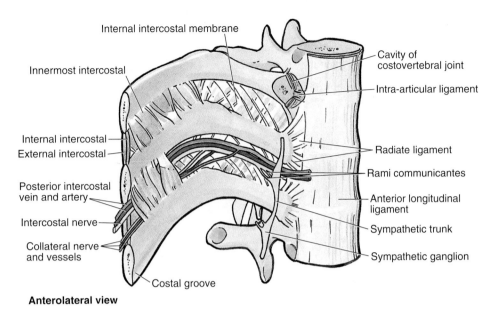

Anterolateral view

Figure 1.10. Dissection of vertebral end of intercostal space. Note the connection of the intercostal nerve to the sympathetic trunk by rami communicantes (communicating branches).

lateral cutaneous branches approximately at the midaxillary line (Fig. 1.9). Anteriorly, the nerves appear on the internal surface of the internal intercostal muscle. Near the sternum, the nerves turn anteriorly, passing between the costal cartilages and entering the subcutaneous tissue as **anterior cutaneous branches.** *Muscular branches* arise all along the course of the intercostal nerves to supply the intercostal, subcostal, transverse thoracic, levator costarum, and serratus posterior muscles (Table 1.2).

Atypical intercostal nerves are the 1st and 2nd and 7th–11th. Intercostal nerves 1 and 2 pass on the internal surfaces of the 1st and 2nd ribs instead of along the inferior margins of the costal grooves. After giving rise to the lateral

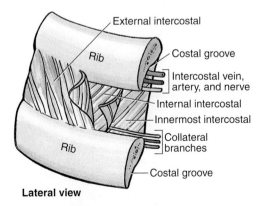

Lateral view

Figure 1.11. Contents of typical intercostal space. Remember the order of the structures in the costal groove, from superior to inferior, as *VAN,* for vein, artery, and nerve.

cutaneous branches, the 7th–11th intercostal nerves continue to supply the abdominal skin and muscles.

Through the posterior ramus and the lateral and anterior cutaneous branches of the anterior ramus, each spinal nerve supplies a stripe-like area of skin extending from the posterior median line to the anterior median line. These band-like skin areas (**dermatomes**) are each supplied by the *sensory fibers* of a single posterior root through the posterior and anterior rami of its spinal nerve (Fig. 1.12). Because any particular area of skin usually receives innervation from two adjacent nerves, considerable *overlapping of adjacent dermatomes* occur. Therefore, complete loss of sensation usually does not occur unless two or more intercostal nerves are anesthetized. The muscles supplied by the *motor fibers* of the posterior and anterior rami of each pair of thoracic spinal nerves constitutes a **myotome** (Fig. 1.12A).

Rami communicantes, or communicating branches, connect each intercostal and subcostal nerve to the ipsilateral **sympathetic trunk** (Fig. 1.10). Presynaptic fibers leave the initial portions of the anterior ramus of each thoracic (and upper lumbar) nerve by means of a white communicating ramus and pass to a **sympathetic ganglion.** Postsynaptic fibers distributed to the body wall and limbs pass from the ganglia of the sympathetic trunk via gray communicating rami to join the anterior ramus of the nearest spinal nerve, including all the intercostal nerves. Sympathetic nerve fibers are distributed through the branches of all spinal nerves (anterior and posterior rami) to reach the blood vessels, sweat glands, smooth muscle of the body wall and limbs.

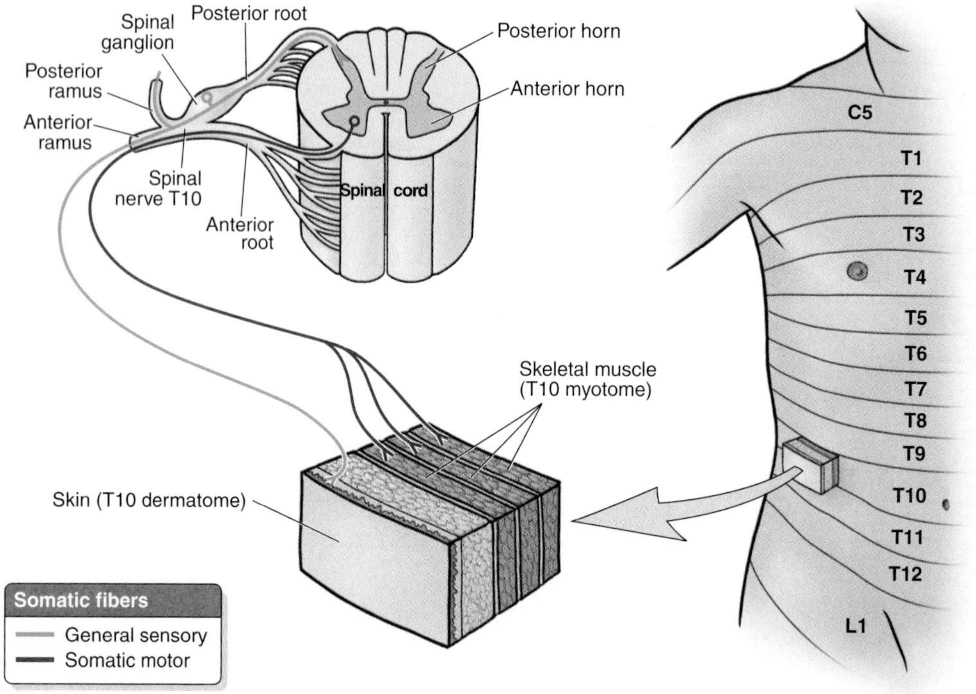

Spinal ganglion
Posterior root
Posterior horn
Posterior ramus
Anterior ramus
Anterior horn
Spinal nerve T10
Spinal cord
Anterior root

C5
T1
T2
T3
T4
T5
T6
T7
T8
T9
T10
T11
T12
L1

Skeletal muscle (T10 myotome)

Skin (T10 dermatome)

Somatic fibers
General sensory
Somatic motor

Figure 1.12. Dermatomes and myotomes of the trunk. Note the relationship between the area of skin (dermatome) and skeletal muscle (myotome) innervated by a spinal nerve or segment of the spinal cord. The dermatomes of the thorax (T1–T12) are shown at the right.

Herpes Zoster Infection

Herpes zoster (*shingles*)—a viral disease of spinal ganglia—is a *dermatomally distributed skin lesion*. The *herpes virus* invades a spinal ganglion and is transported along the axon to the skin, where it produces an infection that causes a sharp burning pain in the dermatome supplied by the involved nerve. A few days later, the skin of the dermatome becomes red and vesicular eruptions appear (Fig B1.4).

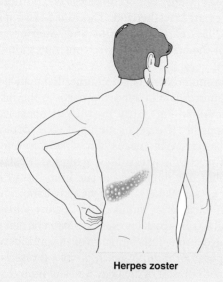

Herpes zoster

Figure B1.4.

Intercostal Nerve Block

Local anesthesia of an intercostal space is produced by injecting a local anesthetic agent around the intercostal nerves. This procedure, *an intercostal nerve block,* involves infiltration of the anesthetic around the intercostal nerve and its collateral branches (Fig. B1.5). Because any particular area of skin usually receives innervation from two adjacent nerves, considerable overlapping of contiguous dermatomes occurs. Therefore, complete loss of sensation usually does not occur, unless two or more intercostal nerves in adjacent intercostal spaces are anesthetized.

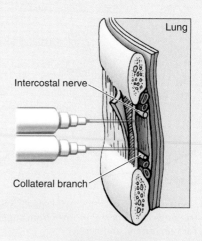

Lung

Intercostal nerve

Collateral branch

Figure B1.5.

Surface Anatomy of Thoracic Wall

Several bony landmarks and imaginary lines facilitate anatomical descriptions, identification of thoracic areas, and location of lesions such as a bullet wound:

- **Anterior median (midsternal) line** indicates the intersection of the median plane with the anterior chest wall (Fig. SA1.1A).

- **Midclavicular lines** pass through the midpoints of the clavicles, parallel to the anterior median line (Fig. SA1.1A).
- **Anterior axillary line** runs vertically along the anterior axillary fold, which is formed by the border of the pectoralis major as it spans from the thorax to the humerus (arm bone) (Fig. SA1.1B).

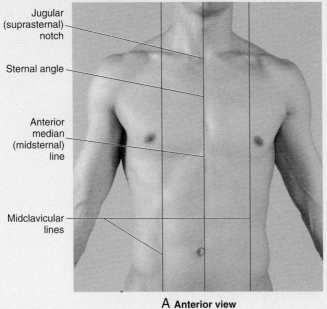

Jugular (suprasternal) notch
Sternal angle
Anterior median (midsternal) line
Midclavicular lines

A **Anterior view**

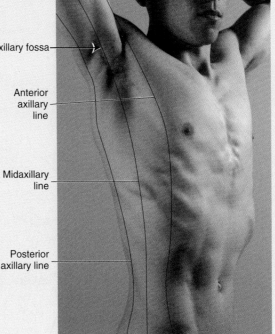

Axillary fossa
Anterior axillary line
Midaxillary line
Posterior axillary line

B **Anterolateral view**

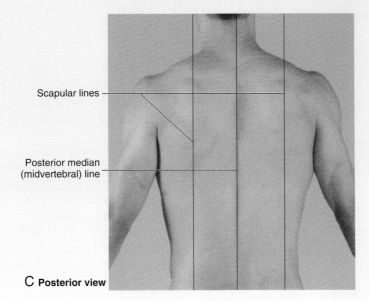

Scapular lines
Posterior median (midvertebral) line

C **Posterior view**

Figure SA1.1.

continued >

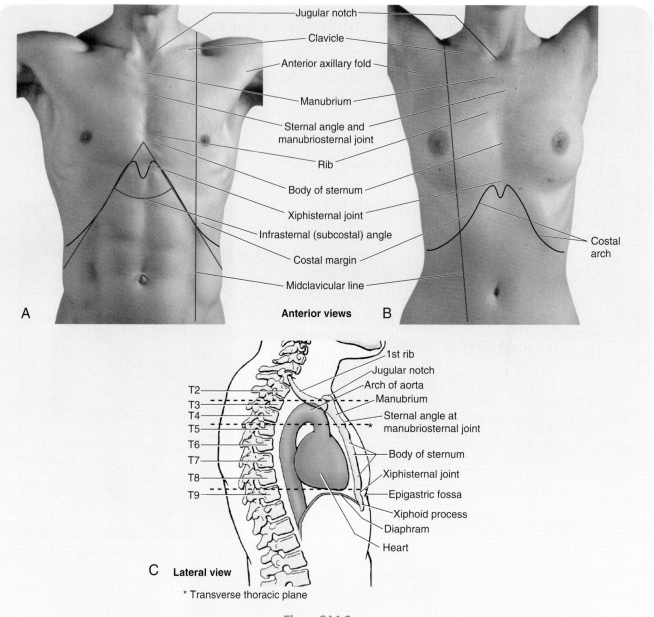

Figure SA1.2.

- **Midaxillary line** runs from the apex (deepest part) of the axilla, parallel to the anterior axillary line (Fig. SA1.1*B*).
- **Posterior axillary line,** also parallel to the anterior axillary line, is drawn vertically along the posterior axillary fold formed by the latissimus dorsi and teres major muscles as they span from the back to the humerus (Fig. SA1.1*B*).
- **Posterior median (midvertebral) line** is a vertical line at the intersection of the median plane with the vertebral column. (Fig. SA1.1*C*).

- **Scapular lines** are parallel to the posterior median line and cross the inferior angles of the scapulae (Fig. SA1.1*C*).

Additional lines (not illustrated) are extrapolated along borders of bony formations—for example, the parasternal line (G. *para,* adjacent to).

The **clavicles** lie subcutaneously, forming bony ridges at the junction of the thorax and neck (Fig. SA1.2). They can be palpated easily throughout their length, especially where their medial ends articulate with the manubrium.

continued >

The **sternum** also lies subcutaneously in the anterior median line and is palpable throughout its length. The *manubrium of the sternum:*

- Lies at the level of the bodies of **T3 and T4 vertebrae.**
- Is anterior to the **arch of the aorta.**
- Has a **jugular notch** that can be palpated between the prominent sternal ends of the clavicles.
- Has a **sternal angle** where it articulates with the sternal body at the level of the **T4–T5 IV disc** and the space between the 3rd and 4th spinous processes.

The **sternal angle** is a palpable landmark that lies at the level of the 2nd pair of costal cartilages. The main bronchi pass inferolaterally from the bifurcation of the trachea at the level of the sternal angle. The sternal angle also demarcates the division between the superior and inferior mediastina and the beginning of the arch of the aorta. The **superior vena cava** passes inferiorly deep to the manubrium, projecting as much as a fingerbreadth to the right of this bone.

The 1st rib cannot be palpated because it lies deep to the clavicle; thus **count the ribs and intercostal spaces anteriorly** by sliding the fingers laterally from the sternal angle onto the 2nd costal cartilage. Start counting with rib 2 and count the ribs and spaces by moving the fingers inferolaterally. The 1st intercostal space is inferior to the 1st rib; likewise, the other spaces lie inferior to the similarly numbered ribs.

The **body of the sternum,** lies anterior to the right border of the heart and vertebrae T5–T9. The **xiphoid process** lies in a slight depression (the **epigastric fossa)** where the converging costal margins form the **infrasternal angle.** This angle is used in *cardiopulmonary resuscitation* (CPR) for locating the proper hand position on the inferior part of the body of the sternum. The **costal margins,** formed by the medial borders of the 7th–10th costal cartilages, are easily palpable where they extend inferolaterally from the **xiphisternal joint.** This articulation, often seen as a ridge, is at the level of the inferior border of the T9 vertebra.

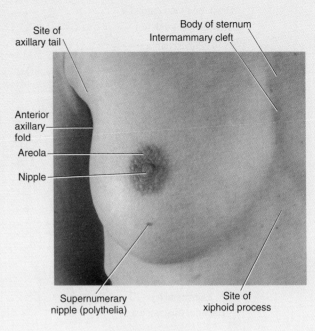

Figure SA1.3.

Breasts are the most prominent surface features of the anterior thoracic wall, especially in women. Their flattened superior surfaces show no sharp demarcation from the anterior surface of the thoracic wall; however, laterally and inferiorly their borders are well defined (Fig. SA1.3). The cleavage in the anterior median line—the **intermammary cleft**—is between the breasts. The **nipple** in the midclavicular line is surrounded by a slightly raised and circular pigmented area—the **areola.** The color of the areola vary with the woman's complexion; they darken during pregnancy and retain this color thereafter. The nipple in men lies anterior to the 4th intercostal space, about 10 cm from the anterior median line. The position of the nipple in women is inconstant and so is not reliable as a surface landmark. ●

Vasculature of Thoracic Wall

The **arterial supply to the thoracic wall** is derived from the **thoracic aorta** through the posterior intercostal and subcostal arteries, the **subclavian artery** through the internal thoracic and supreme intercostal arteries, and the **axillary artery** through the superior and lateral thoracic arteries (Figs. 1.9 and 1.13*A;* Table 1.3). With the exception of the 10th and 11th intercostal spaces, each intercostal space is supplied by three arteries: a large posterior intercostal artery (and its collateral branch) and a small pair of anterior intercostal arteries.

The **veins of the thoracic wall** accompany the intercostal arteries and nerves and lie most superior in the costal grooves (Figs. 1.10 and 1.13*B*). There are 11 posterior intercostal veins and one subcostal vein on each side. The posterior intercostal veins anastomose with the anterior

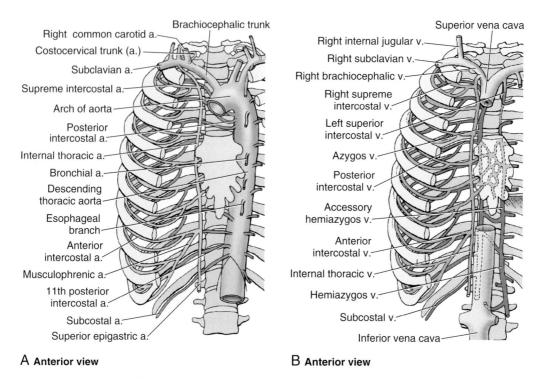

A Anterior view

B Anterior view

Figure 1.13. Arteries and veins of thoracic wall.

intercostal veins, tributaries of the internal thoracic veins. Most posterior intercostal veins end in the *azygos/hemiazygos venous system* (discussed later in this chapter), which conveys venous blood to the superior vena cava.

Endothoracic Fascia

The **endothoracic fascia** is a thin fibroareolar layer between the internal aspect of the thoracic cage and the lining of the pleural cavities (parietal pleura) (Fig. 1.14). This fascia invests the underlying internal and innermost intercostals and the subcostal and transverse thoracic muscles. It blends with the periosteum of the ribs and sternum and perichondrium of the costal cartilages. The endothoracic fascia provides a cleavage plane, allowing the surgeon to separate the parietal pleura from the thoracic wall, providing access to intrathoracic structures.

Table 1.3 Arterial Supply to the Thoracic Wall

Artery	Origin	Course	Distribution
Posterior intercostals	Supreme intercostal arteries (intercostal spaces 1 and 2) and thoracic aorta (remaining intercostal spaces)	Pass between internal and innermost intercostal muscles	Intercostal muscles and overlying skin, parietal pleura
Anterior intercostals	Internal thoracic arteries (intercostal spaces 1–6) and musculophrenic arteries (intercostal spaces 7–9)		
Internal thoracic	Subclavian artery	Passes inferiorly, lateral to sternum, between costal cartilages and internal intercostal muscles to divide into superior epigastric and musculophrenic arteries	By way of anterior intercostal arteries to intercostal spaces 1–6 and musculophrenic arteries to intercostal spaces 7–9
Subcostal	Thoracic aorta	Courses along interior border of 12th rib	Muscles of anterolateral abdominal wall and overlying skin

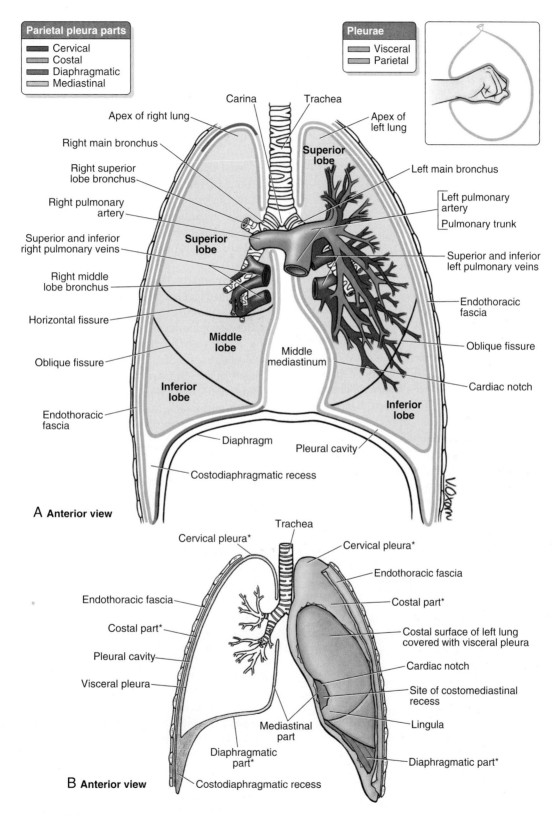

Parietal pleura parts
- Cervical
- Costal
- Diaphragmatic
- Mediastinal

Pleurae
- Visceral
- Parietal

Carina

Trachea

Apex of right lung

Apex of left lung

Right main bronchus

Superior lobe

Right superior lobe bronchus

Left main bronchus

Right pulmonary artery

Left pulmonary artery

Pulmonary trunk

Superior and inferior right pulmonary veins

Superior lobe

Superior and inferior left pulmonary veins

Right middle lobe bronchus

Endothoracic fascia

Horizontal fissure

Middle lobe

Oblique fissure

Middle mediastinum

Oblique fissure

Inferior lobe

Cardiac notch

Inferior lobe

Endothoracic fascia

Diaphragm

Pleural cavity

Costodiaphragmatic recess

A **Anterior view**

Trachea

Cervical pleura*

Cervical pleura*

Endothoracic fascia

Endothoracic fascia

Costal part*

Costal part*

Costal surface of left lung covered with visceral pleura

Pleural cavity

Cardiac notch

Visceral pleura

Site of costomediastinal recess

Lingula

Mediastinal part

Diaphragmatic part*

Diaphragmatic part*

B **Anterior view**

Costodiaphragmatic recess

Figure 1.14. Lungs and pleurae. A. The lungs and pleural cavity are shown. ***Inset:*** A fist invaginating an underinflated balloon demonstrates the relationship of the lung (represented by fist) to the walls of the pleural sac (parietal and visceral layers of pleura). The cavity of the pleural sac (pleural cavity) is comparable to the cavity of the balloon. **B.** The parts of the parietal pleura and recesses of the pleural cavities are shown. *Parts of pariental pleura.

Thoracic Cavity and Viscera

The thoracic cavity, the space enclosed by the thoracic walls, has three compartments (Fig. 1.14A):

- Two lateral compartments—the **pulmonary cavities**—that contain the lungs and pleurae (lining membranes).
- One central compartment—the **mediastinum**—that contains all other thoracic structures: heart, thoracic parts of the great vessels, thoracic part of the trachea, esophagus, thymus, and other structures (e.g., lymph nodes).

The pulmonary cavities are completely separate from each other and, with the lungs and pleurae, occupy the majority of the thoracic cavity. The mediastinum extends from the superior thoracic aperture to the diaphragm.

Pleurae and Lungs

To visualize the relationship of the pleurae and lungs, push your fist into an underinflated balloon (Fig. 1.14A). The part of the balloon wall adjacent to the skin of your fist (which represents the lung) is comparable to the *visceral pleura;* the remainder of the balloon represents the *parietal pleura.* The cavity between the layers of the balloon is analogous to the *pleural cavity.* At your wrist (*root of lung*), the inner and outer walls of the balloon are continuous, as are the visceral and parietal layers of pleura, together forming a *pleural sac.* Note that the lung is outside of but surrounded by the pleural sac, just as your fist is surrounded by but outside of the balloon.

PLEURAE

Each lung is invested by and enclosed in a serous pleural sac that consists of two continuous membranes—the pleurae (Fig. 1.14):

- The **visceral pleura** (pulmonary pleura) covers the lungs and is adherent to all its surfaces, including the surfaces within the horizontal and oblique fissures; it cannot be dissected from the lungs.
- The **parietal pleura** lines the pulmonary cavities, adhering to the thoracic wall, the mediastinum, and the diaphragm.

The root of the lung is enclosed within the area of continuity between the visceral and parietal layers of pleura the **pleural sleeve.** Inferior to the root of the lung, this continuity between parietal and visceral pleura forms the **pulmonary ligament** extending between the lung and the mediastinum. (Fig. 1.15).

The **pleural cavity**—the potential space between the visceral and the parietal layers of pleura—contains a capillary layer of **serous pleural fluid,** which lubricates the pleural surfaces and allows the layers of pleura to slide smoothly over each other during respiration. Its surface tension also provides the cohesion that keeps the lung surface in contact with the thoracic wall; consequently, the lung expands and fills with air when the thorax expands while still allowing sliding to occur, much like a layer of water between two glass plates.

The parietal pleura consists of four parts (Fig. 1.14):

- **Costal part** (pleura) covers the internal surfaces of the thoracic wall (sternum, ribs,costal cartilages, intercostal muscles and membranes, and side of thoracic vertebrae) and is separated from the wall by *endothoracic fascia.*
- **Mediastinal part** (pleura) covers the lateral aspects of the mediastinum (the central compartment of the thoracic cavity).
- **Diaphragmatic part** (pleura) covers the superior or thoracic surface of the diaphragm on each side of the mediastinum.
- **Cervical pleura** extends through the superior thoracic aperture into the root of the neck 2–3 cm superior to the level of the medial third of the clavicle at the level of the neck of the 1st rib, forming a cup-shaped dome over the apex of the lung. It is reinforced by a fibrous extension of the endothoracic fascia, the *suprapleural membrane* (Sibson fascia) spanning between the 1st rib and C7 vertebra.

The relatively abrupt lines along which the parietal pleura changes direction from one wall of the pleural cavity to another are the **lines of pleural reflection.**

- The **sternal line of pleural reflection** is sharp or abrupt and occurs where the costal pleura becomes continuous with the mediastinal pleura anteriorly.
- The **costal line of pleural reflection** is also sharp and occurs where the costal pleura becomes continuous with the diaphragmatic pleura inferiorly.
- The **vertebral line of pleural reflection** is a much rounder, gradual reflection where the costal pleura becomes continuous with the mediastinal pleura posteriorly.

The lungs do not completely occupy the pleural cavities during expiration; thus the peripheral diaphragmatic pleura is in contact with the lowermost part of the costal pleura. The potential pleural spaces here are the **costodiaphragmatic recesses,** the pleural-lined "gutters" that surround the upward convexity of the diaphragm inside the thoracic wall (Fig. 1.14). Similar but smaller pleural recesses are located posterior to the sternum where the costal pleura is in contact with the mediastinal pleura. The potential spaces here are the **costomediastinal recesses** (Fig. 1.14B); the left recess is potentially larger (less occupied) because of the cardiac notch in the left lung. The inferior borders of the lungs move farther into the pleural recesses during deep inspiration and retreat from them during expiration.

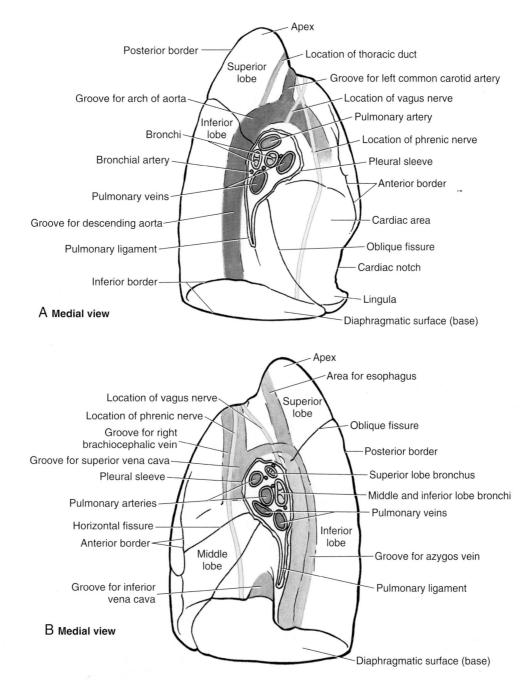

Apex

Posterior border

Superior
lobe

Location of thoracic duct

Groove for left common carotid artery

Groove for arch of aorta

Location of vagus nerve

Inferior
lobe

Pulmonary artery

Bronchi

Location of phrenic nerve

Bronchial artery

Pleural sleeve

Pulmonary veins

Anterior border

Groove for descending aorta

Cardiac area

Pulmonary ligament

Oblique fissure

Cardiac notch

Inferior border

Lingula

A Medial view

Diaphragmatic surface (base)

Apex

Area for esophagus

Location of vagus nerve

Superior
lobe

Location of phrenic nerve

Oblique fissure

Groove for right
brachiocephalic vein

Posterior border

Groove for superior vena cava

Superior lobe bronchus

Pleural sleeve

Middle and inferior lobe bronchi

Pulmonary arteries

Pulmonary veins

Horizontal fissure

Inferior
lobe

Anterior border

Middle
lobe

Groove for azygos vein

Groove for inferior
vena cava

Pulmonary ligament

B Medial view

Diaphragmatic surface (base)

Figure 1.15. Mediastinal surfaces of lungs. Both the left (**A**) and right (**B**) lungs are shown. Observe the somewhat pear-shaped depression, the hilum (doorway) of the lung, near the center of this surface. Embalmed lungs have impressions of the structures in contact with them (e.g., aorta and superior vena cava).

LUNGS

The lungs are the vital organs of respiration. Their main function is to oxygenate the blood by bringing inspired air into close relation with the venous blood in the pulmonary capillaries. Although cadaveric lungs may be shrunken, firm to the touch, and discolored in appearance, healthy lungs in living people are normally light, soft, and spongy. They are also elastic and recoil to about one third their size when the thoracic cavity is opened.

The **root of the lung** is formed by the structures entering and emerging from the lung at its hilum (Fig. 1.15). The root of the lung connects the lung with the heart and trachea. If the root is sectioned before the branching of the

Pulmonary Collapse

If a sufficient amount of air enters the pleural cavity, the surface tension adhering visceral to parietal pleura (lung to thoracic wall) is broken, and the lung collapses because of its inherent elasticity (elastic recoil). When a lung collapses, the pleural cavity—normally a potential space (Fig. B1.6, *purple*)—becomes a real space. The pleural cavity is located between the parietal pleura (*blue*) and the visceral pleura (*red*). One lung may be collapsed after surgery, for example, without collapsing the other because the pleural sacs are separate.

Pneumothorax, Hydrothorax, Hemothorax, and Chylothorax

Entry of air into the pleural cavity—*pneumothorax*—resulting from a penetrating wound of the parietal pleura or rupture of a lung from a bullet, for example, results in partial collapse of the lung. Fractured ribs may also tear the parietal pleura and produce pneumothorax. This may also occur as a result of leakage from the lung through an opening in the visceral pleura. The accumulation of a significant amount of fluid in the pleural cavity—*hydrothorax*—may result from *pleural effusion* (escape of fluid into the pleural cavity). With a chest wound, blood may also enter the pleural cavity (*hemothorax*); this condition results more often from injury to a major intercostal vessel than from laceration of a lung.

Lymph from a torn thoracic duct may also enter the pleural cavity (*chylothorax*). Chyle, a pale white or yellow lymph fluid in the thoracic duct containing fat absorbed by the intestines (see Chapter 2).

Pleuritis

During inspiration and expiration, the normally moist, smooth pleurae make no sound detectable by *auscultation* (listening to breath sounds); however, inflammation of the pleurae—*pleuritis* (pleurisy)—makes the lung surfaces rough. The resulting friction (*pleural rub*) may be heard with a stethoscope. Acute pleuritis is marked by sharp, stabbing pain, especially on exertion, such as climbing stairs, when the rate and depth of respiration may be increased even slightly.

Thoracocentesis

Sometimes it is necessary to insert a hypodermic needle through an intercostal space into the pleural cavity—the potential space between the parietal pleura lining the pulmonary cavity and the visceral pleura covering the lung—to obtain a sample of pleural fluid or to remove blood or pus. To avoid damage to the intercostal nerve and vessels, the needle is inserted superior to the rib, high enough to avoid the collateral branches (Fig. B1.7).

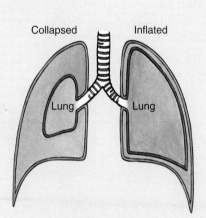

Figure B1.6

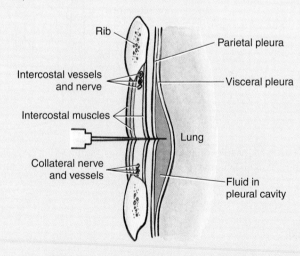

Figure B1.7. Technique for thoracocentesis.

main bronchus and pulmonary artery, its general arrangement is

- Pulmonary artery, superiormost on the left (the superior lobar bronchus may be superiormost on the right).
- Superior and inferior pulmonary veins, anteriormost and inferiormost, respectively.
- Bronchus, against and approximately in the middle of the posterior boundary, with bronchial vessels immediately surrounding.

The root is enclosed within the area of continuity between the parietal and the visceral layers of pleura—the *pleural sleeve* or mesopneumonium (mesentery of the lung). The *hilum of the lung* is the area on the medial surface of each lung the point at which the structures forming the root—the main bronchus, pulmonary vessels, bronchial vessels, lymphatic vessels, and nerves—enter and leave the lung.

The **horizontal and oblique fissures** divide the lungs into lobes (Table 1.4). *The right lung has three lobes, the left lung has two.* The right lung is larger and heavier than the left, but it is shorter and wider because the right dome of the diaphragm is higher and the heart and pericardium bulge more to the left. The anterior margin of the right lung is relatively straight, whereas this margin of the left lung has a **cardiac notch**. The cardiac notch primarily indents the anteroinferior aspect of the superior lobe of the left lung. This often creates a thin, tongue-like process of the superior lobe—the **lingula** (Fig. 1.14*B*), which extends below the

Table 1.4 Lobes and Fissures of the Lungs

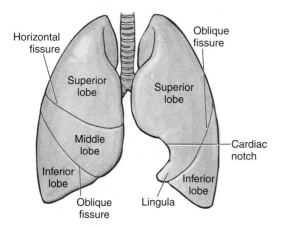

Right lung (three lobes)

Superior (upper) lobe is separated by horizontal fissure from middle lobe, which is separated by oblique fissure from inferior (lower) lobe

Left lung (two lobes)

Superior (upper) lobe is separated by oblique fissure from inferior (lower) lobe

cardiac notch and slides in and out of the costomediastinal recess during inspiration and expiration. Each lung has (Figs. 1.14 and 1.15):

- **An apex:** blunt superior end of the lung ascending above the level of the 1st rib into the root of the neck; covered by cervical pleura.
- **Three surfaces:** *costal surface,* adjacent to the sternum, costal cartilages, and ribs; *mediastinal surface,* including the hilum of the lung and related medially to the mediastinum and posteriorly to sides of the vertebrae; and *diaphragmatic surface,* resting on the convex dome of the diaphragm.
- **Three borders:** *anterior border,* where the costal and mediastinal surfaces meet anteriorly and overlap the heart (the *cardiac notch* indents this border of the left lung); *inferior border,* which circumscribes the diaphragmatic surface of the lung and separates the diaphragmatic surface from the costal and mediastinal surfaces; and *posterior border,* where the costal and mediastinal surfaces meet posteriorly (it is broad and rounded and lies adjacent to the thoracic region of the vertebral column).

TRACHEA AND BRONCHI

The two **main bronchi** (primary bronchi), one to each lung, pass inferolaterally from the **bifurcation of the trachea** to the lungs at the level of the sternal angle to the hila of the lungs (Figs. 1.16 and 1.17*A*). The walls of the trachea and bronchi are supported by C-shaped rings of hyaline cartilage.

- The **right main bronchus** is wider, shorter, and runs more vertically than the left main bronchus as it passes directly to the hilum of the lung.
- The **left main bronchus** passes inferolaterally, inferior to the arch of the aorta and anterior to the esophagus and thoracic aorta, to reach the hilum of the lung.

The main bronchi enter the hila of the lungs and branch in a constant fashion within the lungs to form the **bronchial tree.** Each main bronchus divides into **lobar bronchi** (secondary bronchi), two on the left and three on the right, each of which supplies a lobe of the lung. Each lobar bronchus divides into **segmental bronchi** (tertiary bronchi) that supply the bronchopulmonary segments (Fig. 1.17*B* & *C*). Each **bronchopulmonary segment** is pyramidal, with its apex directed toward the root of the lung and its base at the pleural surface and is named according to the segmental bronchus that supplies it. Each bronchopulmonary segment is supplied independently by a segmental bronchus and a tertiary branch of the pulmonary artery and is drained by intersegmental parts of the pulmonary veins. Beyond the segmental bronchi, there are 20–25 generations of branches that end in

Surface Anatomy of Pleurae and Lungs

The cervical pleurae and apices of the lungs pass through the superior thoracic aperture into the root of the neck superior and posterior to the clavicles. The anterior borders of the lungs lie adjacent to the anterior line of reflection of the parietal pleura between the 2nd and 4th costal cartilages (Fig SA1.4). Here the margin of the left pleural reflection moves laterally and then inferiorly at the cardiac notch to reach the level of the 6th costal cartilage. The anterior border of the left lung is more deeply indented by its cardiac notch. On the right side, the pleural reflection continues inferiorly from the 4th to the 6th costal cartilage, paralleled closely by the anterior border of the right lung. Both pleural reflections pass laterally and reach

the midclavicular line at the level of the 8th costal cartilage, the 10th rib at the midaxillary line, and the 12th rib at the scapular line, proceeding toward the spinous process of the T12 vertebra. Thus the parietal pleura extends approximately two ribs inferior to the lung. The *oblique fissure of the lungs* extends from the level of the spinous process of the T2 vertebra posteriorly to the 6th costal cartilage anteriorly, which coincides approximately with the medial border of the scapula when the upper limb is elevated above the head (causing the inferior angle to be rotated laterally). The *horizontal fissure of the right lung* extends from the oblique fissure along the 4th rib and costal cartilage anteriorly.

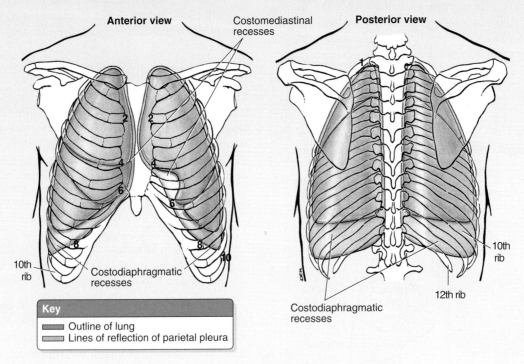

Figure SA1.4.

terminal bronchioles (Fig. 1.18). Each terminal bronchiole gives rise to several generations of **respiratory bronchioles** and each respiratory bronchiole provides 2–11 **alveolar ducts**, each of which gives rise to 5–6 **alveolar sacs**. The **pulmonary alveolus** is the basic structural unit of gas exchange in the lung.

VASCULATURE AND NERVES OF LUNGS AND PLEURAE

Each lung has a large **pulmonary artery** supplying blood to it and two **pulmonary veins** draining blood from it (Fig. 1.19). The right and left pulmonary arteries arise from the **pulmonary trunk** at the level of the sternal angle. The

Auscultation and Percussion of Lungs

Auscultation of the lungs (assessing air flow through the tracheobronchial tree into the lung with a stethoscope) and *percussion of the lungs* (tapping the chest over the lungs with the finger) always include the root of the neck to detect sounds in the apices of the lungs. Percussion helps establish whether the underlying tissues are air-filled (resonant sound), fluid-filled (dull sound), or solid (flat sound). When physicians refer to the base of a lung, they are usually not referring to its diaphragmatic surface (base). They are referring to the inferior part of the posterior costal surface of the inferior lobe. To auscultate this area, physicians apply a stethoscope to the inferoposterior aspect of the thoracic wall at the level of the T10 vertebra.

Variation in Lobes of Lungs

Occasionally, an extra fissure divides a lung or a fissure is absent. For example, the left lung sometimes has three lobes and the right lung only two. The most common "accessory" lobe is the *azygos lobe,* which appears in the right lung in approximately 1% of people. In these cases, the azygos vein arches over the apex of the right lung and not over the right hilum, isolating the medial part of the apex as an azygos lobe.

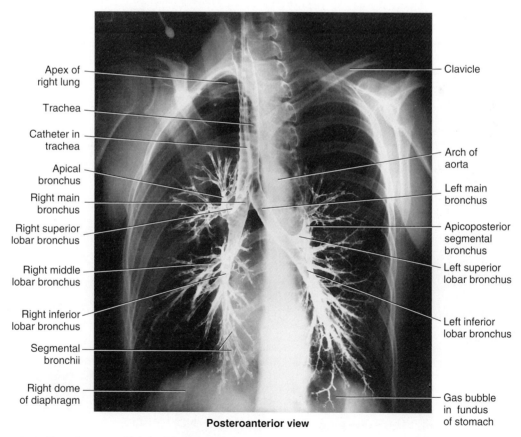

Apex of right lung

Trachea

Catheter in trachea

Apical bronchus

Right main bronchus

Right superior lobar bronchus

Right middle lobar bronchus

Right inferior lobar bronchus

Segmental bronchii

Right dome of diaphragm

Clavicle

Arch of aorta

Left main bronchus

Apicoposterior segmental bronchus

Left superior lobar bronchus

Left inferior lobar bronchus

Gas bubble in fundus of stomach

Posteroanterior view

Figure 1.16. Bronchogram. Slightly oblique, posteroanterior bronchogram of right and left bronchial tree is shown.

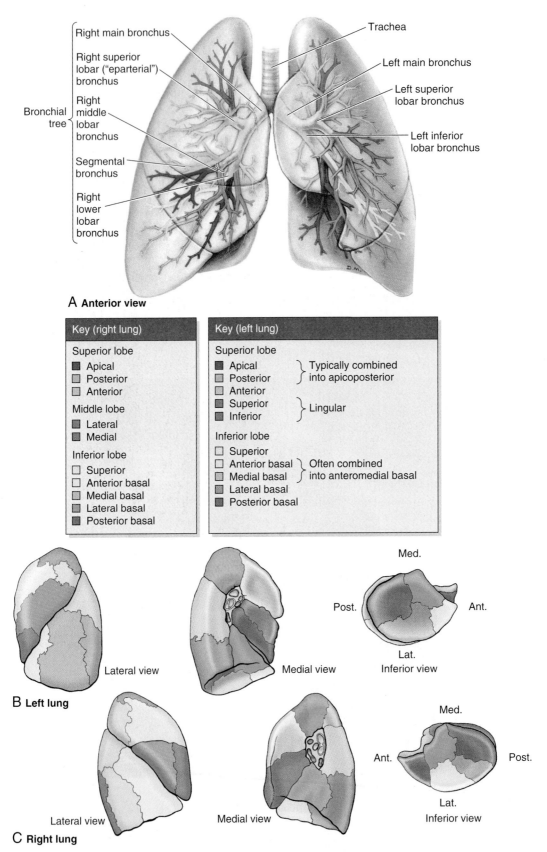

A Anterior view

Key (right lung)	Key (left lung)

Key (right lung)

Superior lobe
- ■ Apical
- □ Posterior
- □ Anterior

Middle lobe
- ■ Lateral
- ■ Medial

Inferior lobe
- □ Superior
- □ Anterior basal
- ■ Medial basal
- ■ Lateral basal
- ■ Posterior basal

Key (left lung)

Superior lobe
- ■ Apical   } Typically combined
- ■ Posterior   } into apicoposterior
- □ Anterior
- ■ Superior   } Lingular
- ■ Inferior   }

Inferior lobe
- □ Superior
- □ Anterior basal } Often combined
- ■ Medial basal   } into anteromedial basal
- ■ Lateral basal
- ■ Posterior basal

Med.

Post.   Ant.

Lat.
Inferior view

Lateral view   Medial view

B Left lung

Med.

Ant.   Post.

Lat.
Inferior view

Lateral view   Medial view

C Right lung

Figure 1.17. Bronchi and bronchopulmonary segments. A. The segmental (tertiary) bronchi are indicated by colors (see key). The bronchopulmonary segments of the left (**B**) and right (**C**) lungs are identified.

Aspiration of Foreign Bodies

Because the right bronchus is wider and shorter and runs more vertically than the left bronchus, aspirated foreign bodies are more likely to enter and lodge in it or one of its branches. A potential hazard encountered by dentists is an aspirated foreign body, such as a piece of tooth, filling material, or a small instrument. Such objects are also most likely to enter the right main bronchus.

Lung Resections

Knowledge of the anatomy of the bronchopulmonary segments is essential for precise interpretations of diagnostic images of the lungs and for surgical resection (removal) of diseased segments. When resecting a bronchopulmonary segment, surgeons follow the interlobar veins to pass between the segments. Bronchial and pulmonary disorders such as tumors or abscesses (collections of pus) often localize in a bronchopulmonary segment, which may be surgically resected. During the treatment of lung cancer, the surgeon may remove a whole lung (**pneumonectomy**), a lobe (**lobectomy**), or one or more bronchopulmonary segments (**segmentectomy**). Knowledge and understanding of the bronchopulmonary segments and their relationship to the bronchial tree are also essential for planning drainage and clearance techniques used in physical therapy for enhancing drainage from specific areas (e.g., in patients with pneumonia or cystic fibrosis).

Bronchoscopy

When examining the bronchi with a **bronchoscope**—an endoscope for inspecting the interior of the tracheobronchial tree for diagnostic purposes—one can observe

a ridge, the **carina,** between the orifices of the main bronchi (Fig. B1.8). The carina is a cartilaginous projection of the last tracheal ring. If the tracheobronchial lymph nodes in the angle between the main bronchi are enlarged because cancer cells have metastasized from a bronchogenic carcinoma, for example, the carina is distorted, widened posteriorly, and immobile.

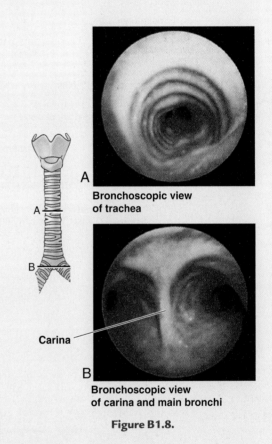

Bronchoscopic view of trachea

Carina

Bronchoscopic view of carina and main bronchi

Figure B1.8.

pulmonary arteries *carry poorly oxygenated ("venous") blood to the lungs for oxygenation.* The pulmonary arteries pass to the corresponding root of the lung and give off a branch to the superior lobe before entering the hilum. Within the lung, each artery descends posterolateral to the main bronchus and divides into **lobar** and **segmental arteries.** Consequently, an arterial branch goes to each lobe and bronchopulmonary segment of the lung, usually on the anterior aspect of the corresponding bronchus. The **pulmonary veins,** two on each side, *carry well-oxygenated ("ar-*terial") blood from the lungs to the left atrium of the heart.* Beginning in the pulmonary capillaries, the veins unite into larger and larger vessels. Intrasegmental veins drain blood from adjacent bronchopulmonary segments into the intersegmental veins in the septa, which separate the segments. A main vein drains each bronchopulmonary segment, usually on the anterior surface of the corresponding bronchus.

The *veins from the parietal pleura join the systemic veins in* adjacent parts of the thoracic wall. The *veins from the visceral pleura drain into the pulmonary veins.*

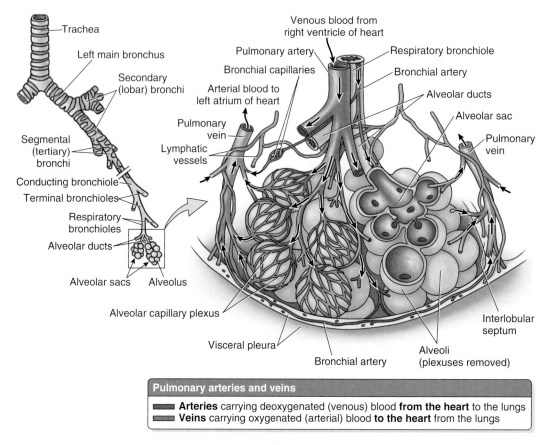

Trachea

Left main bronchus

Secondary (lobar) bronchi

Segmental (tertiary) bronchi

Conducting bronchiole

Terminal bronchioles

Respiratory bronchioles

Alveolar ducts

Alveolar sacs   Alveolus

Venous blood from right ventricle of heart

Pulmonary artery

Bronchial capillaries

Arterial blood to left atrium of heart

Pulmonary vein

Lymphatic vessels

Respiratory bronchiole

Bronchial artery

Alveolar ducts

Alveolar sac

Pulmonary vein

Alveolar capillary plexus

Visceral pleura

Bronchial artery

Alveoli (plexuses removed)

Interlobular septum

Pulmonary arteries and veins

▬ **Arteries** carrying deoxygenated (venous) blood **from the heart** to the lungs
▬ **Veins** carrying oxygenated (arterial) blood **to the heart** from the lungs

Figure 1.18. Internal structure of lungs.

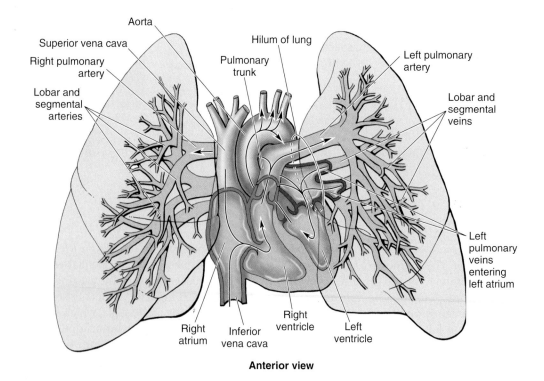

Aorta

Superior vena cava

Right pulmonary artery

Lobar and segmental arteries

Hilum of lung

Pulmonary trunk

Left pulmonary artery

Lobar and segmental veins

Left pulmonary veins entering left atrium

Right atrium

Inferior vena cava

Right ventricle

Left ventricle

Anterior view

Figure 1.19. Pulmonary circulation.

The **bronchial arteries** supply blood to the structures making up the root of the lungs, the supporting tissues of the lung, and the visceral pleura (Figs. 1.15, 1.18, and 1.20). The left bronchial arteries arise from the thoracic aorta; however, the right bronchial artery may arise from:

- A superior posterior intercostal artery.
- A common trunk from the thoracic aorta with the right 3rd posterior intercostal artery.
- A left superior bronchial artery.

The small bronchial arteries provide branches to the superior esophagus and then pass along the posterior aspects of the main bronchi, supplying them and their branches as far distally as the respiratory bronchioles. The distalmost branches of the bronchial arteries anastomose with branches of the pulmonary arteries in the walls of the bronchioles and in the visceral pleura.

The **bronchial veins** drain only part of the blood supplied to the lungs by the bronchial arteries, primarily that distributed to or near the more proximal part of the root of the lungs (Fig. 1.20*B*). The remainder of the blood is drained by the pulmonary veins. The right bronchial vein drains into the **azygos vein**, and the left bronchial vein drains into the **accessory hemiazygos vein** or the left superior intercostal vein.

The **lymphatic plexuses in the lungs** communicate freely (Fig. 1.20*C*).

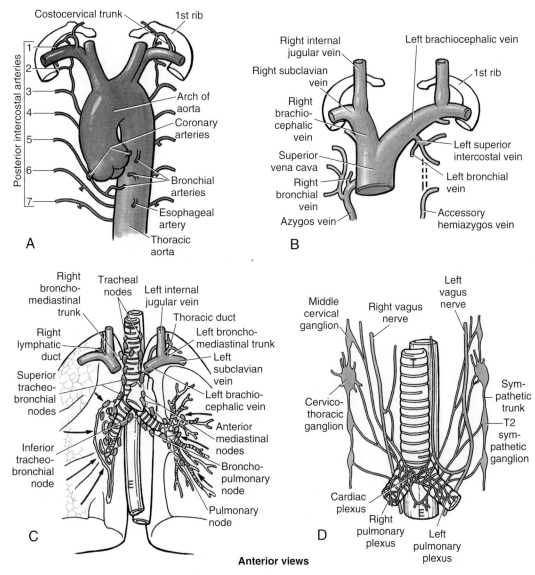

Figure 1.20. Vasculature and nerves of lungs and pleurae. The arteries (**A**), veins (**B**) are shown. **C.** *Arrows* indicate the direction of lymph flow; those on the right show the flow from the superficial pulmonary lymphatic plexuses, and those on the left indicate flow from the deep pulmonary plexuses. **D.** Innervation of the lungs is demonstrated. *E,* esophagus; *T,* trachea; *orange,* sympathetic; *green,* parasympathetic; *blue,* plexus.

Pulmonary Embolism

Obstruction of a pulmonary artery by a **blood clot** (*embolism*) is a common cause of morbidity (sickness) and mortality (death). An embolus in a pulmonary artery forms when a blood clot, fat globule, or air bubble travels in the blood to the lungs from a leg vein. The **embolus** passes through the right side of the heart to a lung through a pulmonary artery. The embolus may block a pulmonary artery—*pulmonary embolism*—or one of its branches. The immediate result is partial or complete obstruction of blood flow to the lung. The obstruction results in a sector of lung that is ventilated but not perfused with blood. When a large embolus occludes a pulmonary artery, the person suffers **acute respiratory distress** because of a major decrease in the oxygenation of blood owing to blockage of blood flow through the lung. A medium-size embolus may block an artery supplying a bronchopulmonary segment, producing a **pulmonary infarct**, an area of necrotic (dead) lung tissue.

The **superficial lymphatic plexus** lies deep to the visceral pleura and drains the lung parenchyma (tissue) and visceral pleura. Lymphatic vessels from the plexus drain into the **bronchopulmonary (hilar) lymph nodes** in the hilum of the lung.

The **deep lymphatic plexus** is located in the submucosa of the bronchi and in the peribronchial connective tissue. It is largely concerned with draining structures that form the root of the lung. Lymphatic vessels from this plexus drain into the **pulmonary lymph nodes** located along the lobar bronchi. At the hilum of the lung, they drain into bronchopulmonary (hilar) lymph nodes (Fig 1.20C).

Lymph from the superficial and deep plexuses drains from the bronchopulmonary lymph nodes to the superior and inferior **tracheobronchial lymph nodes**, superior and inferior to the bifurcation of the trachea, respectively. Lymph from the tracheobronchial lymph nodes passes to the **right** and **left bronchomediastinal lymph trunks**. These trunks usually terminate on each side at the *venous angles* (junction of the subclavian and internal jugular veins); however, the right bronchomediastinal trunk may first merge with other lymphatic trunks, converging here to form the **right lymphatic duct**. The left bronchomediastinal trunk may terminate in the **thoracic duct**. The superficial (subpleural) lymphatic plexus drains lymph from the *visceral pleura*. Lymph from the *parietal pleura* drains into the lymph nodes of the thoracic wall (intercostal, parasternal, mediastinal, and phrenic). A few lymphatic vessels from the cervical pleura drain into the axillary lymph nodes.

The **nerves of the lungs and visceral pleura** derive from the pulmonary plexuses located anterior and (mainly) posterior to the roots of the lungs (Fig. 1.20*D*). These nerve networks contain parasympathetic fibers from the **vagus nerves** (CN X) and sympathetic fibers from the sympathetic trunks. *Parasympathetic ganglion cells*—cell bodies of postsynaptic parasympathetic neurons—are in the **pulmonary plexuses** and along the branches of the bronchial tree. The parasympathetic fibers from CN X are motor to the smooth muscle of the bronchial tree (*bronchoconstrictor*), inhibitory to the pulmonary vessels (*vasodilator*), and secretory to the glands of the bronchial tree (*secretomotor*). The visceral afferent fibers of CN X are distributed to the:

- Bronchial mucosa and are probably concerned with tactile sensation for cough reflexes.
- Bronchial muscles, possibly involved in stretch reception.
- Interalveolar connective tissue, in association with Herring-Breuer reflexes (mechanism that tends to limit respiratory excursions).
- Pulmonary arteries serving pressor receptors (blood pressure) and pulmonary veins serving chemoreceptors (blood gas levels).

Sympathetic ganglion cells—cell bodies of postsynaptic sympathetic neurons—are in the **paravertebral sympathetic ganglia** of the sympathetic trunks. The sympathetic fibers are inhibitory to the bronchial muscle (bronchodilator), motor to the pulmonary vessels (vasoconstrictor), and inhibitory to the alveolar glands of the bronchial tree.

Mediastinum

The mediastinum, occupied by the viscera between the pulmonary cavities, is the central compartment of the thoracic cavity (Fig. 1.21). It is covered on each side by mediastinal pleura and contains all the thoracic viscera and structures, except the lungs. The mediastinum extends from the superior thoracic aperture to the diaphragm inferiorly and from the sternum and costal cartilages anteriorly to the bodies of the thoracic vertebrae posteriorly. The mediastinum in living persons is a highly mobile region because it consists primarily of hollow (liquid or air-filled) visceral structures united only by loose connective tissue, often infiltrated with fat. The major structures in the mediastinum are also surrounded by blood and lymphatic vessels, lymph nodes,

Injury to Pleurae

The visceral pleura is insensitive to pain because its inner-vation is autonomic (motor and visceral afferent). The autonomic nerves reach the visceral pleura in company with the bronchial vessels. The visceral pleura receives no nerves of general sensation. *The parietal pleura is sensitive to pain,* particularly the costal pleura, because it is richly supplied by branches of the somatic intercostal and phrenic nerves. Irritation of the parietal pleura produces local pain and referred pain to the areas sharing innervation by the same segments of the spinal cord. Irritation of the costal and peripheral parts of the diaphragmatic pleura results in local pain and referred pain along the intercostal nerves to the thoracic and abdominal walls. Irritation of the mediastinal and central diaphragmatic areas of the parietal pleura results in pain that is referred to the root of the neck and over the shoulder (C3–C5 dermatomes).

Inhalation of Carbon Particles

Lymph from the lungs carries **phagocytes,** cells possessing the property of ingesting carbon particles from inspired air. In many people, especially cigarette smokers, these particles color the surface of the lungs and associated lymph nodes a mottled gray to black. *Smokers' cough* results from inhalation of irritants in tobacco.

Bronchogenic Carcinoma

Bronchogenic carcinoma (CA) is a common type of lung cancer that arises from the epithelium of the bronchial tree. *Lung cancer* is mainly caused by cigarette smoking. Bronchogenic CA usually metastasizes widely because of the arrangement of the lymphatics. The tumor cells probably enter the systemic circulation by invading the wall of a sinusoid or venule in the lung and are transported through the pulmonary veins, left heart, and aorta to all parts of the body, especially the cranium and brain.

nerves, and fat. The looseness of the connective tissue and the elasticity of the lungs and parietal pleura on each side of the mediastinum enable it to accommodate movement, as well as volume and pressure changes in the thoracic cavity, such as those resulting from movements of the diaphragm, thoracic wall, and tracheobronchial tree during respiration, contraction (beating) of the heart and pulsations of the

great arteries, and passage of ingested substances through the esophagus. The connective tissue here becomes more fibrous and rigid with age; hence the mediastinal structures become less mobile.

The mediastinum is artificially divided into superior and inferior parts for purposes of description.

- The **superior mediastinum** extends inferiorly from the superior thoracic aperture to the horizontal plane (transverse thoracic plane) passing through the sternal angle and the IV disc of the T4–T5 vertebra (Fig. 1.21). It contains the superior vena cava (SVC), brachiocephalic veins, arch of the aorta, thoracic duct, trachea, esophagus, thymus, vagus nerves, left recurrent laryngeal nerve, and phrenic nerves.
- The **inferior mediastinum**, between the transverse thoracic plane and the diaphragm, is further subdivided by the pericardium into the **anterior mediastinum** containing remnants of the thymus, lymph nodes, fat, and connective tissue; **middle mediastinum** containing the pericardium, heart, roots of the great vessels, arch of azygos vein, and main bronchi; and **posterior mediastinum** containing the esophagus, thoracic aorta, azygos and hemiazygos veins, thoracic duct, vagus nerves, sympathetic trunks, and splanchnic nerves.

The anterior and middle mediastinum are described first, followed by the superior and posterior mediastinum because many structures (e.g., the esophagus) pass vertically

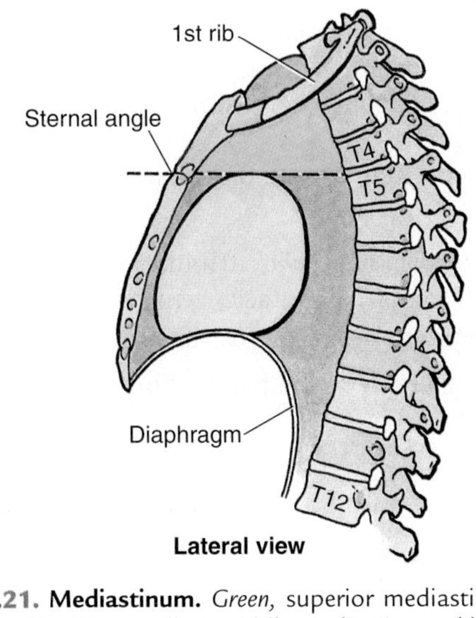

Figure 1.21. Mediastinum. *Green,* superior mediastinum; *purple,* anterior mediastinum; *yellow,* middle mediastinum; *blue,* posterior mediastinum.

through the superior and posterior mediastinum and, therefore, lie in more than one mediastinal compartment.

Anterior Mediastinum

The anterior mediastinum, the smallest subdivision of the mediastinum, lies between the body of the sternum and the transverse thoracic muscles anteriorly and the pericardium posteriorly (Fig. 1.21). The anterior mediastinum is continuous with the superior mediastinum at the sternal angle and is limited inferiorly by the diaphragm. The anterior mediastinum consists of loose connective tissue (*sternopericardial ligaments,* fibrous bands that pass from the pericardium to the sternum), fat, lymphatic vessels, a few lymph nodes, and branches of the internal thoracic vessels. In infants and children, the anterior mediastinum contains the inferior part of the thymus.

Middle Mediastinum

The middle mediastinum contains the pericardium, heart, the ascending aorta, pulmonary trunk, SVC, arch of azygos vein, and main bronchi.

PERICARDIUM

The pericardium is a double-walled fibroserous membrane that encloses the heart and the roots of its great vessels (Table 1.5). This conical **pericardial sac** lies posterior to the body of the sternum and the 2nd–6th costal cartilages at the level of the T5–T8 vertebrae. The tough external fibrous layer of the sac—the **fibrous pericardium**—is continuous with (blends with) the central tendon of the diaphragm (Fig. 1.22A). The internal surface of the fibrous pericardium is lined with a glistening serous membrane, the **parietal layer of serous pericardium.** This layer is reflected onto the heart and great vessels as the **visceral layer of serous pericardium.**

The *pericardial sac* is influenced by movements of the heart and great vessels, sternum, and diaphragm because the fibrous pericardium is:

- Fused with the tunica adventitia of the great vessels entering and leaving the heart.
- Attached to the posterior surface of the sternum by sternopericardial ligaments.
- Fused with the central tendon of the diaphragm.

The **fibrous pericardium** protects the heart against sudden overfilling because it is unyielding and closely related to the great vessels that pierce it superiorly and posteriorly (Fig. 1.22B). The ascending aorta carries the pericardium superiorly beyond the heart to the level of the sternal angle.

The **pericardial cavity** is the potential space between the opposing layers of the parietal and visceral layers of serous

pericardium (Table 2.5). It normally contains a thin film of serous fluid that enables the heart to move and beat in a frictionless environment.

The visceral layer of serous pericardium forms the **epicardium,** the external layer of the heart wall, and reflects from the heart and great vessels to become continuous with the parietal layer of serous pericardium, where:

- The aorta and pulmonary trunk leave the heart; a finger can be inserted into the **transverse pericardial sinus** located posterior to these large vessels and anterior to the SVC (Fig. 1.22C)
- The SVC, inferior vena cava (IVC), and pulmonary veins enter the heart; these vessels are partly covered by serous pericardium, which forms the **oblique pericardial sinus** (Fig. 1.22C), a wide recess posterior to the heart. The oblique sinus can be entered inferiorly and will admit several fingers; however, the fingers cannot pass around any of these vessels because the sinus is a blind recess (cul-de-sac).

These pericardial sinuses form during development of the heart as a consequence of folding of the primordial heart tube (Fig. 1.23). As the heart tube folds, its venous end moves posterosuperiorly so that the venous end of the tube lies adjacent to the arterial end, separated by the transverse pericardial sinus. As these vessels expand and move apart, the pericardium is reflected around them to form the boundaries of the oblique pericardial sinus.

The **arterial supply of the pericardium** is mainly from the **pericardiacophrenic artery** (Fig. 1.22A), a branch of the **internal thoracic artery,** which may accompany or parallel the phrenic nerve to the diaphragm. Smaller contributions of blood to the pericardium come from the *musculophrenic artery,* a terminal branch of the internal thoracic artery; the *bronchial, esophageal,* and *superior phrenic arteries* from the thoracic aorta; and the *coronary arteries* supplying only the visceral layer of serous pericardium (Fig. 1.13A).

The **venous drainage of the pericardium** is from the (Fig. 1.13B):

- *Pericardiacophrenic veins,* tributaries of the brachiocephalic (or internal thoracic) veins.
- Variable tributaries of azygos venous system.

The **nerve supply of the pericardium** is from the (Figs. 1.20D and 1.22A):

- *Phrenic nerves* (C3–C5)—a primary source of sensory fibers; pain sensations conveyed by these nerves are commonly referred to the skin (C3–C5 dermatomes) of the top of the shoulder of the same side.
- *Vagus nerves* (CN X)—function uncertain.
- *Sympathetic trunks*—vasomotor.

Table 1.5 Layers of the Pericardium and Heart

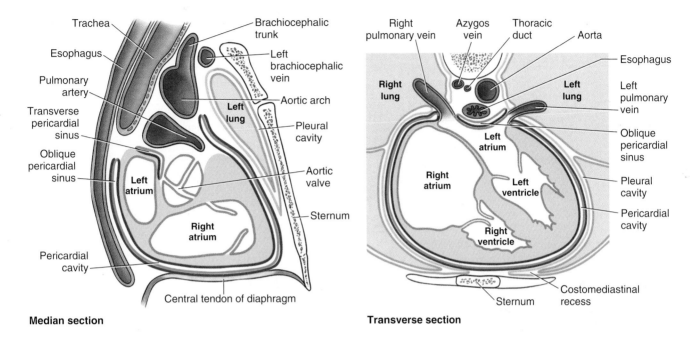

Median section

Transverse section

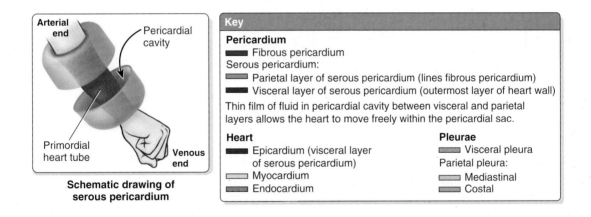

Schematic drawing of serous pericardium

Key

Pericardium

Fibrous pericardium

Serous pericardium:

Parietal layer of serous pericardium (lines fibrous pericardium)

Visceral layer of serous pericardium (outermost layer of heart wall)

Thin film of fluid in pericardial cavity between visceral and parietal layers allows the heart to move freely within the pericardial sac.

Heart

Epicardium (visceral layer of serous pericardium)

Myocardium

Endocardium

Pleurae

Visceral pleura

Parietal pleura:

Mediastinal

Costal

Heart and Great Vessels

The heart, slightly larger than a clenched fist, is a double self-adjusting muscular pump, the parts of which work in unison to propel blood to the body (Fig. 1.24). The right side of the heart receives poorly oxygenated blood from the body through the SVC and IVC and pumps it through the pulmonary trunk to the lungs for oxygenation. The left side of the heart receives well-oxygenated blood from the lungs through the pulmonary veins and pumps it into the aorta for distribution to the body.

STRUCTURE OF THE HEART AND CARDIAC CYCLE

The heart has four chambers: **right** and **left atria** and **right** and **left ventricles.** The atria are receiving chambers that pump blood into the ventricle (the discharging chambers). The synchronous pumping actions of the heart's two

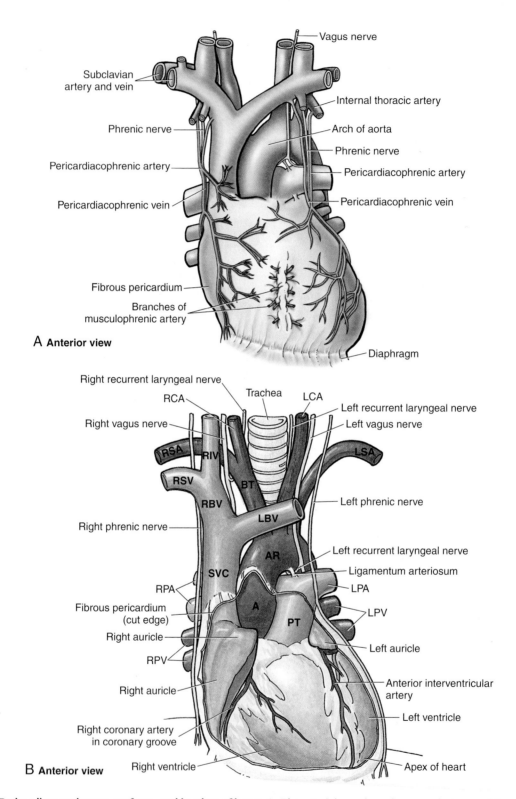

Figure 1.22. Pericardium and parts, surfaces, and borders of heart. A. The arterial supply and venous drainage of the pericardium are shown. **B.** The sternocostal surface of the heart is shown.

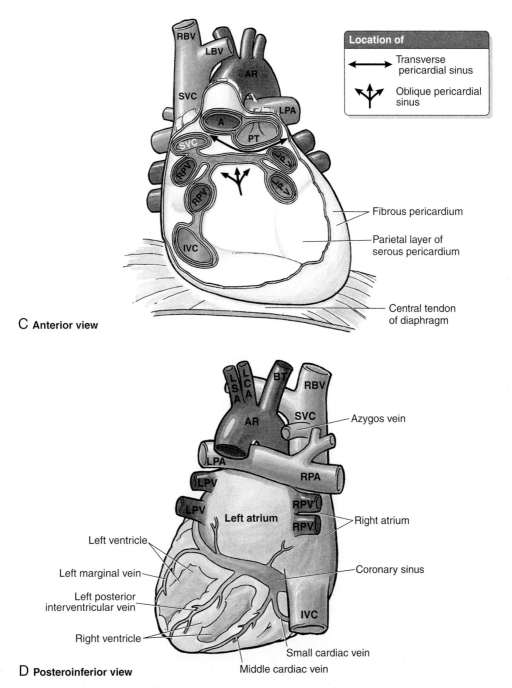

Figure 1.22. *(continued)* **C.** The interior of the pericardial sac is shown after the heart has been removed. **D.** The base and diaphragmatic surface of the heart are illustrated. *A,* aorta; *AR,* arch of aorta; *BT,* brachiocephalic trunk; *IVC,* inferior vena cava; *LBV,* left brachiocephalic vein; *LCA,* left common carotid artery; *LPA,* left pulmonary artery; *LPV,* left pulmonary vein; *LSA,* left subclavian artery; *PT,* pulmonary trunk; *RBV,* right brachiocephalic vein; *RCA,* right common carotid artery; *RIV,* right internal jugular vein; *RPA,* right pulmonary artery; *RPV,* right pulmonary vein; *SVC,* superior vena cava.

atrioventricular (AV) pumps (right and left chambers) constitute the **cardiac cycle** (Fig. 1.24). The cycle begins with a period of ventricular elongation and filling (**diastole**) and ends with a period of ventricular shortening and emptying (**systole**). Two *heart sounds,* resulting from valve closures, can be heard with a stethoscope: a *lub* sound as the blood is transferred (sucked) from the atria to the ventricles and a *dub* sound as the ventricles contract and expel blood from the heart. The heart sounds are produced by the snapping shut of the one-way valves that normally keep blood from flowing backward during contractions of the heart.

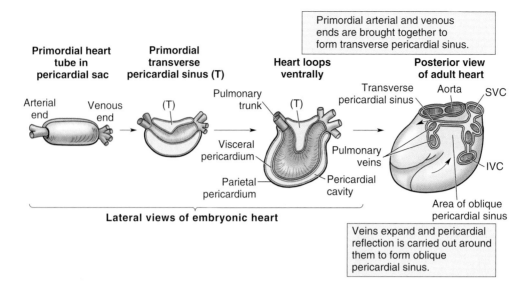

Primordial arterial and venous ends are brought together to form transverse pericardial sinus.

Figure 1.23. Development of heart and pericardium. The primordial heart tube invaginates the double-layered pericardial sac (somewhat like placing a hot dog in a bun). The primordial heart then loops ventrally, bringing the primordial arterial and venous ends of the heart together and creating the transverse pericardial sinus between them. The veins expand and move apart. The pericardium is reflected around them to form the boundaries of the oblique pericardial sinus. ***IVC,*** inferior vena cava; ***SVC,*** superior vena cava.

Surgical Significance of the Transverse Pericardial Sinus

The transverse pericardial sinus is especially important to cardiac surgeons. After the pericardial sac has been opened anteriorly, a finger can be passed through the transverse pericardial sinus posterior to the aorta and pulmonary trunk (Fig. B1.9). By passing a surgical clamp or placing a ligature around these vessels, inserting the tubes of a coronary bypass machine, and then tightening the ligature, surgeons can stop or divert the circulation of blood in these large arteries while performing cardiac surgery, such as coronary artery bypass grafting. Cardiac surgery is performed while the patient is on cardiopulmonary bypass.

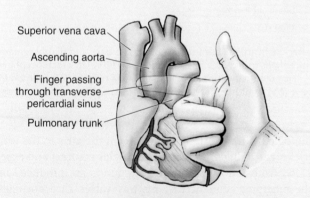

Superior vena cava

Ascending aorta

Finger passing through transverse pericardial sinus

Pulmonary trunk

Figure B1.9

Pericarditis, Pericardial Effusion, and Cardiac Tamponade

Inflammation of the pericardium (***pericarditis***) usually causes chest pain. Normally, the layers of serous pericardium make no detectable sound during auscultation. However, pericarditis makes the surfaces rough and the resulting friction, ***pericardial friction rub,*** sounds like the rustle of silk when listening with a stethoscope. Certain inflammatory diseases may also produce pericardial effusion (passage of fluid from the pericardial capillaries into the pericardial cavity). As a result, the heart becomes compressed (unable to expand and fill fully) and ineffectual.

   Cardiac tamponade (heart compression) is a potentially lethal condition because the fibrous pericardium is tough and inelastic. Consequently, heart volume is increasingly compromised by the fluid outside the heart but inside the pericardial cavity. When there is a slow increase in the size of the heart, ***cardiomegaly***, the pericardium allows the enlargement of heart to occur without compression. Stab wounds that pierce the heart causing blood to enter the pericardial cavity (***hemopericardium***) also risk producing cardiac tamponade. Hemopericardium may also result from perforation of a weakened area of heart muscle after a heart attack. As blood accumulates, the heart is compressed and circulation fails. ***Pericardiocentesis*** (drainage of serous fluid from pericardial cavity) is usually necessary to relieve the cardiac tamponade. To remove the excess fluid, a wide-bore needle may be inserted through the left 5th or 6th intercostal space near the sternum.

Levels of Viscera in Mediastinum

The level of the viscera relative to the mediastinal subdivisions depends on the position of the person. When a person is lying supine, the level of the viscera relative to the subdivisions of the mediastinum are as shown in the figures in this text. Anatomical descriptions traditionally describe the level of the viscera as if the person were in this position—that is, lying in bed or on the operating or dissection table. In this position, the abdominal viscera push the mediastinal structures superiorly. However, in the standing position, the levels of the viscera are as shown in Figure B1.10. This occurs because the soft structures in the mediastinum (especially the pericardium and its contents), the heart and great vessels, and the abdominal viscera supporting them sag inferiorly under the influence of gravity. This movement of mediastinal structures must be considered during physical and radiological examinations.

Mediastinoscopy

Using a *mediastinoscope,* surgeons can see much of the mediastinum and conduct minor surgical procedures. They insert the endoscope through a small incision in the root of the neck, just superior to the manubrium near the jugular notch. During mediastinoscopy, surgeons may view or biopsy mediastinal lymph nodes to determine if cancer cells have metastasized to them from a bronchogenic carcinoma, for example. The mediastinum can also be explored and biopsies taken by removing part of a costal cartilage.

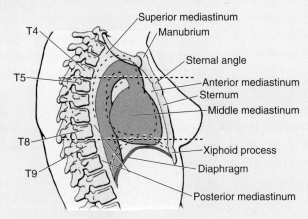

Figure B1.10. Thoracic viscera. The supine position is indicated by the *broken lines*; and the standing position, by the *solid figure.*

The wall of each chamber of the heart consists of three layers from superficial to deep (Table 1.5):

- **Epicardium,** a thin external layer (mesothelium) formed by the visceral layer of serous pericardium.
- **Myocardium,** a thick middle layer composed of cardiac muscle.
- **Endocardium,** a thin internal layer (endothelium and subendothelial connective tissue) or lining membrane of the heart that also covers its valves.

When the ventricles contract, they produce a wringing motion because of the double helical orientation of the cardiac muscle fibers in the myocardium (Torrent-Guasp et al., 2001). This motion initially ejects the blood from the ventricles as the outer (basal) spiral contracts, first narrowing and then shortening the heart, reducing the volume of the ventricular chambers. Continued sequential contraction of the inner (apical) spiral elongates the heart, followed by widening as the myocardium briefly relaxes, increasing the volume of the chambers to draw blood from the atria (Fig. 1.25A). The muscle fibers are anchored to the **fibrous skeleton of the heart** (Fig. 1.25B).

The fibrous framework of dense collagen forms four **fibrous rings**, which surround the orifices of the valves, right and left **fibrous trigones** (formed by connecting the rings, and the membranous parts of the interatrial and interventricular septa). The fibrous skeleton of the heart:

- Keeps the orifices of the AV and semilunar valves patent and from being overly distended by the volume of blood pumping through them.
- Provides attachments for the leaflets and cusps of the valves.
- Provides attachment for the myocardium, which when uncoiled forms a continuous ventricular myocardial band that originates mainly from the fibrous ring of the pulmonary valve and inserts primarily into the fibrous ring of the aortic valve (Torrent-Guasp et al., 2001) (Fig.1.25A).
- Forms an electrical "insulator" by separating the myenterically conducted impulses of the atria and ventricles so that they contract independently and by surrounding and providing passage for the initial part of the AV bundle (part of the conducting system of the heart).

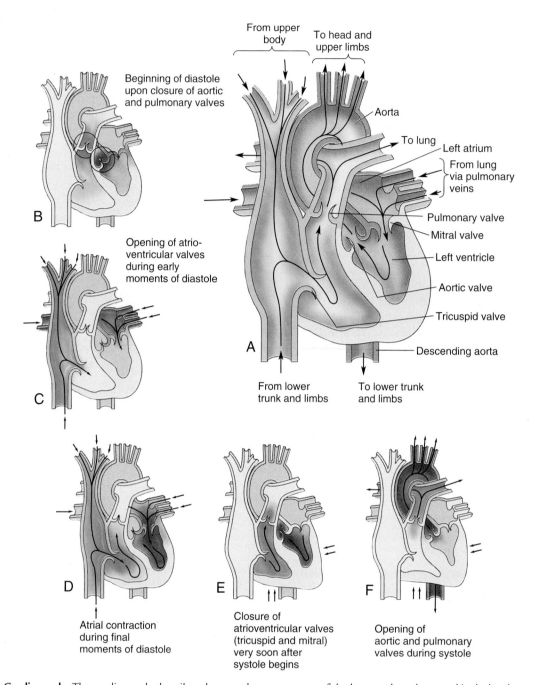

Beginning of diastole upon closure of aortic and pulmonary valves

B

From upper body

To head and upper limbs

Aorta

To lung

Left atrium

From lung via pulmonary veins

Pulmonary valve

Mitral valve

Left ventricle

Aortic valve

Tricuspid valve

A

Descending aorta

From lower trunk and limbs

To lower trunk and limbs

Opening of atrio-ventricular valves during early moments of diastole

C

Atrial contraction during final moments of diastole

D

Closure of atrioventricular valves (tricuspid and mitral) very soon after systole begins

E

Opening of aortic and pulmonary valves during systole

F

Figure 1.24. Cardiac cycle. The cardiac cycle describes the complete movement of the heart or heartbeat and includes the period from the beginning of one heartbeat to the beginning of the next one. The cycle consists of *diastole* (ventricular relaxation and filling) and *systole* (ventricular contraction and emptying). The right heart (*blue*) is the pump for the pulmonary circuit; the left heart (*red*) is the pump for the systemic circuit.

ORIENTATION OF THE HEART

The heart and roots of the great vessels within the pericardial sac are related anteriorly to the sternum, costal cartilages, and the medial ends of the 3rd–5th ribs on the left side. The heart and pericardial sac are situated obliquely, about two thirds to the left and one third to the right of the median plane. The heart is shaped like a tipped-over, three-sided pyramid with an apex, base, and four surfaces.

The **apex of the heart** (Fig. 1.22A):

- Is directed anteriorly and to the left and is formed by the inferolateral part of the left ventricle.
- Is located posterior to the left 5th intercostal space in adults, usually 9 cm from the median plane.
- Is where the sounds of mitral valve closure are maximal (**apex beat**); the apex underlies the site where the heartbeat may be auscultated on the thoracic wall.

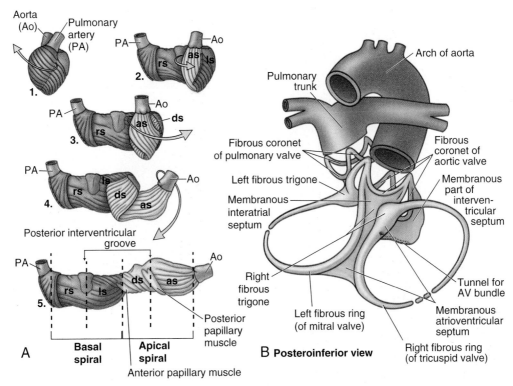

Figure 1.25. Arrangement of myocardium and fibrous skeleton of heart. A. The helical (double spiral) arrangement of the myocardium is shown. The basal spiral (*dark brown*) forms the outer wall of the right ventricle (right segment, *rs*) and the external layer of the outer wall of the left ventricle (left segment, *ls*). The apical spiral is deeper (*light brown*) and forms the internal layer of the outer wall of the left ventricle, consisting of a descending segment (*ds*) and an ascending segment (*as*). The crisscrossing of the *as* and *ds* fibers make up the interventricular septum. **B.** The fibrous skeleton is composed of four fibrous rings—each encircling a valve, two trigones, and the membranous parts of the interatrial (not shown) and interventricular septa. *AV,* atrioventricular.

The **base of the heart** (Fig. 1.22*C*):

- Is the heart's posterior aspect.
- Is formed mainly by the left atrium, with a lesser contribution by the right atrium.
- Faces posteriorly toward the bodies of vertebrae T6–T9, and is separated from them by the pericardium, oblique pericardial sinus, esophagus, and aorta.
- Extends superiorly to the bifurcation of the pulmonary trunk and inferiorly to the coronary groove.
- Receives the pulmonary veins on the right and left sides of its left atrial portion and the superior and inferior venae cavae at the superior and inferior ends of its right atrial portion.

The **four surfaces of the heart** are the (Fig. 1.22*A & C*):

- **Anterior (sternocostal) surface,** formed mainly by the right ventricle.
- **Diaphragmatic (inferior) surface,** formed mainly by the left ventricle and partly by the right ventricle; it is related to the central tendon of the diaphragm.
- **Left pulmonary surface,** formed mainly by the left ventricle; it forms the cardiac impression of the left lung.

- **Right pulmonary surface,** formed mainly by the right atrium.

The heart appears trapezoidal in both anterior and posterior views. The **four borders of the heart** are the (Fig. 1.26):

- **Right border** (slightly convex), formed by the right atrium and extending between the SVC and the IVC.
- **Inferior border** (nearly horizontal), formed mainly by the right ventricle and only slightly by the left ventricle.
- **Left border** (oblique), formed mainly by the left ventricle and slightly by the left auricle.
- **Superior border,** formed by the right and left atria and auricles in an anterior view; the ascending aorta and pulmonary trunk emerge from the superior border, and the SVC enters its right side. Posterior to the aorta and pulmonary trunk and anterior to the SVC, the superior border forms the inferior boundary of the transverse pericardial sinus.

CHAMBERS OF THE HEART

Right Atrium. The right atrium forms the right border of the heart and receives venous blood from the SVC, IVC,

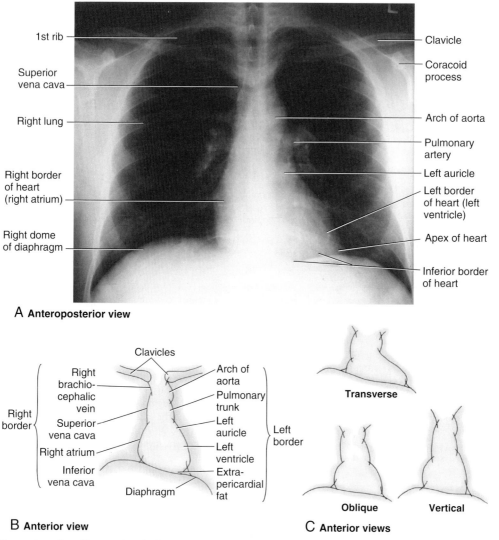

A Anteroposterior view

B Anterior view

C Anterior views

Figure 1.26. Radiograph and cardiovascular shadows. A. A radiograph of the heart is shown. **B.** The composition of the margins of the cardiovascular shadow (cardiac silhouette) are identified. **C.** Common types of cardiovascular shadows are defined.

and coronary sinus (Figs. 1.22*A* & *C* and 1.27). The ear-like **right auricle** is a small, conical muscular pouch that projects from the **right atrium,** increasing the capacity of the atrium as it overlaps the ascending aorta. The primordial atrium is represented in the adult by the right auricle. The definitive atrium is enlarged by incorporation of most of the embryonic venous sinus (L. *sinus venosus*). The **coronary sinus** lies in the posterior part of the coronary groove and receives blood from the cardiac veins. The coronary sinus is also a derivative of the embryonic venous sinus. The part of the venous sinus incorporated into the primordial atrium becomes the smooth-walled **sinus venarum** of the adult right atrium. The separation between the primordial atrium and the sinus venarum is indicated externally by the **sulcus terminalis** (terminal groove) and internally by the

crista terminalis (terminal crest). The **interior of the right atrium** has (Fig. 1.27):

- A smooth, thin-walled posterior part (the **sinus venarum**), on which the SVC, IVC, and coronary sinus open, bringing poorly oxygenated blood into the heart.
- A rough, muscular wall composed of **pectinate muscles** (L. *musculi pectinati*).
- The **opening of the SVC** into its superior part, at the level of the right 3rd costal cartilage.
- The **opening of the IVC** into the inferior part, almost in line with the SVC at approximately the level of the 5th costal cartilage.
- The **opening of the coronary sinus** between the right AV orifice and the IVC orifice.

Percussion of Heart

Percussion defines the density and size of the heart. The classical percussion technique is to create vibration by tapping the chest with a finger while listening and feeling for differences in sound wave conduction. Percussion is performed at the 3rd, 4th, and 5th intercostal spaces from the left anterior axillary line to the right anterior axillary line. Normally the percussion note changes from resonance to dullness (because of the presence of the heart) approximately 6 cm lateral to the left border of the sternum. The character of the sound changes as different areas of the chest are tapped.

Radiographs of Thorax

Anteroposterior chest films show the contour of the heart and great vessels—the *cardiovascular silhouette* or cardiac shadow (Fig. 1.26). The silhouette contrasts with the clearer areas occupied by the air-filled lungs because the heart and great vessels are full of blood. The silhouette becomes longer and narrower during inspiration because the fibrous pericardium is attached to the diaphragm, which descends during inspiration.

Atrial Septal Defects

Congenital anomalies of the interatrial septum—usually related to incomplete closure of the oval foramen—are *atrial septal defects* (ASDs). A probe-size patency (defect) appears in the superior part of the oval fossa in 15–25% of people. These small ASDs, by themselves, are usually of no clinical significance; however, large ASDs allow oxygenated blood from the lungs to be shunted from the left atrium through the defect into the right atrium, causing enlargement of the right atrium and ventricle and dilation of the pulmonary trunk.

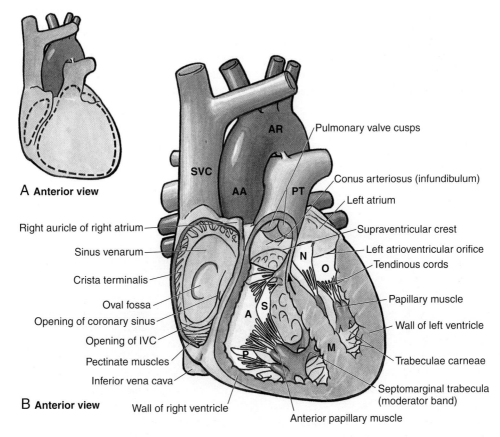

Figure 1.27. Interior of heart. A. The *dashed lines* indicate where the heart's wall has been removed in part **B. B.** Observe the features of each chamber. Note the three cusps of the tricuspid valve—*A*, anterior; *P*, posterior; *S*, septal—and the two cusps of the mitral valve—*N*, anterior; *O*, posterior. *AA,* ascending aorta; *AR,* arch of aorta, *IVC,* inferior vena cava; *M*, muscular part of interventricular septum; *PT,* pulmonary trunk; *SVC,* superior vena cava, *arrow,* membranous part of interventricular septum.

- A **right AV orifice** through which the right atrium discharges the poorly oxygenated blood into the right ventricle.
- The **interatrial septum**, separating the atria, has an oval, thumbprint-size depression, the **oval fossa** (L. *fossa ovalis*), a remnant of the oval foramen and its valve in the fetus (Moore and Persaud, 2003).

Right Ventricle. The right ventricle forms the largest part of the anterior surface of the heart, a small part of the diaphragmatic surface, and almost the entire inferior border of the heart. Superiorly it tapers into an arterial cone, the **conus arteriosus** (infundibulum), which leads into the pulmonary trunk (Fig. 1.27). The interior of the right ventricle has irregular muscular elevations called **trabeculae carneae.** A thick muscular ridge, the **supraventricular crest**, separates the ridged muscular wall of the inflow part of the chamber from the smooth wall of the conus arteriosus or outflow part of the right ventricle. The inflow part of the right ventricle receives blood from the right atrium through the **right AV (tricuspid) orifice**, located posterior to the body of the sternum at the level of the 4th and 5th intercostal spaces. The right AV orifice is surrounded by a fibrous ring (part of the fibrous skeleton of heart) that resists the dilation that might otherwise result from blood being forced through it at varying pressures (Fig. 1.24).

The **tricuspid valve** guards the right AV orifice (Figs. 1.27, 1.28, and 1.29A). The bases of the valve cusps are attached to the fibrous ring around the orifice. **Tendinous cords** (L. *chordae tendineae*) attach to the free edges and ven-

tricular surfaces of the anterior, posterior, and septal cusps—much like the cords attached to a parachute. Because the cords are attached to adjacent sides of two cusps, they prevent separation of the cusps and their inversion when tension is applied to the cords throughout ventricular contraction (systole)—that is, the cusps of the tricuspid valve are prevented from prolapsing (being driven into right atrium) as ventricular pressure rises. Thus regurgitation of blood (backward flow of blood) from the right ventricle into the right atrium is blocked by the valve cusps. The **papillary muscles** form conical projections with their bases attached to the ventricular wall and tendinous cords arising from their apices. There are usually three papillary muscles (anterior, posterior, and septal) in the right ventricle that correspond in name to the cusps of the tricuspid valve. The papillary muscles begin to contract before contraction of the right ventricle, tightening the tendinous cords and drawing the cusps together. Contraction is maintained throughout systole.

The **interventricular septum**, composed of membranous and muscular parts, is a strong, obliquely placed partition between the right and the left ventricles (Fig. 1.27), forming part of the walls of each. The superoposterior *membranous part of the IV septum is thin* and is continuous with the fibrous skeleton of the heart. The *muscular part of the IV septum is thick* and bulges into the cavity of the right ventricle because of the higher blood pressure in the left ventricle. The **septomarginal trabecula** (moderator band) is a curved muscular bundle that runs from the inferior part of the interventricular septum to the base of the anterior papillary muscle. This

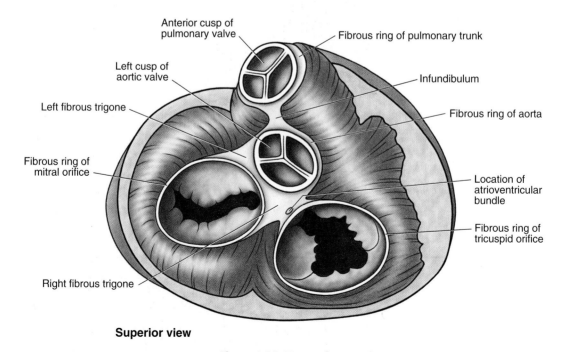

Superior view

Figure 1.28. Heart valves.

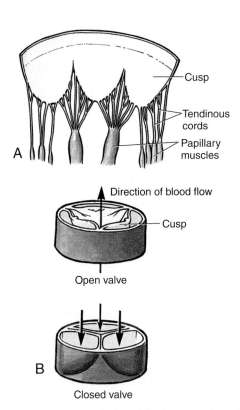

Figure 1.29. Pulmonary and tricuspid valves. A. Tricuspid valve is shown spread out. **B.** Blood flow through the pulmonary valve is demonstrated.

trabecula is important because it carries part of the **right bundle of the AV bundle** of the conducting system of the heart to the anterior papillary muscle (discussed later in this chapter). This "short cut" across the chamber of the ventricle seems to facilitate conduction time, allowing coordinated contraction of the anterior papillary muscle.

When the right atrium contracts, blood is forced through the **right AV orifice** into the right ventricle, pushing the cusps of the tricuspid valve aside like curtains. The inflow of blood into the right ventricle (*inflow tract*) enters posteriorly, and the outflow of blood into the pulmonary trunk (*outflow tract*) leaves superiorly and to the left. Consequently, the blood takes a U-shaped path through the right ventricle. The inflow (AV) orifice and outflow (pulmonary) orifice are approximately 2 cm apart.

The **pulmonary valve** at the apex of the **conus arteriosus** is at the level of the left 3rd costal cartilage (Figs. 1.28 and 1.29 *B*). Each of the semilunar **cusps of the pulmonary valve** (anterior, right, and left) is concave when viewed superiorly. The *pulmonary sinuses* are the spaces at the origin of the pulmonary trunk between the dilated wall of the vessel and each cusp of the pulmonary valve. The blood in the pulmonary sinuses prevents the cusps from sticking to the wall of the pulmonary trunk and failing to close.

Left Atrium. The left atrium forms most of the base of the heart (Fig. 1.22 *C*). The pairs of valveless right and left **pulmonary veins** enter the left atrium. The left auricle forms the superior part of the left border of the heart and overlaps the pulmonary trunk. The **interior of the left atrium** has

- A larger smooth-walled part and a smaller muscular auricle containing pectinate muscles.
- Four pulmonary veins (two superior and two inferior) entering its posterior wall.
- A slightly thicker wall than that of the right atrium.
- An interatrial septum that slopes posteriorly and to the right.
- A left AV orifice through which the left atrium discharges the oxygenated blood it receives from the pulmonary veins into the left ventricle.

Ventricular Septal Defects

The membranous part of the IV septum develops separately from the muscular part and has a complex embryological origin. Consequently, this part is the common site of *ventricular septal defects*. These congenital anomalies rank first on all lists of cardiac defects. Isolated VSDs account for approximately 25% of all forms of congenital heart disease (Moore and Persaud, 2003). The size of the defect varies from 1 to 25 mm. A VSD causes a left-to-right shunt of blood through the defect. A large shunt increases pulmonary blood flow, which causes pulmonary disease (*hypertension,* or increased blood pressure) and may cause cardiac failure.

Pulmonary Stenosis

In *pulmonary valve stenosis* (narrowing), the valve cusps are fused, forming a dome with a narrow central opening. In *infundibular pulmonary stenosis,* the conus arteriosus is underdeveloped, producing a restriction of right ventricular outflow. Both types of pulmonary stenosis may occur together. The degree of hypertrophy of the right ventricle is variable.

The smooth-walled part of the left atrium is formed by absorption of parts of the embryonic pulmonary veins, whereas the rough-walled part, mainly in the auricle, represents the remains of the left part of the primordial atrium.

Left Ventricle. The left ventricle forms the apex of the heart, nearly all of its left (pulmonary) surface and border, and most of the diaphragmatic surface (Fig. 1.22A & C). Because arterial pressure is much higher in the systemic than in the pulmonary circulation, the **left ventricle** performs more work than the right ventricle.

The **interior of the left ventricle** has (Fig. 1.27)

- A double-leaflet **mitral valve** that guards the left AV orifice.
- Walls that are two to three times as thick as that of the right ventricle.
- A conical cavity that is longer than that of the right ventricle.
- Walls that are covered with thick muscular ridges, **trabeculae carneae**, that are finer and more numerous than those in the right ventricle.
- Anterior and posterior **papillary muscles** that are larger than those in the right ventricle.
- A smooth-walled, non-muscular, superoanterior outflow part the **aortic vestibule** leading to the aortic orifice and aortic valve.
- An **aortic orifice** that lies in its right posterosuperior part and is surrounded by a fibrous ring to which the right, posterior, and left cusps of the **aortic valve** are attached.

The **mitral valve** closing the orifice between the left atrium and left ventricle has two cusps, anterior and posterior (Figs. 1.28 and 1.30). The mitral valve is located poste-

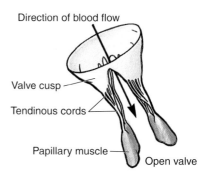

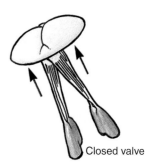

Figure 1.30. Mitral valve. The mitral valve closes the orifice between the left atrium and the left ventricle.

rior to the sternum at the level of the 4th costal cartilage. Each of its cusps receives **tendinous cords** from more than one papillary muscle. These muscles and their cords support the mitral valve, allowing the cusps to resist the pressure developed during contractions (pumping) of the left ventricle. The tendinous cords become taut, just before and during systole, preventing the cusps from being forced into the left atrium. The **ascending aorta**, begins at the aortic orifice.

Strokes or Cardiovascular Accidents

Thrombi (clots) form on the walls of the left atrium in certain types of heart disease. If these thrombi detach or pieces break off, they pass into the systemic circulation and occlude peripheral arteries. Occlusion of an artery in the brain results in a stroke or *cerebrovascular accident* (CVA), which may affect, for example, vision, cognition, or sensory or motor function of parts of the body previously controlled by the now-damaged area of the brain.

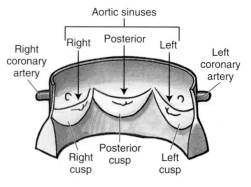

Figure 1.31. Aortic valve. The aortic valve is shown spread out. It is between the left ventricle and the ascending aorta.

The **aortic valve**, obliquely placed, is located posterior to the left side of the sternum at the level of the 3rd intercostal space. The **aortic sinuses** are the spaces at the origin of the ascending aorta between the dilated wall of the vessel and each cusp of the aortic (semilunar) valve (Fig. 1.31). The mouth of the right coronary artery is in the **right aortic sinus**; the mouth of the left coronary artery is in the **left aortic sinus**; and no artery arises from the **posterior aortic (non-coronary) sinus**.

ARTERIAL SUPPLY OF HEART

The coronary arteries supply the myocardium and epicardium and course just deep to the epicardium, normally embedded in fat. The *right* and *left* coronary arteries arise from the corresponding **aortic sinuses** at the proximal part of the ascending aorta (Figs. 1.31 and 1.32; Table 1.6), just superior to the **aortic valve**. The endocardium receives oxygen and nutrients directly from the chambers of the heart.

The **right coronary artery** (RCA) arises from the *right aortic sinus* of the ascending aorta and runs in the coronary groove (sulcus). Near its origin, the RCA usually gives off an ascending **sinuatrial (SA) nodal branch** (Fig. 1.32A) that supplies the *SA node,* (part of the cardiac conducting system). The RCA then descends in the coronary groove and gives off the **right marginal branch**, which supplies the

right border of the heart as it runs toward (but does not reach) the apex of the heart. After giving off this branch, the RCA turns to the left and continues in the coronary groove on the posterior aspect of the heart. At the **crux** (cross) of the heart, the junction of the septa and walls of the four heart chambers, the RCA gives rise to the **AV nodal branch**, which supplies the *AV node* (part of the cardiac conducting system). The RCA then gives off the large posterior IV branch that descends in the posterior IV groove toward the apex of the heart (Fig. 1.32B). The **posterior IV branch** supplies both ventricles and sends perforating **interventricular septal branches** to the IV septum. The terminal (left ventricular) branch of the RCA then continues for a short distance in the coronary groove. Typically, the RCA supplies:

- The right atrium.
- Most of right ventricle.
- Part of left ventricle (diaphragmatic surface).
- Part of IV septum (usually posterior third).
- The SA node (in approximately 60% of people).
- The AV node (in approximately 80% of people).

The **left coronary artery** (LCA) arises from the *left aortic sinus* of the ascending aorta and passes between the left auricle and the left side of the pulmonary trunk in the coronary groove. In approximately 40% of people, the **SA nodal branch** arises from the circumflex branch of the LCA and ascends on the posterior surface of the left atrium to the SA

Valvular Heart Disease

Disorders involving the valves of the heart disturb the pumping efficiency of the heart. *Valvular heart disease* produces either stenosis (narrowing) or insufficiency. **Stenosis** is the failure of a valve to open fully, slowing blood flow from a chamber. **Valvular insufficiency** or **regurgitation,** on the other hand, is failure of the valve to close completely, usually owing to nodule formation on (or scarring and contraction of) the cusps so that the edges do not meet or align. This allows a variable amount of blood (depending on the severity) to flow back into the chamber it was just ejected from. Both stenosis and insufficiency result in an increased workload for the heart. Restriction of high pressure blood flow (stenosis) or passage of blood through a narrow opening into a larger vessel or chamber (stenosis and regurgitation) produce turbulence. Turbulence sets up *eddies* (small whirlpools) that produce vibrations that are

audible as *murmurs.* Superficial vibratory sensations—*thrills*—may be felt on the skin over an area of turbulence.

Because valvular diseases are mechanical problems, damaged or defective cardiac valves are often replaced surgically in a procedure called *valvuloplasty.* Most commonly, artificial valve prosthesis made of synthetic materials are used in these valve replacement procedures, but xenografted valves (valves transplanted from other species, such as pigs) are also used.

A *prolapsed mitral valve* is an insufficient or incompetent valve in which one or both leaflets are enlarged, redundant or "floppy," and extending back into the left atrium during systole. As a result, blood regurgitates into the left atrium when the left ventricle contracts, producing a characteristic murmur.

Aortic valve stenosis is the most frequent valve abnormality and results in *left ventricular hypertrophy.* The great majority of aortic stenosis is a result of degenerative calcification.

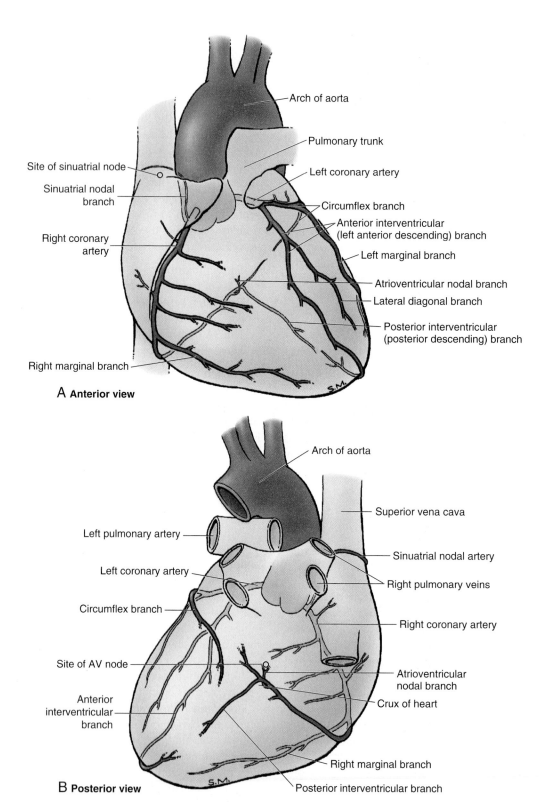

Figure 1.32. Arterial supply of heart. *AV,* atrioventricular.

Table 1.6 Arterial Supply of Heart

Artery/Branch	Origin	Course	Distribution	Anastomoses
Right coronary	Right aortic sinus	Follows coronary (AV) groove between atria and ventricles	Right atrium, SA and AV nodes, and posterior part of IV septum	Circumflex and anterior IV branches (left coronary artery)
SA nodal	Right coronary artery near its origin (in 60%)	Ascends to SA node	Pulmonary trunk and SA node	
Right marginal	Right coronary artery	Passes to inferior margin of heart and apex	Right ventricle and apex of heart	IV branches
Posterior IV	Right coronary artery (in 67%)	Runs in posterior IV groove to apex of heart	Right and left ventricles and posterior third of septum	Anterior IV branches of left coronary artery (at apex)
AV nodal	Right coronary artery near origin of posterior IV artery	Passes to AV node	AV node	
Left coronary	Left aortic sinus	Runs in AV groove and gives off anterior IV and circumflex branches	Most of left atrium and ventricle, IV septum, and AV bundles; may supply AV node	Right coronary artery
Anterior IV (LAD)	Left coronary artery	Passes along anterior IV groove to apex of heart	Right and left ventricles; anterior two thirds IV septum	Posterior IV branch of left coronary artery
Circumflex	Left coronary artery	Passes to left in AV groove and runs to posterior surface of heart	Left atrium and left ventricle	Right coronary artery
Left marginal	Circumflex branch	Follows left border of heart	Left ventricle	IV branches
Posterior IV	Left coronary artery (in 33%)	Runs in posterior IV groove to apex of heart	Right and left posterior third of IV septum	Anterior IV branch of left coronary artery

AV, atrioventricular; *IV,* interventricular; *LAD,* left anterior descending artery; *SA,* sinuatrial.

node. At the left end of the coronary groove, located just left of the pulmonary trunk (Fig. 1.32), the LCA divides into two branches, an **anterior IV branch** (left anterior descending [LAD] branch) and a **circumflex branch**. The anterior IV branch passes along the IV groove to the apex of the heart. Here it turns around the inferior border of the heart and anastomoses with the posterior IV branch of the right coronary artery. The anterior IV branch supplies both ventricles and the IV septum (Table 2.6).

In many people, the anterior IV artery gives rise to a **lateral (diagonal) branch**, which descends on the anterior surface of the heart. The smaller **circumflex branch of the LCA** follows the coronary groove around the left border of the heart to the posterior surface of the heart. The **left marginal artery**, a branch of the circumflex branch, follows the left margin of the heart and supplies the left ventricle. The circumflex branch of the LCA terminates in the coronary groove on the posterior aspect of the heart before reaching the crux, but in about one third of hearts it continues as the posterior IV branch **Typically, the LCA supplies**

- The left atrium.
- Most of left ventricle.
- Part of right ventricle.

- Most of IV septum (usually its anterior two thirds), including the AV bundle of conducting tissue, through its perforating IV septal branches.
- The SA node (in approximately 40% of people).

VENOUS DRAINAGE OF HEART

The heart is drained mainly by veins that empty into the **coronary sinus** and partly by small veins that empty directly into the chambers of the heart. The **coronary sinus**, the main vein of the heart, is a wide venous channel that runs from left to right in the posterior part of the coronary groove. The coronary sinus receives the **great cardiac vein** at its left end and the **middle** and **small cardiac veins** at its right end. The **left posterior ventricular vein** and **left marginal vein** also open into the coronary sinus. The small **anterior cardiac veins** empty directly into the right atrium (Fig. 1.33) and the **smallest cardiac veins** (L. *venae cordis minimae*) are minute vessels that begin in the capillary beds of the myocardium and open directly into the chambers of the heart, chiefly the atria. Although called veins, they are valveless communications with the capillary beds of the myocardium and may carry blood from the heart chambers to the myocardium.

Variations of Coronary Arteries

Variations in the branching patterns of the coronary arteries are common. In the most common right dominant pattern, the RCA and LCA share approximately equally in the blood supply to the heart. In approximately 15% of hearts, the LCA is dominant in that the posterior IV branch is a branch of the circumflex artery. There is codominance in about 18% of people, in which branches of both the RCA and LCA reach the crux and give rise to branches that course in or near the posterior IV groove. A few people have only a single coronary artery. In other people, the circumflex artery arises from the right aortic sinus. The branches of coronary arteries are considered to be end arteries—ones that supply regions of the myocardium without functional overlap from other large branches. However, anastomoses exist between small branches of the coronary arteries. The potential for development of collateral circulation likely exists in most hearts.

Myocardial Infarction

With sudden occlusion of a major artery by an embolus, the region of myocardium supplied by the occluded vessel becomes infarcted (rendered virtually bloodless) and soon degenerates. An area of myocardium that has undergone necrosis is a *myocardial infarct* (MI). The most common cause of *ischemic heart disease* (*ischemia*-lacking adequate blood supply) *is coronary insufficiency,* resulting from *atherosclerosis of*

the coronary arteries (*arteriosclerosis*—hardening of the arteries—characterized by lipid deposits in the medium and large arteries, causing narrowing of arterial lumens). A person with coronary arterial disease often suffers from *angina pectoris* (usually pain in the substernal region and down the medial side of the left arm and forearm). In a coronary bypass graft, a segment of an artery or vein is connected to the ascending aorta or to the proximal part of a coronary artery and then to the coronary artery distal to the stenosis (Fig. B1.11).

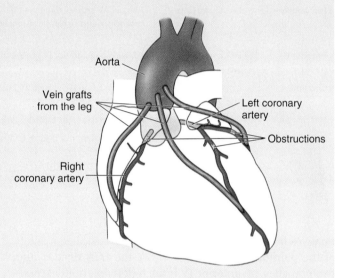

Figure B1.11. Triple coronary bypass.

LYMPHATIC DRAINAGE OF THE HEART

Lymphatic vessels in the myocardium and subendocardial connective tissue pass to the *subepicardial lymphatic plexus.* Vessels from this plexus pass to the coronary groove and follow the coronary arteries. A single lymphatic vessel, formed by the union of various vessels from the heart, ascends between the pulmonary trunk and the left atrium and ends in the **inferior tracheobronchial lymph nodes,** usually on the right side (Fig. 1.20C).

CONDUCTING SYSTEM OF THE HEART

The impulse-conducting system, which coordinates the cardiac cycle (Fig. 1.24), consists of cardiac muscle cells and highly specialized conducting fibers for initiating impulses and conducting them rapidly through the

heart (Fig. 1.34). Nodal tissue initiates the heartbeat and coordinates the contractions of the four heart chambers. The **SA node** initiates and regulates the impulses for contraction, giving off an impulse about 70 times per minute in most people. The SA node, *the pacemaker of the heart,* is located anterolaterally just deep to the epicardium at the junction of the SVC and right atrium near the superior end of the sulcus terminalis. The **AV node** is a smaller collection of nodal tissue located in the posteroinferior region of the interatrial septum near the opening of the coronary sinus. The signal generated by the SA node passes through the walls of the right atrium propagated by the cardiac muscle (*myogenic conduction*), which transmits the signal rapidly from the SA node to the AV node. The AV node then distributes the signal to the ventricles through the **AV bundle.** Sympathetic stimulation speeds

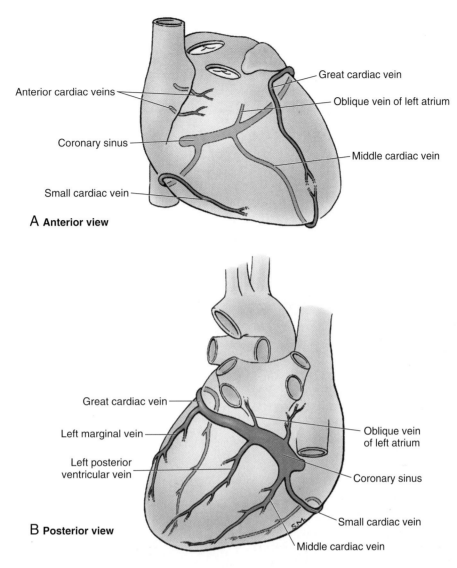

Figure 1.33. Venous drainage of heart.

up conduction and parasympathetic stimulation slows it down.

The *AV bundle,* the only bridge of conduction between the atrial and the ventricular myocardium, passes from the AV node through the fibrous skeleton of the heart and along the membranous part of the IV septum. At the junction of the membranous and muscular parts of the septum, the AV bundle divides into **right** and **left bundle branches.** The bundles proceed on each side of the muscular IV septum deep to the endocardium and then ramify into **subendocardial branches** (Purkinje fibers), which extend into the walls of the respective ventricles. The subendocardial branches of the right bundle stimulate the muscle of the IV septum, the anterior papillary muscle (through the **septomarginal trabecula**), and the wall of the right ventricle. The subendocardial branches of the left bundle stimulate the IV septum, the anterior and posterior papillary muscles, and the wall of the left ventricle.

Summary of Conducting System of Heart

* The SA node initiates an impulse that is rapidly conducted to cardiac muscle fibers in the atria, causing them to contract.
* The impulse spreads by myogenic conduction, which rapidly transmits the impulse from the SA node to the AV node.
* The signal is distributed from the AV node through the AV bundle and the right and left bundle branches, which pass on each side of the IV septum to supply subendocardial branches to the papillary muscles and the walls of the ventricles.

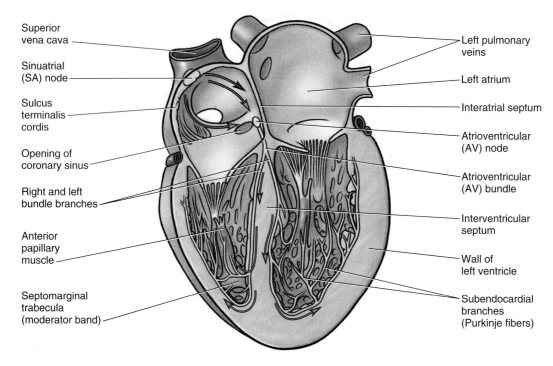

Superior vena cava

Sinuatrial (SA) node

Sulcus terminalis cordis

Opening of coronary sinus

Right and left bundle branches

Anterior papillary muscle

Septomarginal trabecula (moderator band)

Left pulmonary veins

Left atrium

Interatrial septum

Atrioventricular (AV) node

Atrioventricular (AV) bundle

Interventricular septum

Wall of left ventricle

Subendocardial branches (Purkinje fibers)

Figure 1.34. Conducting system of heart. Arrows indicate the flow of impulses initiated at the SA node.

Injury to Conducting System of Heart

Damage to the conducting system, often resulting from ischemia caused by *coronary artery disease,* produces disturbances of cardiac muscle contraction. Because the anterior IV branch (LAD branch) supplies the AV bundle in most people and because branches of the RCA supply both the SA and the AV nodes, parts of the conducting system of the heart are likely to be affected by their occlusion. Damage to the AV node or bundle results in a *heart block* because the atrial excitation does not reach the ventricles. As a result, the ventricles begin to contract independently at their own rate (25–30 times per minute), which is slower than the lowest normal rate of 40–45 times per minute. Damage to one of the bundle branches results in a *bundle branch block,* in which excitation passes along the unaffected branch and causes a

normally timed systole of that ventricle only. The impulse then spreads to the other ventricle, producing a late asynchronous contraction. In a ventricular septal defect, the AV bundle usually lies in the margin of the VSD. This must be preserved during surgical repair of the defect.

Electrocardiography

The passage of impulses over the heart from the SA node can be amplified and recorded as an *electrocardiogram* (ECG). Functional testing of the heart includes exercise tolerance tests (treadmill stress tests). These tests are important in detecting the cause of heartbeat irregularities. Heart rate, ECG, and blood pressure readings are monitored as the patient does increasingly demanding exercise on a treadmill.

INNERVATION OF THE HEART

The heart is supplied by autonomic nerve fibers from superficial and deep **cardiac plexuses** (Fig. 1.20*D*). These nerve networks lie anterior to the bifurcation of the trachea, and posterior to the ascending aorta. The **sympathetic supply of the heart** is from presynaptic fibers with cell bodies in the intermediolateral cell columns (lateral horns) of the superior five or six thoracic segments of the spinal cord and from postsynaptic sympathetic fibers with cell bodies in the cervical and superior thoracic paravertebral ganglia of the sympathetic trunks. The postsynaptic fibers end in the SA and AV nodes and in relation to the terminations of parasympathetic fibers on the coronary arteries. Sympathetic stimulation of the nodal tissue increases the heart's rate and the force of its contractions. Sympathetic stimulation (indirectly) produces dilation of the coronary arteries by inhibiting their constriction. This supplies more oxygen and nutrients to the myocardium during periods of increased activity.

The **parasympathetic supply of the heart** is from presynaptic fibers of the *vagus nerves* (CN X). Postsynaptic parasympathetic cell bodies (intrinsic ganglia) are located near the SA and AV nodes and along the coronary arteries.

Parasympathetic stimulation slows the heart rate, reduces the force of the contraction, and constricts the coronary arteries, saving energy between periods of increased demand.

Superior Mediastinum

The superior mediastinum is located superior to the transverse thoracic plane passing through the sternal angle and the junction (IV disc) of vertebrae T4 and T5 (Fig. 1.35). From anterior to posterior, **the main contents of the superior mediastinum** are (Fig. 1.36)

- Thymus, a primary lymphoid organ.
- Great vessels related to the heart and pericardium:
  - Brachiocephalic veins.
  - Superior part of SVC.
  - Arch of aorta and roots of its major branches:
    - Brachiocephalic trunk.
    - Left common carotid artery.
    - Left subclavian artery.
- Vagus and phrenic nerves.
- Cardiac plexus of nerves.
- Left recurrent laryngeal nerve.
- Trachea.
- Esophagus.
- Thoracic duct.

THYMUS

The thymus, a lymphoid organ, is located in the lower part of the neck and the anterior part of the superior mediastinum. It lies posterior to the manubrium of the sternum and extends into the anterior mediastinum, anterior to the

Cardiac Referred Pain

The heart is insensitive to touch, cutting, cold, and heat; however, ischemia and the accumulation of metabolic products stimulate pain endings in the myocardium. The afferent pain fibers run centrally in the middle and inferior cervical branches and especially in the thoracic cardiac branches of the sympathetic trunk. The axons of these primary sensory neurons enter spinal cord segments T1–T4 or T5, especially on the left side. Cardiac referred pain is a phenomenon whereby noxious stimuli originating in the heart are perceived by the person as pain arising from a superficial part of the body—the skin on the medial aspect of the left upper limb, for example. Visceral pain is transmitted by visceral afferent fibers accompanying sympathetic fibers and is typically referred to somatic structures or areas such as the upper limb having afferent fibers with cell bodies in the same spinal ganglion, and central processes that enter the spinal cord through the same posterior roots.

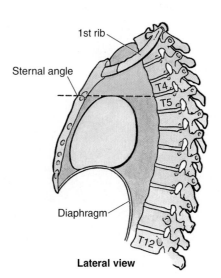

Figure 1.35. Mediastinum. The mediastinum is divided into superior (*green*) and inferior parts. The inferior mediastinum is divided into three parts: anterior (*purple*), middle (*yellow*), and posterior (*blue*).

Surface Anatomy of Heart

The heart and great vessels are approximately in the middle of the thorax, surrounded laterally and posteriorly by the lungs and bounded anteriorly by the sternum and the central part of the thoracic cage (Fig. SA1.5A). The *outline of the heart* can be traced on the anterior surface of the thorax by using these guidelines (Fig. SA1.5C):

• The *superior border* corresponds to a line connecting the inferior border of the 2nd left costal cartilage to the superior border of the 3rd right costal cartilage.

• The *right border* corresponds to a line drawn from the 3rd right costal cartilage to the 6th right costal cartilage; this border is slightly convex to the right.

• The *inferior border* corresponds to a line drawn from the inferior end of the right border to a point in the 5th intercostal space close to the left midclavicular line; the left end of this line corresponds

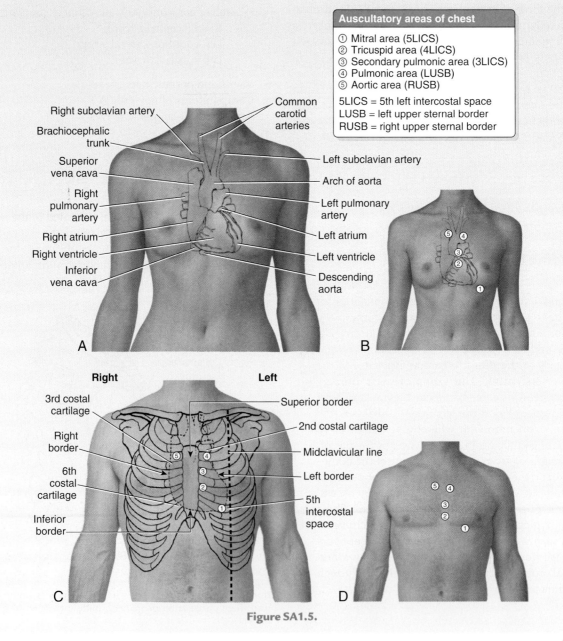

Auscultatory areas of chest

① Mitral area (5LICS)
② Tricuspid area (4LICS)
③ Secondary pulmonic area (3LICS)
④ Pulmonic area (LUSB)
⑤ Aortic area (RUSB)

5LICS = 5th left intercostal space
LUSB = left upper sternal border
RUSB = right upper sternal border

Figure SA1.5.

continued >

to the location of the apex of the heart and the apex beat.

- The *left border* corresponds to a line connecting the left ends of the lines representing the superior and inferior borders.
- The valves are located posterior to the sternum; however, the sounds produced by them are projected to the **auscultatory areas: pulmonary, aortic, mitral, and tricuspid** (Fig. SA1.5*B* & *D*).

The *apex beat* is an impulse that results from the apex being forced against the anterior thoracic wall when the left ventricle contracts. The *location of the apex beat* (mitral area) varies in position and may be located in the 4th or 5th intercostal spaces, 6–10 cm from the midline of the thorax.

Clinicians' interest in the surface anatomy of the heart and cardiac valves results from their need to listen to valve sounds. Because the auscultatory areas are wide apart as possible, the sounds produced at any given valve may be distinguished from those produced at other valves. Blood tends to carry the sound in the direction of its flow. Each area is situated superficial to the chamber or vessel into which the blood has passed and in a direct line with the valve orifice. ●

pericardium. After puberty, the thymus undergoes gradual involution and is largely replaced by fat. A rich *arterial supply to the thymus* derives mainly from the anterior intercostal and anterior mediastinal branches of the **internal thoracic arteries**. The **veins of the thymus** end in the left brachiocephalic, internal thoracic, and inferior thyroid veins. The **lymphatic vessels of the thymus** end in the parasternal, brachiocephalic, and tracheobronchial lymph nodes (Fig. 1.20*C*).

GREAT VESSELS IN THE MEDIASTINUM

The *brachiocephalic veins* form posterior to the sternoclavicular joints by the union of the internal jugular and subclavian veins (Fig. 1.37). At the level of the inferior border of the 1st right costal cartilage, the brachiocephalic veins unite to form the SVC. The **left brachiocephalic vein** is more than twice as long as the right brachiocephalic vein because it passes from the left to the right side, passing across the anterior aspects of the roots of the three major branches of the arch of the aorta, and shunting blood from the head, neck, and left upper limb to the right atrium. The origin

of the **right brachiocephalic vein** (by union of the right internal jugular and subclavian veins—the right venous angle) receives lymph from the **right lymphatic duct**, and the origin of the left brachiocephalic vein (by union of the lef internal jugular and subclavian veins—the left "venous angle") receives lymph from the **thoracic duct** (Fig. 1.42).

The **SVC** returns blood from all structures superior to the diaphragm, except the lungs and heart. It passes inferiorly and ends at the level of the 3rd costal cartilage, where it enters the right atrium. The SVC lies in the right side of the superior mediastinum, anterolateral to the trachea and posterolateral to the ascending aorta (Fig. 1.37). The **right phrenic nerve** lies between the SVC and the mediastinal pleura. The terminal half of the SVC is in the middle mediastinum, where it lies beside the ascending aorta and forms the posterior boundary of the transverse pericardial sinus (Fig. 1.22). The **arch of the aorta**, the curved continuation of the ascending aorta, begins posterior to the second right sternocostal joint at the level of the sternal angle and arches superoposteriorly and to the left (Figs. 1.36 and 1.37; Table 1.7). The aortic arch ascends anterior to the right pulmonary artery and the bifurcation of the trachea, reaching its apex at the left side of the trachea and esophagus as it passes over the root of the left lung. The arch descends on the left side of the body of the T4 vertebra and ends by becoming the **thoracic aorta** posterior to the second left sternocostal joint.

The **ligamentum arteriosum**, the remnant of the fetal ductus arteriosus, passes from the root of the left pulmonary artery to the inferior surface of the arch of the aorta. The **left recurrent laryngeal nerve** hooks beneath the arch immediately lateral to the ligamentum arteriosum and then ascends between the trachea and esophagus (Fig. 1.37). **The branches of the arch of the aorta** are the:

- Brachiocephalic trunk.
- Left common carotid artery.
- Left subclavian artery.

The **brachiocephalic trunk**, the first and largest branch of the arch, arises posterior to the manubrium, where it lies anterior to the trachea and posterior to the left brachiocephalic vein. It ascends superolaterally to reach the right side of the trachea and the right sternoclavicular joint, where it divides into the right common carotid and right subclavian arteries. The **left common carotid artery**, the second branch of the aortic arch, arises posterior to the manubrium, slightly posterior and to the left of the brachiocephalic trunk. It ascends anterior to the left subclavian artery and at first anterior to the trachea and then is to its left. It enters the neck by passing posterior to the left sternoclavicular joint. The **left subclavian artery**, the third branch of the aortic arch, arises from the posterior

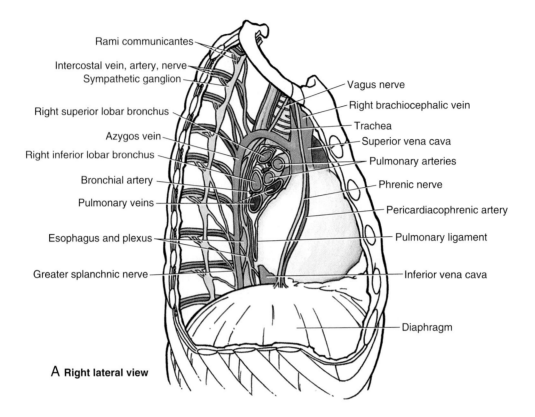

Rami communicantes

Intercostal vein, artery, nerve

Sympathetic ganglion

Right superior lobar bronchus

Azygos vein

Right inferior lobar bronchus

Bronchial artery

Pulmonary veins

Esophagus and plexus

Greater splanchnic nerve

Vagus nerve

Right brachiocephalic vein

Trachea

Superior vena cava

Pulmonary arteries

Phrenic nerve

Pericardiacophrenic artery

Pulmonary ligament

Inferior vena cava

Diaphragm

A Right lateral view

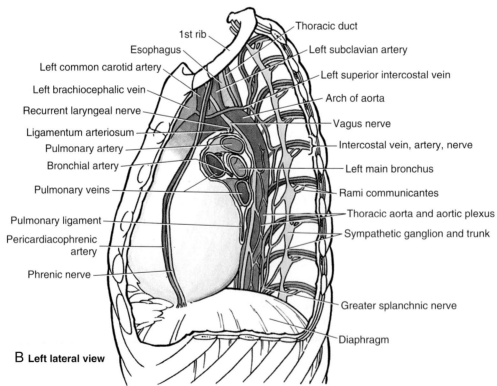

1st rib

Esophagus

Left common carotid artery

Left brachiocephalic vein

Recurrent laryngeal nerve

Ligamentum arteriosum

Pulmonary artery

Bronchial artery

Pulmonary veins

Pulmonary ligament

Pericardiacophrenic artery

Phrenic nerve

Thoracic duct

Left subclavian artery

Left superior intercostal vein

Arch of aorta

Vagus nerve

Intercostal vein, artery, nerve

Left main bronchus

Rami communicantes

Thoracic aorta and aortic plexus

Sympathetic ganglion and trunk

Greater splanchnic nerve

Diaphragm

B Left lateral view

Figure 1.36. Dissections of mediastinum.

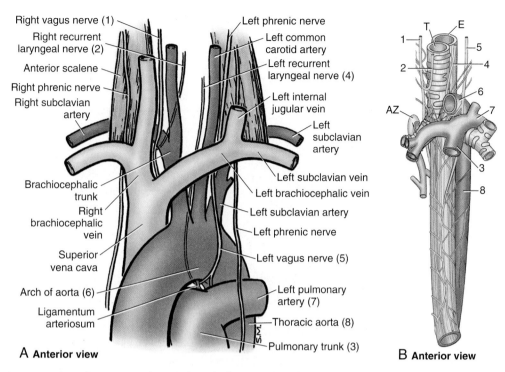

Figure 1.37. Great vessels and nerves. A. The vessels in the lower neck and superior mediastinum are shown. **B.** Note the relationships of the trachea (**T**), esophagus (**E**), and azygos vein (**AZ**).

part of the arch, just posterior to the left common carotid artery. It ascends lateral to the trachea and the left common carotid artery through the superior mediastinum. The left subclavian artery has no branches in the mediastinum. As it leaves the thorax and enters the root of the neck, it passes posterior to the left sternoclavicular joint and lateral to the left common carotid artery.

NERVES IN THE SUPERIOR MEDIASTINUM

The **vagus nerves** (CN X) arise bilaterally from the medulla of the brain, exit the cranium, and descend through the neck posterolateral to the common carotid arteries. Each nerve enters the superior mediastinum posterior to the respective sternoclavicular joint and brachiocephalic vein (Figs. 1.37, 1.38, and 1.39; Table 1.8). The **right vagus nerve** enters the

Table 1.7 The Aorta and Its Branches in the Thorax

Artery	Origin	Course	Branches
Ascending aorta	Aortic orifice of left ventricle	Ascends ~5 cm to sternal angle, where it becomes arch of aorta	Right and left coronary arteries
Arch of aorta	Continuation of ascending aorta	Arches posteriorly on left side of trachea and esophagus and superior to left main bronchus	Brachiocephalic, left common carotid, left subclavian arteries
Thoracic aorta	Continuation of arch of aorta	Descends in posterior mediastinum to left of vertebral column; gradually shifts to right to lie in median plane at aortic hiatus	Posterior intercostal arteries, subcostal, some phrenic arteries, and visceral branches (e.g., esophageal)
Posterior intercostal	Posterior aspect of thoracic aorta	Pass laterally and then anteriorly, parallel to ribs	Lateral and anterior cutaneous branches
Bronchial (1–2 branches)	Anterior aspect of aorta or posterior intercostal artery	Run with tracheobronchial tree	Bronchial and peribronchial tissue, visceral pleura
Esophageal (4–5 branches)	Anterior aspect of thoracic aorta	Run anteriorly to esophagus	To esophagus
Superior phrenic (vary in number)	Anterior aspect of thoracic aorta	Arise at aortic hiatus and pass to superior aspect of diaphragm	To diaphragm

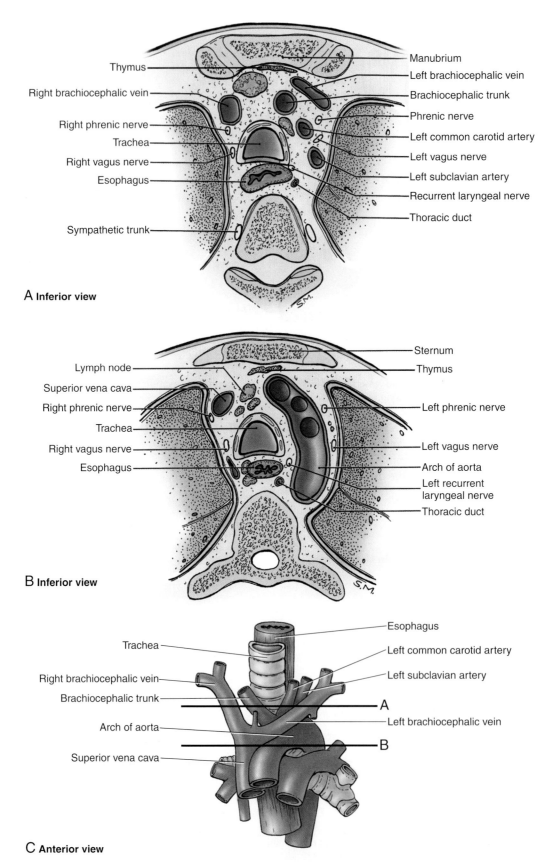

A **Inferior view**

B **Inferior view**

C **Anterior view**

Figure 1.38. Superior mediastinum. Transverse sections superior to (**A**) and at the level of (**B**) the arch of the aorta are shown. **C.** *Solid lines* indicate the level of the sections shown in parts *A* and *B*.

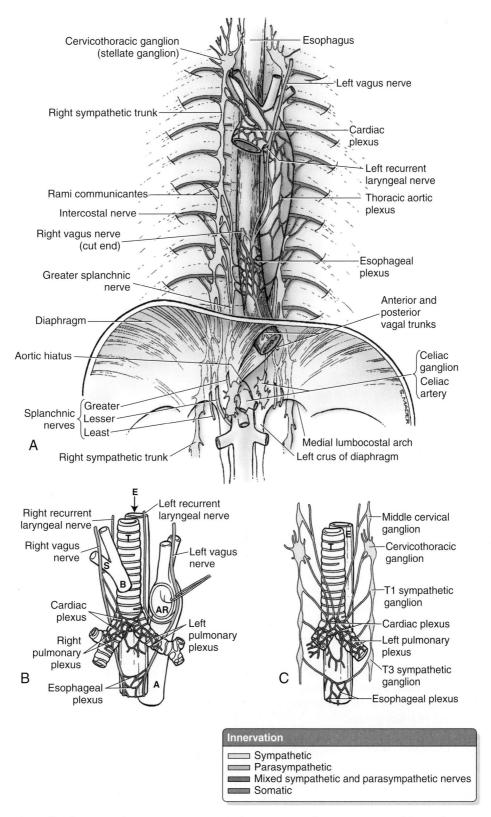

Figure 1.39. Nerves in mediastinum. A. The autonomic nerves in the superior and posterior parts of the mediastinum are shown. **B.** The parasympathetic nerves are identified. **C.** The sympathetic nerves are shown. **A,** aorta; **AR,** arch of aorta; **B,** right brachiocephalic artery; **E,** esophagus; **S,** right subclavian artery; **T,** trachea.

Table 1.8 Nerves of the Thorax

Nerve	Origin	Course	Distribution
Vagus (CN X)	8–10 rootlets from medulla of brainstem	Enters superior mediastinum posterior to sternoclavicular joint and brachiocephalic vein; gives rise to recurrent laryngeal nerve; continues into abdomen	Pulmonary plexus, esophageal plexus, and cardiac plexus
Phrenic	Anterior rami of C3–C5 nerves	Passes through superior thoracic aperture and runs between mediastinal pleura and pericardium	Central portion of diaphragm
Intercostals (1–11)	Anterior rami of T1–T11 nerves	Run in intercostal spaces between internal and innermost layers of intercostal muscles	Muscles in and skin over intercostal space; lower nerves supply muscles and skin of anterolateral abdominal wall
Subcostal	Anterior ramus of T12 nerve	Follows inferior border of 12th rib and passes into abdominal wall	Abdominal wall and skin of gluteal region
Recurrent laryngeal	Vagus nerve	On right, loops around subclavian artery; on left, runs around arch of aorta and ascends in tracheoesophageal groove	Intrinsic muscles of larynx (except cricothyroid); sensory inferior to level of vocal folds
Cardiac plexus	Cervical and cardiac branches of vagus nerve and sympathetic trunk	From arch of aorta and posterior surface of heart, fibers extend along coronary arteries and to SA node	Impulses pass to SA node; parasympathetic fibers slow rate; reduce force of heartbeat, and constrict coronary arteries; sympathetic fibers have opposite effect
Pulmonary plexus	Vagus nerve and sympathetic trunk	Forms on root of lung and extends along bronchial subdivisions	Parasympathetic fibers constrict bronchioles; sympathetic fibers dilate them; afferents convey reflexes
Esophageal plexus	Vagus nerve, sympathetic ganglia and greater splanchnic nerve	Distal to tracheal bifurcation, vagus and sympathetic nerves form the plexus around esophagus	Vagal and sympathetic fibers to smooth muscle and glands of inferior two thirds of esophagus

thorax anterior to the right subclavian artery, where it gives rise to the **right recurrent laryngeal nerve** (Fig. 1.37). This nerve hooks inferior to the right subclavian artery and ascends between the trachea and the esophagus to supply the larynx. The right vagus nerve runs posteroinferiorly through the superior mediastinum on the right side of the trachea. It then passes posterior to the right brachiocephalic vein, SVC, and root of the right lung. Here it breaks up into a number of branches that contribute to the **pulmonary plexus** (Fig. 1.39B). Usually, the right vagus nerve leaves the pulmonary plexus as a single nerve and passes to the esophagus, where it again breaks up and contributes fibers to the **esophageal plexus** (Fig. 1.39C). The right vagus nerve also gives rise to nerves that contribute to the **cardiac plexus.**

The **left vagus nerve** descends in the neck and enters the thorax and mediastinum between the left common carotid and the left subclavian arteries and posterior to the left brachiocephalic vein (Fig. 1.37). When it reaches the left side of the arch of the aorta, the left vagus nerve diverges posteriorly from the left phrenic nerve. It is separated laterally from the phrenic nerve by the left superior intercostal

Injury to the Recurrent Laryngeal Nerves

The recurrent laryngeal nerves supply all the intrinsic muscles of the larynx, except one. Consequently, any investigative procedure or disease process in the superior mediastinum may involve these nerves and affect the voice. Because the left recurrent laryngeal nerve hooks around the arch of the aorta and ascends between the trachea and the esophagus, it may be involved when there is a bronchial or esophageal carcinoma, enlargement of mediastinal lymph nodes, or an aneurysm of the arch of the aorta. In the latter condition, the nerve may be stretched by the dilated arch of the aorta.

vein. As the left vagus nerve curves medially at the inferior border of the arch of the aorta, it gives off the **left recurrent laryngeal nerve** (Figs. 1.37 and 1.39*A* & *B*). This nerve passes inferior to the arch of the aorta just posterolateral to the **ligamentum arteriosum** and ascends to the larynx in the groove between the trachea and the esophagus. The left vagus nerve continues on to pass posterior to the root of the left lung, where it breaks up into many branches, which contribute to the **pulmonary and cardiac plexuses.** The nerve leaves these plexuses as a single trunk and passes to the esophagus, where it joins fibers from the right vagus in the **esophageal plexus.**

The **phrenic nerves** are the sole motor supply to the diaphragm (Figs. 1.36 and 1.37); approximately one third of their fibers are sensory to the diaphragm. Each phrenic nerve enters the superior mediastinum between the subclavian artery and the origin of the brachiocephalic vein (Table 2.8). The **right phrenic nerve** passes along the right side of the right brachiocephalic vein, SVC, and pericardium over the right atrium. It also passes anterior to the root of the right lung and descends on the right side of the IVC to the diaphragm, which it penetrates or passes through the caval opening (foramen). The **left phrenic nerve** descends between the left subclavian and the left common carotid arteries. It crosses the left surface of the arch of the aorta anterior to the left vagus nerve and passes over the left superior intercostal vein. It then descends anterior to the root of the left lung and runs along the pericardium, superficial to the left atrium and ventricle of the heart, where it penetrates the diaphragm to the left of the pericardium.

TRACHEA

The trachea descends anterior to the esophagus and enters the superior mediastinum, inclining a little to the right of the median plane (Fig. 1.40). The posterior surface of the trachea is flat where its cartilaginous "rings" are incomplete and where it is related to the esophagus. The trachea ends at the level of the sternal angle by dividing into the right and left main bronchi.

ESOPHAGUS

The esophagus is a fibromuscular tube that extends from the pharynx to the stomach. It is usually flattened anteroposteriorly (Fig. 1.41). The esophagus enters the superior mediastinum between the trachea and the vertebral column, where it lies anterior to the bodies of vertebrae T1–T4. Initially, the esophagus inclines to the left but is moved by the aortic arch to the median plane opposite the root of the left lung. The **thoracic duct** usually lies on the left side of the esophagus and deep to the aortic arch (Fig. 1.42). Inferior to the arch, the esophagus inclines to the left

as it approaches and passes through the esophageal hiatus in the diaphragm.

Posterior Mediastinum

The **posterior mediastinum** is located anterior to vertebrae T5–T12, posterior to the pericardium and diaphragm, and between the parietal pleura of the two lungs (Fig. 1.35). The posterior mediastinum contains the (Fig. 1.40):

- Thoracic aorta.
- Thoracic duct.
- Posterior mediastinal lymph nodes (e.g., tracheobronchial nodes).
- Azygos and hemiazygos veins.
- Esophagus.
- Esophageal plexus.
- Thoracic sympathetic trunks.
- Thoracic splanchnic nerves.

THORACIC AORTA

The thoracic aorta, the thoracic part of the descending aorta, is the continuation of the **arch of the aorta** (Figs. 1.36*B* and 1.37, Table 2.7). It begins on the left side of the inferior border of the body of T4 vertebra and descends in the posterior mediastinum on the left sides of T5–T12 vertebrae. As it descends, it approaches the median plane and displaces the esophagus to the right. The **thoracic aortic plexus,** an autonomic nerve network, surrounds it (Fig. 1.39*A*). The thoracic aorta lies posterior to the root of the left lung, the pericardium, and the esophagus. Its name is changed to *abdominal aorta* anterior to the inferior border of the T12 vertebra and enters the abdomen through the **aortic hiatus** (opening) in the diaphragm (Figs. 1.38 and 1.41). The **thoracic duct** and azygos vein descend on the right side of the thoracic aorta and accompany it through this hiatus (Fig. 1.42).

The branches of the thoracic aorta are bronchial, pericardial, posterior intercostals, superior phrenic, esophageal, mediastinal, and subcostal (Fig. 1.43). The **bronchial arteries** consist of one right and two small left vessels. The bronchial arteries supply the trachea, bronchi, lung tissue, and lymph nodes. The **pericardial arteries** send twigs to the pericardium. The **posterior intercostal arteries** (nine pairs) pass into the 3rd–11th intercostal spaces. The **superior phrenic arteries** pass to the posterior surface of the diaphragm, where they anastomose with the musculophrenic and pericardiacophrenic branches of the internal thoracic artery. Usually, two **esophageal arteries** supply the middle third of the esophagus. The **mediastinal arteries** are small and supply the lymph nodes and other tissues of the posterior mediastinum. The **subcostal arteries**

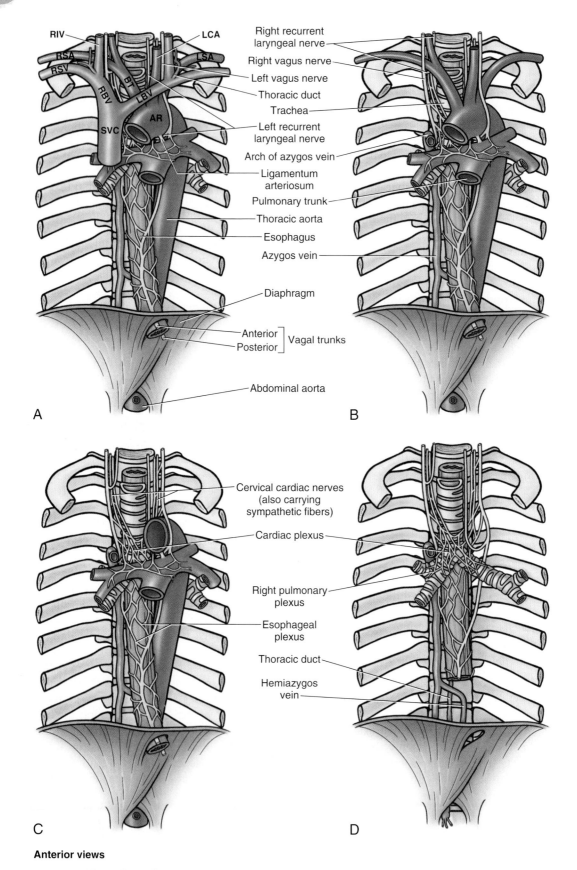

Anterior views

Figure 1.40. Structures of superior and posterior mediastinum. A–D. The structures of the mediastinum are revealed by different levels of dissection. *AR,* aortic arch; *BT,* brachiocephalic trunk; *LBV,* left brachiocephalic vein; *LCA,* left common carotid artery; *LSA,* left subclavian artery; *RBV,* right brachiocephalic vein; *RIV,* right internal jugular vein; *RSA,* right subclavian artery; *RSV,* right subclavian vein; *SVC,* superior vena cava.

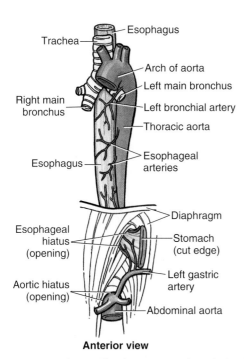

Figure 1.41. Posterior mediastinum. Note the relationships between the trachea, esophagus, and aorta.

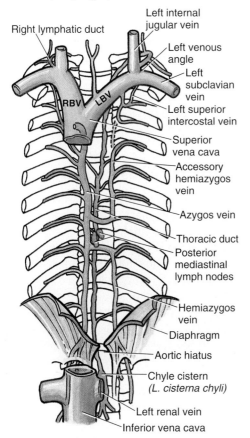

Figure 1.42. Azygos system of veins and thoracic duct. *RBV,* right brachiocephalic vein; *LBV,* left brachiocephalic vein.

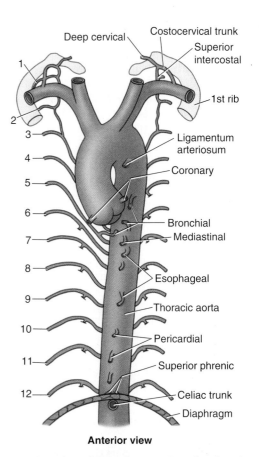

Figure 1.43. Branches of thoracic aorta. Superior phrenic arteries arising from the inferior part of the thoracic aorta supply the diaphragm. *1–12,* posterior intercostal arteries.

that course on the abdominal side of the origin of the diaphragm are in series with the intercostal arteries.

ESOPHAGUS

The esophagus descends into the posterior mediastinum from the superior mediastinum, passing posterior and to the right of the arch of the aorta and posterior to the pericardium and left atrium. The esophagus constitutes the primary posterior relationship of the base of the heart. It then deviates to the left and passes through the **esophageal hiatus** in the diaphragm at the level of the T10 vertebra, anterior to the aorta (Fig. 1.41). The esophagus may have three impressions, or "constrictions," in its thoracic part. These may be observed as narrowings of the lumen in oblique chest radiographs that are taken as barium is swallowed. The esophagus is compressed by three structures: the aortic arch, left main bronchus, and diaphragm. No constrictions are visible in the empty esophagus; however, as it expands during filling, these structures compress its walls.

THORACIC DUCT AND LYMPHATIC TRUNKS

In the posterior mediastinum, the thoracic duct lies on the bodies of the inferior seven thoracic vertebrae (Fig. 1.42). The thoracic duct conveys most lymph of the body to the venous system (that from the lower limbs, pelvic cavity, abdominal cavity, left side of thorax, left side of head, neck, and left upper limb). The thoracic duct originates from the **chyle cistern** (L. *cisterna chyli*) in the abdomen and ascends through the aortic hiatus in the diaphragm. The thoracic duct is usually thin walled and dull white; often, it is beaded because of its numerous valves. It ascends between the thoracic aorta on its left, the azygos vein on its right, the esophagus anteriorly, and the vertebral bodies posteriorly. At the level of the T4–T6 vertebrae, the thoracic duct crosses to the left, posterior to the esophagus, and ascends into the superior mediastinum. The thoracic duct receives branches from the middle and upper intercostal spaces of both sides through several collecting trunks. It also receives branches from posterior mediastinal structures. Near its termination, it often receives the jugular, subclavian, and bronchomediastinal lymphatic trunks. The thoracic duct usually empties into the venous system near the union of the left internal jugular and subclavian veins, the **left venous angle** (Fig. 1.42), or origin of the left brachiocephalic vein.

VESSELS AND LYMPH NODES OF POSTERIOR MEDIASTINUM

The thoracic aorta and its branches were discussed previously. The **azygos system of veins**, on each side of the vertebral column, drains the back and thoracoabdominal walls as well as the mediastinal viscera (Fig. 1.42). The azygos system exhibits much variation, not only in its origin but also in its course, tributaries, anastomoses, and termination. The **azygos vein** and its main tributary, the **hemiazygos vein**, usually arise from "roots" arising from the posterior aspect of the IVC and/or renal vein, respectively, which merge with the ascending lumbar veins. *The azygos vein forms a collateral pathway between the SVC and the IVC and drains blood from the posterior walls of the thorax and abdomen.* The azygos vein ascends in the posterior mediastinum, passing close to the right sides of the bodies of the inferior eight thoracic vertebrae. It arches over the superior aspect of the root of the right lung to join the SVC.

In addition to the **posterior intercostal veins**, the azygos vein communicates with the vertebral venous plexuses that drain the back, vertebrae, and structures in the vertebral canal (see Chapter 4). The azygos vein also receives the mediastinal, esophageal, and bronchial veins. The hemiazygos vein ascends on the left side of the vertebral column, posterior to the thoracic aorta as far as T9. Here it crosses to the right, posterior to the aorta, thoracic duct, and esophagus and joins the azygos vein. The **accessory hemiazygos vein** descends on the left side of the vertebral column from T5–T8 and then crosses over the T7–T8 vertebra posterior to the thoracic aorta and thoracic duct to join the azygos vein. Sometimes, the accessory hemiazygos vein joins the azygos vein and drains with it into the azygos vein.

Posterior mediastinal lymph nodes lie posterior to the pericardium, where they are related to the esophagus and

Laceration of Thoracic Duct

Because the thoracic duct is thin walled and may be colorless, it may not be easily identified. Consequently, it is vulnerable to inadvertent injury during investigative and/or surgical procedures in the posterior mediastinum. Laceration of the thoracic duct results in chyle escaping into the thoracic cavity. Chyle may also enter the pleural cavity, producing *chylothorax*.

Collateral Venous Routes to Heart

The azygos, hemiazygos, and accessory hemiazygos veins offer alternate means of venous drainage from the thoracic, abdominal, and back regions when **obstruction of the IVC** occurs. In some people, an accessory azygos vein parallels the main azygos vein on the right side. Other people have no hemiazygos system of veins. A clinically important variation, although uncommon, is when the azygos system receives all the blood from the IVC, except that from the liver. In these people, the azygos system drains nearly all the blood inferior to the diaphragm, except from the digestive tract. When **obstruction of the SVC** occurs superior to the entrance of the azygos vein, blood can drain inferiorly into the veins of the abdominal wall and return to the right atrium through the IVC and azygos system of veins.

thoracic aorta (Fig. 1.41). There are several nodes posterior to the inferior part of the esophagus and more anterior and lateral to it. The posterior mediastinal lymph nodes receive lymph from the esophagus, the posterior aspect of the pericardium and diaphragm, and the middle posterior intercostal spaces.

NERVES OF POSTERIOR MEDIASTINUM

The sympathetic trunks and their associated ganglia form a major portion of the ANS (Fig. 1.39, Table 2.8). The **thoracic sympathetic trunks** are in continuity with the cervical and lumbar sympathetic trunks. The thoracic sympathetic trunks lie against the heads of the ribs in the superior part of the thorax, the costovertebral joints in the midthoracic level, and the sides of the vertebral bodies in the inferior part of the thorax. The **lower thoracic splanchnic nerves**, also known as greater, lesser, and least splanchnic nerves, are part of the *abdominopelvic splanchnic nerves* because they supply viscera inferior to the diaphragm. They consist of presynaptic fibers from the 5th–12th sympathetic ganglia, which pass through the diaphragm and synapse in prevertebral ganglia in the abdomen. They supply sympathetic innervation for most of the abdominal viscera. These splanchnic nerves are discussed further in Chapter 2.

Medical Imaging of Thorax

The main imaging methods for examination of the thorax are radiography, echocardiography, CT, and MRI. Images from MRI angiography (Fig. 1.44), coronary arteriography (Fig. 1.45), and CT (Fig. 1.46) are presented here. For more imaging modalities, see Moore and Dalley (2005). ●

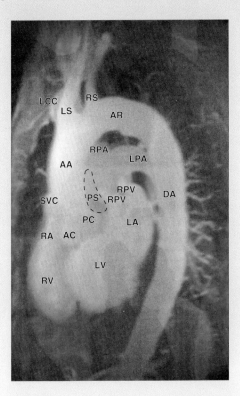

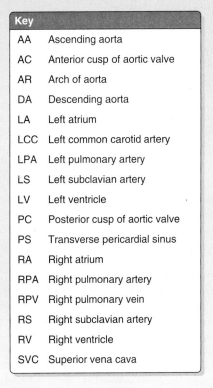

Key	
AA	Ascending aorta
AC	Anterior cusp of aortic valve
AR	Arch of aorta
DA	Descending aorta
LA	Left atrium
LCC	Left common carotid artery
LPA	Left pulmonary artery
LS	Left subclavian artery
LV	Left ventricle
PC	Posterior cusp of aortic valve
PS	Transverse pericardial sinus
RA	Right atrium
RPA	Right pulmonary artery
RPV	Right pulmonary vein
RS	Right subclavian artery
RV	Right ventricle
SVC	Superior vena cava

Figure 1.44. MR angiogram of heart and great vessels.

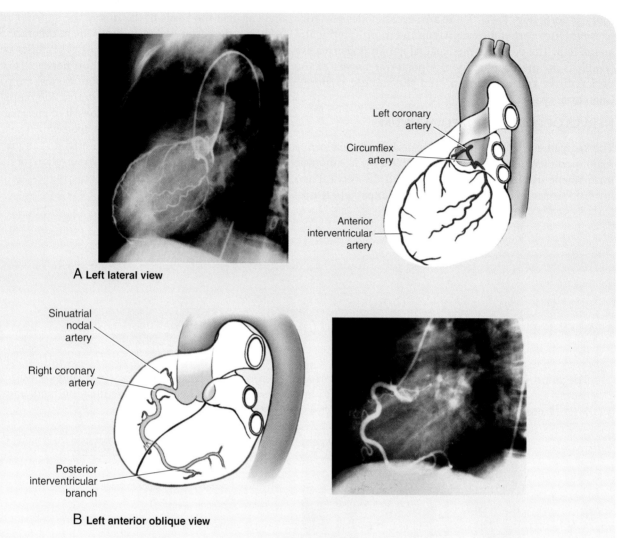

A **Left lateral view**

B **Left anterior oblique view**

Figure 1.45. Coronary arteriograms. Radiopaque dye has been injected into the left (A) and the right (B) coronary arteries.

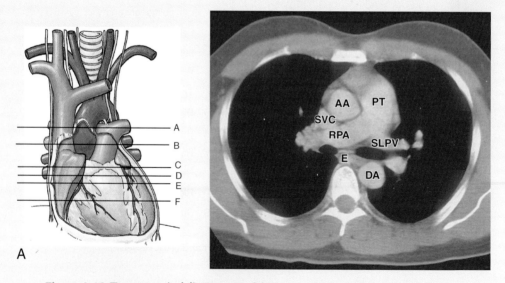

Figure 1.46. Transverse (axial) CT scans of thorax. A. The level of each scan is shown.

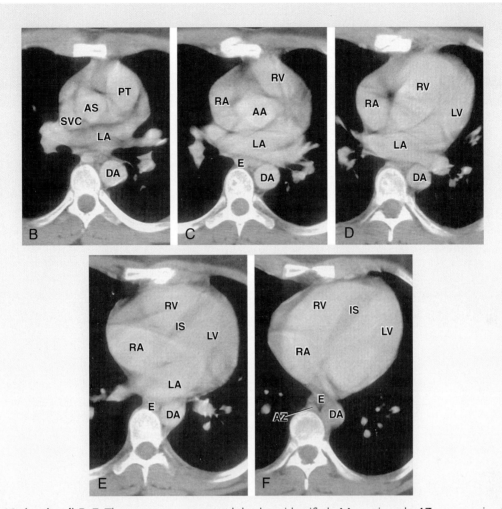

Figure 1.46. *(continued)* **B–F.** The structures seen at each level are identified. ***AA,*** aortic arch; ***AZ,*** azygos vein; ***AS,*** ascending aorta; ***DA,*** descending aorta; ***E,*** esophagus; ***IS,*** interventricular septum; ***LA,*** left atrium; ***LV,*** left ventricle; ***PT,*** pulmonary trunk; ***RA,*** right atrium; ***RPA,*** right pulmonary artery; ***RV,*** right ventricle; ***SVC,*** superior vena cava.

2 Abdomen

The abdomen is the part of the trunk between the thorax and the pelvis (*Fig. 2.1*). It has musculotendinous walls, except posteriorly, where the wall includes the lumbar vertebrae and intervertebral (IV) discs. The abdominal wall encloses the abdominal cavity, containing the peritoneal cavity and housing most of the organs (viscera) of the digestive system and part of the urogenital system.

Abdominal Cavity

The **abdominal cavity** is the space bounded by the abdominal walls, diaphragm, and pelvis. The abdominal cavity forms the major part of the **abdominopelvic cavity**—the combined and continuous abdominal and pelvic cavities (Fig. 2.1). The abdominal cavity is:

- Enclosed anterolaterally by the dynamic musculoaponeurotic abdominal walls.
- Separated superiorly from the thoracic cavity by the diaphragm.
- Undercover of the thoracic cage superiorly extending to the 4th intercostal space.
- Continuous inferiorly with the pelvic cavity.
- Lined with peritoneum, a serous membrane.
- The location of most of the digestive organs, the spleen, the kidneys, and the ureters for most of their course.

Clinicians subdivide the abdominal cavity into nine regions to locate abdominal organs or pain sites: right hypochondriac, right lateral (lumbar), right inguinal (groin), epigastric, umbilical, pubic (hypogastric), left hypochondriac, left lateral (lumbar), and left inguinal (groin). The nine regions are delineated by four planes (Fig. 2.2A):

- Two horizontal:
  - **Subcostal plane,** passing through the inferior border of the 10th costal cartilage on each side.
  - **Transtubercular plane,** passing through the iliac tubercles and the body of the L5 vertebra.
- Two vertical:
  - **Midclavicular planes,** passing from the midpoints of clavicles to the **midinguinal points,** the midpoints of lines joining the *anterior superior iliac spines* and the superior edge of the *pubic symphysis.*

For general clinical descriptions, clinicians use four quadrants of the abdominal cavity: right upper, right lower, left upper, and left lower. The four quadrants are defined by two planes (Fig. 2.2*B*):

- **Transumbilical plane,** passing through the umbilicus and IV disc between the L3 and the L4 vertebrae.
- **Median plane,** passing longitudinally through the body, dividing it into right and left halves.

Anterolateral Abdominal Wall

Although the abdominal wall is continuous, it is subdivided for descriptive purposes into the *anterior wall, right and left*

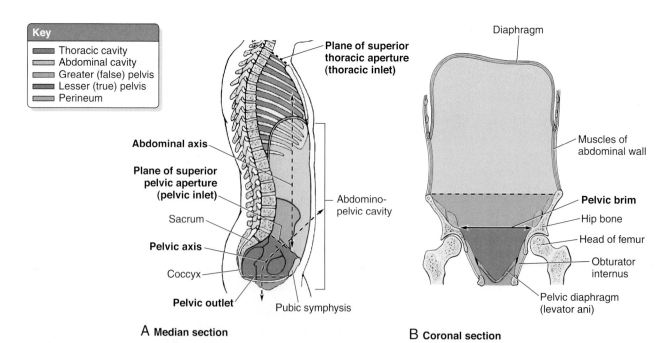

Key
- Thoracic cavity
- Abdominal cavity
- Greater (false) pelvis
- Lesser (true) pelvis
- Perineum

Abdominal axis
Plane of superior pelvic aperture (pelvic inlet)
Sacrum
Pelvic axis
Coccyx
Pelvic outlet

Plane of superior thoracic aperture (thoracic inlet)
Abdomino-pelvic cavity
Pubic symphysis

A Median section

Diaphragm
Muscles of abdominal wall
Pelvic brim
Hip bone
Head of femur
Obturator internus
Pelvic diaphragm (levator ani)

B Coronal section

Figure 2.1. Thoracic and abdominopelvic cavities. A. The pelvic inlet (superior pelvic aperture) is the opening into the lesser pelvis. The pelvic outlet (inferior pelvic aperture) is the lower opening of the lesser pelvis. **B.** Observe that the plane of the pelvic brim (*double-headed arrow*) separates the greater pelvis (part of the abdominal cavity) from the lesser pelvis (the pelvic cavity).

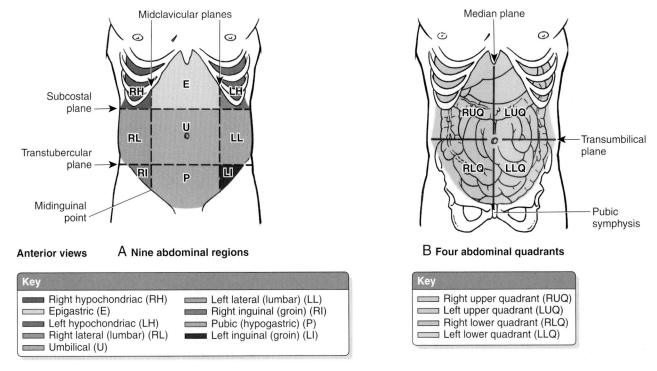

Figure 2.2. Subdivisions of abdomen and reference planes.

lateral walls (*flanks*), and *posterior wall*. The boundary between the anterior and the lateral walls is indefinite. Consequently, the combined term *anterolateral abdominal wall,* extending from the thoracic cage to the pelvis, is often used because some structures, such as the muscles and cutaneous nerves, are in both the anterior and the lateral walls. The anterolateral abdominal wall is bounded superiorly by the cartilages of the 7th–10th ribs and the xiphoid process of the sternum and inferiorly by the inguinal ligament and pelvic bones (Fig. 2.4). The wall consists of skin, subcutaneous tissue (superficial fascia), muscles and their aponeuroses, deep fascia, extraperitoneal fat, and parietal peritoneum (Fig. 2.3). The skin attaches loosely to the subcutaneous tissue except at the umbilicus, where it adheres firmly.

Fascia of Anterolateral Abdominal Wall

The fascial layers from superficial to deep include the **subcutaneous tissue** (superficial fascia), which lies deep to the skin and contains a variable amount of fat (Fig. 2.3*B*). Inferior to the umbilicus, the subcutaneous tissue is composed of two layers: a **superficial fatty layer** (Camper fascia) and a **deep membranous layer** (Scarpa fascia).

The superficial, intermediate, and deep layers of the **investing fascia** cover the external aspects of the three muscle layers of the anterolateral abdominal wall and their aponeuroses. The investing fascias are thin, being represented by the epimysium superficial to or between muscles.

The **endoabdominal fascia** is a membranous sheet of varying thickness that lines the internal aspect of the abdominal wall. Although continuous, different parts of this fascia can be named according to the muscle or aponeurosis it is lining—for example, the portion lining the deep surface of the transverse abdominal muscle or aponeurosis is the **transversalis fascia.**

The **parietal peritoneum** lines the abdominal cavity and is located internal to the transversalis fascia. It is separated from the transversalis fascia by a variable amount of **extraperitoneal fat.**

Muscles of Anterolateral Abdominal Wall

There are five (bilaterally paired) muscles in the anterolateral abdominal wall (Fig. 2.4): three flat muscles and two vertical muscles. Their attachments, nerve supply, and main actions are listed in Table 2.1.

The three flat muscles are the:

- **External oblique**, the superficial muscle: Its fibers pass inferomedially and interdigitate with slips of the serratus anterior. The inferior margin is thickened as an undercurving fibrous band that spans between the anterior superior iliac spine and the pubic tubercle as the **inguinal ligament.**
- **Internal oblique**, the intermediate muscle: Its fibers fan out so that its upper fibers are perpendicular and its lower fibers are parallel to those of the external oblique.

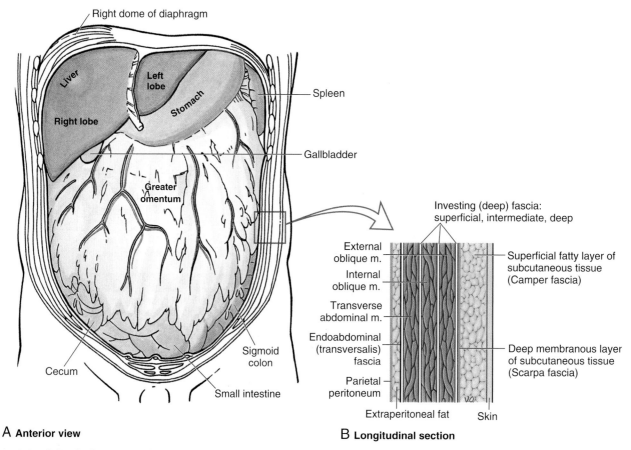

Figure 2.3. Abdominal contents and layers of anterolateral abdominal wall. A. The anterior abdominal wall has been cut away. Note the relationship of the abdominal wall and the superficial abdominal contents. Most of the intestine is covered by the greater omentum. **B.** This section shows the layers of the inferior part of the wall.

- **Transverse abdominal** (L. *transversus abdominis*), the innermost muscle: Its fibers, except for the most inferior ones, run more or less horizontally.

All three flat muscles end anteriorly in a strong sheet-like **aponeurosis**. Between the midclavicular line and the midline, the aponeuroses form the tough **rectus sheath**, enclosing the rectus abdominis. The aponeuroses interweave, forming a midline raphe (G. *rhaphe,* suture, seam), the **linea alba** (L. white line), which extends from the xiphoid process to the pubic symphysis. The interweaving is not only between right and left sides but also between superficial, intermediate, and deep layers. For example, the tendinous fibers of the external oblique that decussate at the linea alba, for the most part, become continuous with the tendinous fibers of the contralateral internal oblique, forming a two-bellied muscle sharing a common central tendon. These two muscles work together to flex and rotate the trunk (torsional movement of trunk).

The two vertical muscles are the:

- **Rectus abdominis,** a long, broad, strap-like muscle that is mostly enclosed in the *rectus sheath* (Figs. 2.4 and 2.5). The

contractile (fleshy) fibers of the rectus do not run the length of the muscle; rather they run between three or more **tendinous intersections** (Fig. 2.4*A*), which are typically located at the level of the xiphoid process, umbilicus, and a level halfway between these points. Each intersection is firmly attached to the anterior layer of the rectus sheath.

- **Pyramidalis,** a small triangular muscle (absent in about 20% of people), lies in the rectus sheath anterior to the inferior part of the rectus abdominis (Fig. 2.4*A*). It ends in the **linea alba** and tenses it.

The **rectus sheath** is formed by the interlaced aponeuroses of the flat abdominal muscles (Fig. 2.5). Until about one third of the distance from the umbilicus to the pubic crest, the rectus abdominis is enveloped by the anterior layer of the rectus sheath (formed by the external oblique aponeurosis and the anterior lamina of the internal oblique aponeurosis) and posterior layer of the rectus sheath (formed by the posterior lamina of the internal oblique aponeurosis and the transverse abdominal aponeurosis). In this region, the aponeuroses of all three muscles, the external and internal oblique and the transverse abdominal,

Clinical Significance of Fascia and Fascial Spaces of the Abdominal Wall

When closing abdominal skin incisions, surgeons include the membranous layer of subcutaneous tissue when suturing because of its strength. Between the membranous layer and the deep fascia covering the rectus abdominis and external oblique muscles is a potential space where fluid may accumulate (e.g., urine from a ruptured urethra). Although no barriers (other than gravity) prevent fluid from spreading superiorly from this space, it cannot spread inferiorly into the thigh because the membranous layer of subcutaneous tissue fuses with the deep fascia of the thigh (fascia lata) along a line inferior and parallel to the inguinal ligament (Fig. B2.1).

The potential or fat-filled space between the endoabdominal fascia and the parietal peritoneum provides a plane that can be opened, enabling the surgeon to approach structures on or in the anterior aspect of the posterior abdominal wall (e.g., kidneys or lumbar vertebrae) without entering the membranous peritoneal sac containing the abdominal viscera. Thus the risk of contamination is minimized.

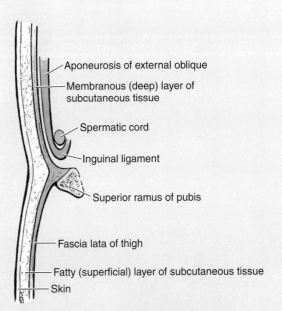

- Aponeurosis of external oblique
- Membranous (deep) layer of subcutaneous tissue
- Spermatic cord
- Inguinal ligament
- Superior ramus of pubis
- Fascia lata of thigh
- Fatty (superficial) layer of subcutaneous tissue
- Skin

Sagittal section of anterior abdominal wall

Figure B2.1.

Table 2.1 Principal Muscles of Anterolateral Abdominal Wall

Muscles[a]	Origin	Insertion	Innervation	Action(s)
External oblique	External surfaces of 5th–12th ribs	Linea alba, pubic tubercle, and anterior half of iliac crest	Thoracoabdominal nerves (T7–T11) and subcostal nerve	Compress and support abdominal viscera; flex and rotate trunk
Internal oblique	Thoracolumbar fascia, anterior two thirds of iliac crest, and lateral half of inguinal ligament	Inferior borders of 10th–12th ribs, linea alba, and pubis via conjoint tendon	Thoracoabdominal anterior rami of inferior six thoracic nerves and first lumbar nerve	
Transverse abdominal	Internal surfaces of 7th–12th costal cartilages, thoracolumbar fascia, iliac crest, and lateral third of inguinal ligament	Linea alba with aponeurosis of internal oblique, pubic crest, and pectin pubis via conjoint tendon		Compresses and supports abdominal viscera
Rectus abdominis	Pubic symphysis and pubic crest	Xiphoid process and 5th–7th costal cartilages	Thoracoabdominal nerves and anterior rami of inferior thoracic nerves	Flexes trunk (lumbar vertebrae) and compresses abdominal viscera;[b] stabilizes and controls tilt of pelvis (antilordosis)

[a]Approximately 80% of people have a *pyramidal muscle,* which is located in the rectus sheath anterior to the most inferior part of the rectus abdominis. It extends from the pubic crest of the hip bone to the linea alba. This small muscle tenses on the linea alba.
[b]In so doing, these muscles act as antagonists of the diaphragm to produce expiration.

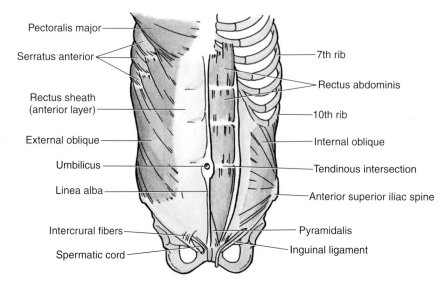

A Anterior view

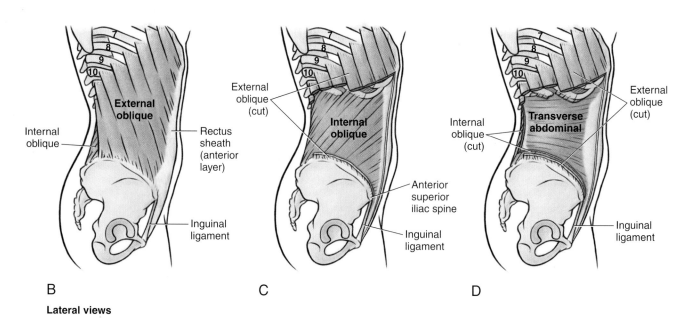

B

C

D

Lateral views

Figure 2.4. Posterior aspect of anterolateral abdominal wall. A. On the right, note the external oblique and intact rectus sheath. On the left, note the internal oblique and opened rectus sheath, revealing the rectus abdominis. The external oblique (**B**), internal oblique (**C**), and transverse abdominal (**D**) muscles are shown.

pass anterior to the rectus abdominis to form the anterior rectus sheath, leaving only the transversalis fascia to cover the rectus abdominis posteriorly. An **arcuate line** often demarcates the transition between the posterior rectus sheath covering the superior three quarters of the rectus abdominis proximally and the transversalis fascia covering the inferior quarter.

The **contents of the rectus sheath** are the rectus abdominis and pyramidalis muscles, the anastomosing superior and inferior epigastric arteries and veins, the lymphatic vessels,

and the distal portions of the anterior rami of spinal nerves T7–T12, which supply the muscle and overlying skin.

FUNCTIONS AND ACTIONS OF THE ANTEROLATERAL ABDOMINAL MUSCLES

The muscles of the anterolateral abdominal wall:

- Form a strong expandable support for the anterolateral abdominal wall.
- Protect the abdominal viscera from injury.

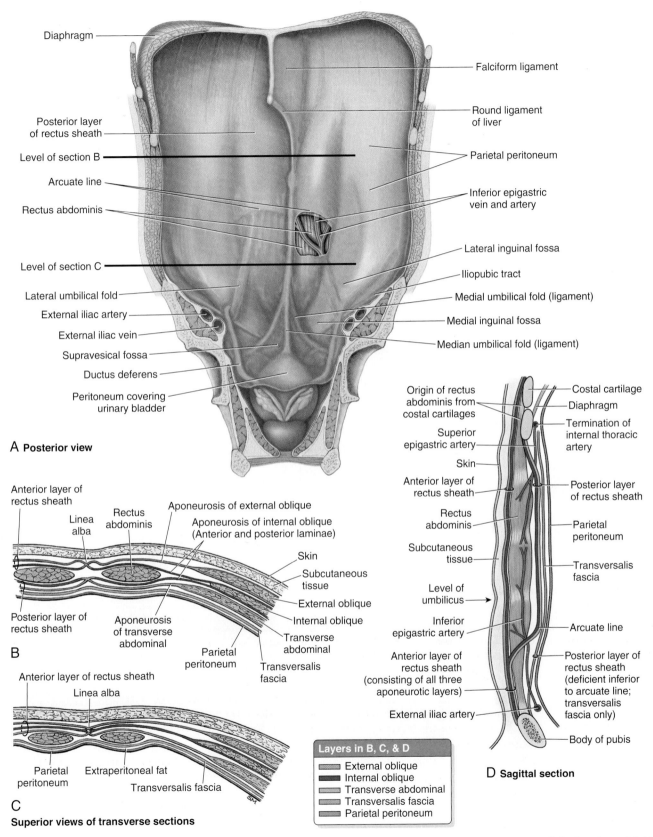

Diaphragm

Falciform ligament

Round ligament of liver

Posterior layer of rectus sheath

Parietal peritoneum

Level of section B

Arcuate line

Inferior epigastric vein and artery

Rectus abdominis

Lateral inguinal fossa

Level of section C

Iliopubic tract

Lateral umbilical fold

Medial umbilical fold (ligament)

External iliac artery

Medial inguinal fossa

External iliac vein

Median umbilical fold (ligament)

Supravesical fossa

Ductus deferens

Peritoneum covering urinary bladder

A Posterior view

Origin of rectus abdominis from costal cartilages

Costal cartilage

Diaphragm

Termination of internal thoracic artery

Superior epigastric artery

Skin

Anterior layer of rectus sheath

Posterior layer of rectus sheath

Rectus abdominis

Parietal peritoneum

Subcutaneous tissue

Transversalis fascia

Level of umbilicus

Inferior epigastric artery

Arcuate line

Anterior layer of rectus sheath (consisting of all three aponeurotic layers)

Posterior layer of rectus sheath (deficient inferior to arcuate line; transversalis fascia only)

External iliac artery

Body of pubis

D Sagittal section

Anterior layer of rectus sheath

Linea alba

Rectus abdominis

Aponeurosis of external oblique

Aponeurosis of internal oblique (Anterior and posterior laminae)

Skin

Subcutaneous tissue

External oblique

Internal oblique

Posterior layer of rectus sheath

Aponeurosis of transverse abdominal

Parietal peritoneum

Transverse abdominal

Transversalis fascia

B

Anterior layer of rectus sheath

Linea alba

Parietal peritoneum

Extraperitoneal fat

Transversalis fascia

C

Superior views of transverse sections

Layers in B, C, & D

External oblique
Internal oblique
Transverse abdominal
Transversalis fascia
Parietal peritoneum

Figure 2.5. Anterolateral abdominal wall. A. This internal view of the infraumbilical part of the wall shows the umbilical peritoneal folds and fossae (supravesical, medial inguinal, and lateral inguinal). Transverse sections of the wall superior to (**B**) and inferior to (**C**) the arcuate line reveal the layers of the rectus sheath. **D.** The rectus sheath is shown in a sagittal section.

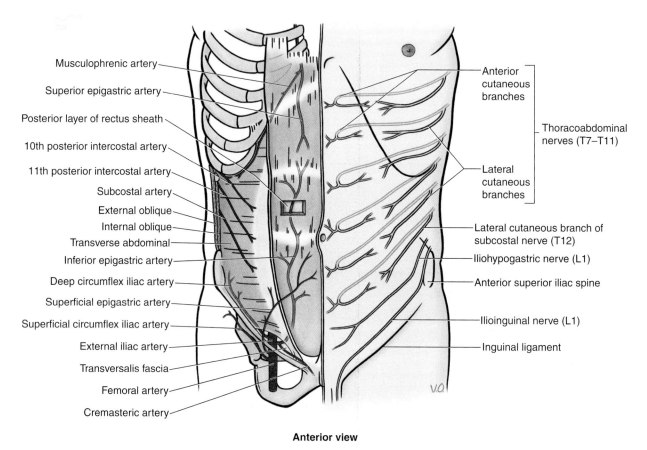

Anterior view

Figure 2.6. Arteries and nerves of anterolateral abdominal wall.

Table 2.2 Nerves of Anterolateral Abdominal Wall

Nerve	Origin	Course	Distribution
Thoracoabdominal (T7–T11)	Continuation of lower intercostal nerves	Run between second and third layers of abdominal muscles; lateral cutaneous and anterior cutaneous branches enter subcutaneous tissue	Muscles of anterolateral abdominal wall and overlying skin
Subcostal (T12)	Anterior ramus of T12 spinal nerve	Runs along inferior border of 12th rib, then onto subumbilical abdominal wall	Muscles of anterolateral abdominal wall and overlying skin superior to iliac crest and inferior to umbilicus
Iliohypogastric (L1)	Anterior ramus of L1 spinal nerve	Pierces transverse abdominal muscle; branches pierce external oblique aponeurosis of inferiormost abdominal wall	Skin overlying iliac crest, upper inguinal and hypogastric regions; internal oblique and transverse abdominal
Ilioinguinal (L1)	Anterior ramus of L1 spinal nerve	Passes between second and third layers of abdominal muscles, then traverses inguinal canal	Skin of scrotum or labium majus, mons pubis, and adjacent medial aspect of thigh; inferiormost internal oblique and transverse abdominal

- Compress the abdominal viscera to maintain or increase intra-abdominal pressure. Compressing the abdominal viscera and increasing intra-abdominal pressure elevates the relaxed diaphragm to expel air during respiration, coughing, voluntary eructation (burping), yelling, and so on. When the diaphragm contracts during inspiration, the anterolateral abdominal wall expands as the muscles relax to make room for the viscera that are pushed inferiorly.
- Produce the force required for defecation (evacuation of fecal material from the rectum), micturition (urination), vomiting, and parturition (childbirth).
- Produce anterior and lateral flexion of the trunk, torsional (rotatory) movements of the trunk and help maintain posture.

Nerves of Anterolateral Abdominal Wall

The skin and muscles of the anterolateral abdominal wall are supplied mainly by the (Fig. 2.6, Table 2.2):

- **Thoracoabdominal nerves:** distal, abdominal parts of the anterior rami of the inferior six thoracic spinal nerves (T7–T11), which have muscular branches and **anterior and lateral cutaneous branches.** The anterior cutaneous branches pierce the rectus sheath a short distance from the median plane, after the rectus abdominis muscle has been supplied. Spinal nerves T7–T9 supply the skin superior to the umbilicus; T10 innervates the skin around the umbilicus.
- **Subcostal nerve:** large anterior ramus of spinal nerve T12.

- **Iliohypogastric and ilioinguinal nerves:** terminal branches of the anterior ramus of spinal nerve L1.
- Spinal nerve T11, plus the cutaneous branches of the subcostal (T12), iliohypogastric, and ilioinguinal (L1) nerves: supply the skin inferior to the umbilicus.

Vessels of Anterolateral Abdominal Wall

The blood vessels of the anterolateral abdominal wall are the (Fig. 2.6, Table 2.3):

- **Superior epigastric vessels** and branches of the **musculophrenic vessels** from the internal thoracic vessels.
- **Inferior epigastric** and **deep circumflex iliac vessels** from the external iliac vessels.
- **Superficial circumflex iliac** and **superficial epigastric vessels** from the femoral artery and great saphenous vein.
- **Posterior intercostal vessels** in the 11th intercostal space and anterior branches of **subcostal vessels.**

The **superior epigastric artery**, the direct continuation of the internal thoracic artery, enters the rectus sheath superiorly through its posterior layer (Fig. 2.4), supplies the upper part of the rectus abdominis, and anastomoses with the inferior epigastric artery. The **inferior epigastric artery** arises from the external iliac artery just superior to the inguinal ligament. It runs superiorly in the transversalis fascia to enter the rectus sheath inferior to the arcuate line. Its branches enter the lower rectus abdominis and anastomose with those of the superior epigastric artery.

Table 2.3 Principle Arteries of Anterolateral Abdominal Wall

Artery	Origin	Course	Distribution
Musculophrenic	Internal thoracic artery	Descends along costal margin	Abdominal wall of hypochondriac region, anterolateral, diaphragm
Superior epigastric	Internal thoracic artery	Descends in rectus sheath deep to rectus abdominis	Rectus abdominis and superior part of anterolateral abdominal wall
10th and 11th posterior intercostal	Aorta	Arteries continue beyond ribs to descend in abdominal wall between internal oblique and transverse abdominal	Abdominal wall, lateral region
Subcostal Inferior epigastric	External iliac artery	Runs superiorly and enters rectus sheath; runs deep to rectus abdominis	Rectus abdominis and medial part of anterolateral abdominal wall
Deep circumflex iliac	External iliac artery	Runs on deep aspect of anterior abdominal wall, parallel to inguinal ligament	Iliacus muscle and inferior part of anterolateral abdominal wall
Superficial circumflex iliac	Femoral artery	Runs in superficial fascia along inguinal ligament	Superficial abdominal wall of inguinal region and adjacent anterior thigh
Superficial epigastric	Femoral artery	Runs in superficial fascia toward umbilicus	Subcutaneous tissue and skin over pubic and inferior umbilical region

Surface Anatomy of Anterolateral Abdominal Wall

The **umbilicus** is where the umbilical cord entered into the fetus and is the reference point for the transumbilical plane (Fig. SA2.1A). It indicates the level of the T10 dermatome and is typically at the level of the IV disc between the L3 and L4 vertebrae; however, its position varies with the amount of fat in the subcutaneous tissue. The **linea alba** is a subcutaneous fibrous band extending from the **xiphoid process** to the **pubic symphysis** that is demarcated by a midline vertical skin groove as far inferiorly as the umbilicus. The pubic symphysis can be felt in the median plane at the inferior end of the linea alba. The bony **iliac crest** at the level of the L4 vertebra can be easily palpated as it extends posteriorly from the **anterior superior iliac spine.**

In an individual with good muscle definition, curved skin grooves, the **semilunar lines** (L. *linae semilunares*) demarcate the lateral borders of the rectus abdominis and rectus sheath. The semilunar lines extend from the inferior costal margin near the 9th costal cartilages to the **pubic tubercles.** Three transverse skin grooves overlie the **tendinous intersections** of the rectus abdominis (Fig. SA2.1B). The interdigitating bellies of the **serratus anterior** and **external oblique muscles** are also visible. The site of the **inguinal ligament** is indicated by a skin crease, the inguinal groove, just inferior and parallel to the ligament, marking the division between the anterolateral abdominal wall and the thigh. ●

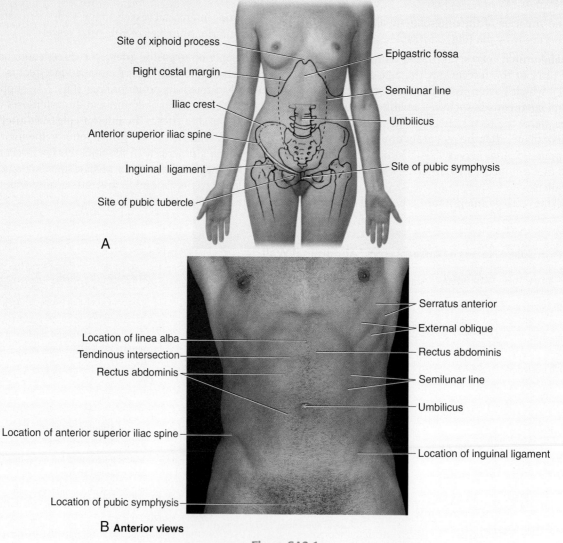

Site of xiphoid process

Right costal margin

Iliac crest

Anterior superior iliac spine

Inguinal ligament

Site of pubic tubercle

Epigastric fossa

Semilunar line

Umbilicus

Site of pubic symphysis

A

Location of linea alba

Tendinous intersection

Rectus abdominis

Location of anterior superior iliac spine

Location of pubic symphysis

Serratus anterior

External oblique

Rectus abdominis

Semilunar line

Umbilicus

Location of inguinal ligament

B Anterior views

Figure SA2.1.

Abdominal Surgical Incisions

Surgeons use various incisions to gain access to the abdominal cavity. The incision that allows adequate exposure and, secondarily, the best possible cosmetic effect, is chosen. The location of the incision also depends on the type of operation, the location of the organ(s), bony or cartilaginous boundaries, avoidance of (especially motor) nerves, maintenance of blood supply, and minimizing injury to muscles and fascia of the wall while aiming for favorable healing. Instead of transecting muscles, causing irreversible necrosis (death) of muscle fibers, the surgeon splits them between their fibers. The rectus abdominis is an exception and can be transected because its

muscle fibers are short and its nerves entering the lateral part of the rectus sheath can be located and preserved. Cutting a motor nerve paralyzes the muscle fibers supplied by it, thereby weakening the anterolateral abdominal wall. However, because of overlapping areas of innervation between nerves in the abdominal wall, one or two small branches of nerves may be cut without a noticeable loss of motor supply to the muscles or loss of sensation to the skin. Some of the most common surgical incisions are illustrated in Figure B2.2.

Incisional Hernia

If the muscular and aponeurotic layers of the abdomen do not heal properly, a hernia may occur through the defect. An incisional hernia is a protrusion of omentum (fold of peritoneum) or an organ through a surgical incision or scar.

Minimally Invasive (Endoscopic) Surgery

Many abdominopelvic surgical procedures are now performed using an endoscope, in which tiny perforations of the abdominal wall allow the entry of remotely operated instruments, replacing the larger conventional incisions. Thus the potential for nerve injury, incisional hernia, or contamination through the open wound and the time required for healing are minimized.

Palpation of Abdomen

Intense guarding, board-like reflexive muscular rigidity that cannot be willfully suppressed, occurs during palpation when an organ (e.g., the appendix) is inflamed and in itself constitutes a clinically significant sign of acute abdomen. The involuntary muscular spasms attempt to protect the viscera from pressure, which is painful when abdominal infection is present. The common nerve supply of the skin and muscular walls explains why these spasms occur.

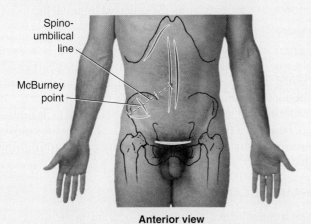

Spino-umbilical line

McBurney point

Anterior view

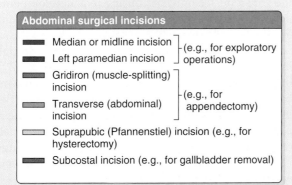

Abdominal surgical incisions

- Median or midline incision ⎤ (e.g., for exploratory
- Left paramedian incision ⎦ operations)
- Gridiron (muscle-splitting) ⎤ incision ⎪
- Transverse (abdominal) ⎬ (e.g., for incision ⎦ appendectomy)
- Suprapubic (Pfannenstiel) incision (e.g., for hysterectomy)
- Subcostal incision (e.g., for gallbladder removal)

Figure B2.2.

The **superficial lymphatic vessels** accompany the subcutaneous veins; those superior to the umbilicus drain mainly to the **axillary lymph nodes**, whereas those inferior to it drain to the **superficial inguinal lymph nodes**. The **deep lymphatic vessels** accompany the deep veins and drain to the external iliac, common iliac, and lumbar (caval and aortic) lymph nodes.

Internal Surface of Anterolateral Abdominal Wall

The internal surface of the anterolateral abdominal wall is covered with transversalis fascia, a variable amount of extraperitoneal fat, and parietal peritoneum (Fig. 2.5*A* & *B*). The infraumbilical part of this surface of the wall exhibits several peritoneal folds, some of which contain remnants of vessels that carried blood to and from the fetus (Moore and Persaud, 2003).

Five umbilical peritoneal folds—two on each side and one in the median plane—pass toward the umbilicus:

* The **median umbilical fold**, extending from the apex of the urinary bladder to the umbilicus, covers the **median umbilical ligament**, the remnant of the *urachus* that joined the apex of the fetal bladder to the umbilicus.
* Two **medial umbilical folds**, lateral to the median umbilical fold, cover the **medial umbilical ligaments**, formed by the occluded parts of the umbilical arteries.
* Two **lateral umbilical folds**, lateral to the medial umbilical folds, cover the **inferior epigastric vessels** and, therefore, bleed if cut.

The depressions lateral to the umbilical folds are *peritoneal fossae,* each of which is a potential site for a hernia. The location of a hernia in one of these fossae determines how the hernia is classified. The shallow fossae between the umbilical folds are the:

* **Supravesical fossae** between the median and the medial umbilical folds, formed as the peritoneum reflects from the anterior abdominal wall onto the bladder. The level of the supravesical fossae rises and falls with filling and emptying of the bladder.
* **Medial inguinal fossae** between the medial and the lateral umbilical folds, areas also commonly called **inguinal triangles** (Hesselbach triangles). These are potential sites for direct inguinal hernias.
* **Lateral inguinal fossae**, lateral to the lateral umbilical folds, include the deep inguinal rings and are potential sites for the most common type of hernia in the lower abdominal wall, the indirect inguinal hernia.

Inguinal Area

The area extends between the anterior superior iliac spine and the pubic tubercle. Anatomically, it is a region where structures exit and enter the abdominal cavity and is, therefore, clinically important because these are potential sites of herniation. Inguinal hernias occur in both sexes, but most (about 86%) occur in males because of the passage of the spermatic cord through the inguinal canal. The migration of the testes from the abdomen into the perineum accounts for many of the structural fea-

tures of the region. Thus the testis and scrotum are usually studied in relation to the anterior abdominal wall and inguinal region.

INGUINAL LIGAMENT AND ILIOPUBIC TRACT

The **inguinal ligament,** the inferiormost part of the external oblique aponeurosis, and the **iliopubic tract,** the thickened inferior margin of the transversalis fascia, extend from the anterior superior iliac spine to the pubic tubercle. Most of the fibers of the inguinal ligament insert into the pubic tubercle, but some fibers:

1. Attach to the superior pubic ramus lateral to the pubic tubercle as the **lacunar ligament** and then continue to run along the pectin pubis as the **pectineal ligament** (of Cooper).
2. Arch superiorly to blend with the contralateral external oblique aponeurosis as the **reflected inguinal ligament.**

The *iliopubic tract* is a fibrous band that runs parallel and posterior (deep) to the inguinal ligament. It is seen in place of the inguinal ligament when the inguinal region is viewed from its internal (posterior) aspect, as through an endoscope (Fig. 2.5*A*). The iliopubic tract reinforces the posterior wall and floor of the inguinal canal as it bridges the structures (hip flexors and much of the neurovascular supply of the lower limb) traversing the **subinguinal space.**

INGUINAL CANAL

The inguinal canal is formed in relation to the descent of the gonad (testes or ovary) during fetal development. The inguinal canal in adults is an approximately 4-cm-long, inferomedially directed oblique passage (between the superficial and the deep inguinal rings) that runs through the inferior part of the anterior abdominal wall (Fig. 2.7). The inguinal canal lies parallel and just superior to the medial half of the inguinal ligament. The main occupant of the inguinal canal is the *spermatic cord* in males and the *round ligament of the uterus* in females. The inguinal canal also contains blood and lymphatic vessels and the ilioinguinal nerve in both sexes. The inguinal canal has an opening at each end.

* The **deep (internal) ring** (internal entrance to the inguinal canal) is an evagination of the transversalis fascia superior to the middle of the inguinal ligament and *lateral to the inferior epigastric vessels* (Fig. 2.7*B*).
* The **superficial (external) inguinal ring** (exit from the inguinal canal) is a slit-like opening between the diagonal fibers of the aponeurosis of the external oblique, superolateral to the pubic tubercle (Fig. 2.7*C*). The lateral and medial margins of the superficial ring formed by the split in the aponeurosis are the **lateral** and **medial crura**

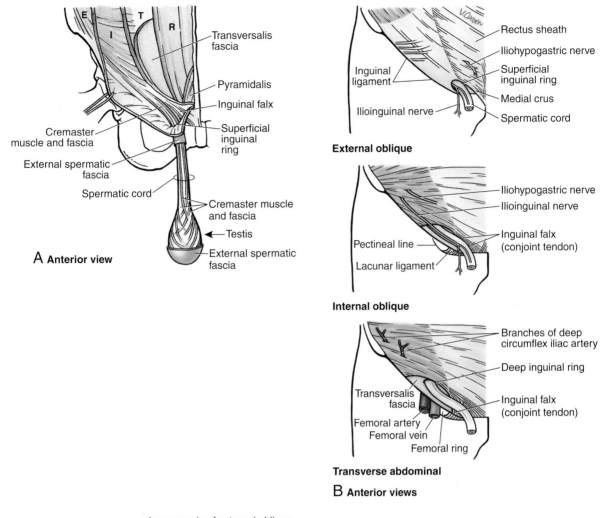

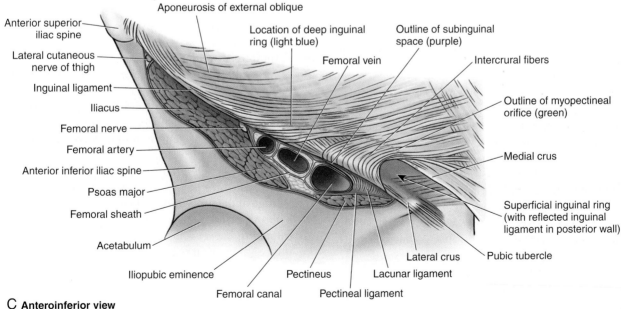

Figure 2.7. Inguinal region. A. The spermatic cord and inguinal canal are shown. *E*, external oblique; *I*, internal oblique; *R*, rectus abdominis; *T*, transverse abdominal. **B.** These progressive dissections of abdominal muscles show the relationships of the inguinal canal. **C.** Inguinal ligament and superficial inguinal ring are shown. Note the lacunar and pectineal ligaments.

(L. leg-like parts). The **intercrural fibers** help prevent the crura from spreading apart.

The deep and superficial inguinal rings do not overlap because of the oblique path of the inguinal canal through the aponeuroses of the abdominal muscles. Consequently, increases in intra-abdominal pressure force the posterior wall of the canal against the anterior wall, closing this passageway, strengthening this potential defect of the abdominal wall. Simultaneous contraction of the external oblique also approximates the anterior wall of the canal to the posterior wall and increases tension on the crura, resisting dilation of the superficial inguinal ring. Contraction of the internal oblique and transverse abdominal muscles makes the roof of the canal descend, which constricts the canal. All these events occur during acts such as sneezing, coughing, and "bearing down" (Valsalva maneuver) to increase intra-abdominal pressure for elimination (e.g., of feces).

The inguinal canal has two walls (anterior and posterior), a roof, and a floor (Fig. 2.7).

- **Anterior wall:** formed by external oblique aponeurosis throughout the length of the canal; the anterior wall of the lateral part of the canal is reinforced by fibers of internal oblique.
- **Posterior wall:** formed by transversalis fascia; the posterior wall of the medial part of the canal is reinforced by merging of the pubic attachments of the internal oblique and transverse abdominal aponeuroses into a common tendon—the **inguinal falx (conjoint tendon).**
- **Roof:** formed laterally by transversalis fascia, centrally by the musculoaponeurotic arches of internal oblique and transverse abdominal muscles, and medially by the medial crus of the external oblique aponeurosis.
- **Floor:** formed laterally by the iliopubic tract, centrally by the superior surface of the inguinal ligament, and medially by the lacunar ligament.

SPERMATIC CORD

The spermatic cord contains structures running to and from the testis and suspends the testis in the scrotum. The spermatic cord begins at the deep inguinal ring lateral to the inferior epigastric vessels, passes through the inguinal canal, exits at the superficial inguinal ring, and ends in the scrotum at the posterior border of the testis (Figs. 2.7A & B and 2.8). Fascial coverings derived from the anterolateral abdominal wall during prenatal development (Table 2.4) include the:

- **Internal spermatic fascia:** derived from the transversalis fascia at the deep inguinal ring.
- **Cremasteric fascia:** derived from the fascia of both the superficial and the deep surfaces of the internal oblique muscle.

- **External spermatic fascia:** derived from the external oblique aponeurosis and its investing fascia

The cremasteric fascia contains loops of the **cremaster muscle,** which is formed by the lowermost fascicles of the internal oblique muscle arising from the inguinal ligament. The cremaster reflexly draws the testis superiorly in the scrotum, particularly when it is cold; in a warm environment, the cremaster relaxes and the testis descends deeply in the scrotum. Both responses occur in an attempt to regulate the temperature of the testis for *spermatogenesis* (formation of sperms), which requires a constant temperature of approximately one degree cooler than core temperature. The cremaster acts with the **dartos muscle,** smooth muscle of the fat-free subcutaneous tissue of the scrotum (dartos fascia), which inserts into the skin. The dartos assists in testicular elevation as it produces contraction of the skin of the scrotum. The cremaster is innervated by the **genital branch of the genitofemoral nerve** (L1, L2), a derivative of the lumbar plexus, whereas the dartos receives autonomic innervation. Although less well developed and usually indistinct, the round ligament of the female receives similar contributions from the layers of the abdominal wall as it traverses the canal.

The **constituents of the spermatic cord** are the (Fig. 2.8):

- **Ductus deferens** (deferent duct, vas deferens), a muscular tube that conveys sperms from the epididymis to the ejaculatory duct. It courses through the substance of the prostate to open into the prostatic part of the urethra.
- **Testicular artery** arising from the aorta (vertebral level L2) and supplying the testis and epididymis.
- **Artery of ductus deferens** arising from the inferior vesical artery.
- **Cremasteric artery** arising from the inferior epigastric artery.
- **Pampiniform venous plexus,** a network formed by up to 12 veins that converge superiorly as the right or left testicular veins.
- **Sympathetic nerve fibers** on arteries and sympathetic and parasympathetic nerve fibers on the ductus deferens.
- **Genital branch of genitofemoral nerve** supplying the cremaster muscle.
- **Lymphatic vessels** draining the testis and closely associated structures to the lumbar lymph nodes (Fig. 2.8C).
- **Vestige of the processus vaginalis,** which may be seen as a fibrous thread in the anterior part of the spermatic cord extending between the abdominal peritoneum and the tunica vaginalis; it may not be detectable.

SCROTUM

The scrotum is a cutaneous sac consisting of two layers: heavily pigmented skin and closely related **dartos fascia,** a

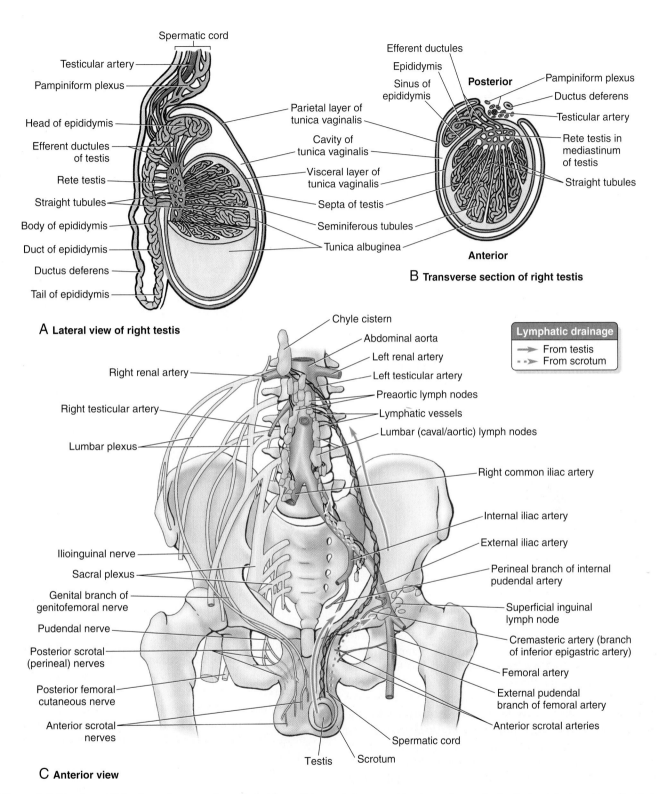

Spermatic cord

Testicular artery

Pampiniform plexus

Head of epididymis

Efferent ductules
of testis

Rete testis

Straight tubules

Body of epididymis

Duct of epididymis

Ductus deferens

Tail of epididymis

Parietal layer of
tunica vaginalis

Cavity of
tunica vaginalis

Visceral layer of
tunica vaginalis

Septa of testis

Seminiferous tubules

Tunica albuginea

A **Lateral view of right testis**

Efferent ductules

Epididymis

Sinus of
epididymis

Posterior

Pampiniform plexus

Ductus deferens

Testicular artery

Rete testis in
mediastinum
of testis

Straight tubules

Anterior

B **Transverse section of right testis**

Chyle cistern

Abdominal aorta

Left renal artery

Left testicular artery

Preaortic lymph nodes

Lymphatic vessels

Lumbar (caval/aortic) lymph nodes

Right renal artery

Right testicular artery

Lumbar plexus

Ilioinguinal nerve

Sacral plexus

Genital branch of
genitofemoral nerve

Pudendal nerve

Posterior scrotal
(perineal) nerves

Posterior femoral
cutaneous nerve

Anterior scrotal
nerves

Right common iliac artery

Internal iliac artery

External iliac artery

Perineal branch of internal
pudendal artery

Superficial inguinal
lymph node

Cremasteric artery (branch
of inferior epigastric artery)

Femoral artery

External pudendal
branch of femoral artery

Anterior scrotal arteries

Spermatic cord

Testis   Scrotum

C **Anterior view**

Lymphatic drainage
→ From testis
⇢ From scrotum

Figure 2.8. Testis, epididymis, and spermatic cord. A. Most of the testis is covered by the tunica vaginalis. **B.** A vertical section of testis is shown. **C.** The blood supply, innervation, and lymphatic drainage are shown. *Arrows,* direction of the flow of lymph to the lymph nodes.

Table 2.4 Corresponding Layers of Anterior Abdominal Wall, Spermatic Cord, and Scrotum

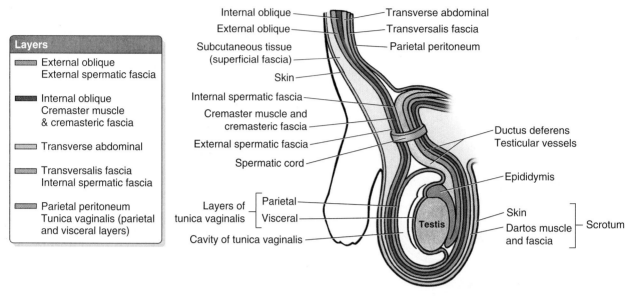

Layers of the Anterior Abdominal Wall	Scrotum and Covering of the Testis	Coverings of the Spermatic Cord
Skin	Skin	Skin continuous with scrotum (and scrotal septum)
Subcutaneous tissue (superficial fascia)	Subcutaneous tissue (dartos fascia) and dartos muscle	
External oblique aponeurosis or muscle	External spermatic fascia	External spermatic fascia
Internal oblique muscle	Cremaster muscle	Cremaster muscle
Fascia of both superficial and deep surfaces of internal oblique muscle	Cremasteric fascia	Cremasteric fascia
Transverse abdominal muscle		
Transversalis fascia	Internal spermatic fascia	Internal spermatic fascia
Extraperitoneal fat		
Peritoneum	Tunica vaginalis (parietal and visceral layers)	Vestige of processus vaginalis

fat-free fascial layer including smooth muscle fibers (dartos muscle) responsible for the rugose (wrinkled) appearance of the scrotum. Because the **dartos muscle** attaches to the skin, its contraction causes the scrotum to wrinkle when cold, which thickens the integumentary layer while reducing the scrotal surface area and assists the cremaster in holding the testes closer to the body, thus reducing heat loss. *Scrotal veins* accompany the arteries. The *lymphatic vessels* drain into the superficial inguinal lymph nodes (Fig. 2.8C).

The arterial supply of the scrotum is from the (Fig. 2.8C):

- **Posterior scrotal branches of the perineal artery,** a branch of the internal pudendal artery.
- **Anterior scrotal branches of the deep external pudendal artery,** a branch of the femoral artery.
- **Cremasteric artery,** a branch of the inferior epigastric artery.

The nerves of the scrotum include the:

- **Genital branch of the genitofemoral nerve** (L1, L2) supplying the anterolateral surface.
- **Anterior scrotal nerves,** branches of the ilioinguinal nerve (L1) supplying the anterior surface.
- **Posterior scrotal nerves,** branches of the perineal branch of the **pudendal nerve** (S2–S4) supplying the posterior surface.
- **Perineal branches of the posterior femoral cutaneous nerve** (S2, S3) supplying the inferior surface.

TESTES

The ovoid testes are suspended in the scrotum by the spermatic cords (Figs. 2.7A and 2.8A). The testes produce sperms (spermatozoa) and hormones, principally testos-

Descent of Gonads

The **fetal testes** descend from the dorsal abdominal wall in the superior lumbar region to the deep inguinal rings during the 9th–12th fetal weeks (Fig. B2.3A–C). This movement probably results from growth of the vertebral column and pelvis. The male *gubernaculum,* attached to the caudal pole of the testis and accompanied by an outpouching of peritoneum, the *processus vaginalis,* projects into the scrotum. The testis descends posterior to the processus vaginalis. The inferior remnant of the processus vaginalis forms the *tunica vaginalis* covering the testis. The ductus deferens, testicular vessels, nerves, and lymphatics accompany the testis. The final descent of the testis usually occurs before or shortly after birth.

The **fetal ovaries** also descend from the dorsal abdominal wall in the superior lumbar region during the 12th week but pass into the lesser pelvis (Fig. B2.3D & E). The female gubernaculum also attaches to the caudal pole of the ovary and projects into the labia majora, attaching en route to the uterus; the part passing from the uterus to the ovary forms the *ovarian ligament,* and the remainder of it becomes the *round ligament of the uterus.* For a complete description of the embryology of the inguinal region, see Moore and Persaud (2003).

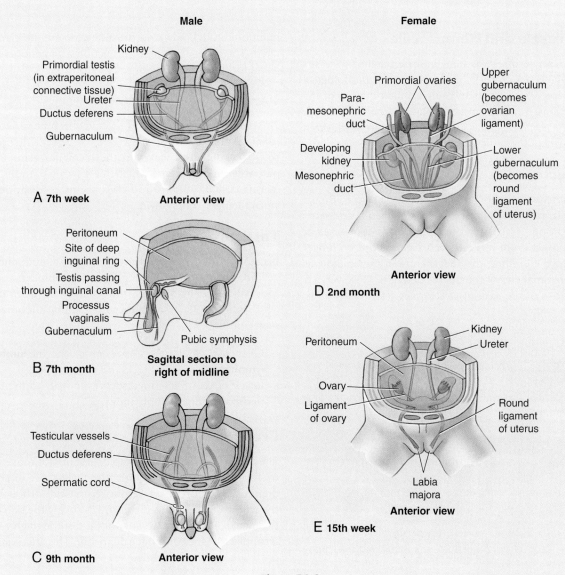

Figure B2.3.

terone. The sperms are formed in the **seminiferous tubules** that are joined by **straight tubules** to the **rete testis.** The testes have a tough outer surface, the **tunica albuginea,** that forms a ridge on its internal, posterior aspect as the **mediastinum of the testis.** The surface of each testis is covered by the visceral layer of the tunica vaginalis, except where the testis attaches to the epididymis and spermatic cord. The **tunica vaginalis** is a closed peritoneal sac surrounding the testis (Table 2.4).

The **visceral layer of the tunica vaginalis,** a glistening, transparent serous membrane, is closely applied to the testis, epididymis, and inferior part of the ductus deferens. The **parietal layer of the tunica vaginalis,** adjacent to the internal spermatic fascia, is more extensive than the visceral

layer and extends superiorly for a short distance into the distal part of the spermatic cord. The small amount of fluid in the cavity of the tunica vaginalis separates the visceral and parietal layers, allowing the testis to move freely within its side of the scrotum.

The **testicular arteries** arise from the abdominal aorta (vertebral level L2) just inferior to the renal arteries (Fig. 2.8C). The long, slender testicular arteries pass retroperitoneally (posterior to the peritoneum) in an oblique direction, crossing over the ureters and the inferior parts of the external iliac arteries. They traverse the inguinal canals, becoming part of the spermatic cords to supply the testes.

The **testicular veins** emerging from the testis and epididymis form the **pampiniform venous plexus,** consisting of

Hydrocele and Hematocele

The presence of excess fluid in a persistent processus vaginalis is a *hydrocele of the testis.* Certain pathological conditions—such as injury and/or inflammation of the epididymis—may also produce a *hydrocele of the spermatic cord.* A *hematocele of the testis* is a collection of blood in the cavity of the tunica vaginalis (Fig. B2.4).

Vasectomy

The *ductus deferens* is ligated bilaterally when sterilizing a man. To perform a vasectomy, also called a *deferentectomy,* the duct is isolated on each side and transected or a small section of it is removed. Sperms can no longer pass to the urethra; they degenerate in the epididymis and proximal end of the ductus deferens. However, the secretions of the *auxiliary genital glands* (seminal glands,

bulbourethral glands, and prostate) can still be ejaculated. The testis continues to function as an endocrine gland for the production of testosterone.

Varicocele

The pampiniform plexus of veins may become varicose (dilated) and tortuous. These varicose vessels often result from defective valves in the testicular vein. The palpable enlargement, which feels like a bundle of worms, usually drains and thus seems to disappear when the person lies down.

Testicular Cancer

Because the testes descend from the dorsal abdominal wall into the scrotum during fetal development, their lymphatic drainage differs from that of the scrotum, which is an outpouching of the anterolateral abdominal skin. Consequently,

* *Cancer of the testis* metastasizes initially to the **lumbar lymph nodes.**
* *Cancer of the scrotum* metastasizes initially to the **superficial inguinal lymph nodes.**

Cremasteric Reflex

The cremasteric reflex is the rapid elevation of the testis on the same side; this reflex is extremely active in children. Contraction of the cremaster muscle—producing the reflex—can be induced by lightly stroking the skin on the medial aspect of the superior part of the thigh with an applicator stick or tongue depressor. This area is supplied by the *ilioinguinal nerve.*

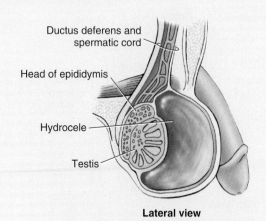

Lateral view

Figure B2.4.

Ductus deferens and spermatic cord
Head of epididymis
Hydrocele
Testis

8–12 anastomosing veins lying anterior to the ductus deferens and surrounding the testicular artery in the spermatic cord (Fig. 2.8A). The pampiniform plexus is part of the thermoregulatory system of the testis, helping to keep this gland at a constant temperature. The **left testicular vein** originates as the veins of the pampiniform plexus coalesce; it empties into the left renal vein. The **right testicular vein** has a similar origin and course but enters the inferior vena cava (IVC).

The *lymphatic drainage of the testis* follows the testicular artery and vein to the **right and left lumbar (caval/aortic)** and **preaortic lymph nodes** (Fig. 2.8C). The *autonomic nerves of the testis* arise as the **testicular plexus of nerves** on the testicular artery, which contains vagal parasympathetic and visceral afferent and sympathetic fibers from the T7 segment of the spinal cord.

EPIDIDYMIS

The epididymis is an elongated structure on the posterior surface of the testis formed by minute convolutions of the **duct of the epididymis**, so tightly compacted that they appear solid (Fig. 2.8A). The testis is covered by the tunica vaginalis, except at its posterior margin where the epididymis lies. The **efferent ductules** transport newly formed sperms from the rete testis to the epididymis, where they are stored until mature. The **rete testis** is a network of

canals at the termination of the seminiferous tubules. The epididymis consists of a:

- **Head:** the superior expanded part composed of lobules formed by the coiled ends of 12–14 efferent ductules.
- **Body:** the convoluted duct of the epididymis.
- **Tail:** continuous with the **ductus deferens**, the duct that transports sperms from the epididymis to the ejaculatory duct for expulsion into the prostatic urethra (see Chapter 3).

Peritoneum and Peritoneal Cavity

The **peritoneum** is a glistening, transparent serous membrane that consists of two continuous layers (Fig. 2.9):

- **Parietal peritoneum,** lining the internal surface of the abdominopelvic wall.
- **Visceral peritoneum,** investing viscera (organs) such as the spleen and stomach.

The peritoneum and viscera are in the abdominopelvic cavity. The relationship of the viscera to the peritoneum is as follows:

- **Intraperitoneal organs** are almost completely covered with visceral peritoneum (e.g., the spleen and stomach);

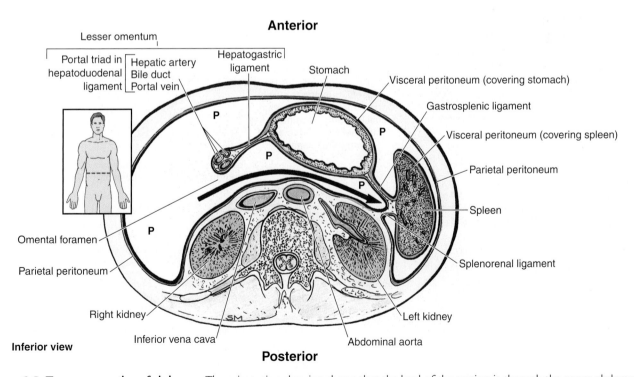

Figure 2.9. Transverse section of abdomen. The orientation drawing shows that the level of the section is through the upper abdomen. Observe the omental foramen and the horizontal extent of the omental bursa (lesser sac). *Arrow* passes from the greater sac through the omental foramen across the full extent of the omental bursa; *P*, peritoneal cavity.

Inguinal Hernias

An inguinal hernia is a protrusion of parietal peritoneum and viscera, such as the small intestine through a normal or abnormal opening from the abdominal cavity. There are two major categories of inguinal hernia: indirect and direct; more than two thirds are indirect hernias. An indirect inguinal hernia can occur in women; however, it is about 20 times more common in males of all ages (Table B2.1).

Table B2.1 Characteristics of Inguinal Hernias

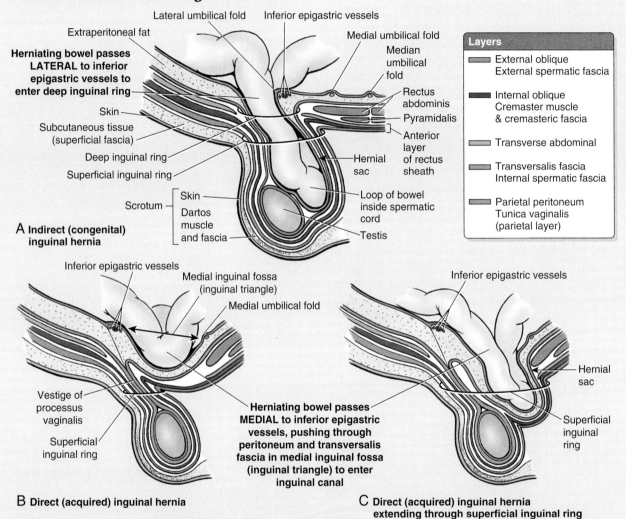

A Indirect (congenital) inguinal hernia

B Direct (acquired) inguinal hernia

C Direct (acquired) inguinal hernia extending through superficial inguinal ring

Characteristics[a]	Direct (Acquired)	Indirect (Congenital)
Predisposing factors	Weakness of anterior abdominal wall in inguinal triangle (e.g., owing to distended superficial ring, narrow inguinal falx, or attenuation of aponeurosis in males > 40 years of age)	Patency of processus vaginalis (complete or at least of superior part) in younger persons, the great majority of whom are males
Frequency	Less common (one third to one quarter of inguinal hernias)	More common (two thirds to three quarters of inguinal hernias)
Coverings at exit from abdominal cavity (A & B)	Peritoneum plus transversalis fascia (lies outside inner one or two fascial coverings of cord)	Peritoneum of persistent processus vaginalis plus all three fascial coverings of cord/round ligament
Course (C)	Usually traverses only medial third of inguinal canal, external and parallel to vestige of processus vaginalis	Traverses inguinal canal (entire canal if it is sufficient size) within processus vaginalis
Exit from anterior abdominal wall	Via superficial ring, lateral to cord; rarely enters scrotum	Via superficial ring inside cord, commonly passing into scrotum/labium majus

[a]Letters in parentheses refer to the figure parts.

Palpation of Superficial Inguinal Ring

The superficial inguinal ring is palpable superolateral to the pubic tubercle and by invaginating the skin of the upper scrotum with the index finger. The examiner's finger follows the spermatic cord superolaterally to the superficial inguinal ring. If the ring is dilated, it may admit the fingertip without causing pain. With the palmar surface of the finger against the anterior abdominal wall, the deep inguinal ring may be felt as a skin depression superior to the inguinal ligament, 2–4 cm superlolateral to the pubic tubercle. Detection of an impulse against the examining finger, when the person coughs, at the superficial ring and a mass at the site of the deep ring suggests an indirect hernia. Palpation of a direct inguinal hernia is performed by placing the index and/or middle finger over the inguinal triangle and asking the person to cough or strain. If a hernia is present, a forceful impulse is felt against the pad of the finger (Fig. B2.5).

Cysts and Hernias of the Canal of Nuck

If the processus vaginalis persists in females, it forms a small peritoneal pouch, the canal of Nuck, in the inguinal canal that may extend to the labium majus. In female infants, such remnants can enlarge and form cysts that have the potential to develop into an indirect inguinal hernia.

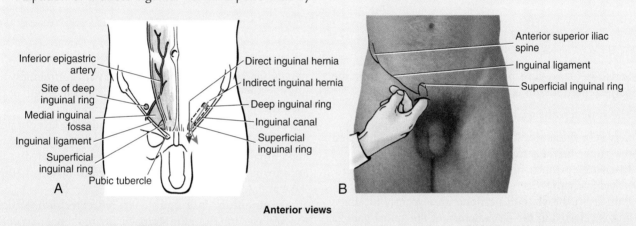

Anterior views

Figure B2.5. Detection of hernias. A. The location of inguinal hernias is shown. **B.** Palpation of the inguinal ring is demonstrated.

intraperitoneal organs have conceptually, if not literally, invaginated into a closed sac, like pressing your fist into an inflated balloon.

- **Extraperitoneal, retroperitoneal, and subperitoneal organs** are outside the peritoneal cavity—external or posterior to the parietal peritoneum—and are only partially covered with peritoneum (usually on one surface). Organs such as the kidneys are between the parietal peritoneum and the posterior abdominal wall and have parietal peritoneum only on their anterior surfaces, often with a considerable amount of intervening fatty tissue (Fig. 2.9).

The **peritoneal cavity** is within the abdominal cavity and continues into the pelvic cavity. It is a potential space of capillary thinness between the parietal and the visceral layers of peritoneum. The peritoneal cavity contains a thin layer of **peritoneal fluid** that keeps the peritoneal surfaces moist. *There are no organs in the peritoneal cavity.* Peritoneal fluid lubricates the peritoneal surfaces, enabling the viscera to move over each other without friction and allowing the movements of digestion. In addition, the fluid contains leukocytes and antibodies that resist infection. The peritoneal cavity is completely closed in males; however, there is a communication pathway in females to the exterior of the body through the uterine tubes, uterine cavity, and vagina (see Chapter 3). This communication constitutes a potential pathway of infection from the exterior.

Peritoneal Vessels and Nerves

The *parietal peritoneum is*

- Served by the same blood and lymphatic vasculature and the same *somatic nerve supply* as the region of the abdominopelvic wall it lines.

Peritonitis

When bacterial contamination occurs or when the gut is traumatically penetrated or ruptured as the result of infection and inflammation, gas, fecal matter, and bacteria enter the peritoneal cavity. The result is infection and inflammation of the peritoneum, called *peritonitis*.

Peritoneal Adhesions

If the peritoneum is damaged, for example, by a stab wound or infected, parts of the inflamed parietal and visceral layers of the peritoneum may adhere, forming an *adhesion* that interferes with the movement of the viscera. The surgical separation of adhesions is *adhesiotomy*.

Ascites and Paracentesis

Under certain pathological conditions such as *peritonitis*, the peritoneal cavity may be distended with abnormal fluid (*ascites*). Widespread *metastases* (spread) of cancer cells to the abdominal viscera cause exudation (escape) of fluid that is often blood stained. Thus the peritoneal cavity may be distended with several liters of abnormal fluid. Surgical puncture of the peritoneal cavity for the aspiration or drainage of fluid is called *paracentesis*.

- Sensitive to pressure, pain, heat, and cold; pain from the parietal peritoneum is generally well localized.

The *visceral peritoneum is*

- Served by the same blood and lymphatic vasculature and the same *visceral nerve supply* as the organs it covers.
- Insensitive to touch, heat, cold, and laceration and is stimulated primarily by stretching and chemical irritation.
- Pain from the visceral peritoneum is poorly localized and is referred to the dermatomes of the spinal ganglia providing the sensory fibers: Pain from the foregut derivatives is usually experienced in the epigastric region; that from the midgut derivatives, in the umbilical region; and that from the hindgut derivatives, in the pubic region.

Peritoneal Formations

Various terms are used to describe the parts of the peritoneum that connect organs with other organs or to the abdominal wall, and to describe the compartments and recesses that are formed as a consequence. The disposition of peritoneum in the adult is easier to understand when developmental changes are considered (for a description of the embryology of the peritoneal cavity and viscera, see Moore and Persaud, 2003, and Moore and Dalley, 2005).

A **mesentery** is a double layer of peritoneum that occurs as a result of the invagination of the peritoneum by an organ and constitutes a continuity of the visceral and parietal peritoneum (e.g., *mesentery of small intestine and transverse mesocolon*) (Figs. 2.10, 2.11*A*, and 2.12). Mesenteries provide a means for neurovascular communication between the organ and the body wall and thus have a core of connective tissue containing blood and lymphatic vessels, nerves, fat, and lymph nodes. Viscera with a mesentery are mobile; the degree of mobility depends on the length of the mesentery.

A **peritoneal ligament** consists of a double layer of peritoneum that connects an organ with another organ or to the abdominal wall. For example, the liver is connected to the anterior abdominal wall by the *falciform ligament* (Figs. 2.5*A* and 2.10*A*).

An **omentum** is a double-layered extension of peritoneum passing from the stomach and proximal part of the duodenum to adjacent organs. The **greater omentum** extends superiorly, latterally to the left, and inferiorly from the greater curvature of the stomach and the proximal part of the duodenum (Fig. 2.10). The greater omentum has three parts:

1. The **gastrophrenic ligament** between the greater curvature of the stomach and the diaphragm.
2. The **gastrosplenic ligament** between the greater curvature of the stomach and the spleen.
3. The **gastrocolic ligament** from the inferior portion of the greater curvature of the stomach. The gastrocolic ligament is the largest part, descending anteriorly and inferiorly beyond the transverse colon and then ascending again posteriorly, fusing with the visceral peritoneum of the transverse colon and the superior layer of its mesentery. The descending and ascending portions of the gastrocolic part of the greater omentum usually fuse together, forming a four-layered fatty "omental apron."

The **lesser omentum** (hepatogastric and hepatoduodenal ligaments) connects the lesser curvature of the stomach

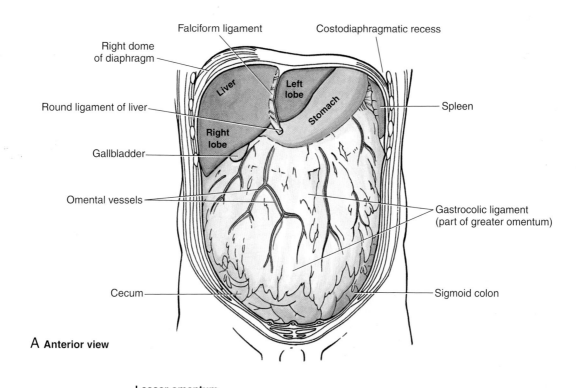

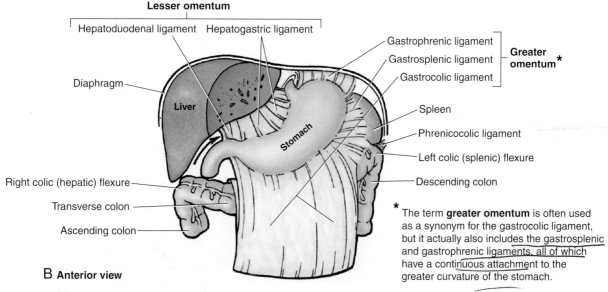

* The term **greater omentum** is often used as a synonym for the gastrocolic ligament, but it actually also includes the gastrosplenic and gastrophrenic ligaments, all of which have a continuous attachment to the greater curvature of the stomach.

Figure 2.10. Abdominal contents and peritoneum. A. The anterior thoracic and abdominal walls have been cut away to show the undisturbed contents. **B.** The stomach, lesser and greater omenta, and associated peritoneal ligaments are shown. *Arrow*, site of omental foramen.

and the proximal part of the duodenum to the liver (Fig. 2.10*B*). The hepatogastric and hepatoduodenal ligaments are continuous parts of the lesser omentum and are separated only for descriptive convenience. The stomach is connected to the liver by the **hepatogastric ligament**, the membranous portion of the lesser omentum. The **hepatoduodenal ligament**, the thickened free edge of the lesser omentum, conducts the *portal triad:* portal vein, hepatic artery, and bile duct.

Every organ must have an area that is not covered with visceral peritoneum to allow the entrance and exit of neurovascular structures. Such areas are called **bare areas** and are formed in relation to the attachments of mesenteries, omenta, and ligaments.

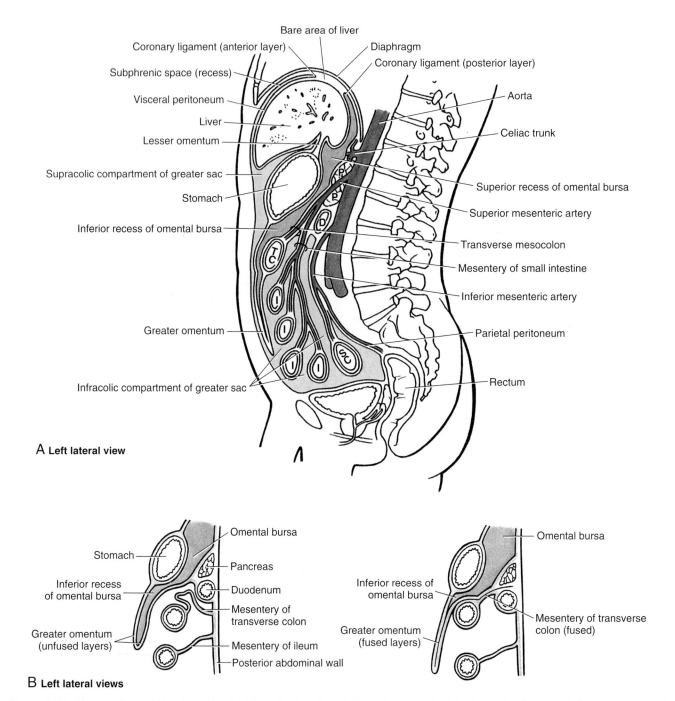

Figure 2.11. **Mesenteries and blood vessels. A.** This sagittal section of the abdomen and pelvis shows the viscera and the arrangement of the peritoneum. *D,* duodenum; *I,* jejunum and ileum; *P,* pancreas; *SC,* sigmoid colon; *TC,* transverse colon. **B.** These sagittal sections through the inferior recess of the omental bursa show the formation of the transverse mesocolon and fusion of the layers of the greater omentum in an infant (left) and an adult (right).

A **peritoneal fold** (e.g., *medial and lateral umbilical folds*) is a reflection of peritoneum that is raised from the body wall by underlying blood vessels, ducts, and obliterated fetal vessels (Fig. 2.5*A*).

A **peritoneal recess**, or fossa, is a pouch or concavity formed by a peritoneal fold (e.g., *inferior recess of the omental bursa* between the layers of the greater omentum (Fig.

2.5*A*) and the *supravesical* and *umbilical fossae* between the umbilical folds) (Fig. 2.11).

Subdivisions of Peritoneal Cavity

The peritoneal cavity is divided into a greater sac and an omental bursa (Figs. 2.11 and 2.12).

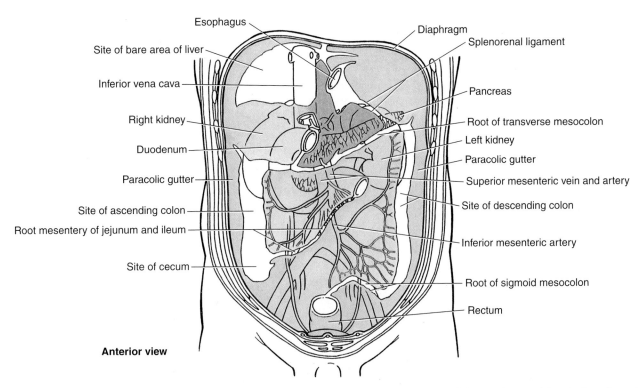

Figure 2.12. Posterior wall of peritoneal cavity. Observe the roots of the peritoneal reflection and the arteries supplying the large intestine. The transverse and sigmoid mesocolons and the mesentry of the jejunum and ileum have been cut at their roots.

- The **greater sac** is the main and larger part of the peritoneal cavity. A surgical incision through the anterolateral abdominal wall enters the greater sac.
- The **omental bursa** (lesser sac) is the smaller part of the peritoneal cavity that lies posterior to the stomach, lesser omentum, and adjacent structures. The omental bursa permits free movement of the stomach on adjacent structures because the anterior and posterior walls of the omental bursa slide smoothly over each other. The omental bursa has two recesses (Fig. 2.11A):
  - A **superior recess,** which is limited superiorly by the diaphragm and the posterior layers of the coronary ligament of the liver.
  - An **inferior recess** between the superior part of the layers of the greater omentum.

Most of the inferior recess of the omental bursa is a potential space sealed off from the main part of the omental bursa posterior to the stomach after adhesion of the anterior and posterior layers of the greater omentum (Fig. 2.11B). The omental bursa communicates with the greater sac through the **omental foramen** (epiploic foramen), an opening situated posterior to the free edge of the lesser omentum forming the hepatoduodenal ligament (Figs. 2.9 and 2.10B). The boundaries of the omental foramen are

- *Anteriorly*—the hepatoduodenal ligament (frce edge of lesser omentum) containing the portal vein, hepatic artery, and bile duct.

- *Posteriorly*—IVC and right crus of diaphragm, covered with parietal peritoneum (they are retroperitoneal).
- *Superiorly*—the liver, covered with visceral peritoneum.
- *Inferiorly*—superior or first part of the duodenum.

The **transverse mesocolon** (mesentery of transverse colon) divides the abdominal cavity into a (Fig. 2.11A):

- **Supracolic compartment,** containing the stomach, liver, and spleen.
- **Infracolic compartment,** containing the small intestine and ascending and descending colon. The infracolic compartment lies posterior to the greater omentum and is divided into *right* and *left infracolic spaces* by the mesentery of the small intestine.

Free communication occurs between the supracolic and the infracolic compartments through the **paracolic gutters,** the grooves between the lateral aspect of the ascending or descending colon and the posterolateral abdominal wall (Fig. 2.12).

Abdominal Viscera

The principal viscera of the abdomen are the esophagus (terminal part), stomach, intestines, spleen, pancreas, liver,

Functions of the Greater Omentum

The large, fat-laden greater omentum usually prevents the visceral peritoneum from adhering to the parietal peritoneum lining the anterolateral abdominal wall. The apron-like greater omentum has considerable mobility and moves around the peritoneal cavity with peristaltic movements of the viscera. It often forms adhesions adjacent to an inflamed organ (e.g., appendix) sometimes walling it off and thereby protecting other viscera from the infected organ.

Spread of Pathological Fluids

Peritoneal recesses are of clinical importance in connection with the spread of pathological fluids, such as pus, a product of inflammation. The recesses determine the extent and direction of the spread of fluids that may enter the peritoneal cavity when an organ is diseased or injured.

gallbladder, kidneys, and suprarenal glands. The esophagus, stomach, and intestine form the **alimentary (digestive) tract.** Food passes from the *mouth* and *pharynx* through the *esophagus* to the *stomach.* Digestion mostly occurs in the stomach and duodenum. **Peristalsis,** a series of ring-like contraction waves that begin around the middle of the stomach and move slowly toward the pylorus, is responsible for mixing of the masticated (chewed) food mass with gastric juices and for emptying the contents of the stomach into the duodenum.

Absorption of chemical compounds occurs principally in the *small intestine,* consisting of the *duodenum, jejunum,* and *ileum* (Fig. 2.13). The stomach is continuous with the duodenum, which receives the openings of the ducts from the *pancreas* and *liver* (major glands of digestive tract). Peristalsis also occurs in the jejunum and ileum, although it is not forceful unless an obstruction is present. The *large intestine* consists of the *cecum,* which receives the terminal part of the ileum, *appendix, colon* (*ascending, transverse, and descending*), *rectum,* and *anal canal* (which ends at the *anus*). Most reabsorption of water occurs in the ascending colon. Feces (stools) are formed in the descending and sigmoid colon and accumulate in the rectum before defecation.

The arterial supply to the abdominal part of the alimentary tract, spleen, pancreas, gallbladder, and liver is from the *abdominal aorta* (Fig. 2.14A). The three major branches of the abdominal aorta are the *celiac trunk* and the *superior* and *inferior mesenteric arteries.*

The *portal vein,* formed by the union of the superior mesenteric and splenic veins (Fig. 2.14B), is the main channel of the *portal venous system,* which collects blood from the abdominal part of the alimentary tract, pancreas, spleen, and most of the gallbladder and carries it to the liver.

Esophagus

The **esophagus** is a muscular tube, approximately 25 cm (10 in.) long with an average diameter of 2 cm, that extends from the pharynx to the stomach (Figs. 2.13 and 2.15). The esophagus:

- Follows the concavity of the vertebral column as it descends through the neck and mediastinum (see Chapter 1).
- Passes through the elliptical *esophageal hiatus* in the muscular right crus of the diaphragm, just to the left of the median plane at the level of the T10 vertebra (Fig. 2.40).
- Terminates at the **esophagogastric junction,** where ingested matter enters the cardial orifice of the stomach (Fig. 2.15B) is located to the left of the midline at the level of the 7th left costal cartilage and the T11 vertebra; the esophagus is retroperitoneal during its short abdominal course.
- Has circular and external longitudinal layers of muscle. In its superior third, the external layer consists of voluntary striated muscle, the inferior third is composed of smooth muscle, and the middle third is made up of both types of muscle.

The esophagogastric junction is marked internally by the abrupt transition from esophageal to gastric mucosa, referred to clinically as the **Z-line** (Fig. 2.15C). Just superior to this junction, the diaphragmatic musculature forming the esophageal hiatus functions as a physiological **inferior esophageal sphincter** that contracts and relaxes. Radiological studies show that food or liquid may be stopped here momentarily and that the sphincter mechanism is normally efficient in preventing reflux of gastric contents into the esophagus.

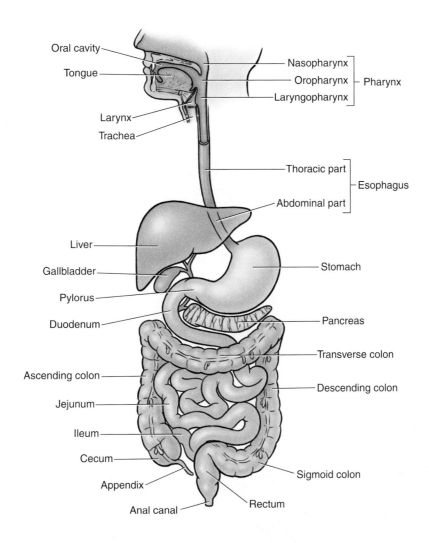

Anterior view; medial view of bisected head

Figure 2.13. Schematic overview of alimentary tract and abdominal viscera.

The abdominal part of the esophagus has its:

- *Arterial supply* from the **left gastric artery** (Fig. 2.14*A*), a branch of the *celiac trunk,* and the **left inferior phrenic artery** (see Chapter 1).
- *Venous drainage* primarily to the *portal venous system* through the **left gastric vein** (Fig. 2.14*B*), while the proximal thoracic part of the esophagus drains primarily into the *systemic venous system* through the **esophageal veins** entering the *azygos vein* (see Chapter 1). However, the veins of the two parts of the esophagus communicate and provide a clinically important portal–systemic anastomosis.
- *Lymphatic drainage* into the **left gastric lymph nodes,** which in turn drain mainly to the **celiac lymph nodes** (Fig. 2.16*C*).
- *Innervation* from the **vagal trunks** (becoming anterior and posterior gastric nerves), the **thoracic sympathetic trunks** via the **greater** (abdominopelvic) **splanchnic nerves,** and the **periarterial plexus** around the left gastric artery and left inferior phrenic artery (Fig. 2.14*A;* see Chapter 1).

Stomach

The **stomach** acts as a food blender and reservoir; its chief function is enzymatic digestion. The *gastric juice* gradually converts a mass of food into a semiliquid mixture, *chyme* (G. juice), which passes into the duodenum.

PARTS AND CURVATURE OF THE STOMACH

The shape of the stomach is dynamic (changing in shape as it functions) and highly variable from person to person. The stomach has four parts and two curvatures (Fig. 2.15):

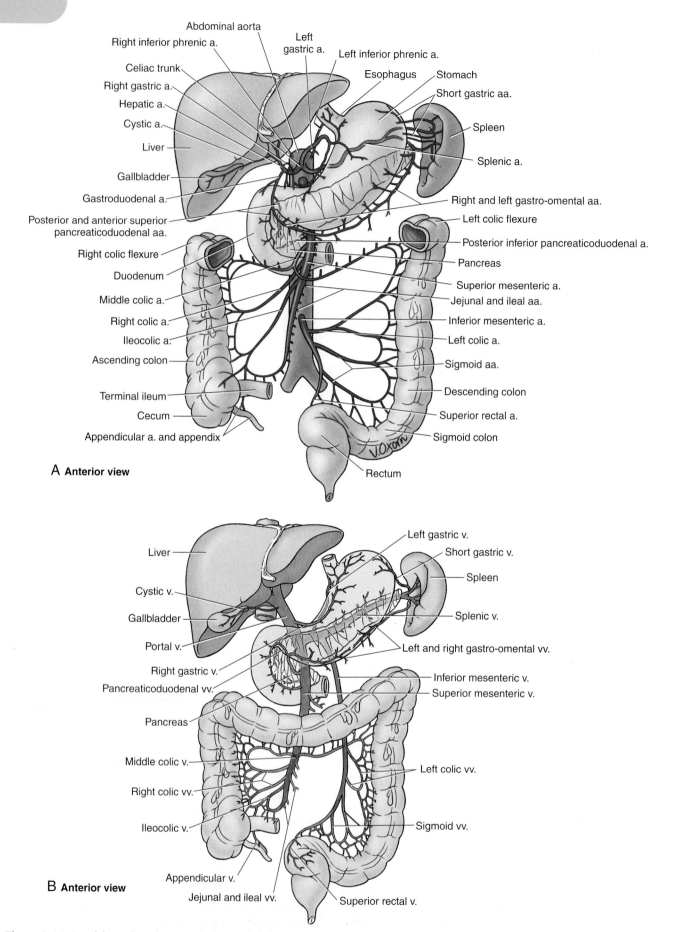

Figure 2.14. Arterial supply and venous drainage of abdominal part of alimentary tract. The arterial supply (**A**) and venous drainage (**B**) are shown. The portal vein drains poorly oxygenated, nutrient-rich blood from the stomach, intestines, spleen, pancreas, and gallbladder to the liver.

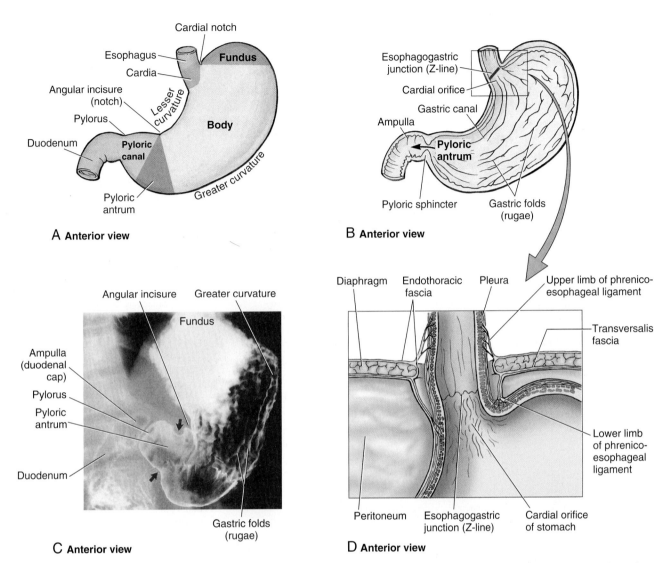

Figure 2.15. Esophagus (terminal part), stomach, and proximal duodenum. A. The areas of the external surface are identified. **B.** The anterior wall has been removed to show the internal surface (mucous membrane). *Arrow*, passes from pyloric antrum through the pyloric canal. **C.** Radiograph of the stomach and duodenum after barium ingestion. *Arrows*, peristaltic wave. **D.** Details of the gastroesophageal junction are shown.

- The **cardia** is the part surrounding the **cardial orifice**, the trumpet-shaped opening of the esophagus into the stomach.
- The **fundus** is the dilated superior part of the stomach that is related to the left dome of the diaphragm and is limited inferiorly by the horizontal plane of the cardial orifice. The superior part of the fundus usually reaches the level of the left 5th intercostal space. The **cardial notch** is between the esophagus and the fundus. The fundus may be dilated by gas, fluid, food, or any combination of these.
- The **body**, the major part of the stomach, lies between the fundus and the pyloric antrum.
- The **pyloric part** of the stomach is the funnel-shaped region; its wide part, the **pyloric antrum**, leads into the **pyloric canal**, its narrow part. The **pylorus**, the distal sphinc-

teric region, is a thickening of the circular layer of smooth muscle, which controls discharge of the stomach contents through the **pyloric orifice** into the duodenum.
- The **lesser curvature** forms the shorter concave border of the stomach; the **angular incisure** (notch) is the sharp indentation approximately two thirds of the distance along the lesser curvature that approximates the junction of the body and pyloric part of the stomach.
- The **greater curvature** forms the longer convex border of the stomach.

INTERIOR OF THE STOMACH

When contracted, the gastric mucosa is thrown into longitudinal **gastric folds**, or **gastric rugae** (Fig. 2.15 *B* & *C*). These

Table 2.5 Arterial Supply to Esophagus, Stomach, Duodenum, Liver, Gallbladder, Pancreas, and Spleen

Artery[a]	Origin	Course	Distribution
Celiac trunk	Abdominal aorta (T12) just distal to aortic hiatus of diaphragm	Soon divides into left gastric, splenic, and common hepatic arteries	Esophagus, stomach, duodenum (proximal to bile duct), liver and biliary apparatus, and pancreas
Left gastric	Celiac trunk	Ascends retroperitoneally to esophageal hiatus, giving rise to an esophageal branch, then runs along lesser curvature of stomach	Distal portion of esophagus and left portion of lesser curvature of stomach
Splenic		Runs retroperitoneally along superior border of pancreas, then passes between layers of splenorenal ligament to hilum of spleen	Body of pancreas, spleen, and greater curvature of stomach; posterior gastric branch supplies posterior wall and fundus of stomach
Left gastro-omental (gastroepiploic)	Splenic artery in hilum of spleen	Passes between layers of gastrosplenic ligament to greater curvature of stomach	Left portion of greater curvature of stomach
Short gastric (n = 4–5)		Pass between layers of gastrosplenic ligament to fundus of stomach	Fundus of stomach
Hepatic[b]	Celiac trunk	Passes retroperitoneally to reach hepatoduodenal ligament and passes between its layers to porta hepatis; divides into right and left hepatic arteries	Liver, gallbladder, stomach, pancreas, duodenum, and respective lobes of liver
Cystic	Right hepatic artery	Arises within hepatoduodenal ligament	Gallbladder and cystic duct
Right gastric	Hepatic artery	Runs along lesser curvature of stomach	Right portion of lesser curvature of stomach
Gastroduodenal		Descends retroperitoneally posterior to gastroduodenal junction	Stomach, pancreas, first part of duodenum, and distal part of bile duct
Right gastro-omental (gastroepiploic)	Gastroduodenal artery	Passes between layers of greater omentum to greater curvature of stomach	Right portion of greater curvature of stomach
Anterior and posterior superior pancreatico-duodenal		Descend on head of pancreas	Proximal portion of duodenum and head of pancreas
Anterior and posterior inferior pancreatico-duodenal	Superior mesenteric artery	Ascend on head of pancreas	Distal portion of duodenum and head of pancreas

[a]For anastomoses, see Figure 2.16.
[b]For descriptive purposes, the hepatic artery is often divided into the common hepatic artery from its origin to the origin of gastroduodenal artery, and the remainder of the vessel is called hepatic artery proper.

are most marked toward the pyloric part and along the greater curvature. A **gastric canal** (furrow) forms temporarily during swallowing between the longitudinal gastric folds along the lesser curvature. Saliva and small quantities of masticated food and other fluids pass through the gastric canal to the pyloric canal when the stomach is mostly empty.

RELATIONS OF THE STOMACH

The stomach is covered by peritoneum, except where blood vessels run along its curvatures and in a small area posterior to the cardial orifice. The two layers of the lesser omentum separate to extend around the stomach and come together again to leave its greater curvature as the greater omentum.

- *Anteriorly,* the stomach is related to the **diaphragm**, the left lobe of the liver, and the anterior abdominal wall (Fig. 2.10A).
- *Posteriorly,* the stomach is related to the **omental bursa** and **pancreas**; the posterior surface of the stomach forms most of the anterior wall of the omental bursa (Figs. 2.11 and 2.12).

The **stomach bed** on which the stomach rests when a person is in the supine position is formed by the structures forming the posterior wall of the omental bursa (Table 2.6). From superior to inferior, the stomach bed is formed by the left dome of the diaphragm, spleen, left kidney and suprarenal gland, splenic artery, pancreas, transverse mesocolon, and colon.

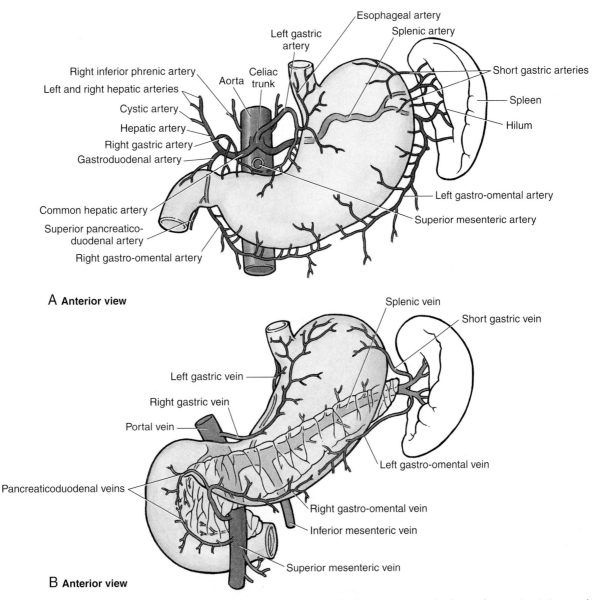

Figure 2.16. Blood vessels, lymphatics, and innervation of stomach, duodenum, pancreas, and spleen. The arteries (**A**); portal venous drainage (**B**) are shown

VASCULATURE AND NERVES OF THE STOMACH

The stomach has

- A rich *arterial supply,* arising from the celiac trunk and its branches (Fig. 2.16A; Table 2.5). Most of the blood is supplied by anastomoses formed along the lesser curvature by the **right** and **left gastric arteries** and, along the greater curvature, by the **right** and **left gastro-omental artery** (gastroepiploic artery). The fundus and upper body of stomach receive blood from the **short** and posterior gastric arteries branches of the splenic artery.
- Gastric *veins* parallel the arteries in position and course (Fig. 2.16B). The **left** and **right gastric veins** drain di-

rectly into the *portal vein.* The **short gastric veins** and the **left gastro-omental veins** drain into the *splenic vein,* which then joins the *superior mesenteric vein* (SMV) to form the portal vein. The **right gastro-omental vein** usually empties into the SMV.

- *Gastric lymphatic vessels* that accompany the arteries along the greater and lesser curvatures (Fig. 2.16C) and drain lymph from its anterior and posterior surfaces toward its curvatures, where the **gastric** and **gastro-omental lymph nodes** are located. The efferent vessels from these nodes via the **pancreaticosplenic**, **pyloric**, and **pancreaticoduodenal lymph nodes** accompany the large arteries to the *celiac lymph nodes.*

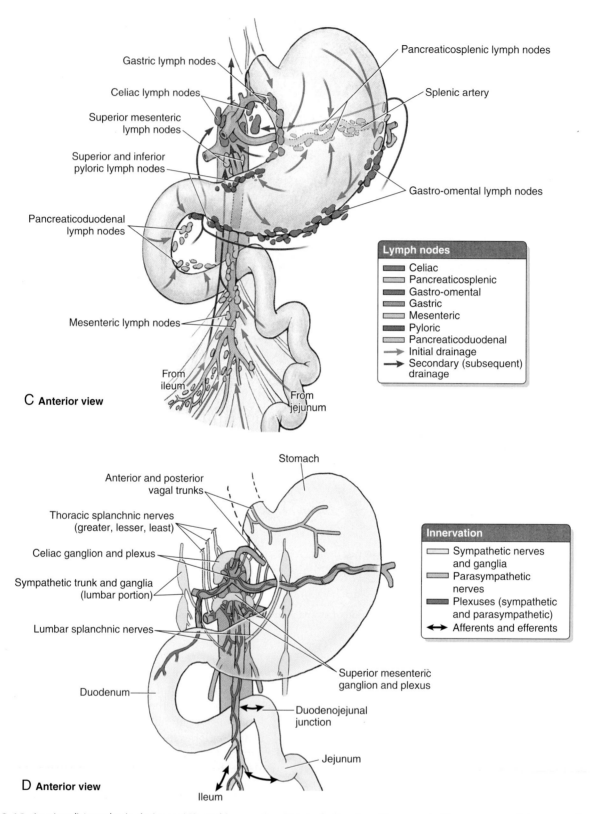

Gastric lymph nodes
Celiac lymph nodes
Superior mesenteric lymph nodes
Superior and inferior pyloric lymph nodes
Pancreaticoduodenal lymph nodes
Mesenteric lymph nodes
From ileum
From jejunum

Pancreaticosplenic lymph nodes
Splenic artery
Gastro-omental lymph nodes

C Anterior view

Lymph nodes
- Celiac
- Pancreaticosplenic
- Gastro-omental
- Gastric
- Mesenteric
- Pyloric
- Pancreaticoduodenal
- → Initial drainage
- → Secondary (subsequent) drainage

Anterior and posterior vagal trunks
Thoracic splanchnic nerves (greater, lesser, least)
Celiac ganglion and plexus
Sympathetic trunk and ganglia (lumbar portion)
Lumbar splanchnic nerves
Duodenum

Stomach
Superior mesenteric ganglion and plexus
Duodenojejunal junction
Jejunum
Ileum

D Anterior view

Innervation
- Sympathetic nerves and ganglia
- Parasympathetic nerves
- Plexuses (sympathetic and parasympathetic)
- ↔ Afferents and efferents

Figure 2.16. *(continued)* Lymphatic drainage (**C**); and innervation (**D**), including the afferent and efferent nerves of the sympathetic and parasympathetic nervous systems, are shown.

Surface Anatomy of Stomach

The *surface markings of the stomach vary* because its size and position change under various circumstances (e.g., after a heavy meal). The surface markings in the supine position include the (Fig. SA2.2):

- **Cardial orifice**, usually lies posterior to the 6th left costal cartilage, 2–4 cm from the median plane at the level of the T10 or T11 vertebra.
- **Fundus**, usually lies posterior to the *5th left rib* in the midclavicular plane.
- **Greater curvature**, passes inferiorly to the left as far as the *10th left costal cartilage* before turning medially to reach the pyloric antrum.

- **Lesser curvature**, passes from the right side of the cardia to the pyloric antrum; the most inferior part of the curvature is marked by the **angular incisure** (Fig. 2.15A), which lies just to the left of the midline.
- **Pyloric part of the stomach**, usually lies at the level of the 9th costal cartilage at the level of the L1 vertebra; the pyloric orifice is approximately 1.25 cm left of the midline.
- **Pylorus**, usually lies on the right side; its location varies from the L2 to the L4 vertebra. ●

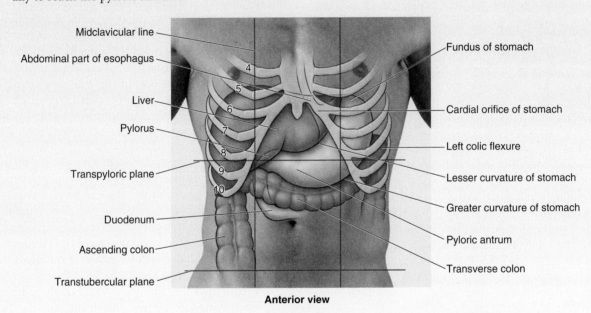

Anterior view

Figure SA2.2.

Carcinoma of Stomach and Gastrectomy

When the body or pyloric part of the stomach contains a malignant tumor, the mass may be palpable. Using *gastroscopy*, physicians can inspect the lining of the air-inflated stomach, enabling them to observe gastric lesions and take biopsies. **Partial gastrectomy** (removal of part of the stomach) may be performed to remove the region of the stomach involved by carcinoma. Because of the anastomoses of the arteries supplying the stomach provide good collateral circulation, one or more arteries may be ligated during this procedure without seriously affecting the blood supply of the remaining part of the stomach. The extensive lymphatic drainage of the stomach and the impossibility of removing all the lymph nodes create a surgical problem. Removal of the aortic and celiac nodes and those around the head of the pancreas is difficult.

- Parasympathetic and sympathetic *innervation.* The **parasympathetic nerve supply** is from the **anterior vagal trunk** (mainly from the left vagus nerve) and **posterior vagal trunk** (mainly from the right vagus nerve) and their branches, which enter the abdomen through the esophageal hiatus (Fig. 2.16D). The **sympathetic nerve supply is** from the T6–T9 segments of the spinal cord, which passes to the **celiac plexus** via the greater splanchnic nerves and is distributed as plexuses around the gastric and gastro-omental arteries.

Small Intestine

The **small intestine**, consisting of the duodenum, jejunum, and ileum, extends from the pylorus of the stomach to the ileocecal junction, where the ileum joins the cecum, the first part of the large intestine (Fig. 2.13).

DUODENUM

The duodenum, the first and shortest (25 cm) part of the small intestine, is also the widest and most fixed part. The duodenum begins at the pylorus on the right side and ends at the **duodenojejunal junction** on the left side. Four parts of the duodenum are described (Table 2.6):

- **Superior (1st) part:** short (approximately 5 cm), mostly horizontal, and lies anterolateral to the body of L1 vertebra.
- **Descending (2nd) part:** longer (7–10 cm) and runs inferiorly along the right sides of the L2 and L3 vertebrae, curving around the head of the pancreas; initially it lies to the right and parallel to the IVC. The *bile duct* and *main pancreatic ducts* via the hepatopancreatic ampulla enter its posteromedial wall (Table 2.6).
- **Horizontal (3rd) part:** 6–8 cm long and crosses anterior to the IVC and aorta and posterior to the superior mesenteric artery (SMA) and SMV at the level of the L3 vertebra.
- **Ascending (4th) part:** short (approximately 5 cm) and begins at the left of the L3 vertebra and rises superiorly as far

as the superior border of the L2 vertebra, 2–3 cm to the left of the midline. It passes on the left side of the aorta to reach the inferior border of the body of the pancreas. Here it curves anteriorly to join the jejunum at the **duodenojejunal junction**, which takes the form of an acute angle—the **duodenojejunal flexure** (Fig. 2.13)—which is supported by the attachment of the **suspensory muscle of the duodenum** (ligament of Treitz).

The suspensory muscle of the duodenum is commonly composed of a slip of skeletal muscle from the diaphragm and a fibromuscular band of smooth muscle from the 3rd and 4th parts of the duodenum. Contraction of this suspensory muscle widens the angle of the duodenojejunal flexure, facilitating movement of the intestinal contents. The suspensory muscle passes posterior to the pancreas and splenic vein and anterior to the left renal vein.

The first 2 cm of the superior part of the duodenum has a mesentery and is mobile. This free part—relatively dilated and smooth walled—is called the **ampulla** or duodenal cap (Fig. 2.15B & C). The distal 3 cm of the superior part and the other three parts of the duodenum have no mesentery and are immobile because they are retroperitoneal (Fig. 2.12). The principal relations of the duodenum are outlined in Table 2.6.

The duodenum has

- *Arterial supply* from two different vessels. An important transition in the blood supply of the alimentary tract occurs over the course of the descending (2nd) part of the duodenum, approximately where the bile duct enters. The basis of this transition is embryological because this is the site of the junction of the foregut and midgut. Consequently, the **duodenal arteries** arise from two different sources: (Figs. 2.16A and 2.23A)
  - Proximally, the abdominal part of the alimentary tract is supplied by the **celiac trunk**, and the 1st and 2nd parts of the duodenum are supplied via the **gastroduodenal artery** and its branch, the **superior pancreaticoduodenal artery.**

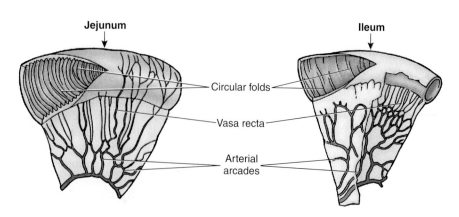

Figure 2.17. Characteristics of jejunum and ileum.

Table 2.6 Relationships of Duodenum, Spleen, and Pancreas

151

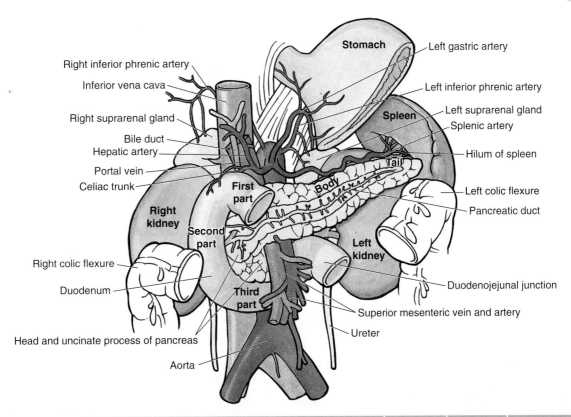

Organ	Anterior	Posterior	Medial	Superior	Inferior	Level
Superior (1st) part of duodenum	Peritoneum Gallbladder Quadrate lobe of liver	Bile duct Gastroduodenal artery Portal vein IVC		Neck of gallbladder	Neck of pancreas	Anterolateral to L1 vertebra
Descending (2nd) part of duodenum	Transverse colon Transverse mesocolon Coils of small intestine	Hilum of right kidney Renal vessels Ureter Psoas major	Head of pancreas Pancreatic duct Bile duct			Right of L2–L3 vertebrae
Horizontal (3rd) part of duodenum	SMA SMV Coils of small intestine	Right psoas major IVC Aorta Right ureter		Head and uncinate process of pancreas SMV SMA		Anterior to L3 vertebra
Ascending (4th) part of duodenum	Beginning of root of mesentery Coils of jejunum	Left psoas major Left margin of aorta	Head of pancreas	Body of pancreas		Left of L3 vertebra
Spleen	Stomach	Left part of diaphragm	Left kidney		Left colic flexure	Left upper quadrant between 9th and 11th ribs
Head of pancreas		IVC Right renal artery and vein				
Neck of pancreas	Pylorus of stomach	SMA SMV				
Body of pancreas	Omental bursa	Aorta SMA Left suprarenal gland Left kidney and renal vessels				L2 vertebra
Tail of pancreas		Left kidney				

IVC, inferior vena cava; *SMA*, superior mesenteric artery; *SMV*, superior mesenteric vein.

Duodenal (Peptic) Ulcers

Most inflammatory erosions of the duodenal wall, *duodenal ulcers,* are in the posterior wall of the superior part of the duodenum within 3 cm of the pylorus. Occasionally, an ulcer perforates the duodenal wall, permitting its contents to enter the peritoneal cavity and produce *peritonitis.* Because the superior part of the duodenum closely relates to the liver and gallbladder, either of them may adhere to and be ulcerated by a duodenal ulcer. *Erosion of the gastroduodenal artery,* a posterior relation of the superior part of the duodenum, by a duodenal ulcer results in severe hemorrhage into the peritoneal cavity.

Table 2.7 Distinguishing Characteristics of Jejunum and Ileum in Living Persons

Characteristic	Jejunum	Ileum
Color	Deeper red	Paler pink
Caliber	2–4 cm	2–3 cm
Wall	Thick and heavy	Thin and light
Vascularity	Greater	Less
Vasa recta	Long	Short
Arcades	A few large loops	Many short loops
Fat in mesentery	Less	More
Circular folds (L. *plicae circulares*)	Large, tall, and closely packed	Low and sparse; absent in distal part
Lymphoid nodules (Peyer patches)	Few	Many

- Distally, a major part of the alimentary canal (extending as far as the left colic flexure) is supplied by the **superior mesenteric artery (SMA)**, and the 3rd and 4th parts of the duodenum are supplied by its branch, the **inferior pancreaticoduodenal artery**. The superior and inferior pancreaticoduodenal arteries form an anastomotic loop between the celiac trunk and the SMA; consequently, there is potential for collateral circulation here.
- *Duodenal veins,* follow the arteries and drain into the **portal vein** (Fig. 2.16*B*); some veins drain directly and others indirectly through the superior mesenteric and splenic veins.
- *Lymphatic vessels,* follow the arteries in a retrograde direction. The *anterior lymphatic vessels* drain into the **pancreaticoduodenal lymph nodes** located along the superior and inferior pancreaticoduodenal arteries, and into the **pyloric lymph nodes**, which lie along the gastroduodenal artery (Fig. 2.16*C*). The *posterior lymphatic vessels* pass posterior to the head of the pancreas and drain into the **superior mesenteric lymph nodes**. Efferent lymphatic vessels from the duodenal lymph nodes drain into the **celiac lymph nodes.**
- *Parasympathetic innervation* from the **vagus** and *sympathetic innervation* from the **greater** and **lesser splanchnic nerves** by way of the **celiac** and **superior mesenteric plexuses** and then via periarterial plexuses extending to the pancreaticoduodenal arteries (Fig. 2.16*D*).

JEJUNUM AND ILEUM

The jejunum begins at the **duodenojejunal junction** and the ileum ends at the **ileocecal junction**, the union of the terminal ileum and cecum (Fig 2.13). Together, the jejunum and ileum are 6–7 m long in cadavers; however, tonic contraction makes them substantially shorter in living persons. The jejunum constitutes approximately two fifths of the length, and the ileum the remainder. The terminal ileum usually lies in the pelvis from which it ascends to end in the medial aspect of the cecum. Although no clear line of demarcation between the jejunum and ileum exists, they have distinctive characteristics for most of their lengths (Table 2.7).

The **mesentery**, a fan-shaped fold of peritoneum, attaches the jejunum and ileum to the posterior abdominal wall. The **root (origin) of the mesentery** (approximately 15 cm long) is directed obliquely, inferiorly, and to the right (Fig. 2.18). It extends from the duodenojejunal junction on the left side of the L2 vertebra to the ileocolic junction and the right sacroiliac joint. The root of the mesentery crosses (successively) the ascending and horizontal parts of duodenum, abdominal aorta, inferior vena cava, right ureter, right psoas major muscle, and right testicular or ovarian vessels.

The jejunum and ileum have:

- *Arterial supply* from the SMA (Fig. 2.19*A;* Table 2.8). The **SMA** runs between the layers of the mesentery and sends many branches to the jejunum and ileum. The arteries unite to form loops or arches—**arterial arcades**—that give rise to straight arteries—the **vasa recta** (Fig. 2.17).
- *Venous drainage* from the SMV (Fig. 2.16*B*). The **SMV** lies anterior and to the right of the SMA in the root of the mesentery. The SMV ends posterior to the neck of the pancreas, where it unites with the splenic vein to form the portal vein.
- Specialized *lymphatic vessels,* called **lacteals**, in the intestinal villi that absorb fat and drain into the lymphatic plexuses in the walls of the jejunum and ileum. The lymphatic plexuses drain into lymphatic vessels between the layers of the mesentery and then sequentially through

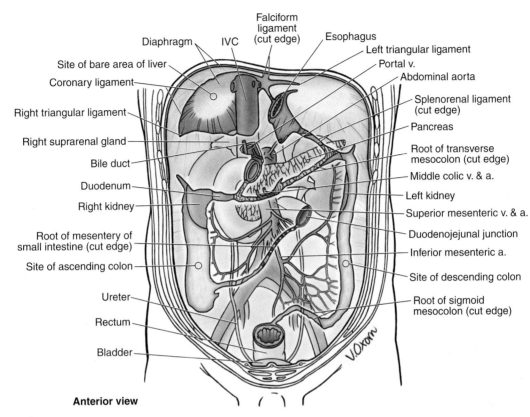

Diaphragm
Falciform ligament (cut edge)
IVC
Esophagus
Site of bare area of liver
Left triangular ligament
Coronary ligament
Portal v.
Right triangular ligament
Abdominal aorta
Right suprarenal gland
Splenorenal ligament (cut edge)
Bile duct
Pancreas
Duodenum
Root of transverse mesocolon (cut edge)
Right kidney
Middle colic v. & a.
Root of mesentery of small intestine (cut edge)
Left kidney
Site of ascending colon
Superior mesenteric v. & a.
Ureter
Duodenojejunal junction
Rectum
Inferior mesenteric a.
Bladder
Site of descending colon
Root of sigmoid mesocolon (cut edge)

Anterior view

Figure 2.18. Posterior wall of peritoneal cavity. The arteries supplying the large intestine are shown. The transverse and sigmoid mesocolons and the mesentry of the jejunum and ileum have been cut at their roots. *IVC*, inferior vena cava.

Table 2.8 Arterial Supply to Intestines

Artery	Origin	Course	Distribution
Superior mesenteric	Abdominal aorta (L1)	Runs in root of mesentery to ileocecal junction	Part of gastrointestinal tract derived from midgut
Intestinal (*n* = 15–18)		Passes between two layers of mesentery	Jejunum and ileum
Middle colic	Superior mesenteric artery	Ascends retroperitoneally and passes between layers of transverse mesocolon	Transverse colon
Right colic		Passes retroperitoneally to reach ascending colon	Ascending colon
Ileocolic	Terminal branch of superior mesenteric artery	Runs along root of mesentery and divides into ileal and colic branches	Ileum, cecum, and ascending colon
Appendicular	Ileocolic artery	Passes between layers of mesoappendix	Appendix
Inferior mesenteric	Abdominal aorta (L3)	Descends retroperitoneally to left of abdominal aorta	Descending colon
Left colic		Passes retroperitoneally toward left to descending colon	
Sigmoid (*n* = 3–4)	Inferior mesenteric artery	Passes retroperitoneally toward left to descending colon	Descending and sigmoid colon
Superior rectal	Terminal branch of inferior mesenteric artery	Descends retroperitoneally to rectum	Proximal part of rectum
Middle rectal	Internal iliac artery	Passes retroperitoneally to rectum	Midpart of rectum
Inferior rectal	Internal pudendal artery	Crosses ischioanal fossa to reach rectum	Distal part of rectum and anal canal

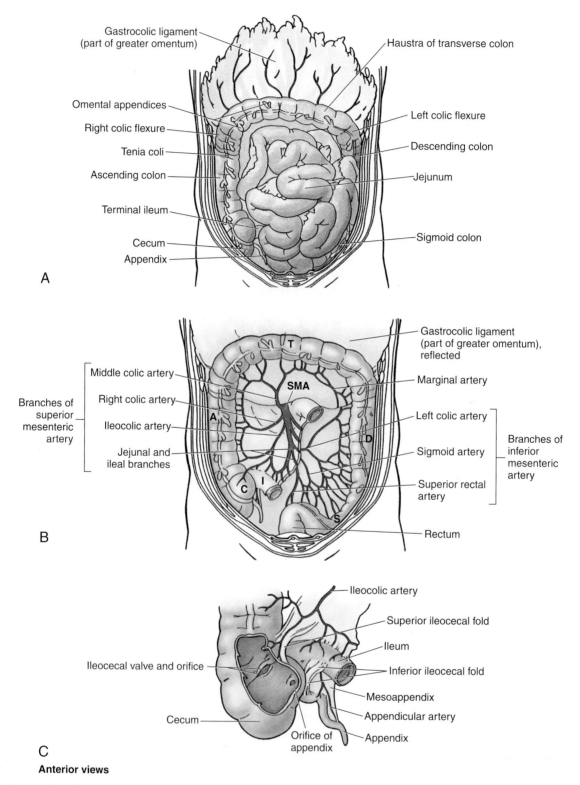

Anterior views

Figure 2.19. Small and large intestine, arteries, and mesenteries. A. The greater omentum has been pulled superiorly to show the intestine. **B.** Most of the small intestine has been removed to show the blood supply of the large intestine. *A*, ascending colon; *C*, cecum; *D*, descending colon; *I*, terminal ileum; *S*, sigmoid colon; *SMA*, superior mesenteric artery; *T*, transverse colon. **C.** The blood supply of the cecum and appendix are shown. A window has been cut in the wall of the cecum to expose the ileocecal orifice and the orifice of the appendix.

three groups of lymph nodes (Fig. 2.16C): **juxta-intestinal lymph nodes** (close to the intestinal wall), **mesenteric lymph nodes** (scattered among the arterial arcades), and **superior central nodes** (along the proximal part of the SMA). Efferent lymphatic vessels from these nodes drain into the **superior mesenteric lymph nodes.** Lymphatic vessels from the terminal ileum follow the ileal branch of the ileocolic artery to the **ileocolic lymph nodes.**

- *Sympathetic and parasympathetic innervation.*
  - In general, sympathetic stimulation reduces motility of the intestine, and secretion and acts as a vasoconstrictor, reducing or stopping digestion and making blood (and energy) available for "fleeing or fighting." Parasympathetic stimulation increases motility of the intestine and secretion, restoring digestive activity after a sympathetic reaction. The SMA and its branches are surrounded by a dense **perivascular nerve plexus** through which the nerve fibers are conducted to the parts of the intestine supplied by the SMA. The **sympathetic fibers** originate in the T8–T10 segments of the spinal cord and reach the **superior mesenteric nerve plexus** through the *sympathetic trunks* and *thoracic abdominopelvic (greater, lesser and least) splanchnic nerves* (Figs. 2.16D and 2.20). The presynaptic sympathetic fibers synapse on cell bodies of postsynaptic sympathetic neurons in the *celiac and superior mesenteric (prevertebral) ganglia.*
  - The **parasympathetic fibers** derive from the **posterior vagal trunk.** The presynaptic parasympathetic fibers synapse with postsynaptic parasympathetic neurons in

the *myenteric and submucous plexuses* in the intestinal wall. The small intestine also has *sensory (visceral afferent) fibers.* The intestine is insensitive to most pain stimuli, including cutting and burning; however, it is sensitive to sudden distention ("gas pains") and transient ischemia from abnormally long contractions that are perceived as **colic** (spasmodic abdominal pains).

Large Intestine

The **large intestine** consists of the *cecum, colon (ascending, transverse, descending,* and *sigmoid), rectum,* and *anal canal* (Fig. 2.19A–C). The large intestine can be distinguished from the small intestine by:

- **Teniae coli:** three thickened bands of longitudinal muscle fibers.
- **Haustra:** sacculations or pouches of the colon between the teniae.
- **Omental appendices:** small, fatty appendices (projections) of colon.
- **Caliber:** the internal diameter is much larger.

The three teniae coli make up most of the longitudinal muscle of the large intestine, except in the rectum. Because the teniae are shorter than the large intestine, the colon has the typical sacculated shape formed by the haustra. The teniae begin at the base of the appendix and run the length of the large intestine, merging at the rectosigmoid junction into a continuous layer around the rectum.

CECUM AND APPENDIX

The **cecum,** the first part of the large intestine that is continuous with the ascending colon, is a blind intestinal pouch in the right lower quadrant where it lies in the iliac fossa inferior to the junction of the terminal ileum and cecum. The cecum is usually almost entirely enveloped by peritoneum and can be lifted freely; however, *the cecum has no mesentery* (Fig. 2.12). The ileum enters the cecum obliquely and partly invaginates into it, forming folds superior and inferior to the **ileal orifice** (Fig. 2.19B). These folds form the **ileocecal valve.**

The vermiform (L. worm-like) **appendix,** a blind intestinal diverticulum, extends from the posteromedial aspect of the cecum inferior to the ileocecal junction. The appendix varies in length and has a short triangular mesentery, the **mesoappendix,** which derives from the posterior side of the mesentery of the terminal ileum. The mesoappendix attaches to the cecum and the proximal part of the appendix. The position of the appendix is variable, but it is usually retrocecal (posterior to cecum). The base of the appendix most often lies deep to a point that is one third of the way along the oblique line joining the right anterior superior iliac spine to the umbilicus (*spinoumbilical* or *McBurney point*).

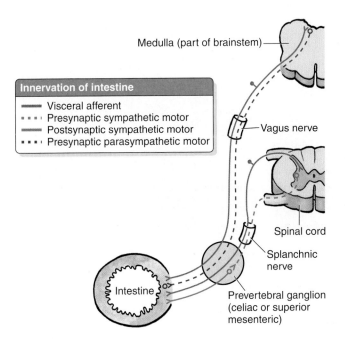

Medulla (part of brainstem)

Innervation of intestine
— Visceral afferent
- - - Presynaptic sympathetic motor
— Postsynaptic sympathetic motor
- - - Presynaptic parasympathetic motor

Vagus nerve

Spinal cord

Splanchnic nerve

Intestine

Prevertebral ganglion (celiac or superior mesenteric)

Figure 2.20. Innervation of intestine.

Overview of Embryological Rotation of the Midgut

The primordial gut consists of the *foregut* (esophagus, stomach, pancreas, duodenum, liver, and biliary ducts), *midgut* (small intestine distal to the bile duct, cecum, appendix, ascending colon, and most of the transverse colon) and *hindgut* (distal transverse colon, descending and sigmoid colon and rectum). For 4 weeks, the rapidly growing midgut, supplied by the SMA, is herniated into

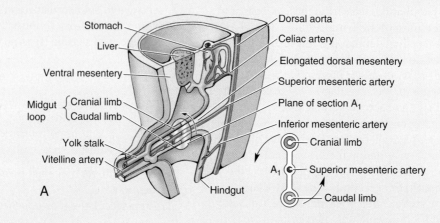

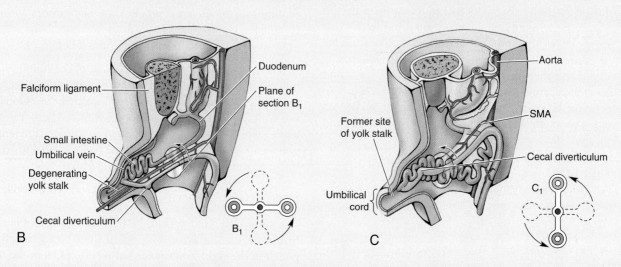

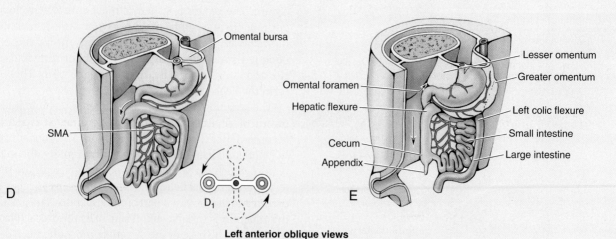

Left anterior oblique views

Figure B2.6.

the proximal part of the umbilical cord (Fig. B2.6A). It is attached to the yolk sac by the yolk stalk. As it returns to the abdominal cavity, the midgut rotates 270° around the axis of the SMA (Fig. B2.6B & C). As the parts of the intestine reach their definitive positions, their mesenteric attachments undergo modifications. Some mesenteries shorten and others disappear (Fig. B2.6D & E). Malrotation of the midgut results in several congenital anomalies, such as volvulus (twisting) of the intestine.

Ileal Diverticulum

An *ileal diverticulum* (of Meckel) is a congenital anomaly that occurs in 1–2% of people. A remnant of the proximal part of the embryonic yolk stalk, the diverticulum usually appears as a finger-like pouch (3–6 cm long). It is always on the antimesenteric border of the ileum—the border of the intestine opposite the mesenteric attachment. An ileal diverticulum may become inflamed and produce pain mimicking the pain produced by appendicitis.

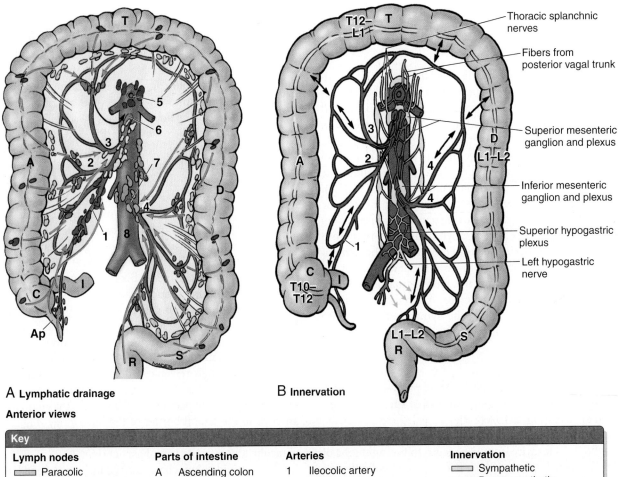

A **Lymphatic drainage**

B **Innervation**

Anterior views

Key							
Lymph nodes		**Parts of intestine**		**Arteries**		**Innervation**	
▭	Paracolic	A	Ascending colon	1	Ileocolic artery	▭	Sympathetic
▭	Superior mesenteric	Ap	Appendix	2	Right colic artery	▭	Parasympathetic
▭	Inferior mesenteric	C	Cecum	3	Middle colic artery	▬	Plexuses (sympathetic
▬	Intermediate colic	D	Descending colon	4	Left colic artery		and parasympathetic)
▬	Ileocolic	I	Terminal ileum	5	Celiac trunk	◄►	Afferents and efferents
▬	Lateral aortic	R	Rectum	6	Superior mesenteric artery	→	Pelvic splanchnic (S2–S4)
▬	Epicolic	S	Sigmoid colon	7	Inferior mesenteric artery		
▬	Appendicular	T	Transverse colon	8	Aorta		
▬	Celiac						
→	Direction of flow of lymph						

Figure 2.21. Lymphatic drainage and innervation of large intestine.

Appendicitis

Acute inflammation of the appendix is a common cause of an *acute abdomen* (severe abdominal pain arising suddenly). Digital pressure over the McBurney point registers the maximum abdominal tenderness. The pain of appendicitis usually commences as a vague pain in the periumbilical region because afferent pain fibers enter the spinal cord at the T10 level. Later, severe pain in the right lower quadrant results from irritation of the parietal peritoneum lining the posterior abdominal wall.

The cecum is supplied by the **ileocolic artery**, the terminal branch of the SMA. The appendix is supplied by the **appendicular artery**, a *branch* of the ileocolic artery (Fig. 2.19*B* & *C;* Table 2.8). A tributary of the SMV, the **ileocolic vein**, drains blood from the cecum and appendix (Fig. 2.14). The **lymphatic vessels** from the cecum and appendix pass to lymph nodes in the mesoappendix and to the **ileocolic lymph nodes** that lie along the ileocolic artery (Fig. 2.21*A*). Efferent lymphatic vessels pass to the **superior mesenteric lymph nodes**. The *nerve supply to the cecum and appendix* derives from sympathetic and parasympathetic nerves from the **superior mesenteric plexus** (Fig. 2.21*B*). The **sympathetic nerve fibers** originate in the lower thoracic part of the spinal cord (T10–T12), and the **parasympathetic nerve fibers** derive from the **vagus nerves**. Afferent nerve fibers from the appendix accompany the sympathetic nerves to the T10 segment of the spinal cord.

COLON

The colon is described as having four parts—ascending, transverse, descending, and sigmoid—that succeed one another in an arch (Fig. 2.19*A* & *B*).

The **ascending colon** passes superiorly on the right side of the abdominal cavity from the cecum to the right lobe of the liver, where it turns to the left as the **right colic flexure** (hepatic flexure). The ascending colon, narrower than the cecum, lies retroperitoneally along the right side of the posterior abdominal wall. The ascending colon is covered by peritoneum anteriorly and on its sides; however, in approximately 25% of people it has a short mesentery. The ascending colon is separated from the anterolateral abdominal wall by the greater omentum. The ascending colon has a vertical groove lined with parietal peritoneum (the **right paracolic gutter**) on its lateral aspect (Fig. 2.12). The *arterial*

supply to the ascending colon and right colic flexure is from branches of the SMA—the **ileocolic** and **right colic arteries** (Fig. 2.19*B;* Table 2.8). Tributaries of the SMV, the **ileocolic** and **right colic veins**, drain blood from the ascending colon. The **lymphatic vessels** first pass to the **epicolic and paracolic lymph nodes**, next to the **ileocolic** and intermediate **right colic lymph nodes**, and from them to the **superior mesenteric nodes** (Fig. 2.21*A*). The **nerves to the ascending colon** derive from the **superior mesenteric plexus** (Fig. 2.21*B*).

The **transverse colon**, the largest and most mobile part of the large intestine, crosses the abdomen from the right colic flexure to the left colic flexure, where it bends inferiorly to become the descending colon (Fig. 2.19*A*). The **left colic flexure** (splenic flexure)—usually more superior, more acute, and less mobile than the right colic flexure—lies anterior to the inferior part of the left kidney and attaches to the diaphragm through the **phrenicocolic ligament** (Fig. 2.10*B*). The mesentery of the transverse colon, the *transverse mesocolon,* loops down, often inferior to the level of the iliac crests, and is adherent to the posterior wall of the omental bursa. The **root of the transverse mesocolon** lies along the inferior border of the pancreas and is continuous with the parietal peritoneum posteriorly (Fig. 2.18). The *arterial supply of the transverse colon* is mainly from the **middle colic artery** (Fig. 2.19*B;* Table 2.8), a branch of the SMA; however, it may also be supplied to variable degrees by the *right* and *left colic arteries* via anastomoses. *Venous drainage of the transverse colon* is through the **SMV**. *Lymphatic drainage* is to the **middle colic lymph nodes**, which in turn drain to the **superior mesenteric lymph nodes** (Fig. 2.21*A*). The *nerves of the transverse colon* arise from the **superior mesenteric plexus** and follow the right and middle colic arteries (Fig. 2.21*B*). These nerves transmit sympathetic and parasympathetic (vagal) nerve fibers. The nerves that derive from the **inferior mesenteric plexus** follow the left colic artery.

The **descending colon** passes retroperitoneally from the left colic flexure into the left iliac fossa, where it is continuous with the sigmoid colon. Peritoneum covers the colon anteriorly and laterally and binds it to the posterior abdominal wall. Although retroperitoneal, the descending colon, especially in the iliac fossa, has a short mesentery in approximately 33% of people. As it descends, the colon passes anterior to the lateral border of the left kidney (Fig. 2.18). As with the ascending colon, the descending colon has a **paracolic gutter** on its lateral aspect (Fig. 2.12).

The **sigmoid colon**, characterized by its S-shaped loop of variable length, links the descending colon and the rectum (Fig. 2.19*A*). The sigmoid colon extends from the iliac fossa to the third sacral segment, where it joins the rectum. The termination of the teniae coli indicates the *rectosigmoid junction.* The sigmoid colon usually has a long mesentery (*sigmoid mesocolon*) and, therefore, has considerable freedom of movement, especially its middle part. The **root of the sigmoid mesocolon** has an inverted V-shaped attachment (Fig. 2.18), extending first medially and superiorly along the external iliac vessels and then medially and inferiorly from the bifurcation of the common iliac vessels to the anterior aspect of the sacrum. The *left ureter* and the division of the left common iliac artery lie retroperitoneally posterior to the apex of the root of the sigmoid mesocolon.

The second important transition in the blood supply to the abdominal portion of the alimentary tract occurs approximately at the left colic flexure. Proximal to this point (back to mid-duodenum), the blood is supplied to the alimentary tract by the **SMA** (embryonic midgut); distal to this point, blood is supplied by the **inferior mesenteric artery** (IMA) (embryonic hindgut). The *arterial supply of the descending and sigmoid colon* is from the **left colic** and **sigmoid arteries,** branches of the IMA (Fig. 2.19*B*; Table 2.8). The left colic and sigmoid arteries pass to the left where they divide into ascending and descending branches. Usually all or most of the branches of the arteries supplying blood to the colon (ileocolic; right, middle, and left colic; and sigmoid arteries) anastomose with each other as they approach the colon, thus forming a continuous anastomotic channel, the **marginal artery,** which may provide important collateral circulation (Fig. 2.19*B*).

The **IMV** returns blood from the descending and sigmoid colon, flowing usually into the splenic vein and then the portal vein on its way to the liver (Fig. 2.14*B*). The *lymphatic vessels from the descending and sigmoid colon* pass to the **epicolic** and **paracolic lymph nodes** and then through the **intermediate colic lymph nodes** along the left colic artery (Fig. 2.21*A*). Lymph from these nodes passes to **inferior mesenteric lymph nodes** that lie around the IMA; however, lymph from the left colic flexure also drains to the *superior mesenteric lymph nodes.* Note.

The **sympathetic nerve supply** of the descending and sigmoid colon is from the lumbar part of the sympathetic trunk via **lumbar (abdominopelvic) splanchnic nerves,** the **superior mesenteric plexus,** and the **periarterial plexuses on the IMA** and its branches (Fig. 2.21*B*). The **parasympathetic nerve supply** is from the **pelvic splanchnic nerves** via *not vagus* the inferior hypogastric (pelvic) plexus and nerves, which ascend retroperitoneally from the plexus, independent of the arterial supply. Proximal to the middle of the sigmoid colon the visceral afferents conveying pain pass retrogradely with sympathetic fibers to thoracolumbar spinal sensory ganglia, whereas those carrying reflex information travel with the parasympathetic fibers to vagal sensory ganglia. Distal to the middle of the sigmoid colon, the visceral afferents follow the parasympathetic fibers retrogradely to the sensory ganglia of spinal nerves S2–S4.

RECTUM AND ANAL CANAL

The rectum, the fixed terminal part of the large intestine, is continuous with the sigmoid colon at the level of the S3 vertebra. The junction is at the lower end of the mesentery of the sigmoid colon (Fig. 2.18). The rectum is continuous in-

Colitis, Colectomy, and Ileostomy

Chronic inflammation of the colon (*ulcerative colitis, Crohn disease*) is characterized by severe inflammation and ulceration of the colon and rectum. In some patients, a *colectomy* is performed, during which the terminal ileum and colon as well as the rectum and anal canal are removed. An *ileostomy* is then constructed to establish an artificial cutaneous opening between the ileum and the skin of the anterolateral abdominal wall.

Colonoscopy

The interior of the colon can be observed with an elongated *endoscope,* usually a fiberoptic *colonoscope.* The endoscope is a tube that inserts into the colon through the anus and rectum. Most tumors of the large intestine occur in the rectum; approximately 12% of them appear near the rectosigmoid junction.

feriorly with the anal canal. These parts of the large intestine are described with the pelvis in Chapter 3.

Spleen

The **spleen,** a mobile ovoid lymphatic organ, lies intraperitoneally in the left upper quadrant (Table 2.6). The spleen is entirely surrounded by peritoneum except at the **hilum** (Fig. 2.9), where the splenic branches of the splenic artery and vein enter and leave. It is associated posteriorly with the left 9th–11th ribs and separated from them by the diaphragm and the **costodiaphragmatic recess,** the cleft-like extension of the pleural cavity between the diaphragm and the lower part of the thoracic cage (Fig. 2.10*A*). The spleen normally does not descend inferior to the costal (rib) region; it rests on the left colic flexure. The spleen varies considerably in size, weight, and shape; however, it is usually about 12 cm long and 7 cm wide, roughly the size and shape of a clenched fist.

The **diaphragmatic surface of the spleen** is convexly curved to fit the concavity of the diaphragm. The anterior and superior borders of the spleen are sharp and often notched, whereas its posterior and inferior borders are rounded. The spleen contacts the posterior wall of the stomach and is connected to its greater curvature by the **gastrosplenic ligament** and to the left kidney by the **splenorenal ligament** (Figs. 2.9 and 2.10*B*). These ligaments, containing splenic vessels, are attached to the hilum of the spleen on its medial aspect. Except at the hilum where these peritoneal reflections occur, the spleen is intimately covered with peritoneum. The **hilum of the spleen** is often in contact with the tail of the pancreas and constitutes the left boundary of the omental bursa.

The **splenic artery,** the largest branch of the celiac trunk, follows a tortuous course posterior to the omental bursa, anterior to the left kidney, and along the superior border of the pancreas (Fig. 2.16*A*). Between the layers of the splenorenal ligament, the splenic artery divides into five or more branches that enter the hilum of the spleen, dividing it into two to three vascular segments. The **splenic vein** is formed by several tributaries that emerge from the hilum (Fig. 2.16*B*). It is joined by the IMV and runs posterior to the body and tail of the pancreas throughout most of its course. The splenic vein unites with the SMV posterior to the neck of the pancreas to form the **portal vein.**

The *splenic lymphatic vessels* leave the lymph nodes in the hilum and pass along the splenic vessels to the **pancreaticosplenic lymph nodes** (Fig. 2.22*A*). These nodes relate to the posterior surface and superior border of the pancreas. The **nerves of the spleen** derive from the **celiac plexus** Fig. 2.22*B*). They are distributed mainly along branches of the splenic artery and are vasomotor in function.

Pancreas

The **pancreas,** an elongated accessory digestive gland, lies retroperitoneally and transversely across the posterior ab-

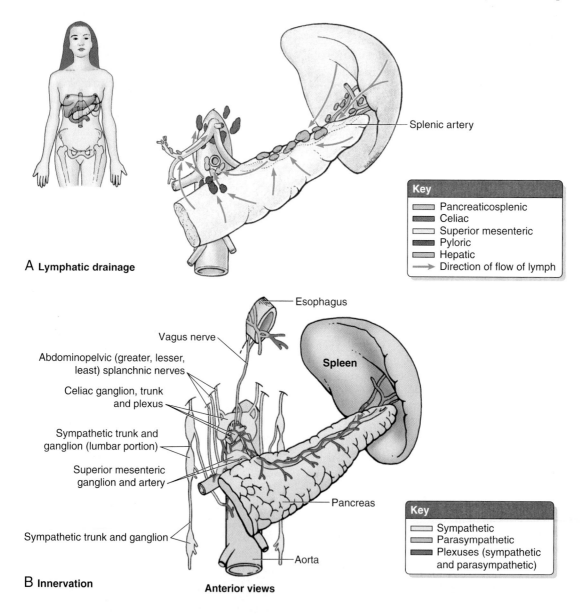

A **Lymphatic drainage**

Splenic artery

Key
	Pancreaticosplenic
	Celiac
	Superior mesenteric
	Pyloric
	Hepatic
→	Direction of flow of lymph

Esophagus

Vagus nerve

Abdominopelvic (greater, lesser, least) splanchnic nerves

Celiac ganglion, trunk and plexus

Sympathetic trunk and ganglion (lumbar portion)

Superior mesenteric ganglion and artery

Sympathetic trunk and ganglion

Spleen

Pancreas

Aorta

B **Innervation**

Anterior views

Key
	Sympathetic
	Parasympathetic
	Plexuses (sympathetic and parasympathetic)

Figure 2.22. Spleen and pancreas.

Surface Anatomy of Spleen and Pancreas

The **spleen** lies superficially in the left upper abdominal quadrant between the 9th and the 11th ribs (Fig. SA2.3). Its convex, costal surface fits the inferior surface of the diaphragm and the curved bodies of the ribs. In the supine position, the long axis of the spleen is roughly parallel to the long axis of the 10th rib. The spleen is seldom palpable through the anterolateral abdominal wall unless it is enlarged. The **neck of the pancreas** overlies the L1 and L2 vertebrae in the transpyloric plane. Its head is to the right and inferior to this plane, and its body and tail are to the left and superior to this level. Because the pancreas is deep in the abdominal cavity, posterior to the stomach and omental bursa, it is usually not palpable.

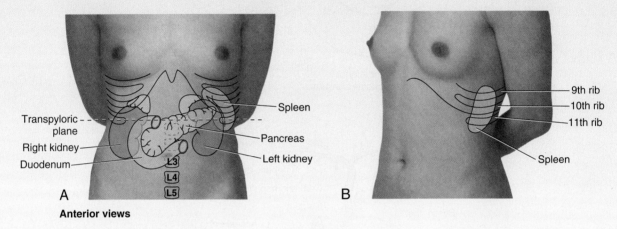

Transpyloric plane
Right kidney
Duodenum
L3
L4
L5

Spleen
Pancreas
Left kidney

A   **Anterior views**

9th rib
10th rib
11th rib
Spleen

B

Figure SA2.3.

Rupture of Spleen

Although well protected by the 9th–12th ribs, the spleen is the most frequently injured organ in the abdomen. Severe blows on the left side may fracture one or more ribs, resulting in sharp bone fragments that can lacerate the spleen. Blunt trauma to other regions of the abdomen that cause a sudden, marked increase in intra-abdominal pressure (e.g., by impalement on the steering wheel of a car) can also rupture the spleen because its capsule is thin and its parenchyma (essential substance) is soft and pulpy. If ruptured, the spleen bleeds profusely. Rupture of the spleen causes severe intraperitoneal hemorrhage and shock. Repair of a ruptured spleen is difficult; consequently, *splenectomy* (removal of spleen) or *subtotal (partial) splenectomy* (removal of one or more segments of the spleen) is often performed to prevent the patient from bleeding to death. Even total splenectomy usually does not produce serious side effects, especially in adults, because most of its functions are assumed by other reticuloendothelial organs (e.g., liver and bone marrow), but there is greater susceptibility to certain bacterial infections.

dominal wall, posterior to the stomach between the duodenum on the right and the spleen on the left (Figs. 2.17 and 2.19). The root of the transverse mesocolon lies along its anterior margin. The pancreas produces an exocrine secretion (*pancreatic juice* from the acinar cells) that enters the duodenum and endocrine secretions (*glucagon* and *insulin* from the pancreatic islets [of Langerhans]) that enter the blood.

For descriptive purposes, the pancreas is divided into four parts: head, neck, body, and tail (Fig. 2.17).

- The **head of the pancreas**, the expanded part of the gland, is embraced by the C-shaped curve of the duodenum. The **uncinate process**, a projection from the inferior part of the head, extends medially to the left, posterior to the SMA.

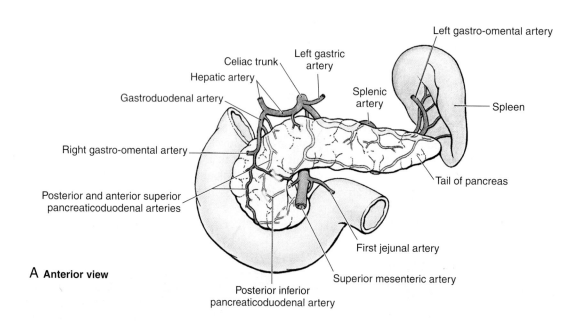

A **Anterior view**

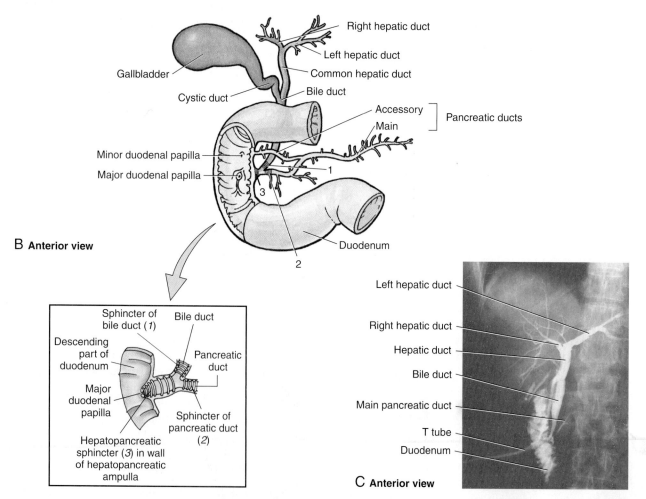

B **Anterior view**

C **Anterior view**

Figure 2.23. Pancreas and biliary system. A. The pancreatic arteries are shown. **B.** The extrahepatic bile passages and pancreatic ducts are shown. *Inset,* The sphincters are illustrated. **C.** Endoscopic retrograde cholangiography and pancreatography reveals the bile and pancreatic ducts.

- The **neck of the pancreas** is short and overlies the superior mesenteric vessels, which form a groove in its posterior aspect.
- The **body of the pancreas** continues from the neck and lies to the left of the SMA and SMV.
- The **tail of the pancreas** is closely related to the hilum of the spleen and the left colic flexure (Table 2.6). The tail is relatively mobile and passes between the layers of the **splenorenal ligament** with the splenic vessels.

The **pancreatic duct** begins in the tail of the pancreas and runs through the parenchyma (substance) of the gland to the head, where it turns inferiorly and merges with the bile duct (Fig. 2.23 *B* & *C*; Table 2.5).

The **bile duct** (common bile duct) crosses the posterosuperior surface of the head of the pancreas or is embedded in its substance. The pancreatic and bile ducts unite to form a short, dilated **hepatopancreatic ampulla** (Fig. 2.23 *B*), which opens into the descending part of the duodenum at the summit of the **major duodenal papilla**. The **sphincter of the pancreatic duct** (around the terminal part of the pancreatic duct), the **sphincter of the bile duct** (around the termination of the bile duct), and the **hepatopancreatic sphincter** (sphincter of Oddi) (around the hepatopancreatic ampulla) are smooth-muscle sphincters that control the flow of bile and pancreatic juice into the duodenum. The **accessory pancreatic duct** drains the uncinate process and the inferior part of the head of the pancreas and opens into the duodenum at the **minor duodenal papilla** (Fig. 2.23 *B*). Usually, the accessory duct communicates with the main pancreatic duct but in some people it is a separate duct.

The **pancreatic arteries** derive mainly from the branches of the splenic artery (Fig. 2.23 *A*; Table 2.5). The anterior and posterior **superior pancreaticoduodenal arteries**, branches of the gastroduodenal artery, and the anterior and posterior **inferior pancreaticoduodenal arteries**, branches of the SMA, supply the head. The **pancreatic veins** are tributaries of the splenic and superior mesenteric parts of the portal vein; however, most of them empty into the **splenic vein** (Fig. 2.16 *B*). The *pancreatic lymphatic vessels* follow the blood vessels (Fig. 2.22 *A*). Most of them end in the **pancreaticosplenic nodes** that lie along the splenic artery, but some vessels end in the **pyloric lymph nodes**. Efferent vessels from these nodes drain to the **superior mesenteric lymph nodes** or to the **celiac lymph nodes** via the **hepatic lymph nodes**.

The *nerves of the pancreas* are derived from the **vagus** and **abdominopelvic splanchnic nerves** passing through the diaphragm (Fig. 2.22 *B*; Table 2.7). The **parasympathetic** and **sympathetic nerve fibers** reach the pancreas by passing along the arteries from the **celiac plexus** and **superior mesenteric plexuses**. In addition to the sympathetic fibers that pass to blood vessels, sympathetic and parasympathetic fibers are distributed to pancreatic acinar cells and islets. The parasympathetic fibers are secretomotor, but pancreatic secretion is primarily mediated by hormones, secretin and cholecystokinin formed in the duodenum and proximal intestine.

Liver

The **liver**, the largest internal organ and largest gland in the body, weighs about 1500 g (Fig. 2.24 *A*). The diaphragm

Rupture of Pancreas

Pancreatic injury can result from sudden, severe, forceful compression of the abdomen such as the force of impalement on steering wheel in an automobile accident. Because the pancreas lies transversely, the vertebral column acts like an anvil and the traumatic force may rupture the pancreas. Rupture of the pancreas frequently tears its duct system, allowing pancreatic juice to enter the parenchyma of the gland and to invade adjacent tissues. Digestion of pancreatic and other tissues by pancreatic juice is painful.

Pancreatic Cancer

Cancer involving the pancreatic head accounts for most cases of extrahepatic obstruction of the biliary system. Because of the posterior relationships of the pancreas, cancer of the head often compresses and obstructs the bile duct and/or the hepatopancreatic ampulla. This condition causes *obstructive jaundice*, resulting in the retention of bile pigments, enlargement of the gallbladder, and jaundice (yellow staining of most body tissues). Cancer of the neck and body of the pancreas may cause portal or IVC obstruction because the pancreas overlies these large veins.

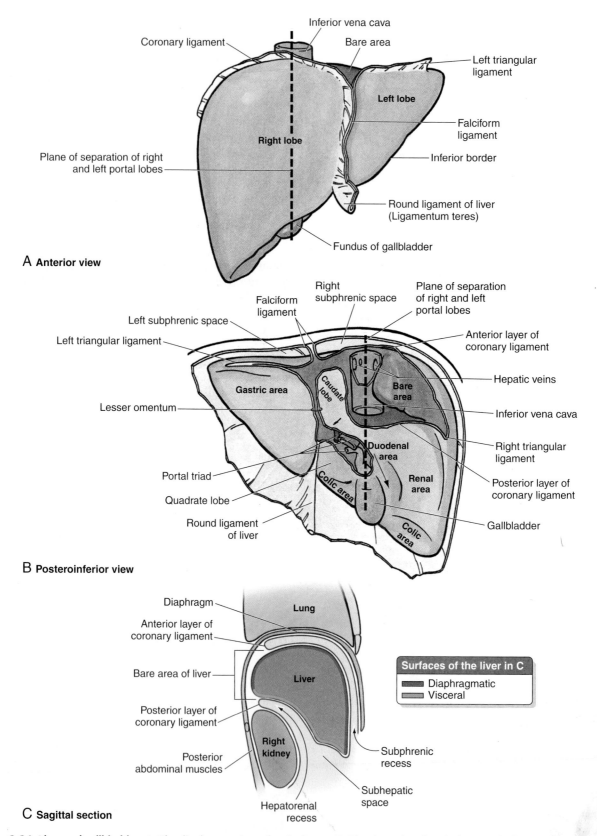

Figure 2.24. Liver and gallbladder. A. The diaphragmatic surface is shown. **B.** The visceral surface is shown. The bare area is demarcated by the reflection of peritoneum from the diaphragm to the liver as the anterior (upper) and posterior (lower) layers of the coronary ligament. These layers meet at the right to form the right triangular ligament and diverge toward the left to enclose the bare area. The anterior layer of the coronary ligament is continuous on the left with the right layer of the falciform ligament, and the posterior layer is continuous with the right layer of the lesser omentum. The left layers of the falciform ligament and lesser omentum meet to form the left triangular ligament. **C.** The surfaces and recesses are identified.

separates the liver from the pleura, lungs, pericardium, and heart. With the exception of lipids, every substance absorbed by the alimentary tract is received first by the liver. In addition to its many metabolic activities, the liver stores glycogen and secretes bile.

SURFACES OF LIVER

The liver has a convex **diaphragmatic surface** (anterior, superior, and some posterior), and a relatively flat, concave **visceral surface** (posteroinferior), which are separated anteriorly by the sharp **inferior border** (Fig. 2.24A). The diaphragmatic surface is smooth and dome shaped, where it is related to the concavity of the inferior surface of the diaphragm. **Subphrenic spaces** (recesses), superior extensions of the peritoneal cavity, are located between the anterior and the superior aspects of the liver and the diaphragm (Fig. 2.24C). The subphrenic spaces are separated by the **falciform ligament**, which extends between the liver and the anterior abdominal wall, into right and left recesses.

The **hepatorenal recess** (Morrison pouch) of the subhepatic space is a deep recess of the peritoneal cavity on the right side inferior to the liver and anterior to the kidney and suprarenal gland. The hepatorenal recess is a gravity-dependent part of the peritoneal cavity when a person is in the supine position; fluid draining from the omental bursa flows into this recess. The hepatorenal recess communicates anteriorly with the right subphrenic space. The diaphragmatic surface is covered with peritoneum, except posteriorly in the **bare area of the liver**, where it lies in direct contact with the diaphragm (Fig. 2.24). The **visceral surface of the liver** is covered with peritoneum, except at the *bed of the gallbladder* and the *porta hepatis*. The **porta hepatis** is a transverse fissure in the middle visceral surface of the liver (Fig. 2.26) that gives passage to the portal vein, hepatic artery, hepatic nerve plexus, hepatic ducts, and lymphatic vessels. The visceral surface of the liver is related to the:

- Right side of the anterior aspect of the stomach—*gastric* and *pyloric areas.*

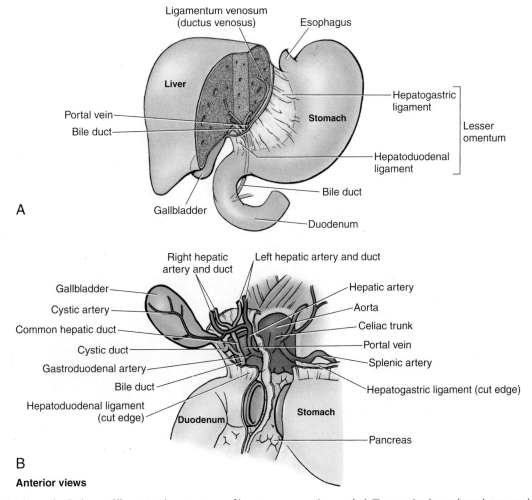

A

B

Anterior views

Figure 2.25. Peritoneal relations of liver. A. The structure of lesser omentum is revealed. Two sagittal cuts have been made through the liver, and these cuts have been joined by a coronal cut. **B.** Portal triad (bile duct, hepatic artery, and portal vein) within the hepatoduodenal ligament is shown.

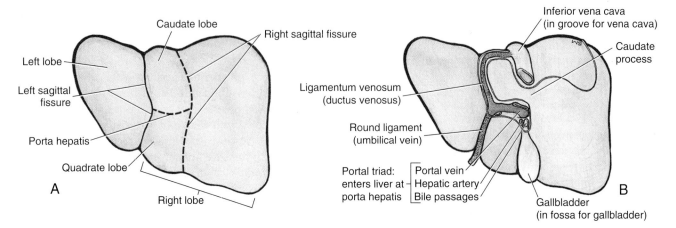

Figure 2.26. Anatomical lobes of liver. A. The lobes and fissures are identified. **B.** The structures of the visceral surface are shown. The round ligament (ligamentum teres) is the occluded remains of the fetal umbilical vein. The ligamentum venosum is the fibrous remnant of the fetal ductus venosus.

- Superior part of the duodenum—*duodenal area.*
- Lesser omentum.
- Gallbladder—fossa for gallbladder.
- Right colic flexure and right transverse colon—*colic area.*
- Right kidney and suprarenal gland—*renal* and *suprarenal areas.*

The **lesser omentum**, enclosing the **portal triad** (portal vein, hepatic artery, and bile duct), passes from the liver to the lesser curvature of the stomach and the first 2 cm of the superior part of the duodenum (Fig. 2.25A). The thickened free edge of the lesser omentum extending between the porta hepatis and the duodenum is the **hepatoduodenal lig-**

Surface Anatomy of Liver

The liver lies mainly in the right upper quadrant where it is hidden and protected by the thoracic cage and diaphragm (Fig. SA2.4). The normal liver lies deep to ribs 7–11 on the right side and crosses the midline toward the left nipple. The liver is located more inferiorly when one is erect because of gravity. Its sharp inferior border follows the right costal margin. When the person is asked to inspire deeply, the liver may be palpated because of the inferior movement of the diaphragm and liver.

Subphrenic Abscesses

Peritonitis may result in the formation of abscesses (localized collections of pus) in various parts of the peritoneal cavity. A common site for an abscess is in the subphrenic spaces. Subphrenic abscesses occur much more frequently on the right side because of the frequency of ruptured appendices and perforated duodenal ulcers. Because the right and left subphrenic recesses are continuous with the hepatorenal recess (Fig. 2.24C), pus from a subphrenic abscess may drain into one of the hepatorenal recesses, especially when the individual is bedridden. A subphrenic abscess is often drained by an incision inferior to, or through, the bed of the 12th rib.

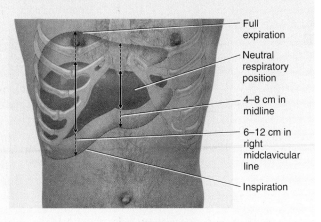

Figure SA2.4.

ament (Fig. 2.25 B); it encloses the structures that pass through the porta hepatis (Fig. 2.26 B).

LOBES AND SEGMENTS OF LIVER

Anatomically, based only on external features, the liver is described as having four "lobes": right, left, caudate, and quadrate; however, functionally, in terms of blood supply and glandular secretion, the liver is divided into independent right and left livers—portal lobes (Fig. 2.24). The anatomical large **right lobe** is separated from the smaller **left lobe** by the falciform ligament and the left sagittal fissure. On the visceral surface, the right and left sagittal fissures and porta hepatis demarcate the **caudate lobe** (posterior and superior) and **quadrate lobe** (anterior and inferior)—both are parts of right lobe. The **right sagittal fissure** is the continuous groove formed by the fossa for the gallbladder anteriorly and the groove for the inferior vena cava posteriorly. The **left sagittal fissure** is the continuous groove formed anteriorly by the **fissure for the round ligament** (L. *ligamentum teres*) and posteriorly by the **fissure for the ligamentum venosum**. The **round ligament of the liver** is the obliterated remains of the umbilical vein (Fig. 2.26), which carried well-oxygenated blood from the placenta to the fetus. The **ligamentum venosum** is the fibrous remnant of the fetal ductus venosus that shunted blood from the umbilical vein to the IVC, short-circuiting the liver (Moore and Persaud, 2003).

The division between **right** and **left livers** (parts or portal lobes) is approximated by the sagittal plane passing through the gallbladder fossa and the fossa for the IVC on the visceral surface of the liver and an imaginary line over the diaphragmatic surface that runs from the fundus of

Hepatic Lobectomies and Segmentectomy

When it was discovered that the right and left hepatic arteries and ducts, as well as branches of the right and left portal veins, do not communicate significantly, it became possible to perform *hepatic lobectomies*—removal of the right or left (part of the) liver—with a minimal amount of bleeding. If a severe injury or tumor involves one segment or adjacent segments, it may be possible to resect (remove) only the affected segment(s): *segmentectomy*. The intersegmental hepatic veins serve as guides to the interlobular planes.

the gallbladder to the IVC (Fig. 2.24). The left liver includes the anatomical caudate lobe and most of the quadrate lobe. The right and left livers are more equal in mass than the anatomical lobes, but the right lobe is still somewhat larger. Each portal lobe has its own blood supply from the hepatic artery and portal vein and its own venous and biliary drainage. The portal lobes of the liver are further subdivided into eight **segments** (Fig. 2.27). The segmentation is based on the principal branches of the right and left hepatic arteries, portal veins, and hepatic ducts. Each segment is supplied by a branch of the right or left hepatic artery and portal vein and drained by a branch of the right or left hepatic duct. *Intersegmental hepatic veins* pass between and thus further demarcate segments on their way to the IVC.

VASCULATURE AND NERVES OF LIVER

The liver receives blood from two sources (Figs. 2.25 B and 2.27 A): the portal vein (75–80%) and the hepatic artery (20–25%). The **portal vein** carries poorly oxygenated blood from the abdominopelvic portion of the gastrointestinal tract. The **hepatic artery,** a branch of the celiac trunk, carries well-oxygenated blood from the aorta. At or close to the porta hepatis, the hepatic artery and portal vein terminate by dividing into right and left branches, which supply the right and left livers, respectively. Within each lobe, the primary branches of the portal vein and hepatic artery are consistent enough to form **vascular segments** (Fig 2.27). Between the segments are the **right, intermediate (middle),** and **left hepatic veins,** which drain parts of adjacent segments. The hepatic veins open into the IVC just inferior to the diaphragm (Fig. 2.24 B). The attachment of these veins to the IVC helps hold the liver in position.

The liver is a major lymph-producing organ; between one quarter and one half of the lymph received by the thoracic duct comes from the liver. The **lymphatic vessels of the liver** occur as superficial lymphatics in the subperitoneal fibrous capsule of the liver (Glisson capsule), which form its outer surface, and as *deep lymphatics* in the connective tissue that accompany the ramifications of the portal triad and hepatic veins. Superficial lymphatics from the anterior aspects of the diaphragmatic and visceral surfaces and the deep lymphatic vessels accompanying the portal triads converge toward the porta hepatis and drain to the **hepatic lymph nodes** scattered along the hepatic vessels and ducts in the lesser omentum (Fig. 2.28 A). Efferent lymphatic vessels from these lymph nodes drain into the **celiac lymph nodes,** which in turn drain into the **chyle cistern** (L. *cisterna chyli*) at the inferior end of the thoracic duct. Superficial lymphatics from the posterior aspects of the diaphragmatic and visceral surfaces of the liver drain toward the bare area of the liver. Here, they drain into **phrenic lymph nodes** or join deep lymphatics that have

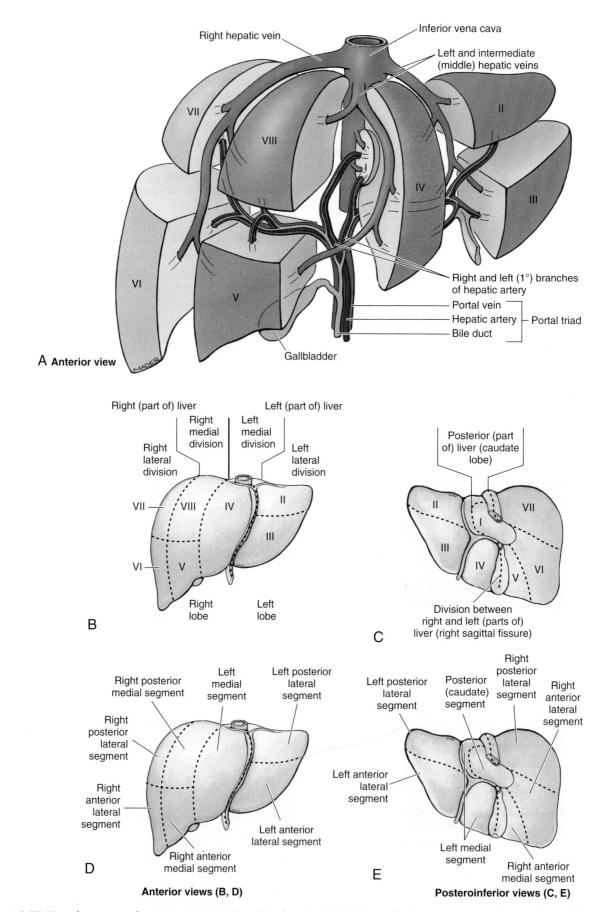

Right hepatic vein

Inferior vena cava

Left and intermediate (middle) hepatic veins

VII

VIII

I

II

IV

III

VI

V

Right and left (1°) branches of hepatic artery

Portal vein
Hepatic artery — Portal triad
Bile duct

Gallbladder

A **Anterior view**

Right (part of) liver

Left (part of) liver

Right medial division

Left medial division

Right lateral division

Left lateral division

VII — VIII   IV   II

III

VI — V

Right lobe

Left lobe

B

Posterior (part of) liver (caudate lobe)

II   I   VII

III

IV   V   VI

Division between right and left (parts of) liver (right sagittal fissure)

C

Right posterior medial segment

Left medial segment

Left posterior lateral segment

Right posterior lateral segment

Right anterior lateral segment

Left anterior lateral segment

Right anterior medial segment

D

Anterior views (B, D)

Left posterior lateral segment

Posterior (caudate) segment

Right posterior lateral segment

Right anterior lateral segment

Left anterior lateral segment

Left medial segment

Right anterior medial segment

E

Posteroinferior views (C, E)

Figure 2.27. Hepatic segmentation. Segmentation is based on the principal divisions of the hepatic artery and portal vein and the accompanying hepatic duct.

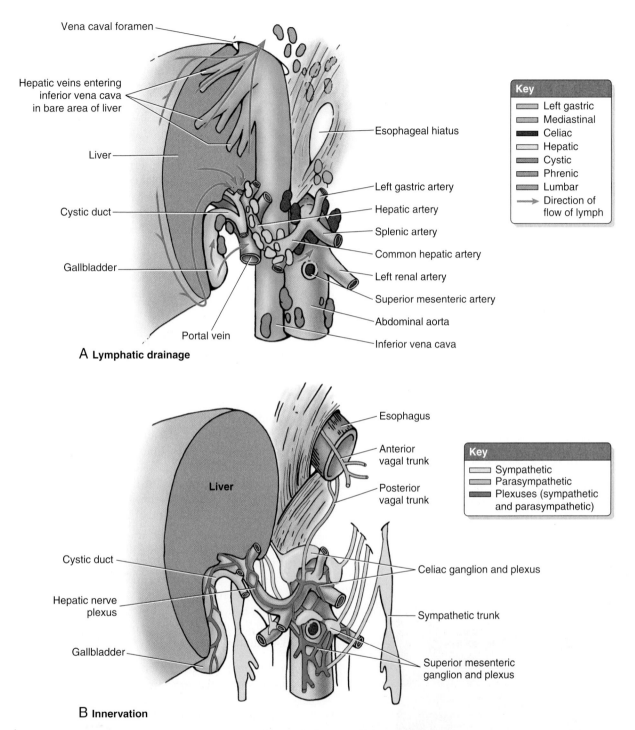

A **Lymphatic drainage**

Vena caval foramen

Hepatic veins entering inferior vena cava in bare area of liver

Liver

Cystic duct

Gallbladder

Portal vein

Esophageal hiatus

Left gastric artery

Hepatic artery

Splenic artery

Common hepatic artery

Left renal artery

Superior mesenteric artery

Abdominal aorta

Inferior vena cava

Key
- Left gastric
- Mediastinal
- Celiac
- Hepatic
- Cystic
- Phrenic
- Lumbar
- → Direction of flow of lymph

B **Innervation**

Esophagus

Anterior vagal trunk

Posterior vagal trunk

Liver

Cystic duct

Hepatic nerve plexus

Gallbladder

Celiac ganglion and plexus

Sympathetic trunk

Superior mesenteric ganglion and plexus

Key
- Sympathetic
- Parasympathetic
- Plexuses (sympathetic and parasympathetic)

Figure 2.28. Lymphatic drainage and innervation of liver.

accompanied the hepatic veins converging on the IVC and then pass with this large vein through the diaphragm to drain into the **posterior mediastinal lymph nodes.** Efferent vessels from these nodes join the right lymphatic and thoracic ducts. A few lymphatic vessels also drain to the left gastric nodes, along the falciform ligament to the parasternal lymph nodes and along the round ligament of the liver

to the lymphatics of the anterior abdominal wall. The **nerves of the liver** derive from the **hepatic nerve plexus** (Fig. 2.28B), the largest derivative of the celiac plexus. The hepatic plexus accompanies the branches of the hepatic artery and portal vein to the liver. It consists of *sympathetic fibers* from the **celiac plexus** and *parasympathetic fibers* from the anterior and posterior **vagal trunks.**

Liver Biopsy

Hepatic tissue may be obtained for diagnostic purposes by liver biopsy. The *needle puncture* is commonly made through the right 10th intercostal space in the midaxillary line. Before the physician takes the biopsy, the person is asked to hold his or her breath in full expiration to reduce the *costodiaphragmatic recess* and to lessen the possibility of damaging the lung and contaminating the pleural cavity.

Rupture of Liver

Although less so than the spleen, the liver is vulnerable to rupture because it is large, fixed in position, and friable. Often the liver is torn by a fractured rib that perforates the diaphragm. Because of the liver's great vascularity and friability, liver lacerations often cause considerable hemorrhage and right upper quadrant pain.

Cirrhosis of Liver

There is progressive destruction of hepatocytes in cirrhosis of the liver and replacement of them by fibrous tissue. This tissue surrounds the intrahepatic blood vessels and biliary ducts, making the liver firm and impeding circulation of blood through it. Cirrhosis, the most common of many causes of *portal hypertension,* frequently develops in chronic alcoholics (Fig. B2.7).

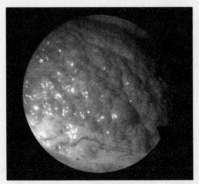

Cirrhosis of liver

Figure B2.7.

Biliary Ducts and Gallbladder

Bile is produced continuously in the liver and stored in the gallbladder. In addition to storing bile, the gallbladder concentrates it by absorbing water and salts. When fat enters the duodenum, the gallbladder sends concentrated bile through the cystic and bile ducts to the duodenum. Bile emulsifies the fat so it can be absorbed in the distal intestine. The hepatocytes (liver cells) secrete bile into the **bile canaliculi** formed between them (Fig. 2.29A). The canaliculi drain into the small *interlobular biliary ducts* and then into large collecting bile ducts of the intrahepatic portal triad, which merge to form the right and left hepatic ducts. The **right** and **left hepatic ducts** drain the right and left livers (portal lobes), respectively. Shortly after leaving the porta hepatis, the right and left hepatic ducts unite to form the **common hepatic duct**, which is joined on the right side by the **cystic duct** to form the **bile duct** (Fig. 2.29B & C).

BILE DUCT

The bile duct (formerly, common bile duct) forms in the free edge of the lesser omentum by the union of the *cystic duct* and *common hepatic duct* (Figs. 2.25 and 2.29B). The bile duct descends posterior to the superior part of the duodenum and lies in a groove on the posterior surface of the head of the pancreas. On the left side of the descending part of the duodenum, the bile duct comes into contact with the **main pancreatic duct** (Fig. 2.23B & C). The two ducts run obliquely through the wall of this part of the duodenum, where they unite to form the **hepatopancreatic ampulla** (ampulla of Vater). The distal end of the ampulla opens into the duodenum through the **major duodenal papilla.** The muscle around the distal end of the bile duct is thickened to form the **sphincter of the bile duct.** When this sphincter contracts, bile cannot enter the ampulla and/or the duodenum; hence bile backs up and passes along the cystic duct to the *gallbladder* for concentration and storage.

The arteries supplying the bile duct include the (Figs. 2.23A and 2.25B):

- **Posterior superior pancreaticoduodenal artery** and **gastroduodenal artery**, supplying the retroduodenal part of the duct.
- **Cystic artery**, supplying the proximal part of the duct.
- **Right hepatic artery**, supplying the middle part of the duct.

The veins from the proximal part of the bile duct and the hepatic ducts generally enter the liver directly. The **posterior superior pancreaticoduodenal vein** drains the distal part of the bile duct and empties into the **portal vein** or one of its tributaries (Fig. 2.30A). The *lymphatic vessels from the bile duct* pass to the **cystic lymph node** near the neck of the gallbladder, the **node of the omental foramen** and the **hepatic lymph**

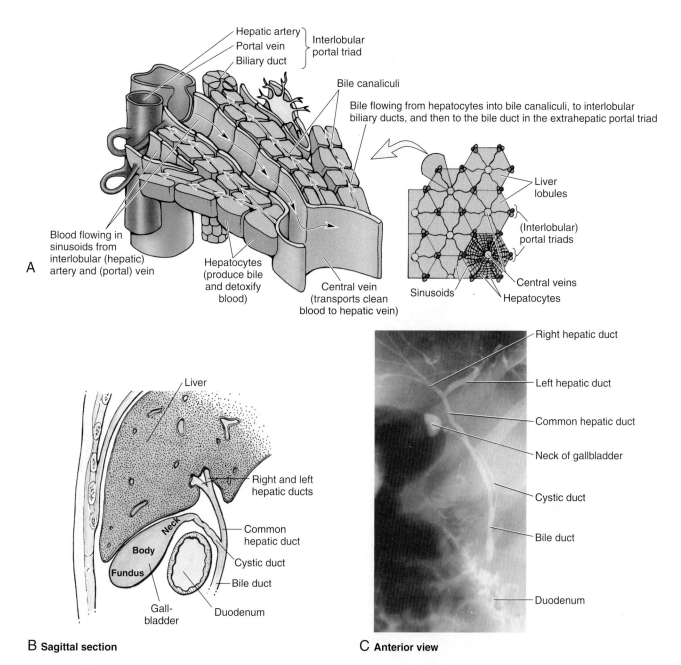

Figure 2.29. Biliary ducts and gallbladder. A. The flow of blood and bile in the liver is demonstrated. This small part of a liver lobule shows the components of the interlobular portal triad and the positioning of the sinusoids and bile canaliculi. *Right:* The cut surface of the liver shows the hexagonal pattern of the lobes. **B.** The extrahepatic bile passages and gallbladder are identified. **C.** An endoscopic retrograde cholangiography shows the gallbladder and biliary passages. The cystic duct usually lies on the right of the common hepatic duct and joins it just superior to the first part of the duodenum.

nodes (Fig. 2.28*A*). Efferent lymphatic vessels from the bile duct pass to the **celiac lymph nodes.**

GALLBLADDER

The pear-shaped **gallbladder** (7–10 cm long) lies in the **gallbladder fossa** on the visceral surface of the liver (Fig. 2.24*B*). Peritoneum completely surrounds the fundus of the gallbladder and binds its body and neck to the liver.

The hepatic surface of the gallbladder attaches to the liver by connective tissue of the fibrous capsule of the liver. The gallbladder has three parts (Fig. 2.29*B*):

• The **fundus,** the wide end, projects from the inferior border of the liver and is usually located at the tip of the right 9th costal cartilage in the midclavicular line.
• The **body** contacts the visceral surface of the liver, the transverse colon, and the superior part of the duodenum.

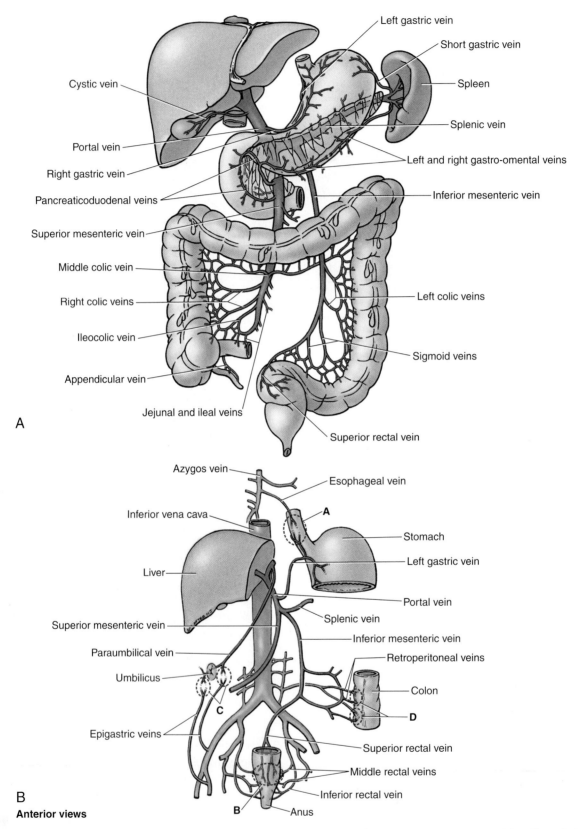

Figure 2.30. Portal venous system. A. The venous system is demonstrated. **B.** Portal-systemic anastomoses provide collateral circulation in cases of obstruction in the liver or portal vein. *Darker blue,* portal tributaries; *lighter blue,* systemic tributaries; *A,* anastomoses between esophageal veins; *B,* anastomoses between rectal veins; *C,* anastomoses between the paraumbilical veins (portal) and small epigastric veins of the anterior abdominal wall; *D,* anastomoses between the twigs of colic veins (portal) and the retroperitoneal veins.

• The **neck** of the gallbladder is narrow, tapered, and directed toward the porta hepatis.

The neck makes an S-shaped bend and joins the **cystic duct.** Internally, the mucosa of the neck spirals into a fold, the **spiral valve,** which keeps the cystic duct open so that bile can easily divert into the gallbladder when the distal end of the bile duct is closed by the sphincter of the bile duct and/or the hepatopancreatic sphincter, or when bile passes to the duodenum as the gallbladder contracts. The **cystic duct** (approximately 4 cm long) connects the *neck of the gallbladder* to the common hepatic duct. The cystic duct passes between the layers of the lesser omentum, usually parallel to the **common hepatic duct,** which it joins to form the bile duct.

The **cystic artery,** which supplies the gallbladder and cystic duct, commonly arises from the **right hepatic artery** in the angle between the common hepatic duct and the cystic duct (Fig. 2.25*B*). Variations in the origin and course of the cystic artery are common. The **cystic veins** draining the biliary ducts and the neck of the gallbladder may pass to the liver directly or drain through the portal vein to the liver (Fig. 2.30*A*). The veins from the fundus and body pass directly into the visceral surface of the liver and drain into the hepatic sinusoids. The *lymphatic drainage of the gallbladder* is to the **hepatic lymph nodes** (Fig. 2.28*A*), often by way of the **cystic lymph node** located near the neck of the gallbladder. Efferent lymphatic vessels from these nodes pass to the **celiac lymph nodes.** The *nerves to the gallbladder and cystic duct* pass along the cystic artery from the **celiac nerve plexus** (sympathetic and visceral [pain] afferents), the **vagus nerve** (parasympathetic), and the **right phrenic nerve** (somatic afferent fibers) (Fig. 2.28*B*).

Impaction of Gallstones

Gallstones are concretions (L. *caculi,* pebbles) in the gallbladder, hepatic ducts, cystic duct, or bile duct. The distal end of the hepatopancreatic ampulla is the narrowest part of the biliary passages and is the common site for impaction of a gallstone. Gallstones may produce **biliary colic** (pain in the epigastric region). When the gallbladder relaxes, the stone in the cystic duct may pass back into the gallbladder. If a stone blocks the cystic duct, *cholecystitis* (inflammation of gallbladder) occurs because of bile accumulation, causing enlargement of the gallbladder. Pain develops in the epigastric region and later shifts to the right hypochondriac region at the junction of the 9th costal cartilage and the lateral border of the rectus sheath. Inflammation of the gallbladder may cause pain in the posterior thoracic wall or right shoulder as a result of irritation of the diaphragm. If bile cannot leave the gallbladder, it enters the blood and causes *obstructive jaundice* (see clinical correlation [blue] box "Pancreatic Cancer," in this chapter).

Portal–Systemic Anastomoses

The communications between the portal venous system and the systemic venous system are important clinically in the advent of an intrahepatic or extrahepatic portal venous block. When portal circulation through the liver is obstructed because of liver disease or physical pressure from a tumor, for example, blood from the alimentary tract can still reach the right side of the heart through the IVC by way of several collateral routes. These alternate routes are available because the portal vein and its tributaries have no valves; hence blood can flow in a reverse direction to the IVC.

Portal Hypertension

When scarring and fibrosis from cirrhosis of the liver obstruct the portal vein, pressure rises in the portal vein and its tributaries, producing **portal hypertension.** At the sites of anastomoses between portal and systemic veins, portal hypertension produces enlarged varicose veins and blood flow from the portal to the systemic system of veins. The veins may become so dilated that their walls rupture, resulting in hemorrhage. Bleeding from *esophageal varices* (dilated esophageal veins) at the distal end of the esophagus is often severe and may be fatal. A common method for reducing portal hypertension is to divert blood from the portal venous system to the systemic venous system by creating a communication between the portal vein and the IVC or by joining the splenic and left renal veins—a **portacaval anastomosis** or **portosystemic shunt.**

Portal Vein and Portal–Systemic Anastomoses

The **portal vein** is the main channel of the **portal venous system** (Fig. 2.30*A*). It collects poorly oxygenated but nutrient-rich blood from the abdominal part of the alimentary tract, including the gallbladder, pancreas, and spleen and carries it to the liver. Within the liver, its branches are distributed in a segmental pattern and end in expanded capillaries, the **venous sinusoids of the liver** (Fig. 2.29*A*).

Portal–systemic anastomoses, in which the portal venous system communicates with the systemic venous system, are in the following locations (Fig. 2.30*B*):

- Between the **esophageal veins** draining into either the **azygos vein** (systemic system) or the **left gastric vein** (portal system); when dilated these are *esophageal varices.*
- Between the **rectal veins,** the inferior and middle veins draining into the IVC (systemic system) and the superior rectal vein continuing as the inferior mesenteric vein (portal system); when abnormally dilated these are *hemorrhoids.*
- **Paraumbilical veins** of the anterior abdominal wall (portal system) anastomosing with **superficial epigastric veins** (systemic system); when dilated these veins produce *caput medusae*—varicose veins radiating from the

umbilicus. These dilated veins were called caput medusae because of their resemblance to the serpents on the head of Medusa, a character in Greek mythology.
- Twigs of **colic veins** (portal system) anastomosing with retroperitoneal veins (systemic system).

Kidneys, Ureters, and Suprarenal Glands

The *kidneys* lie retroperitoneally on the posterior abdominal wall, one on each side of the vertebral column (Fig. 2.31). These urinary organs remove excess water, salts, and wastes of protein metabolism from the blood while returning nutrients and chemicals to the blood. The kidneys convey the waste products from the blood into the urine, which drains through the ureters to the urinary bladder. The *ureters* run inferiorly from the kidneys, passing over the pelvic brim at the bifurcation of the common iliac arteries. They then run along the lateral wall of the pelvis and enter the *urinary bladder.* The superomedial aspect of each kidney normally contacts a suprarenal gland. A weak fascial septum separates these glands from the kidneys. The *suprarenal glands* function as part of the endocrine system, completely separate in function from the kidneys so they are not attached to each other. They secrete corticosteroids and androgens and make epinephrine and norepinephrine hormones.

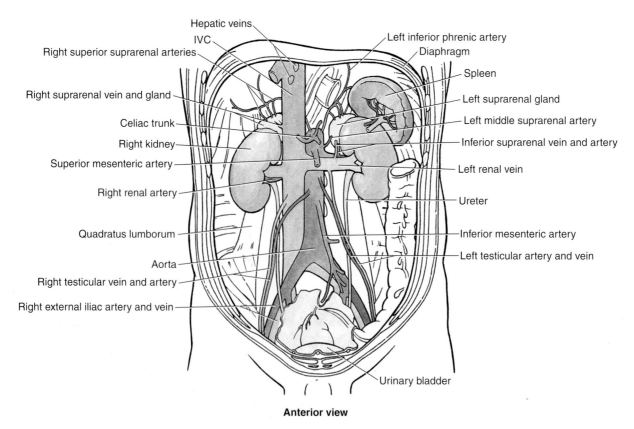

Anterior view

Figure 2.31. Retroperitoneal viscera and vessels of posterior abdominal wall. *IVC,* inferior vena cava.

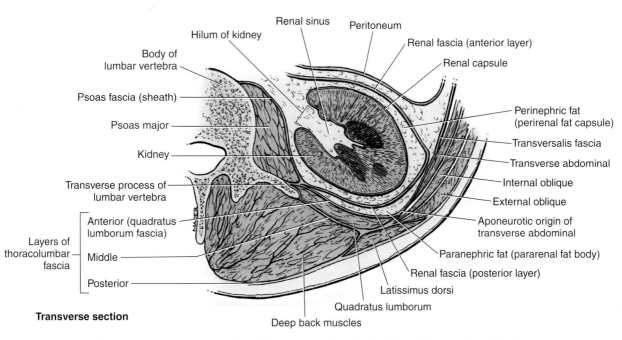

Figure 2.32. Transverse section of kidney. Note the relationships of the muscle and fascia.

RENAL FASCIA AND FAT

Perinephric fat (perirenal fat capsule) surrounds the kidneys and suprarenal glands and is continuous with the fat in the renal sinus (Fig. 2.32). The kidneys, suprarenal glands, and perinephric fat surrounding them are enclosed (except inferiorly) by a membranous layer of **renal fascia.** Inferomedially, the renal fascia is prolonged along the ureters as **periureteric fascia.** External to the renal fascia is the **paranephric fat (pararenal fat body)**, the extraperitoneal fat of the lumbar region that is most obvious posterior to the kidney. The renal fascia sends collagen bundles through the paranephric fat. Movement of the kidneys occurs during respiration and when changing from supine to erect positions; normal renal mobility is about 3 cm. Supe-

riorly, the renal fascia is continuous with diaphragmatic fascia on the inferior surface of the diaphragm. Inferiorly, the anterior and posterior layers of renal fascia are loosely united, if attached at all.

KIDNEYS

The **kidneys** lie on the posterior abdominal wall at the level of the T12–L3 vertebrae. The *right kidney* lies at a slightly lower level than the *left kidney,* probably owing to its relationship to the liver. Each kidney has anterior and posterior surfaces, medial and lateral margins, and superior and inferior poles (Fig. 2.33). The lateral margin is convex, and the medial margin is concave where the renal sinus and renal pelvis are located, giving the kidney a somewhat kidney bean–shaped appearance. At the concave medial margin of each kidney is a vertical cleft, the **renal hilum.** The hilum is the entrance to the space within the kidney, the **renal sinus,** which is occupied mostly by fat in which the renal pelvis, calices, vessels, and nerves are embedded. At the hilum, the **renal vein** is anterior to the **renal artery,** which is anterior to the **renal pelvis.**

Superiorly, the kidneys are related to the diaphragm, which separates them from the pleural cavities and the 12th pair of ribs. More inferiorly, the posterior surface of the kidney is related to the quadratus lumborum muscle (Fig. 2.31). The subcostal nerve and vessels and the iliohypogastric and ilioinguinal nerves descend diagonally across the posterior surfaces of the kidneys (Fig. 2.42). The liver, duodenum, and ascending colon are anterior to the right kidney. The left kidney is related to the stomach, spleen, pancreas, jejunum, and descending colon (Table 2.6).

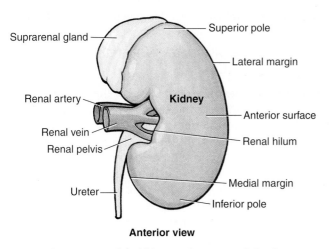

Figure 2.33. Right kidney and suprarenal gland.

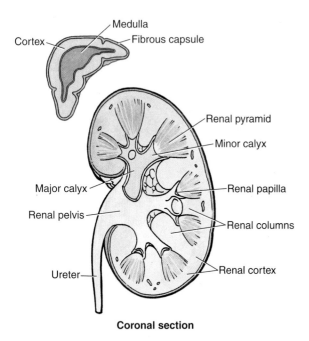

Coronal section

Figure 2.34. Internal features of kidney and suprarenal gland.

Perinephric Abscess

The attachments of the renal fascia determine the path of extension of a *perinephric abscess*. For example, the fascia at the renal hilum firmly attaches to the renal vessels and ureter, usually preventing spread of pus to the contralateral side. However, pus from an abscess (or blood from an injured kidney) may force its way into the pelvis between the loosely attached anterior and posterior layers of the pelvic fascia.

Renal Transplantation

Renal transplantation is now an established operation for the treatment of selected cases of chronic renal failure. The site for the transplanted kidney is in the iliac fossa of the greater pelvis (see Chapter 3), where it is firmly supported and where only short lengths of renal vessels and ureters are required for transplantation. The renal artery and vein are joined to the adjacent external iliac artery and vein, respectively; and the ureter is sutured into the nearby urinary bladder.

URETERS

The **ureters** are muscular ducts with narrow lumina that carry urine from the kidneys to the urinary bladder (Fig. 2.31). The superior expanded end of the ureter, the **renal pelvis**, is formed through the merging of two or three **major calices** (calyces), each of which was formed by the merging of two or three **minor calices** (Fig. 2.34). Each minor calyx is indented by the apex of the **renal pyramid**—the **renal papilla**. The abdominal parts of the ureters adhere closely to the parietal peritoneum and are retroperitoneal throughout their course. The ureters run inferomedially along the transverse processes of the lumbar vertebrae and cross the external iliac artery just beyond the bifurcation of the common iliac artery. They then run along the lateral wall of the pelvis to enter the urinary bladder. The ureters are normally constricted to a variable degree in three places: (1) at the junction of the ureters and renal pelves, (2) where the ureters cross the brim of the pelvic inlet, and (3) during their passage through the wall of the urinary bladder (Fig. 2.36). These constricted areas are potential sites of obstruction by ureteric (kidney) stones.

SUPRARENAL GLANDS

The **suprarenal (adrenal) glands** are located between the superomedial aspects of the kidneys and the diaphragmatic crura (Figs. 2.31 and 2.33), where they are surrounded by connective tissue containing considerable perinephric fat. The glands are enclosed by renal fascia by which they are attached to the *crura of the diaphragm* (see Fig. 2.40*B*); however, they are separated from the kidneys by fibrous tissue. The shape and relations of the suprarenal glands differ on the two sides.

- The pyramidal-shaped right gland lies anterior to the diaphragm and makes contact with the IVC anteromedially and the liver anterolaterally.
- The crescent-shaped left gland is related to the spleen, stomach, pancreas, and the left crus of the diaphragm.

Each suprarenal gland has two parts: the **suprarenal cortex** and **suprarenal medulla** (Fig. 2.34). These parts have different embryological origins and different functions. (Moore and Persaud, 2003). The suprarenal cortex secretes corticosteroids and androgens, and the medulla secretes epinephrine (adrenalin) and norepinephrine (noradrenalin).

VASCULATURE OF KIDNEYS, URETERS, AND SUPRARENAL GLANDS

The **renal arteries** arise at the level of the IV disc between the L1 and the L2 vertebrae (Fig. 2.31). The longer **right renal artery** passes posterior to the IVC. Typically, each artery divides close to the hilum into five **segmental arteries** that are end arteries—that is, they do not anastomose (Fig. 2.35). Segmental arteries are distributed to the **segments of the kidney.** Several veins drain the kidney and unite in a variable fashion to form the renal vein. The **renal veins** lie anterior to the renal arteries, and the longer left renal vein passes anterior to the aorta. Each renal vein drains into the IVC. The **arteries to the ureters** arise mainly from three

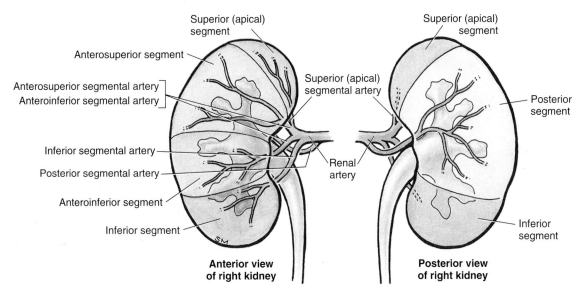

Figure 2.35. Segments and segmental arteries of kidneys. Only the superior and inferior arteries supply the whole thickness of the kidney.

sources (Fig. 2.31): the *renal artery, testicular or ovarian arteries,* and *abdominal aorta.* The **veins of the ureters** drain into the renal and testicular or ovarian veins.

The endocrine function of the suprarenal glands makes their abundant blood supply necessary. The **suprarenal arteries** arise from three sources (Fig. 2.31):

- **Superior suprarenal arteries** (six to eight) from the *inferior phrenic artery.*
- **Middle suprarenal arteries** (one or more) from the *abdominal aorta* near the origin of the SMA.
- **Inferior suprarenal arteries** (one or more) from the *renal artery.*

The venous drainage of the suprarenal gland is into a large **suprarenal vein** (Fig. 2.41*B*). The **short right suprarenal vein** drains into the IVC, whereas the longer **left suprarenal vein,** often joined by the inferior phrenic vein, empties into the left renal vein.

The **renal lymphatic vessels** follow the renal veins and drain into the **lumbar lymph nodes** (Fig. 2.36*A*). Lymphatic vessels from the superior part of the ureter may join those from the kidney or pass directly to the lumbar (caval and aortic) nodes. Lymphatic vessels from the middle part of the ureter usually drain into the **common iliac lymph nodes,** whereas vessels from its inferior part drain into the common, external, or internal **iliac lymph nodes.** The **suprarenal lymphatic vessels** arise from a plexus deep to the capsule of the gland and from one in its medulla. The lymph passes to the **lumbar lymph nodes.**

NERVES OF KIDNEYS, URETERS, AND SUPRARENAL GLANDS

The nerves to the kidneys and ureters arise from the **renal nerve plexus** and consist of sympathetic, parasympathetic, and visceral afferent fibers (Fig. 2.36*B*). The renal nerve

Accessory Renal Vessels

During their "ascent" to their final site, the embryonic kidneys receive their blood supply and venous drainage from successively more superior vessels. Usually, the inferior vessels degenerate as superior ones take over the blood supply and venous drainage. Failure of some of these vessels to degenerate results in *accessory (or polar) renal arteries and veins.* Variations in the number and position of these vessels occur in about 25% of people (Moore and Dalley, 2005).

Renal and Ureteric Calculi

Excessive distention of the ureter owing to a **renal calculus** (kidney stone) causes severe intermittent pain, *ureteric colic,* as it is gradually forced down the ureter by waves of contraction. The calculus may cause complete or intermittent obstruction of urinary flow (Fig. 2.36*A*). Depending on the level of obstruction, the pain may be referred to the lumbar (loin) or inguinal regions (groin), proximal anterior aspect of thigh, or external genitalia and/or testis. The pain is referred to the cutaneous areas innervated by the spinal cord segments and sensory ganglia, which supply the ureter—mainly T11–L2. Ureteric calculi can be observed and removed with a *nephroscope.* Another technique, *lithotripsy,* focuses a shock wave through the body that breaks the stones into fragments, which then pass with the urine.

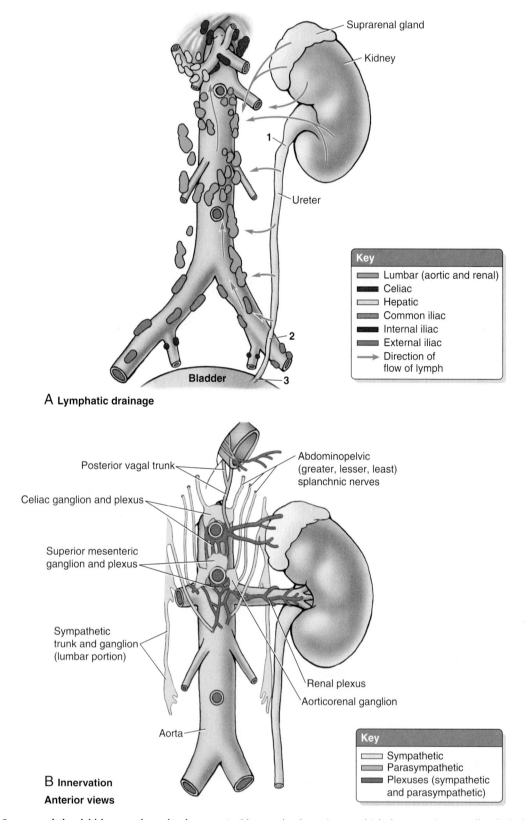

A Lymphatic drainage

Key
- Lumbar (aortic and renal)
- Celiac
- Hepatic
- Common iliac
- Internal iliac
- External iliac
- → Direction of flow of lymph

B Innervation

Anterior views

Key
- Sympathetic
- Parasympathetic
- Plexuses (sympathetic and parasympathetic)

Figure 2.36. Suprarenal gland, kidney, and proximal ureter. A. Observe the three sites at which the ureter is normally relatively constricted: (**1**) the junction of the renal pelvis and ureter, (**2**) as the ureter crosses the external iliac vessels and pelvic brim, and (**3**) as it penetrates the wall of the urinary bladder. **B.** Innervation is demonstrated.

Surface Anatomy of Kidneys and Ureters

The hilum of the left kidney lies near the transpyloric plane, approximately 5 cm from the median plane (Fig. SA2.5). The transpyloric plane passes through the superior pole of the right kidney, which is approximately 2.5 cm lower than the left pole. Posteriorly, the superior parts of the kidneys lie deep to the 11th and 12th ribs. The levels of the kidneys change during respiration and with changes in posture by 2–3 cm in a vertical direction. The kidneys may be impalpable. In lean adults, the inferior pole of the right kidney is palpable by bimanual examination as a firm, smooth, somewhat rounded mass that descends during inspiration. The left kidney is usually not palpable unless it is enlarged or displaced. The ureters occupy a sagittal plane that intersects the tips of the transverse processes of the lumbar vertebrae.

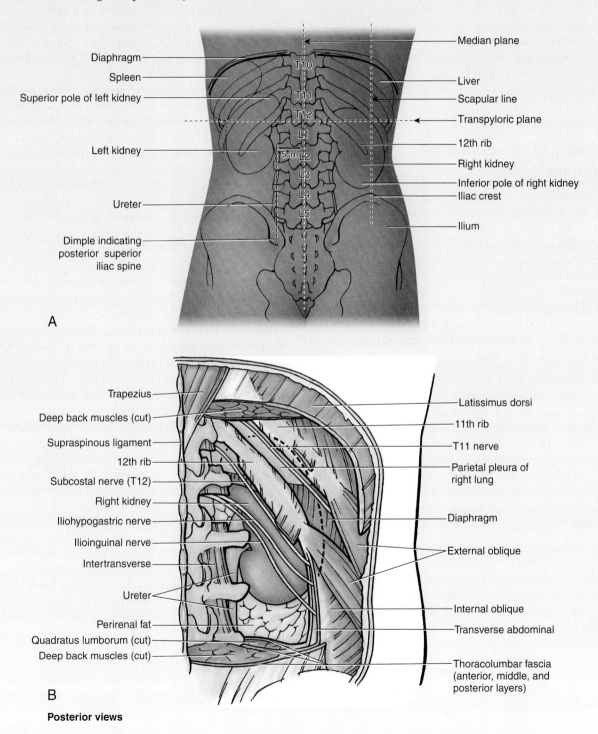

A

Median plane
Diaphragm
Spleen
Superior pole of left kidney
Liver
Scapular line
Transpyloric plane
Left kidney
12th rib
Right kidney
Inferior pole of right kidney
Iliac crest
Ureter
Ilium
Dimple indicating posterior superior iliac spine

T10 T11 T12 L1 L2 L3 L4 L5
5cm

B

Trapezius
Deep back muscles (cut)
Supraspinous ligament
12th rib
Subcostal nerve (T12)
Right kidney
Iliohypogastric nerve
Ilioinguinal nerve
Intertransverse
Ureter
Perirenal fat
Quadratus lumborum (cut)
Deep back muscles (cut)

Latissimus dorsi
11th rib
T11 nerve
Parietal pleura of right lung
Diaphragm
External oblique
Internal oblique
Transverse abdominal
Thoracolumbar fascia (anterior, middle, and posterior layers)

Posterior views

Figure SA2.5.

plexus is supplied by fibers from the abdominopelvic (especially the least) splanchnic nerves (Table 2.9). The nerves to the abdominal part of the ureters derive from the renal, abdominal aortic, and superior hypogastric plexuses. Visceral afferent fibers conveying pain sensations follow the sympathetic fibers retrograde to spinal ganglia and cord segments T11–L2. The **suprarenal glands** have a rich nerve supply from the **celiac plexus** and **abdominopelvic** (greater, lesser, and least) **splanchnic nerves.** The nerves are mainly myelinated presynaptic sympathetic fibers that derive from the lateral horn of the spinal cord and traverse the paravertebral and prevertebral ganglia, without synapse, to be distributed to the chromaffin cells in the suprarenal medulla (see Fig. 2.39).

Summary of Innervation of Abdominal Viscera

The autonomic nerves of the abdomen consist of several different splanchnic nerves and one cranial nerve (the vagus, CNX) which deliver presynaptic sympathetic and parasympathetic fibers, respectively, to the abdominal aortic plexus and its associated sympathetic ganglia. The periarterial extensions of these plexuses deliver postsynaptic sympathetic fibers and the continuation of the parasympathetic fibers to the abdominal viscera, where intrinsic parasympathetic ganglia are located (Figs. 2.37 and 2.38; Table 2.9).

The sympathetic part of the autonomic nervous system in the abdomen consists of:

- *Abdominopelvic splanchnic* nerves consisting of *lower thoracic splanchnic nerves* (greater, lesser, and least) from the thoracic part of the sympathetic trunks and *lumbar splanchnic nerves* from the lumbar part of the sympathetic trunks.
- Prevertebral sympathetic ganglia.
- *Abdominal aortic plexus* and its extensions, the periarterial plexuses. The plexuses are mixed, shared with the parasympathetic nervous system and visceral afferent fibers.

The **abdominopelvic splanchnic nerves** convey presynaptic sympathetic fibers to the abdominopelvic cavity (Fig. 2.38). These presynaptic sympathetic fibers originate from cell bodies in the intermediolateral cell column, or lateral horn, of the gray matter of spinal cord segments T7–L2 or L3. The fibers pass successively through the anterior roots, anterior rami, and white communicating branches of thoracic and upper lumbar spinal nerves to reach the sympathetic trunks. They pass through the paravertebral ganglia of the sympathetic trunks without synapsing to enter the abdominopelvic splanchnic nerves, which convey them to the prevertebral ganglia of the abdominal cavity. The abdominopelvic splanchnic nerves include the lower thoracic splanchnic nerves and the lumbar splanchnic nerves.

The **lower thoracic splanchnic nerves** are the main source of presynaptic sympathetic fibers serving abdominal viscera (Figs. 2.37 and 2.38; Table 2.9). The **greater splanchnic nerve** (from the sympathetic trunk from the T5–T9 or T10 vertebral levels), **lesser splanchnic nerve** (from the T10–T11 levels), and **least splanchnic nerve** (from the T12 level) are the specific thoracic splanchnic nerves that arise from the thoracic part of the sympathetic trunks and pierce the corresponding crus of the diaphragm to convey the presynaptic sympathetic fibers to the celiac, superior mesenteric, and aorticorenal (prevertebral) sympathetic ganglia, respectively.

The **lumbar splanchnic nerves** arise from the abdominal part of the sympathetic trunks. Medially, the lumbar sympathetic trunks give off three to four lumbar splanchnic nerves, which pass to the **intermesenteric, inferior mesenteric,** and **superior hypogastric plexuses,** conveying presynaptic sympathetic fibers to the associated prevertebral ganglia of those plexuses (Figs. 2.37 and 2.38; Table 2.9).

The cell bodies of postsynaptic sympathetic neurons constitute the major prevertebral ganglia that cluster around the roots of the major branches of the abdominal aorta—the *celiac, aorticorenal, superior mesenteric,* and *inferior mesenteric ganglia*—and minor, unnamed prevertebral ganglia that occur within the intermesenteric and superior hypogastric plexuses. The synapse between presynaptic and postsynaptic neurons occurs in the prevertebral ganglia. Postsynaptic sympathetic nerve fibers pass from the prevertebral ganglia to the abdominal visceral through the periarterial plexuses associated with the branches of the abdominal aorta. Sympathetic innervation in the abdomen, as elsewhere, is primarily involved in producing vasoconstriction. In regard to the alimentary tract, it acts to inhibit (slow down or stop) peristalsis. The sympathetic supply to the suprarenal gland is an exception. The secretory cells of the medulla are postsynaptic sympathetic neurons that lack axons or dendrites. Consequently, the **suprarenal medulla** is supplied directly by presynaptic sympathetic neurons (Fig. 2.39).

Visceral afferent fibers conveying pain sensations accompany the sympathetic (visceral motor) fibers. The pain impulses pass retrogradely to those of the motor fibers along the splanchnic nerves to the sympathetic trunk. The fibers then pass through white communicating branches to the anterior rami of the spinal nerves, and then enter the posterior root to the spinal sensory ganglia and spinal cord. The stomach (foregut) receives information from the T6–T9 levels; the small intestine through the transverse colon (midgut), from the T8–T12 levels; and the descending colon (hindgut), from the T12–L2 levels. Starting from the midpoint of the sigmoid colon, visceral pain fibers run with parasympathetic fibers to the S2–S4 sensory ganglia and spinal cord. These are the same spinal cord segments involved in the sympathetic innervation of those portions of the gastrointestinal tract.

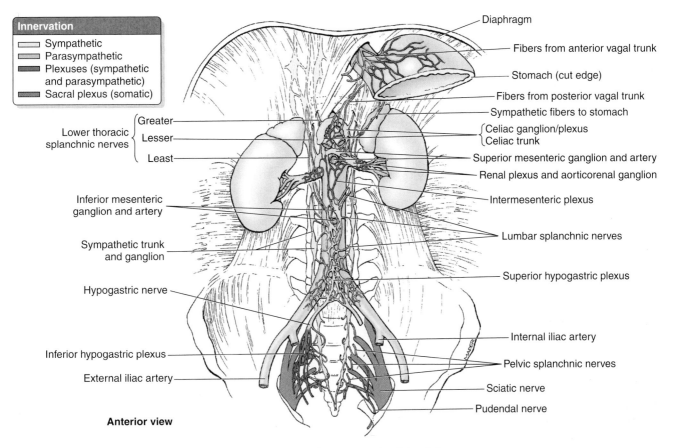

Innervation

☐ Sympathetic
☐ Parasympathetic
☐ Plexuses (sympathetic and parasympathetic)
☐ Sacral plexus (somatic)

Diaphragm
Fibers from anterior vagal trunk
Stomach (cut edge)
Fibers from posterior vagal trunk
Sympathetic fibers to stomach
{ Celiac ganglion/plexus
{ Celiac trunk
Superior mesenteric ganglion and artery
Renal plexus and aorticorenal ganglion
Intermesenteric plexus
Lumbar splanchnic nerves
Superior hypogastric plexus
Internal iliac artery
Pelvic splanchnic nerves
Sciatic nerve
Pudendal nerve

Lower thoracic splanchnic nerves { Greater — Lesser — Least
Inferior mesenteric ganglion and artery
Sympathetic trunk and ganglion
Hypogastric nerve
Inferior hypogastric plexus
External iliac artery
Anterior view

Figure 2.37. Autonomic nerve supply of the abdomen.

Table 2.9 Splanchnic Nerves

Splanchnic Nerves	Autonomic Fiber Type[a]	System	Origin	Destination
A. Cardiopulmonary (cervical and upper thoracic)	Postsynaptic		Cervical and superior thoracic sympathetic trunk	Thoracic cavity (viscera superior to level of diaphragm)
B. Abdominopelvic			Lower thoracic and abdominal sympathetic trunk	Abdominopelvic cavity (prevertebral ganglia serving viscera below level of diaphragm)
1. Lower thoracic	Presynaptic	Sympathetic	Thoracic sympathetic trunk	Abdominal prevertebral ganglia
a. Greater			T5–T9 (T10) level	Celiac ganglia
b. Lesser			T10–T11 level	Aorticorenal
c. Least			T12 level	Other abdominal prevertebral ganglia
2. Lumbar	Presynaptic		Abdominal sympathetic trunk	Superior and inferior mesenteric ganglia and inter-mesenteric hypogastric plexuses
3. Sacral	Presynaptic		Pelvic (sacral) sympathetic trunk	Pelvic prevertebral ganglia
C. Pelvic	Presynaptic	Parasympathetic	Anterior rami of S2–S4 spinal nerves	Intrinsic ganglia of descending and sigmoid colon, rectum, and pelvic viscera

[a]Splanchnic nerves also convey visceral afferent fibers.

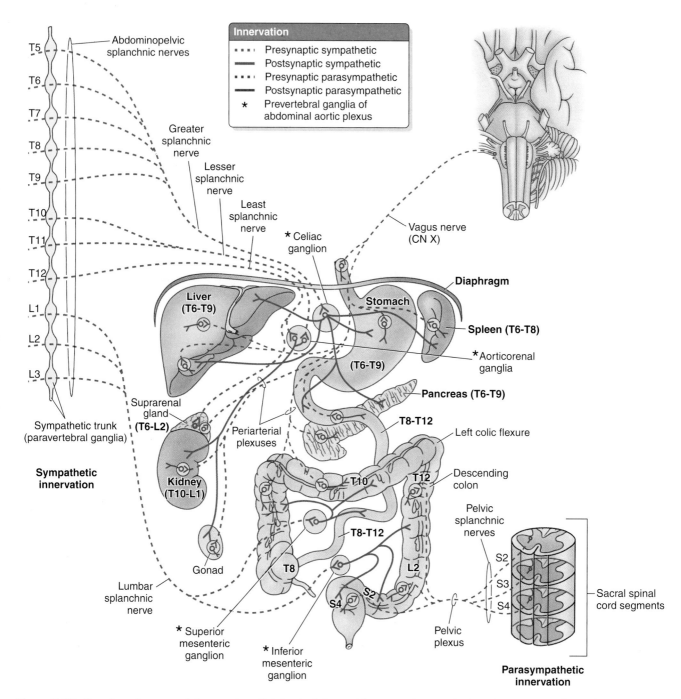

Figure 2.38. Overview of autonomic innervation of abdominal viscera. The approximate spinal cord segments and spinal sensory ganglia involved in sympathetic and visceral afferent innervation of the abdominal visera are listed on each organ.

The **parasympathetic part of the autonomic nervous system in the abdomen** consists of the (Figs. 2.37 and 2.38; Table 2.9):

- *Anterior and posterior vagal trunks.*
- *Pelvic splanchnic nerves.*
- *Abdominal (para-aortic) autonomic nerve plexuses* and their extensions, the periarterial plexuses; the nerve

plexuses are mixed—that is, are shared with the sympathetic nervous system and visceral afferent fibers.
- *Intrinsic (enteric) parasympathetic ganglia.*

The **anterior and posterior vagal trunks** are the continuation of the left and right vagus nerves, which emerge from the esophageal plexus and pass through the esophageal hiatus on the anterior and posterior aspects of

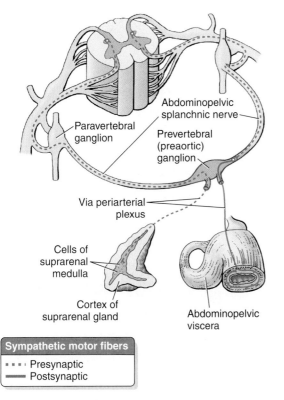

Figure 2.39. Sympathetic motor innervation of suprarenal gland and abdominopelvic viscera.

(labels in figure:)
Paravertebral ganglion
Abdominopelvic splanchnic nerve
Prevertebral (preaortic) ganglion
Via periarterial plexus
Cells of suprarenal medulla
Cortex of suprarenal gland
Abdominopelvic viscera

Sympathetic motor fibers
• • • • Presynaptic
——— Postsynaptic

the esophagus and stomach. The vagus nerves convey presynaptic parasympathetic and visceral afferent fibers (mainly for unconscious sensations associated with reflexes) to the abdominal aortic plexuses and the periarterial plexuses.

The **pelvic splanchnic nerves** are distinct from other splanchnic nerves in that they:

- Have nothing to do with the sympathetic trunks.
- Derive directly from anterior rami of spinal nerves S2–S4.
- Convey presynaptic parasympathetic fibers to the inferior hypogastric (pelvic) plexus.

Presynaptic fibers terminate on the isolated and widely scattered cell bodies of the postsynaptic neurons lying on or within the abdominal viscera, constituting intrinsic ganglia. The presynaptic parasympathetic, and visceral afferent reflex fibers conveyed by the vagus nerves extend to intrinsic ganglia of the lower esophagus, stomach, small intestine (including the duodenum), ascending and most of the transverse colon; those conveyed by the pelvic splanchnic nerves supply the descending and sigmoid parts of the colon, rectum, and pelvic organs. In terms of the alimentary tract, the vagus nerves provide parasympathetic innervation of the smooth muscle and glands of the

gut as far as the left colic flexure; the pelvic splanchnic nerves provide the remainder.

The **abdominal autonomic plexuses** are networks consisting of both sympathetic and parasympathetic fibers that surround the abdominal aorta and its major branches. The celiac, superior mesenteric, and inferior mesenteric plexuses are interconnected. The **prevertebral sympathetic ganglia** are scattered among the celiac and mesenteric plexuses. The **intrinsic parasympathetic ganglia**, such as the *myenteric plexus* (Auerbach plexus) in the muscular coat of the stomach and intestine, are in the walls of the viscera.

The **celiac plexus**, surrounding the root of the celiac trunk, contains right and left *celiac ganglia* (approximately 2 cm long) that unite superior and inferior to the celiac trunk (Fig. 2.37). The *parasympathetic root of the celiac plexus* is a branch of the *posterior vagal trunk,* which contains fibers from the right and left vagus nerves. The *sympathetic roots of the celiac plexus* are the greater and lesser splanchnic nerves.

The **superior mesenteric plexus** and ganglion or ganglia surround the origin of the SMA. The plexus has one median and two lateral branches. The median branch is from the celiac plexus, and the lateral branches arise from the lesser and least splanchnic nerves, sometimes with a contribution from the first lumbar ganglion of the sympathetic trunk. The **inferior mesenteric plexus** surrounds the inferior mesenteric artery and gives off shoots to its branches. It receives a medial root from the intermesenteric plexus and lateral roots from the lumbar ganglia of the sympathetic trunks. An *inferior mesenteric ganglion* may also appear just inferior to the root of the inferior mesenteric artery.

The **intermesenteric plexus** is part of the aortic plexus of nerves between the superior and the inferior mesenteric arteries. It gives rise to renal, testicular or ovarian, and ureteric plexuses. The **superior hypogastric plexus** is continuous with the intermesenteric plexus and inferior mesenteric plexus and lies anterior to the inferior part of the abdominal aorta and its bifurcation. Right and left **hypogastric nerves** join the superior hypogastric plexus to the **inferior hypogastric plexus**. The superior hypogastric plexus supplies *ureteric* and *testicular plexuses* and a plexus on each common iliac artery. The right and left **inferior hypogastric plexuses** are formed by hypogastric nerves from the superior hypogastric plexus. The right and left plexuses are situated on the sides of the rectum, uterine cervix, and urinary bladder. The plexuses receive small branches from the superior sacral sympathetic ganglia and the sacral parasympathetic outflow from the S2–S4 spinal nerves (**pelvic parasympathetic splanchnic nerves**). Extensions of the inferior hypogastric plexus send autonomic fibers along the blood vessels, which form visceral plexuses on the walls of the pelvic viscera (e.g., *the rectal and vesical plexuses*).

Visceral Referred Pain

Pain arising from a viscus such as the stomach varies from dull to severe; however, the pain is poorly localized; it radiates to the dermatome level that receives visceral sensory fibers from the organ concerned (Table B2.2).

Table B2.2 Visceral Referred Pain

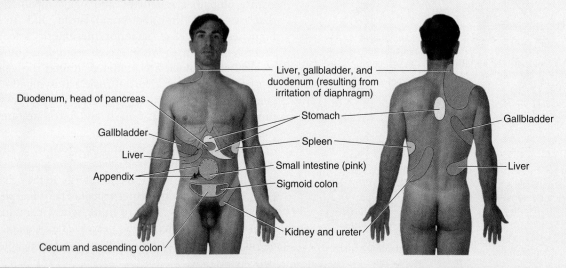

Origin	Nerve Supply	Spinal Cord[a]	Referred Site and Clinical Example
Stomach	Anterior and posterior vagal trunks; presynaptic sympathetic fibers reach celiac and other ganglia through greater splanchnic nerves	T6–T9 or T10	Epigastric and left hypochondriac regions (e.g., gastric peptic ulcer)
Duodenum	Vagus nerves; presynaptic sympathetic fibers reach celiac and superior mesenteric ganglia through greater splanchnic nerves	T5–T9 or T10	Epigastric region (e.g., duodenal peptic ulcer); right shoulder (if ulcer perforates)
Pancreatic head	Vagus and thoracic splanchnic nerves	T8–T9	Inferior part of epigastric region (e.g., pancreatitis)
Small intestine (jejunum and ileum)	Posterior vagal trunks; presynaptic sympathetic fibers reach celiac ganglion through greater splanchnic nerves	T5–T9	Periumbilical region (e.g., acute intestinal obstruction)
Colon	Vagus nerves; presynaptic sympathetic fibers reach celiac, superior mesenteric, and inferior mesenteric ganglia through greater splanchnic nerves; parasympathetic supply to distal colon derived from pelvic splanchnic nerves through hypogastric nerves and inferior hypogastric plexus	T10–T12 (proximal colon) L1–L3 (distal colon)	Hypogastric region (e.g., ulcerative colitis); left lower quadrant (e.g., sigmoiditis)
Spleen	Celiac plexus, especially from greater splanchnic nerve	T6–T8	Left hypochondriac region (e.g., splenic infarct)
Appendix	Sympathetic and parasympathetic nerves from superior mesenteric plexus; afferent nerve fibers accompany sympathetic nerves to T10 segment of spinal cord	T10	Periumbilical region and later to right lower quadrant (e.g., appendicitis)
Gallbladder and liver	Nerves derived from celiac plexus (sympathetic), vagus nerve (parasympathetic), and right phrenic nerve (sensory)	T6–T9	Epigastric region and right hypochondriac region; may cause pain on posterior thoracic wall or right shoulder owing to diaphragmatic irritation
Kidneys and ureters	Nerves arise from renal plexus and consist of sympathetic, parasympathetic, and visceral afferent fibers from thoracic and lumbar splanchnics and vagus nerve	T11–T12	Small of back, flank (lumbar quadrant), extending to groin (inguinal region) and genitals (e.g., renal or ureteric calculi)

[a]Pain is perceived as originating in areas supplied by the somatic nerves entering the spinal cord at the same segment as the sensory nerves from the organ producing the pain.

Diaphragm

The **diaphragm** is a dome-shaped, musculotendinous partition separating the thoracic and abdominal cavities. The diaphragm, the chief muscle of inspiration, forms the convex floor of the thoracic cavity and the concave roof of the abdominal cavity (Fig. 2.40). The diaphragm descends during inspiration; however, only its central part moves because its periphery, as the fixed origin of the muscle, attaches to the inferior margin of the thoracic cage and the superior lumbar vertebrae. The diaphragm curves superiorly into **right** and **left domes**; normally, the right dome is higher than the left owing to the presence of the liver. During expiration, the right dome reaches as high as the 5th rib and the left dome ascends to the 5th intercostal space. The level of the domes of the diaphragm varies according to the phase of respiration (inspiration or expiration), posture (e.g., supine or standing), and size and degree of distention of the abdominal viscera.

The muscular part of the diaphragm is situated peripherally with fibers that converge radially on the trifoliate central aponeurotic part, the **central tendon.** This tendon has no bony attachments and is incompletely divided into three leaves, resembling a wide cloverleaf. Although it lies near the center of the diaphragm, the central tendon is closer to the anterior part of the thorax. The superior aspect of the central tendon is fused with the inferior surface of the fibrous pericardium (Fig. 2.41A).The surrounding muscular part of the diaphragm forms a continuous sheet; however, for descriptive purposes it is divided into three parts, based on the peripheral attachments:

- A **sternal part**, consisting of two muscular slips that attach to the posterior aspect of the xiphoid process of the sternum; this part is not always present.
- A **costal part**, consisting of wide muscular slips that attach to the internal surfaces of the inferior six costal cartilages and their adjoining ribs on each side; this part forms the domes of the diaphragm.
- A **lumbar part**, arising from two aponeurotic arches, the *medial* and *lateral arcuate ligaments,* and the three superior lumbar vertebrae; this part forms right and left muscular crura that ascend to the central tendon.

The **crura of the diaphragm** are musculotendinous bundles that arise from the anterior surfaces of the bodies of the superior three lumbar vertebrae, the anterior longitudinal ligament, and the IV discs. The **right crus,** larger and longer than the left crus, arises from the first three of four lumbar vertebrae, whereas the **left crus** arises from only the first two or three. The crura are united by the **median arcuate ligament,** which passes over the anterior surface of the aorta. The diaphragm is also attached on each side to the medial and **lateral arcuate ligaments,** which are thickenings of the fascia covering the psoas and quadratus lumborum muscles, respectively.

Diaphragmatic Apertures

The **diaphragmatic apertures** permit structures (e.g., esophagus, vessels, nerves, and lymphatics) to pass between the thorax and the abdomen (Fig. 2.40). The three large apertures for the IVC, esophagus, and aorta are the caval opening, esophageal hiatus, and aortic hiatus, respectively.

CAVAL OPENING

The **caval opening** is an aperture in the central tendon primarily for the IVC. Also passing through the caval opening are terminal branches of the right phrenic nerve and some lymphatic vessels on their way from the liver to the middle phrenic and mediastinal lymph nodes. The caval opening is located to the right of the median plane at the junction of the tendon's right and middle leaves. The most superior of the three diaphragmatic apertures, the caval opening lies at the level of the IV disc between the T8 and the T9 vertebrae. The IVC is adherent to the margin of the opening; consequently, when the diaphragm contracts during inspiration, it widens the opening and dilates the IVC. These changes facilitate blood flow to the heart through this large vein.

ESOPHAGEAL HIATUS

The **esophageal hiatus** is an oval aperture for the esophagus in the muscle of the right crus of the diaphragm at the level of the T10 vertebra. The fibers of the right crus decussate (cross one another) inferior to the hiatus, forming a muscular sphincter for the esophagus that constricts it when the diaphragm contracts. In 30% of individuals, a superficial muscular bundle from the left crus contributes to the formation of the right margin of the hiatus. The esophageal hiatus also transmits the anterior and posterior vagal trunks, esophageal branches of the left gastric vessels, and a few lymphatic vessels.

AORTIC HIATUS

The **aortic hiatus** is an opening posterior to the diaphragm for the aorta. The aortic hiatus transmits the aorta, azygos vein, and the thoracic duct. Because the aorta does not pierce the diaphragm, blood flow through it is not affected by the muscle's movements during respiration. The aorta passes between the crura of the diaphragm posterior to the median arcuate ligament, which is at the level of the T12 vertebra.

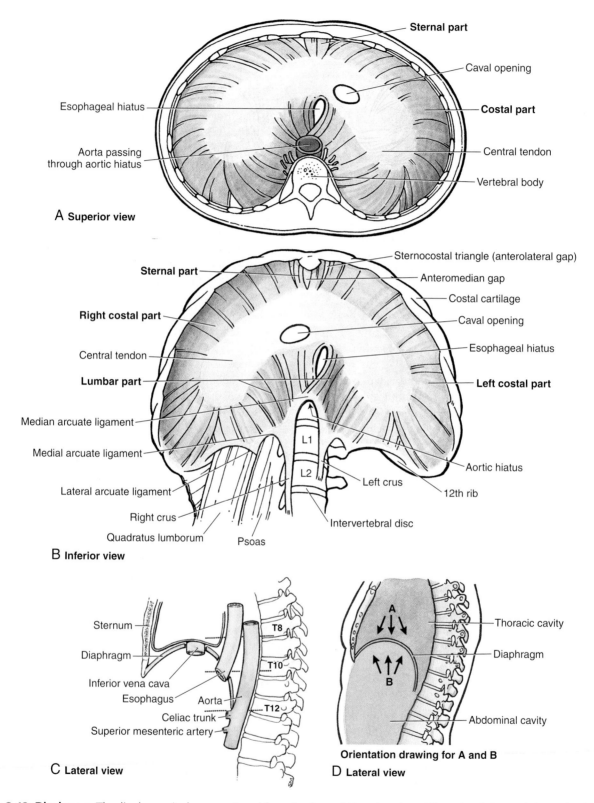

A Superior view

B Inferior view

C Lateral view

Orientation drawing for A and B

D Lateral view

Figure 2.40. Diaphragm. The diaphragm is shown as viewed from the thorax (**A**) and as viewed from the abdomen (**B**). **C.** The diaphragmatic apertures are demonstrated. The *caval foramen* for the IVC is most anterior at the T8 level to the right of the midline. The *esophageal hiatus* is intermediate at the T10 level and to the left of the midline. The *aortic hiatus* is in the midline at the T12 level. (**D**) Orientation drawing for A and B.

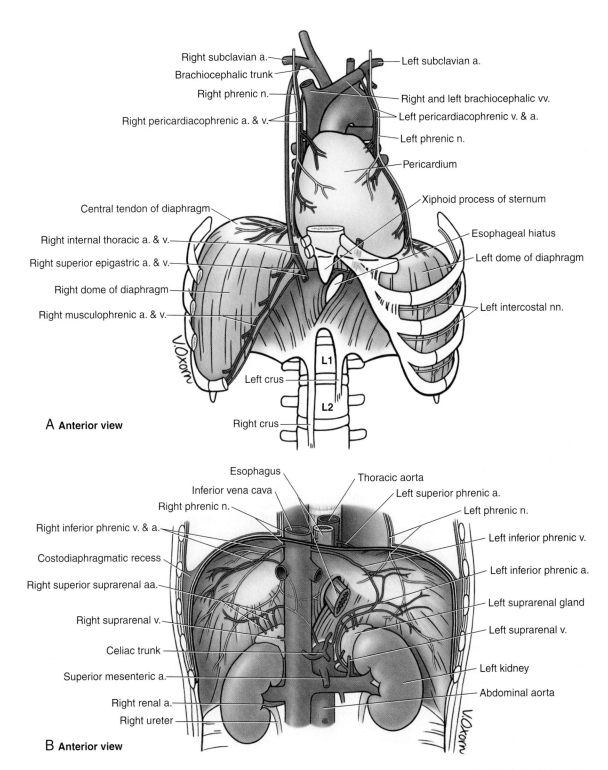

Right subclavian a.
Brachiocephalic trunk
Right phrenic n.
Right pericardiacophrenic a. & v.

Central tendon of diaphragm
Right internal thoracic a. & v.
Right superior epigastric a. & v.
Right dome of diaphragm
Right musculophrenic a. & v.

Left crus
Right crus

A Anterior view

Left subclavian a.
Right and left brachiocephalic vv.
Left pericardiacophrenic v. & a.
Left phrenic n.
Pericardium
Xiphoid process of sternum
Esophageal hiatus
Left dome of diaphragm
Left intercostal nn.

L1
L2

Esophagus
Inferior vena cava
Right phrenic n.
Right inferior phrenic v. & a.
Costodiaphragmatic recess
Right superior suprarenal aa.
Right suprarenal v.
Celiac trunk
Superior mesenteric a.
Right renal a.
Right ureter

B Anterior view

Thoracic aorta
Left superior phrenic a.
Left phrenic n.
Left inferior phrenic v.
Left inferior phrenic a.
Left suprarenal gland
Left suprarenal v.
Left kidney
Abdominal aorta

Figure 2.41. Blood vessels and lymphatics of diaphragm. The arteries and veins of the superior (**A**) and inferior (**B**) surfaces are demonstrated.

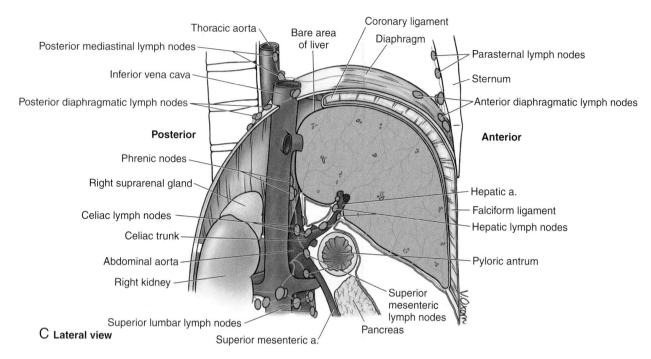

Figure 2.41. *(Continued)* **C.** The lymphatics are shown.

OTHER APERTURES IN DIAPHRAGM

There is a small opening, the **sternocostal triangle (foramen)**, between the sternal and the costal attachments of the diaphragm. This triangle transmits lymphatic vessels from the diaphragmatic surface of the liver and the superior epigastric vessels. The sympathetic trunks pass deep to the medial arcuate ligament. There are two small apertures in each crus of the diaphragm; one transmits the greater and the other the lesser splanchnic nerve.

Vasculature and Nerves of Diaphragm

The **arteries of the diaphragm** form a branch-like pattern on both its superior and inferior surfaces. The arteries supplying the superior surface of the diaphragm are the **pericardiacophrenic and musculophrenic arteries**, branches of internal thoracic artery, and the **superior phrenic arteries** arising from thoracic aorta (Fig. 2.41; Table 2.10). The arteries supplying the inferior surface of the diaphragm are the **inferior phrenic arteries**, which typically are the first

Table 2.10 Vessels and Nerves of Diaphragm

Vessels and Nerves	Superior Surface of Diaphragm	Inferior Surface of Diaphragm
Arterial supply	Superior phrenic arteries from thoracic aorta; musculophrenic and pericardiacophrenic arteries from internal thoracic arteries	Inferior phrenic arteries from abdominal aorta
Venous drainage	Musculophrenic and pericardiacophrenic veins drain into internal thoracic veins; superior phrenic vein (right side) drains into IVC	Inferior phrenic veins: right vein drains into IVC; left vein is doubled and drains into IVC and left suprarenal vein
Lymphatic drainage	Diaphragmatic lymph nodes to phrenic nodes, then to parasternal and posterior mediastinal nodes	Superior lumbar lymph nodes; lymphatic plexuses on superior and inferior surfaces communicate freely
Innervation	*Motor supply:* phrenic nerves (C3–C5) *Sensory supply:* centrally by phrenic nerves (C3–C5); peripherally by intercostal nerves (T5–T11) and subcostal nerves (T12)	

IVC, inferior vena cava.

branches of the abdominal aorta; however, they may arise from the celiac trunk.

The veins draining the superior surface of the diaphragm are the **pericardiacophrenic** and **musculophrenic veins,** which empty into the *internal thoracic veins,* and on the right side, a *superior phrenic vein,* which drains into the IVC. Posteriorly, some veins drain into the *azygos and hemiazygos veins.* The inferior phrenic veins drain blood from the inferior surface of the diaphragm. The **right inferior phrenic vein** usually opens into the IVC, whereas the **left inferior phrenic vein** is usually double, with one branch passing anterior to the esophageal hiatus to end in the IVC and the other, more posterior branch usually joining the left suprarenal vein.

The **lymphatic plexuses** on the thoracic and abdominal surfaces of the diaphragm communicate freely (Fig. 2.41C). The anterior and posterior **diaphragmatic lymph nodes** are on the thoracic surface of the diaphragm. Lymph from these nodes drains into the *parasternal, posterior mediastinal,* and *phrenic lymph nodes.* Lymph vessels from the abdominal surface of the diaphragm drain into the anterior diaphragmatic, phrenic, and *superior lumbar (caval/aortic) lymph nodes.* Lymphatic vessels are dense on the inferior surface of the diaphragm, constituting the primary means for absorption of peritoneal fluid and substances introduced by intraperitoneal (I.P.) injection.

The entire motor supply to the diaphragm is from the **right** and **left phrenic nerves,** each of which is distributed to half of the diaphragm and arises from the anterior rami of the C3–C5 segments of the spinal cord. The phrenic nerves also supply sensory fibers (pain and proprioception) to most of the diaphragm. Peripheral parts of the diaphragm receive their sensory nerve supply from the **intercostal nerves** (lower six or seven) and the **subcostal nerves.**

ACTIONS OF THE DIAPHRAGM

When the diaphragm contracts, its domes move inferiorly so that the convexity of the diaphragm is somewhat flattened. Although this movement is often described as the "descent of the diaphragm," only the domes of the diaphragm descend; its periphery remains attached to the ribs and cartilages of the inferior six ribs. As the diaphragm descends, it pushes the abdominal viscera inferiorly. This increases the volume of the thoracic cavity and decreases the intrathoracic pressure, resulting in air being taken into the lungs. In addition, the volume of the abdominal cavity decreases slightly and the intra-abdominal pressure increases somewhat. Movements of the diaphragm are also important in circulation because the increased intra-abdominal pressure and decreased intrathoracic pressure help return venous blood to the heart. When the diaphragm contracts, compressing the abdominal viscera, blood in the IVC is forced superiorly into the heart.

Referred Pain from Diaphragm

Pain from the diaphragm radiates to two different areas because of the difference in the sensory nerve supply of the diaphragm. Pain resulting from irritation of the diaphragmatic pleura or diaphragmatic peritoneum is referred to the shoulder region, the area of skin supplied by the C3–C5 segments of the spinal cord. These segments also contribute anterior rami to the phrenic nerves. Irritation of peripheral regions of the diaphragm, innervated by the inferior intercostal nerves, is more localized, being referred to the skin over the costal margins of the anterolateral abdominal wall.

Section of Phrenic Nerve

Section of a phrenic nerve in the neck results in complete paralysis and eventual atrophy of the muscular part of the corresponding half of the diaphragm, except in persons who have an accessory phrenic nerve (see Chapter 8). *Paralysis of a hemidiaphragm* can be recognized radiographically by its permanent elevation and paradoxical movement. Instead of descending on inspiration, it is forced superiorly by the increased intra-abdominal pressure secondary to descent of the opposite, unparalyzed hemidiaphragm.

Rupture of Diaphragm and Herniation of Viscera

Rupture of the diaphragm and herniation of viscera can result from a sudden large increase in either the intrathoracic or intra-abdominal pressure—for example, owing to severe trauma during a motor vehicle accident. When a traumatic diaphragmatic hernia occurs, upper abdominal organs (e.g., stomach, small intestine, and transverse colon) may herniate into the thorax through the lumbocostal triangle. This triangle is of variable size and is located between the costal and the lumbar parts of the diaphragm.

Posterior Abdominal Wall

The posterior abdominal wall is composed mainly—from deep (posterior) to superficial (anterior)—of the (Figs. 2.37 and 2.42):

* Five lumbar vertebrae and associated IV discs.
* Posterior abdominal wall muscles—psoas, quadratus lumborum, iliacus, transverse abdominal, and oblique muscles.
* Lumbar plexus, composed of the anterior rami of lumbar spinal nerves.
* Fascia, including thoracolumbar fascia.
* Diaphragm, contributing to the superior part of the posterior wall.
* Fat, nerves, vessels, and lymph nodes.

Fascia of Posterior Abdominal Wall

The posterior abdominal wall is covered with a continuous layer of endoabdominal fascia, which lies between the parietal peritoneum and the muscles. The fascia lining the posterior abdominal wall is continuous with the transversalis fascia that lines the transverse abdominal muscle (Fig. 2.32). It is customary to name the fascia according to the structure it covers. The **psoas fascia** covering the psoas major (psoas sheath) is attached medially to the lumbar vertebrae and pelvic brim. The psoas fascia is thickened superiorly to form the **medial arcuate ligament** and fuses laterally with the quadratus lumborum and thoracolumbar fascia (Fig. 2.40*B*). Inferior to the iliac crest, the psoas fascia is continuous with the part of the iliac fascia covering the iliacus muscle.

The **thoracolumbar fascia** is an extensive fascial complex that has anterior, middle, and posterior layers with muscles enclosed between them (Fig. 2.32). It is thin and transparent where it covers thoracic parts of the deep muscles but is thick and strong in the lumbar region. The **posterior and middle layers of thoracolumbar fascia** enclose the vertical deep back muscles (erector spinae). The lumbar part of this posterior layer, extending between the 12th rib and the iliac crest, attaches laterally to the internal oblique and transverse abdominal muscles. The **anterior layer of the thoracolumbar fascia** (quadratus lumborum fascia) covering the quadratus lumborum muscle attaches to the anterior surfaces of the transverse processes of the lumbar vertebrae, the iliac crest, and the 12th rib and is continuous laterally with the aponeurotic origin of the transverse abdominal muscle. The anterior layer of the thoracolumbar fascia is thickened superiorly to form the **lateral arcuate ligaments** and is adherent inferiorly to the iliolumbar ligaments (Fig. 2.40*B*).

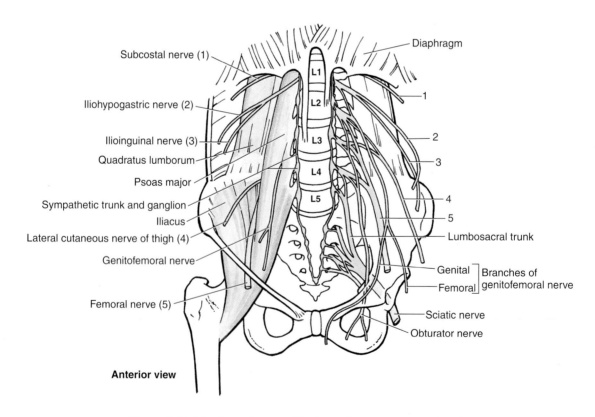

Figure 2.42. Muscles and nerves. *Numbers,* refer to nerves on right side.

Psoas Abscess

An abscess resulting from tuberculosis in the lumbar region tends to spread from the vertebrae into the psoas sheath, where it produces a *psoas abscess*. As a consequence, the psoas fascia thickens to form a strong stocking-like tube. Pus from the psoas abscess passes inferiorly along the psoas within this fascial tube over the pelvic brim and deep to the inguinal ligament. The pus usually surfaces in the superior part of the thigh. Pus can also reach the psoas sheath by passing from the posterior mediastinum when the thoracic vertebrae are diseased.

Posterior Abdominal Pain

The *iliopsoas* has extensive and clinically important relations to the kidneys, ureters, cecum, appendix, sigmoid colon, pancreas, lumbar lymph nodes, and nerves of the posterior abdominal wall. When any of these structures is diseased, movement of the iliopsoas usually causes pain. When intra-abdominal inflammation is suspected, the **iliopsoas test** is performed. The person is asked to lie on the unaffected side and to extend the thigh on the affected side against the resistance of the examiner's hand. Pain resulting from this maneuver is a *positive psoas sign*. An acutely inflamed appendix, for example, will produce a positive sign.

Muscles of Posterior Abdominal Wall

The main paired muscles in the posterior abdominal wall (Fig. 2.42) are the:

- **Psoas major,** passing inferolaterally.
- **Iliacus,** lying along the lateral sides of the inferior part of the psoas major; together the psoas and iliacus form the **iliopsoas.**
- **Quadratus lumborum,** lying adjacent to the transverse processes of the lumbar vertebrae and lateral to the superior parts of the psoas major.

The attachments, nerve supply, and main actions of these muscles are summarized in Table 2.11.

Nerves of Posterior Abdominal Wall

There are somatic and autonomic nerves in the posterior abdominal wall. The somatic nerves will be discussed here.

The **subcostal nerves,** the anterior rami of T12, arise in the thorax, pass posterior to the lateral arcuate ligaments into the abdomen, and run inferolaterally on the anterior surface of the quadratus lumborum muscle (Fig. 2.42). They pass through the transverse abdominal and internal oblique muscles to supply the external oblique and skin of the anterolateral abdominal wall.

Table 2.11 Main Muscles of Posterior Abdominal Wall

Muscle	Superior Attachments	Inferior Attachment(s)	Innervation	Actions
Psoas major[a]	Transverse processes of lumbar vertebrae; sides of bodies of T12–L5 vertebrae and intervening IV discs	By a strong tendon to lesser trochanter of femur	Lumbar plexus via anterior branches of nerves L2–L4	Acting inferiorly with iliacus, flexes thigh Acting superiorly, flexes vertebral column laterally Used to balance the trunk When sitting, acts inferiorly with iliacus to flex trunk
Iliacus[a]	Superior two thirds of iliac fossa, ala of sacrum, and anterior sacroiliac ligaments	Lesser trochanter of femur and shaft inferior to it, and to psoas major tendon	Femoral nerve (L2–L4)	Flexes thigh and stabilizes hip joint Acts with psoas major
Quadratus lumborum	Medial half of inferior border of 12th rib and tips of lumbar transverse processes	Iliolumbar ligament and internal lip of iliac crest	Anterior branches of T12 and L1–L4 nerves	Extends and laterally flexes vertebral column Fixes 12th rib during inspiration

[a]Psoas major and iliacus muscles are often described together as the iliopsoas muscle when flexion of the thigh is discussed (see Chapter 5). *The iliopsoas is the chief flexor of the thigh;* and when thigh is fixed, it is a strong flexor of the trunk (e.g., during sit-ups).
IV, intervertebral.

The **lumbar spinal nerves** pass from the spinal cord through the IV foramina inferior to the corresponding vertebrae, where they divide into posterior and anterior rami. Each ramus contains sensory and motor fibers. The posterior rami pass posteriorly to supply the deep back muscles and skin of the back, whereas the anterior rami pass inferolaterally through the psoas major to supply the skin and muscles of inferiormost trunk and lower limb. The proximal parts of the anterior rami of L1–L2 or L3 give rise to *white communicating* (L. *rami communicantes*) *branches* that convey presynaptic sympathetic fibers to the lumbar sympathetic trunks. The lumbar sympathetic trunks descend on the anterolateral aspects of the bodies of the lumbar vertebrae in a groove formed by the psoas major.

For the innervation of the abdominal wall and lower limbs, synapses occur in the sympathetic ganglia of the sympathetic trunks. Postsynaptic sympathetic fibers then travel via the *gray communicating branches* to the anterior rami. The anterior rami become the thoracoabdominal and subcostal nerves, and the lumbar plexus (somatic nerves) and the accompanying postsynaptic sympathetic fibers stimulate vasomotor, sudomotor, and pilomotor action in the distribution of these nerves. The *lumbar splanchnic nerves* that innervate pelvic viscera are described in Chapter 4.

The **lumbar plexus of nerves** is in the posterior part of the psoas major, anterior to the lumbar transverse processes (Fig. 2.42). This nerve network is composed of the anterior rami of L1–L4 nerves. All rami receive *gray communicating branches* from the sympathetic trunks. The following nerves are **branches of the lumbar plexus**; the three largest are listed first:

- The **obturator nerve** (L2–L4) emerges from the medial border of the psoas major and passes through the pelvis to the medial thigh, supplying the adductor muscles.
- The **femoral nerve** (L2–L4) emerges from the lateral border of the psoas major and innervates the iliacus and passes deep to the inguinal ligament to the anterior thigh, supplying the flexors of the hip and extensors of the knee.
- The **lumbosacral trunk** (L4, L5) passes over the ala (wing) of the sacrum and descends into the pelvis to participate in the formation of the sacral plexus along with the anterior rami of the S1–S4 nerves.
- The **ilioinguinal and iliohypogastric nerves** (L1) arise from the anterior ramus of L1 and enter the abdomen posterior to the medial arcuate ligaments and pass inferolaterally, anterior to the quadratus lumborum. They pierce the transverse abdominal muscles near the anterior superior iliac spines and pass through the internal and external oblique muscles to supply the abdominal muscles and skin of the pubic and inguinal regions.

- The **genitofemoral nerve** (L1, L2) pierces the anterior surface of the psoas major and runs inferiorly on it deep to the psoas fascia; it divides lateral to the common and external iliac arteries into femoral and genital branches.
- The **lateral cutaneous nerve of the thigh** (L2, L3) runs inferolaterally on the iliacus muscle and enters the thigh posterior to the inguinal ligament, just medial to the anterior superior iliac spine; it supplies the skin on the anterolateral surface of the thigh.

Vasculature of Posterior Abdominal Wall

Most arteries supplying the posterior abdominal wall arise from the **abdominal aorta** (Fig. 2.43); however, the **subcostal arteries** arise from the thoracic aorta and distribute inferior to the 12th rib. The abdominal aorta, approximately 13 cm in length, begins at the aortic hiatus in the diaphragm at the level of the T12 vertebra and ends at the level of the L4 vertebra by dividing into two common iliac arteries. The **level of the aortic bifurcation** is 2–3 cm inferior and to the left of the umbilicus at the level of the iliac crests. Four or five pairs of **lumbar arteries** arise from the abdominal aorta and supply the lumbar vertebrae, back muscles, and posterior abdominal wall.

The **common iliac arteries**—terminal branches of the abdominal aorta, diverge and run inferolaterally, following the medial border of the psoas muscles to the pelvic brim. Here each common iliac artery divides into the **internal** and **external iliac arteries**. The internal iliac artery enters the pelvis; its course and branches are described in Chapter 4. The external iliac artery follows the iliopsoas muscle. Just before leaving the abdomen, the external iliac artery gives rise to the **inferior epigastric** and **deep iliac circumflex arteries**, which supply the anterolateral abdominal wall.

From superior to inferior, the important *anterior relations* of the abdominal aorta are the celiac plexus and ganglion, body of pancreas, splenic and left renal veins, horizontal part of the duodenum, and the coils of small intestine (Table 2.6). The left lumbar veins pass *posterior* to the aorta to reach the IVC. On the *right*, the aorta is related to the azygos vein, chyle cistern, right crus of diaphragm, and right celiac ganglion. On the *left*, the aorta is related to the left crus of diaphragm and left celiac ganglion. The branches of the abdominal aorta may be described as visceral or parietal and paired or unpaired (Fig. 2.43).

The **paired visceral branches** (vertebral level of origin) are the:

- Suprarenal arteries (L1).
- Renal arteries (L1).
- Gonadal arteries, the ovarian or testicular arteries (L2).

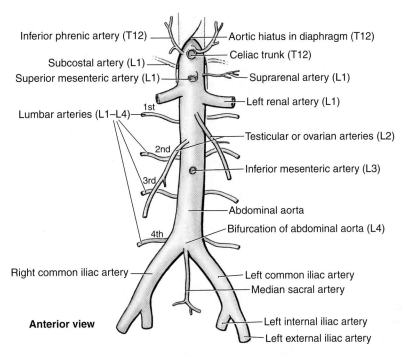

Inferior phrenic artery (T12)
Subcostal artery (L1)
Superior mesenteric artery (L1)
Lumbar arteries (L1–L4)
1st
2nd
3rd
4th
Right common iliac artery
Anterior view

Aortic hiatus in diaphragm (T12)
Celiac trunk (T12)
Suprarenal artery (L1)
Left renal artery (L1)
Testicular or ovarian arteries (L2)
Inferior mesenteric artery (L3)
Abdominal aorta
Bifurcation of abdominal aorta (L4)
Left common iliac artery
Median sacral artery
Left internal iliac artery
Left external iliac artery

Figure 2.43. Abdominal aorta and its branches. The vertebral level is indicated in parentheses.

The **unpaired visceral branches** (vertebral level of origin) are the:

- Celiac trunk (T12).
- Superior mesenteric artery (L1).
- Inferior mesenteric artery (L3).

The **paired parietal branches** are the:

- Inferior phrenic arteries that arise just inferior to the aortic hiatus and supply the inferior surface of the diaphragm and the suprarenal glands.
- Lumbar arteries that pass around the sides of the superior four lumbar vertebrae to supply the posterior abdominal wall.

The **unpaired parietal branch** is the:

- **Median sacral artery,** which arises from the aorta at its bifurcation and descends into the lesser pelvis.

The **veins of the posterior abdominal wall** are tributaries of the **inferior vena cava,** except for the **left testicular** or **ovarian vein,** which enters the **left renal vein** instead of entering the IVC (Fig. 2.44). The IVC, the largest vein in the body, has no valves except for a variable, non-functional one at its orifice in the right atrium of the heart. The IVC returns poorly oxygenated blood from the lower limbs, most of the back, the abdominal walls, and the abdominopelvic viscera. Blood from the viscera passes

through the *portal venous system* and the liver before entering the IVC via the hepatic veins. The IVC begins anterior to L5 vertebra by the union of the common iliac veins. This union occurs approximately 2.5 cm to the right of the median plane, inferior to the bifurcation of the aorta and posterior to the proximal part of the right *common iliac artery.* The IVC ascends on the right side of the bodies of the L3–L5 vertebrae and on the psoas major muscle to the right of the aorta. The IVC leaves the abdomen by passing through the caval opening in the diaphragm to enter the thorax. The tributaries of the IVC correspond to branches of the aorta:

- Common iliac veins, formed by union of external and internal iliac veins.
- The 3rd (L3) and 4th (L4) lumbar veins.
- Right testicular or ovarian veins (the left testicular or ovarian veins usually drain into the left renal vein).
- Right and left renal veins.
- Ascending lumbar veins (the azygos and hemiazygos veins arise, in part, from ascending lumbar veins (see Chapter 1); the ascending lumbar and azygos veins connect the IVC and superior vena cava, either directly or indirectly.
- Right suprarenal vein (the left suprarenal vein usually drains into the left renal vein).
- Inferior phrenic veins.
- Hepatic veins.

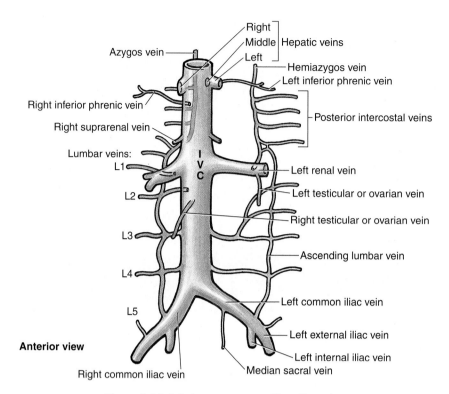

Figure 2.44. Inferior vena cava and its tributaries.

Lymphatics of Posterior Abdominal Wall

Lymphatic vessels and **lymph nodes** lie along the aorta, IVC, and iliac vessels. The **common iliac lymph nodes** receive lymph from the external and internal iliac lymph nodes. Lymph from the common iliac lymph nodes passes to the **lumbar lymph nodes** (Fig. 2.45A). These nodes receive lymph directly from the posterior abdominal wall, kidneys, ureters, testes or ovaries, uterus, and uterine tubes. They also receive lymph from the descending colon, pelvis, and lower limbs through the **inferior mesenteric** and **common iliac lymph nodes**. Efferent lymphatic vessels from the lymph nodes form the right and left **lumbar lymph trunks**. Lymphatic vessels from the intestine, liver, spleen, and pancreas pass along the celiac, superior, and inferior mesenteric arteries to the **preaortic lymph nodes** (celiac and superior and inferior mesenteric nodes) scattered around the origins of these arteries from the aorta. Efferent vessels from these nodes form the **intestinal lymphatic trunks**, which may be single or multiple and participate in the confluence of lymphatic trunks that gives rise to the thoracic duct.

The **chyle cistern** is a thin-walled sac at the inferior end of the **thoracic duct**, variable in size and shape, located anterior to the bodies of the L1 and L2 vertebrae between the right crus of the diaphragm and the aorta (Fig. 2.45B). A pair of **descending thoracic lymphatic trunks** carry lymph from the lower six intercostal spaces on each side. Consequently, essentially all the lymphatic drainage from the lower half of the body (deep lymphatic drainage inferior to the level of the diaphragm and all superficial drainage inferior to the level of the umbilicus) converges in the abdomen to enter the beginning of the thoracic duct. The thoracic duct begins with the convergence of the main lymphatic ducts of the abdomen, which only in a small proportion of individuals takes the form of the commonly depicted, thin-walled sac—the *chyle cistern*. More often there is merely a simple or plexiform convergence at this level of the right and left lumbar lymphatic trunks, the intestinal lymph trunk(s), and a pair of **descending thoracic lymphatic trunks** (which carry lymph from the lower six intercostals spaces). The thoracic duct ascends through the aortic hiatus in the diaphragm into the posterior mediastinum, where it collects more parietal and visceral drainage, particularly from the left upper quadrant of the body, and ultimately ends by entering the venous system at the junction of the **left subclavian and internal jugular veins** (the left venous angle).

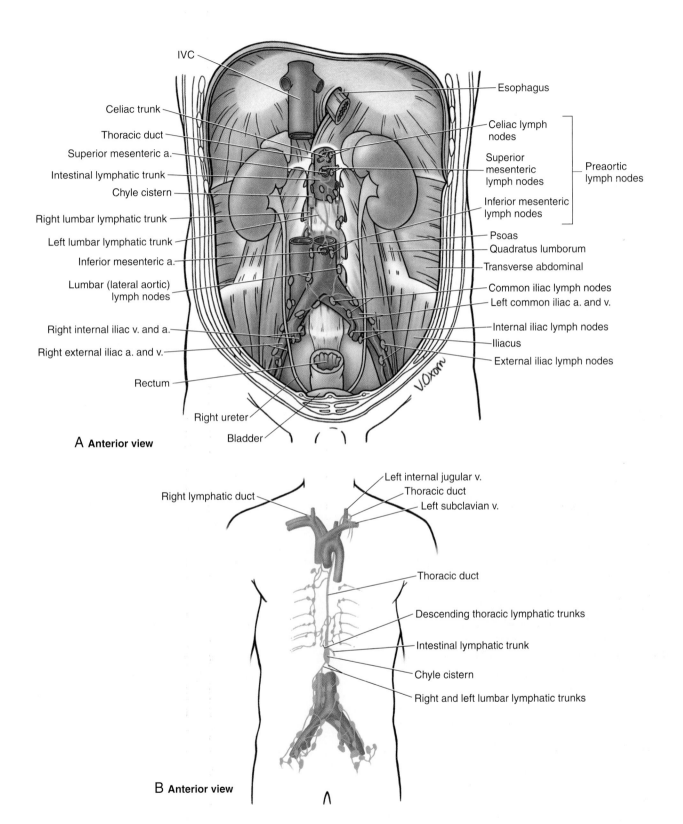

Figure 2.45. Abdominal lymphatic drainage. A. The posterior abdominal wall is shown. **B.** The lymphatic trunks are identified. *IVC,* inferior vena cava.

Abdominal Aortic Aneurysm

Rupture of an aneurysm (localized enlargement) of the abdominal aorta causes severe pain in the abdomen or back. If unrecognized, a ruptured aneurysm has a mortality rate of nearly 90% because of heavy blood loss. Surgeons can repair an aneurysm by opening it, inserting a prosthetic graft (such as one made of Dacron), and sewing the wall of the aneurysmal aorta over the graft to protect it. Aneurysms may also be treated by endovascular catheterization procedures (Fig. B2.8).

Collateral Routes for Abdominopelvic Venous Blood

Three collateral routes, formed by valveless veins of the trunk, are available for venous blood to return to the heart when the IVC is obstructed or ligated.

• The *inferior epigastric veins,* tributaries of the external iliac veins of the inferior caval system, anastomose

in the rectus sheath with *superior epigastric veins,* which drain in sequence through the internal thoracic veins of the superior caval system.

• The *superficial epigastric* or *superficial circumflex iliac veins,* normally tributaries of the great saphenous vein of the inferior caval system, anastomose in the subcutaneous tissues of the anterolateral body wall with one of the tributaries of the axillary vein, commonly the *lateral thoracic vein.* When the IVC is obstructed, this subcutaneous collateral pathway— called the *thoracoepigastric vein*—becomes particularly conspicuous.

• The *epidural venous plexus* inside the vertebral column (see Chapter 4) communicates with the lumbar veins of the inferior caval system, and the tributaries of the azygos system of veins, which is part of the superior caval system.

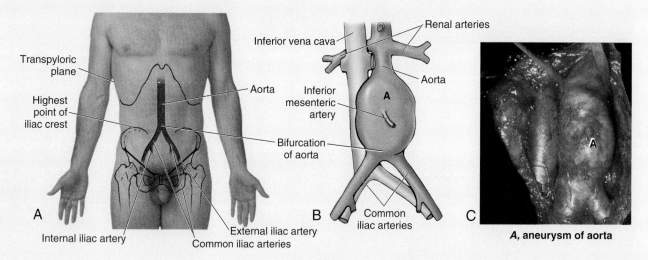

Figure B2.8.

Examples of some of the modalities used in medical imaging of the abdomen follow. Radiographs of the abdomen demonstrate normal and abnormal anatomical relationships, such as those resulting from tu-mors. CT scans (Fig. 2.46), MRI studies (Fig. 2.47), and ultra-sound (Fig. 2.48) are also used to examine the abdominal viscera. MRI studies provide better differentiation than CT scans between soft tissues.

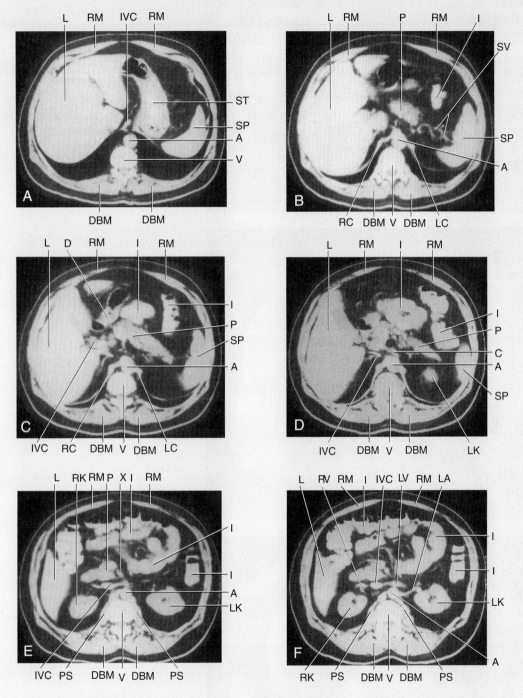

Figure 2.46. CT scans of the abdomen at progressively lower levels showing viscera and blood vessels. *A,* aorta; *C,* celiac trunk; *D,* duodenum; *DBM,* deep back muscles; *I,* intestine, *IVC,* inferior vena cava; *L,* liver; *LA,* left renal artery; *LC,* left crus of diaphragm; *LK,* left kidney; *LV,* left renal vein; *P,* pancreas; *PS,* psoas major; *RC,* right crus of diaphragm; *RK,* right kidney; *RM,* rectus abdominis; *RV,* right renal vein; *SP,* spleen; *ST,* stomach; *SV,* splenic vessels; *V,* vertebral body; *X,* superior mesenteric artery.

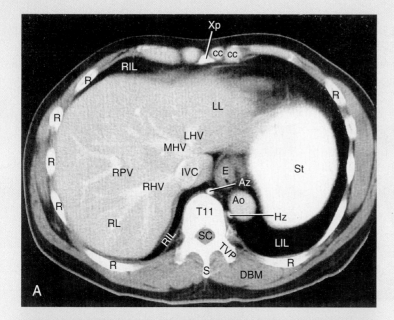

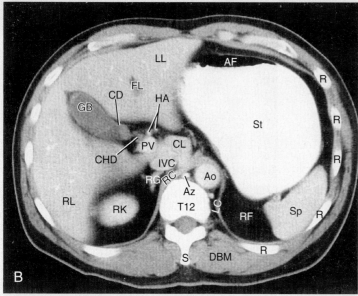

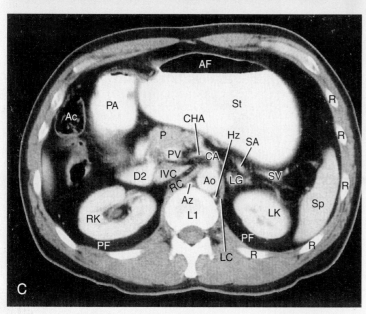

Key	
Ac	Ascending colon
AF	Air-fluid level of stomach
Ao	Aorta
Az	Azygos vein
CA	Celiac artery
cc	Costal cartilage
CD	Cystic duct
CHA	Common hepatic artery
CHD	Common hepatic duct
CL	Caudate lobe of liver
DBM	Deep back muscles
Dc	Descending colon
D2	2nd part of duodenum
D3	3rd part of duodenum
E	Esophagus
FL	Falciform ligament
GB	Gallbladder
HA	Hepatic artery
Hz	Hemiazygos vein
IVC	Inferior vena cava
L1	1st lumbar vertebra
L2	2nd lumbar vertebra
L3	3rd lumbar vertebra
LC	Left crus of diaphragm
LG	Left suprarenal gland
LHV	Left hepatic vein
LIL	Left inferior lobe of lung
LK	Left kidney
LL	Left lobe of liver
LRV	Left renal vein
MHV	Middle hepatic vein

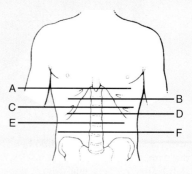

Figure 2.47. Transverse MRI studies of the abdomen.

Key (continued)	
P	Pancreas
PA	Pyloric antrum of stomach
PB	Body of pancreas
PC	Portal confluence
PF	Perirenal fat
PH	Head of pancreas
PS	Psoas
PT	Tail of pancreas
PU	Uncinate process of pancreas
PV	Portal vein
QL	Quadratus lumborum
R	Rib
RA	Rectus abdominis
RC	Right crus of diaphragm
RF	Retroperitoneal fat
RG	Right suprarenal gland
RHV	Right hepatic vein
RIL	Right inferior lobe of lung
RK	Right kidney
RL	Right lobe of liver
RP	Renal pelvis
RPV	Right branch of portal vein
RRA	Right renal artery
RRV	Right renal vein
RU	Right ureter
S	Spinous process
SA	Splenic artery
SC	Spinal cord
SF	Splenic flexure
SI	Small intestine
SMA	Superior mesenteric artery
SMV	Superior mesenteric vein
Sp	Spleen
St	Stomach
SV	Splenic vein
T11	11th thoracic vertebra
T12	12th thoracic vertebra
Tc	Transverse colon
TVP	Transverse process
Xp	Xiphoid process

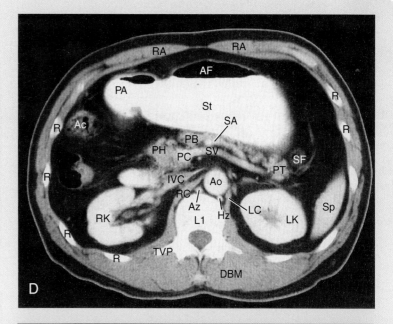

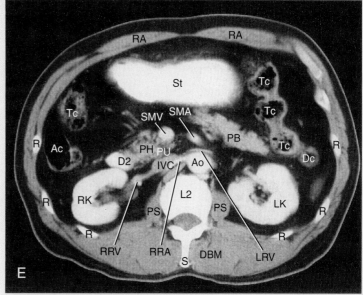

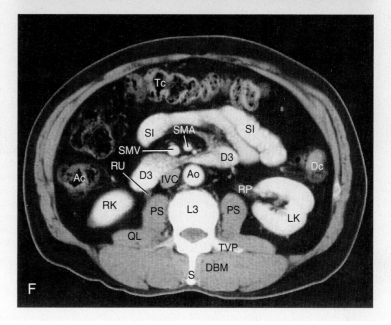

Figure 2.47. *(Continued)*

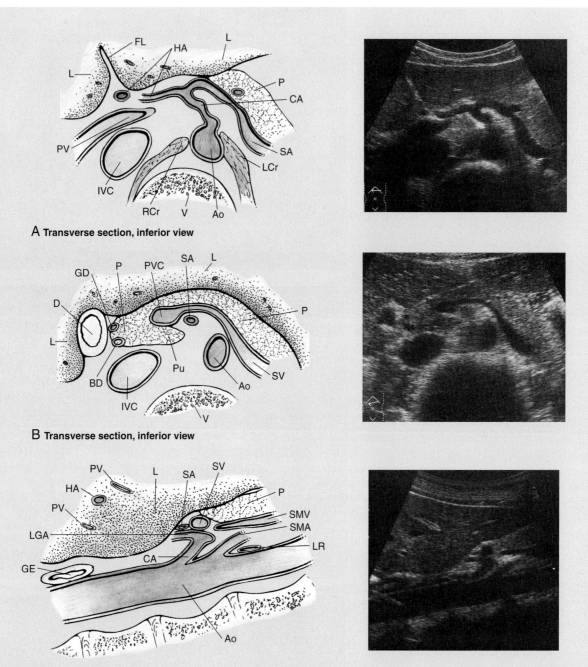

A Transverse section, inferior view

B Transverse section, inferior view

C Median section, right lateral view

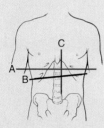

Figure 2.48. Ultrasound scans of the abdomen. A. This section is through the celiac trunk (artery). **B.** This section is through the pancreas. **C.** This section is through the aorta. *Ao,* aorta; *BD,* bile duct; *CA,* celiac artery; *D,* duodenum; *FL,* falciform ligament; *GD,* gastroduodenal artery; *GE,* gastroesophageal junction; *HA,* hepatic artery; *IVC,* inferior vena cava; *L,* liver; *LCr,* left crus of diaphragm; *LGA,* left gastric artery; *LR,* left renal vein; *P,* pancreas; *Pu,* uncinate process of pancreas; *PV,* portal vein; *PVC,* portal venous confluence; *RCr,* right crus of diaphragm; *SA,* splenic artery; *SMA,* superior mesenteric artery; *SMV,* superior mesenteric vein; *SV,* splenic vein; *V,* vertebra.

An image in virtually any plane can be reconstructed after scanning is complete. Abdominal arteriography, radiography after the injection of radiopaque material directly into the bloodstream, detects abnormalities of the abdominal arteries (Fig. 2.49). Angiographic studies may also be performed using MRI.●

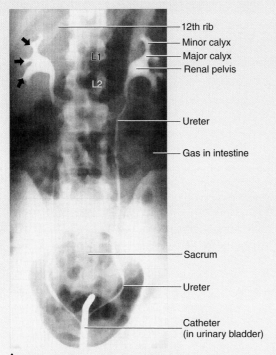

12th rib
Minor calyx
Major calyx
Renal pelvis

Ureter

Gas in intestine

Sacrum

Ureter

Catheter
(in urinary bladder)

A Anteroposterior pyelogram

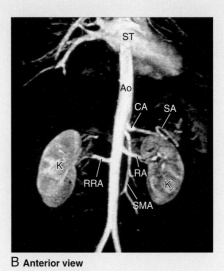

B Anterior view

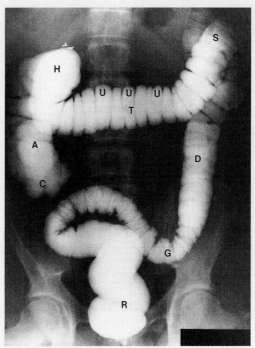

C Posteroanterior radiograph

Figure 2.49. **Abdominal images after introduction of contrast material. A.** A pyelogram is shown **B.** An MR angiogram study is shown. *Ao,* aorta; *CA,* celiac trunk; *K,* kidney; *LRA,* left renal artery; *RRA,* right renal artery; *SA,* splenic artery; *SMA,* superior mesenteric artery; *ST,* stomach. **C.** A single-contrast study of the colon after a barium enema is shown. *A,* ascending colon; *C,* cecum; *D,* descending colon; *G,* sigmoid colon; *H,* hepatic (right colic) flexure; *R,* rectum; *S,* left splenic (right colic) flexure; *T,* transverse colon; *U,* haustra.

3

Pelvis and Perineum

The **pelvis** (L. *basin*) is the part of the trunk inferoposterior to the abdomen and is the area of transition between the trunk and the lower limbs (Fig. 3.1). The pelvis is also the space or compartment surrounded by the *pelvic girdle* (bony pelvis). The bony pelvis is subdivided into *greater* and *lesser pelves*. The greater pelvis is the inferior part of the abdominal cavity between the alae of the ilium, and the lesser pelvis provides the skeletal framework for the pelvic cavity and the perineum. The pelvic cavity contains the urinary bladder, terminal parts of the ureters, pelvic genital organs, rectum, blood vessels, lymphatics, and nerves. The perineum includes the anus and external genitalia, the penis and scrotum of the male and the vulva of the female. The **perineum** refers to the area of the trunk between the thighs and the buttocks, extending from the pubis to the coccyx and to the shallow compartment lying deep to this area and inferior to the pelvic diaphragm.

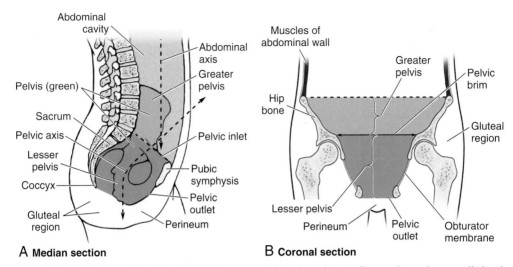

Figure 3.1. Abdominopelvic cavity. A and B. The pelvis is the space within the pelvic girdle, overlapped externally by the abdominal and gluteal (lower limb) regions and the perineum. *Light green,* greater pelvis; *dark green,* lesser pelvis.

Pelvis

The superior boundary of the **pelvic cavity** is the **pelvic inlet**, the superior pelvic aperture (Figs. 3.1 and 3.2). The pelvis is limited inferiorly by the **pelvic outlet**, the inferior pelvic aperture, which is bounded anteriorly by the **pubic symphysis** (L. *symphysis pubis*) and posteriorly by the **coccyx.**

The **pelvic inlet** is bounded by the **linea terminalis** of the pelvis, which is formed by the:

- Superior margin of the pubic symphysis anteriorly.
- Posterior border of the pubic crest.
- Pecten pubis, the continuation of the superior ramus of the pubis, which forms a sharp ridge.
- Arcuate line of the ilium.
- Anterior border of the ala (L. *wing*) of the sacrum.
- Sacral promontory.

The **pelvic outlet** is bounded by the:

- Inferior margin of the pubic symphysis anteriorly.
- Inferior rami of the pubis and ischial tuberosities anterolaterally.
- Sacrotuberous ligaments posterolaterally (Fig. 3.3*B*).
- Tip of the coccyx posteriorly.

Pelvic Girdle

The **pelvic girdle** is a basin-shaped ring of bones that connects the vertebral column to the femurs in the thighs. The main functions of the strong pelvic girdle are to transfer the weight of the upper body from the axial to the lower appendicular skeleton for standing and walking and to withstand compression and other forces resulting from its support of

body weight. The bony pelvis is formed by three bones (Fig. 3.2; Table 3.1):

- Right and left **hip bones:** two large, irregularly shaped bones, each of which forms at puberty by fusion of three bones—*ilium, ischium,* and *pubis.*
- **Sacrum:** formed by the fusion of five originally separate sacral vertebrae.

The hip bones are joined at the *pubic symphysis* anteriorly and to the sacrum posteriorly at the **sacroiliac joints** to form a bony ring, the *pelvic girdle.*

The **ilium** is the superior, flattened, fan-shaped part of the hip bone (Fig. 3.2). The **ala** of the ilium represents the spread of the fan; and the **body** of the ilium, the handle of the fan. The body of the ilium forms the superior part of the **acetabulum,** the cup-shaped depression on the external surface of the hip bone with which the head of the femur articulates. The **iliac crest,** the rim of the ilium, has a curve that follows the contour of the ala between the **anterior** and the **posterior superior iliac spines.** The anterior concave part of the ala forms the **iliac fossa.**

The **ischium** has a body and a ramus (L. *branch*). The **body** of the ischium forms the posterior part of the acetabulum, and the **ramus** forms part of the inferior boundary of the **obturator foramen.** The large posteroinferior protuberance of the ischium is the **ischial tuberosity** (Fig. 3.2). The small pointed posterior projection near the junction of the ramus and body is the **ischial spine.**

The **pubis** is an angulated bone that has the **superior pubic ramus,** which forms the anterior part of the acetabulum, and the **inferior pubic ramus,** which forms part of the inferior boundary of the *obturator foramen.* The superior pubic ramus has an oblique ridge, the **pecten pubis** (pectineal line of pubis), on its superior aspect. A

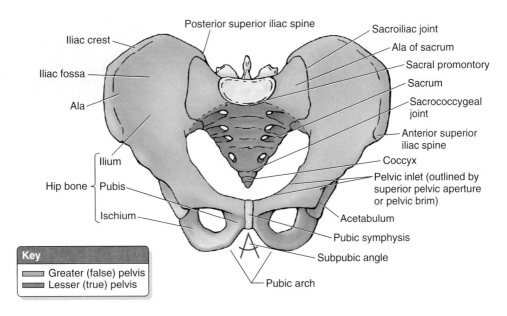

A **Anterior view**

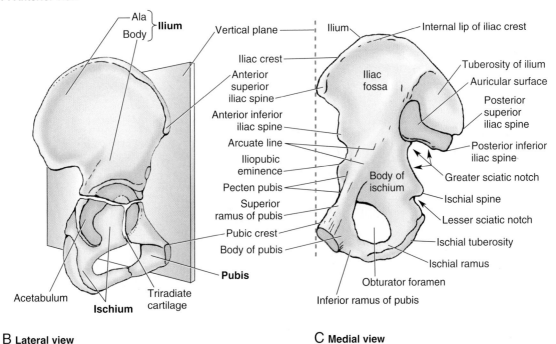

B **Lateral view**   C **Medial view**

Figure 3.2. Bony pelvis. An articulated pelvis (**A**), a child's hip bone (**B**), and an adult's right hip bone (**C**) are shown. Note that in the anatomical position the anterior superior iliac spine and the anterior aspect of the pubis lie in the same vertical plane.

thickening on the anterior part of the **body of the pubis** is the **pubic crest**, which ends laterally as a swelling—the **pubic tubercle** (Figs. 3.3A).

The **pubic arch** is formed by the **ischiopubic rami** (conjoined inferior rami of the pubis and ischium) of the two sides. These rami meet at the *pubic symphysis,* and their inferior borders define the **subpubic angle** (the distance be-

tween the right and the left ischial tuberosities), which can be measured with the fingers in the vagina during a pelvic examination.

The bony pelvis is divided into *greater (false)* and *lesser (true) pelves* by the oblique plane of the **pelvic inlet** (superior pelvic aperture) (Figs. 3.1 and 3.2; Table 3.1). The bony edge (rim) surrounding the pelvic inlet is the **pelvic brim**.

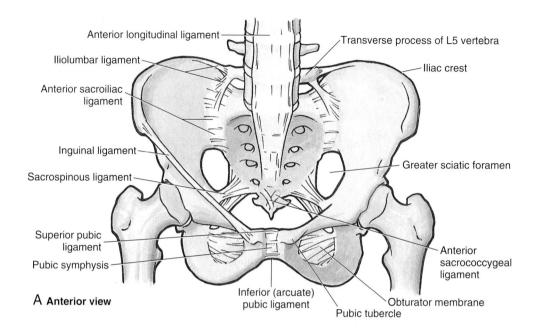

A **Anterior view**

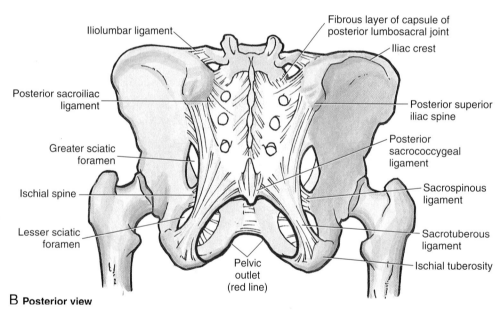

B **Posterior view**

Figure 3.3. Ligaments of pelvis.

The **greater pelvis** (L. *pelvis major*) is:

- Superior to the pelvic inlet.
- Bounded by the abdominal wall anteriorly, the iliac alae laterally, and the L5 and S1 vertebrae posteriorly.
- The location of some abdominal viscera, such as the sigmoid colon and some loops of ileum.

The **lesser pelvis** (L. *pelvis minor*) is:

- Between the *pelvic inlet* and the *pelvic outlet*.
- The location of the pelvic viscera—urinary bladder and reproductive organs, such as the uterus and ovaries.

- Bounded by the pelvic surfaces of the hip bones, sacrum, and coccyx.
- Limited inferiorly by the musculofascial pelvic diaphragm (levatorani) (see Table. 3.2).

Joints and Ligaments of Pelvic Girdle

The primary joints of the pelvis are the *sacroiliac joints* and the *pubic symphysis*, which link the skeleton of the trunk and the lower limb (Fig. 3.2). The *lumbosacral* and *sacrococcygeal* joints are directly related to the pelvic girdle. Strong ligaments support and strengthen these joints (Fig. 3.3).

Table 3.1 Comparison of the Male and Female Pelves

Iliac crest — Ala of sacrum — Promontory of sacrum — Lateral part of sacrum — Acetabulum — Pubic symphysis

Sacroiliac joint — Iliac fossa — Anterior superior iliac spine — Coccyx — Pubis — Obturator foramen

Anterior sacral foramen — Arcuate line of ilium — Pecten pubis — Pubic crest — Ramus of ischium

Body of sacrum — Hip bone — Coccyx — Ischial spine — Superior ramus of pubis — Obturator foramen — Pubic tubercle

∧, subpubic angle and pubic arch.

Bony Pelvis	Male (♂)	Female (♀)
General structure	Thick and heavy	Thin and light
Greater pelvis (pelvis major)	Deep	Shallow
Lesser pelvis (pelvis minor)	Narrow and deep	Wide and shallow
Pelvic inlet (superior pelvic aperture)	Heart shaped	Oval or rounded
Pelvic outlet (inferior pelvic aperture)	Comparatively small	Comparatively large
Pubic arch and subpubic angle	Narrow ($< 70°$)	Wide ($> 80°$)
Obturator foramen	Round	Oval
Acetabulum	Large	Small

Sexual Differences in Bony Pelves

The male and female bony pelves differ in several respects (Table 3.1). These sexual differences are related mainly to the heavier build and larger muscles of men and to the adaptation of the pelvis, particularly the lesser pelvis, in women for childbearing. Hence, the **male pelvis** is heavier and thicker than the female pelvis and usually has more prominent bone markings. In contrast, the **female pelvis** is wider, shallower, and has a larger pelvic inlet and outlet. The shape and size of the pelvic inlet (and the pelvic brim) are significant because it is through this opening that the fetal head enters the lesser pelvis during labor. To determine the capacity of the pelvis for childbirth, the diameters of the lesser pelvis are noted during a pelvic examination. The *ischial spines* face each other and the **interspinous distance** between them is the narrowest part of the pelvic canal (the passageway traversing the pelvic inlet, lesser pelvis, and pelvic outlet through which a baby's head must pass at birth).

Pelvic Fractures

Pelvic fractures can result from direct trauma to the pelvic bones, such as occurs during an automobile accident, or from forces transmitted to these bones from the lower limbs during falls on the feet. Pelvic fractures may cause injury to pelvic soft tissues, blood vessels, nerves, and organs.

SACROILIAC JOINTS

The sacroiliac joints are strong, weightbearing, compound joints, consisting of an anterior synovial joint (between the ear-shaped auricular surfaces of the sacrum and ilium covered with articular cartilage) and a posterior syndesmosis (between the tuberosities of the same bones) (Figs. 3.2 and 3.4). The articular (auricular) surfaces of the synovial joint have irregular but congruent elevations and depressions that interlock. The sacroiliac joints differ from most synovial joints in that limited mobility is allowed, a consequence of their role in transmitting the weight of most of the body to the hip bones. The sacrum is suspended between the iliac bones and is firmly attached to them by posterior and interosseous sacroiliac ligaments. The thin **anterior sacroiliac ligaments** form the anterior part of the fibrous capsule. The **interosseous sacroiliac ligaments** occupy an area of about 10 cm^2 each and are the primary structures involved in transferring the weight of the upper body from the axial skeleton to the two ilia and then to the femurs during standing and to the ischial tuberosities during sitting.

Usually movement is limited to slight gliding and rotary movements, except when subject to considerable force such as occurs after a high jump. Then the weight of the body is transmitted through the sacrum anterior to the rotation axis, tending to push the superior sacrum inferiorly, thereby causing the inferior sacrum to rotate superiorly. This tendency is resisted by the strong **sacrotuberous** and **sacrospinous ligaments**. These ligaments allow only limited upward movement of the inferior end of the sacrum, thus providing resilience to the sacroiliac region when the vertebral column sustains sudden weight increases (Figs. 3.3 and 3.4).

PUBIC SYMPHYSIS

The pubic symphysis is a secondary cartilaginous joint that is formed by the union of the bodies of the pubic bones in the median plane (Figs. 3.2 and 3.3). The fibrocartilaginous **interpubic disc** is generally wider in women than in men. The ligaments joining the pubic bones are thickened superiorly and inferiorly to form the **superior pubic ligament** and the **inferior** (arcuate) **pubic ligament**, respectively. The decussating fibers of tendinous attachments of the rectus abdominis and external oblique muscles also strengthen the pubic symphysis anteriorly.

LUMBOSACRAL JOINTS

The L5 and S1 vertebrae articulate at the anterior **intervertebral joint**, formed by the intervertebral (IV) disc between their bodies and at two posterior **zygapophysial joints** (facet joints) between the articular processes of these vertebrae. The facets on the S1 vertebra face posteromedially, interlocking with the anterolaterally facing inferior articular facets of the L5 vertebra, preventing L5 from sliding anteriorly. **Iliolumbar ligaments** unite the transverse processes of L5 to the ilia (Fig. 3.3).

SACROCOCCYGEAL JOINT

The sacrococcygeal joint is a secondary cartilaginous joint with an IV disc. Fibrocartilage and ligaments join the apex of the sacrum to the base of the coccyx. The anterior

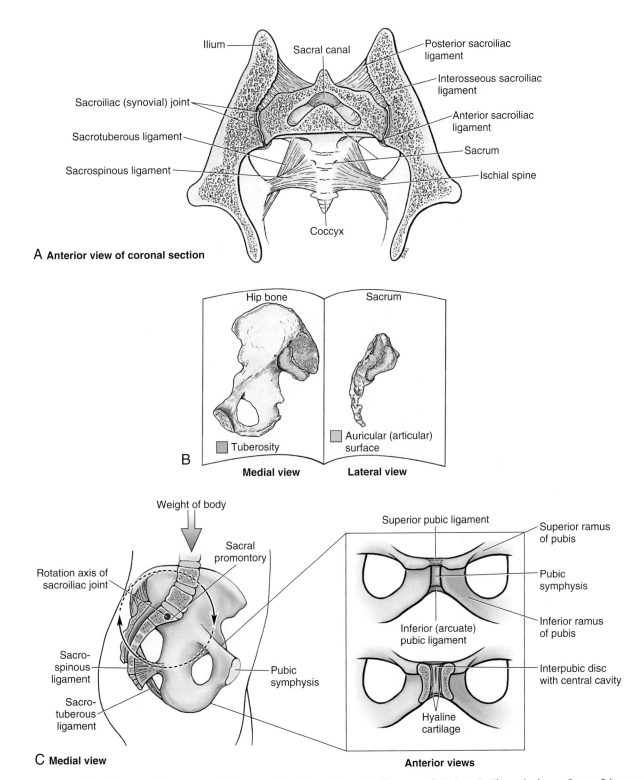

Figure 3.4. Sacroiliac joints and ligaments. A. This coronal section of the pelvis illustrates the joints. **B.** The articular surfaces of the sacroiliac joint are shown. **C.** The pubic symphysis is detailed.

Relaxation of Pelvic Ligaments and Increased Joint Mobility during Pregnancy

During pregnancy, the pelvic joints and ligaments relax and pelvic movements increase. This relaxation during the latter half of pregnancy is caused by the increase in levels of the sex hormones and the presence of the hormone relaxin. The sacroiliac interlocking mechanism is less effective because the relaxation permits greater rotation of the pelvis and contributes to the lordotic posture often assumed during pregnancy with the change in the center of gravity. Relaxation of the sacroiliac joints and pubic symphysis permits as much as a 10–15% increase in diameters (mostly transverse), facilitating passage of the fetus through the pelvic canal. The coccyx is also allowed to move posteriorly.

and posterior **sacrococcygeal ligaments** are long strands that reinforce the joint, much like the anterior and posterior longitudinal ligaments do for superior vertebrae (Fig. 3.3).

Peritoneum and Peritoneal Cavity of Pelvis

The **peritoneum** lining the abdominal cavity continues into the pelvic cavity, reflecting onto the superior aspects of most pelvic viscera (Table 3.2). Only the uterine tubes—except for their ostia, which are open—are intraperitoneal and suspended by a mesentry. The ovaries, although suspended in the peritoneal cavity by a mesentry, are not covered with peritoneum. The peritoneum creates a number of folds and fossae as it reflects onto most of the pelvic viscera.

The peritoneum is not firmly bound to the suprapubic crest, allowing the bladder to expand between the peritoneum and the anterior abdominal wall as it fills.

Walls and Floor of Pelvic Cavity

The pelvic cavity has an *anteroinferior wall,* two *lateral walls,* and a *posterior wall.* Muscles of the pelvic walls are summarized in Table 3.3.

The **anteroinferior pelvic wall:**

- Is formed primarily by the bodies and rami of the pubic bones and the pubic symphysis.
- Participates in bearing the weight of the urinary bladder.

The **lateral pelvic walls:**

- Have a bony framework formed by the hip bones, including the obturator foramen (Fig. 3.2A); the **obturator foramen** is closed by the **obturator membrane** (Fig. 3.3A).
- Are covered and padded by the **obturator internus muscles** (Fig. 3.5B & C). Each obturator internus passes posteriorly from its origin within the lesser pelvis, exits through the lesser sciatic foramen, and turns sharply laterally to attach to the femur (see Chapter 5). The medial surfaces of these muscles are covered by **obturator fascia,** thickened centrally as a **tendinous arch** that provides attachment for the pelvic diaphragm (Fig. 3.5C)
- Have the obturator nerves and vessels and other branches of the internal iliac vessels located on their medial aspects (medial to obturator internus muscles).

The *posterior pelvic wall:*

- Consists of a bony wall and roof in the midline (formed by the sacrum and coccyx) and musculoligamentous posterolateral walls (formed by the sacroiliac joints and their associated ligaments and piriformis muscles).
- Each **piriformis muscle** leaves the lesser pelvis through the *greater sciatic foramen* to attach to the femur (see Chapter 5).
- Is the site of the nerves forming the **sacral plexus;** the piriformis muscles form a "muscular bed" for this nerve network (Table 3.3).

The **pelvic floor** is formed by the funnel-shaped **pelvic diaphragm,** which consists of the *levator ani* and *coccygeus* muscles and the fascias (L. *fasciae*) covering the superior and inferior aspects of these muscles (Table 3.2). The **coccygeus muscles** extend from the ischial spines to the inferior sacrum and coccyx. The **levator ani** is attached to the pubic bones anteriorly, to the ischial spines posteriorly, and to a thickening in the obturator fascia (**tendinous arch of levator ani**) on each side (Fig. 3.5C). The levator ani consists of three parts, each named according to the attachment of its fibers (Table 3.3). The parts of the levator ani are:

- The **puborectalis,** consisting of the thicker, narrower, medial part of the levator ani, which is continuous between the posterior aspects of the right and left pubic bones. It forms a U-shaped muscular sling (puborectal sling) that passes posterior to the anorectal junction. This part plays a major role in maintaining fecal continence.
- The **pubococcygeus** the wider but thinner intermediate part of the levator ani. It arises from the posterior aspect of the body of the pubis and the anterior part of

Table 3.2 **Peritoneal Reflections in the Pelvis**

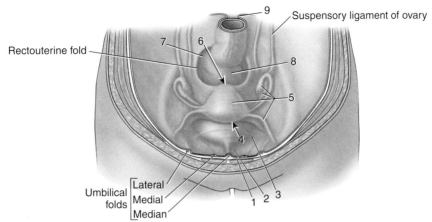

A Anterior view of female

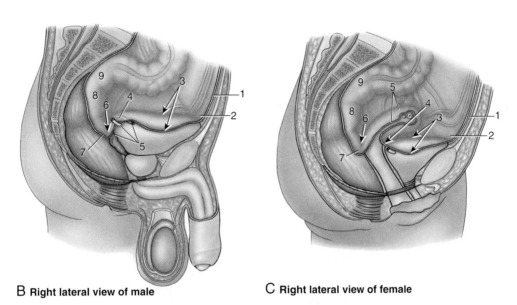

B Right lateral view of male

C Right lateral view of female

Male (Part B)[a]	Female (Parts A & C)[a]
1 Descends anterior abdominal wall (loose attachment allows insertion of bladder as it fills)	1 Descends anterior abdominal wall (loose attachment allows insertion of bladder as it fills)
2 Reflects onto superior surface of bladder, creating **supravesical fossa**	2 Reflects onto superior surface of bladder, creating **supravesical fossa**
3 Covers convex superior surface (roof) of bladder, sloping down sides of roof to ascend lateral wall of pelvis, creating **paravesical fossae** on each side	3 Covers convex superior surface of bladder; slopes down sides of bladder to ascend lateral wall of pelvis, creating **paravesical fossae** on each side
4 Descends posterior surface of bladder as much as 2 cm	4 Reflects from bladder body of uterus forming **vesicouterine pouch**
5 Laterally, forms fold over ureters (**ureteric fold**), ductus deferentes, and superior ends of seminal glands	5 Covers body and fundus of uterus, posterior fornix of vagina; extends laterally from uterus as double fold or mesentery, the **broad ligament** that engulfs uterine tubes, and round ligaments of uterus, and suspends ovaries
6 Reflects from bladder and seminal glands onto rectum, forming **rectovesical pouch**	6 Reflects from vagina onto rectum, forming **rectouterine pouch**
7 Rectovesical pouch extends laterally and posteriorly to form **pararectal fossae** on each side of rectum	7 Rectouterine pouch extends laterally and posteriorly to form **pararectal fossae** on each side of rectum
8 Ascends rectum; from inferior to superior, rectum is subperitoneal and then retroperitoneal	8 Ascends rectum; from inferior to superior, rectum is subperitoneal and then retroperitoneal
9 Engulfs sigmoid colon beginning at rectosigmoid junction	9 Engulfs sigmoid colon beginning at rectosigmoid junction

[a]Numbers refer to the figure.

Table 3.3 Muscles of the Pelvic Walls and Floor

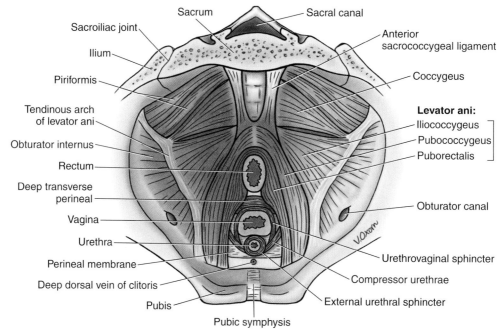

A **Floor of female pelvis, superior view**

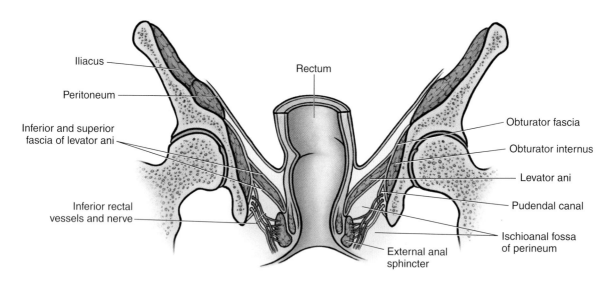

B **Anterior view, coronal section**

Muscle	Proximal Attachment	Distal Attachment	Innervation	Main Action
Levator ani (pubococcygeus and iliococcygeus)	Body of pubis, tendinous arch of obturator fascia, ischial spine	Perineal body, coccyx, anococcygeal ligament, walls of prostate or vagina, rectum, anal canal	Nerve to levator ani (branches of S4), inferior anal (rectal) nerve, coccygeal plexus	Helps support pelvic viscera; resists increases in intra-abdominal pressure
Coccygeus (ischiococcygeus)	Ischial spine	Inferior end of sacrum	Branches of S4 and S5 nerves	Forms small part of pelvic diaphragm that supports pelvic viscera; flexes coccyx

Table 3.3 Muscles of the Pelvic Walls and Floor (continued)

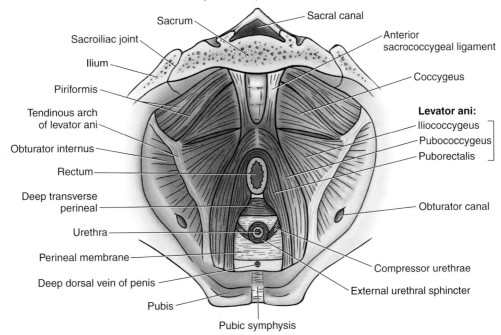

C Floor of male pelvis, superior view

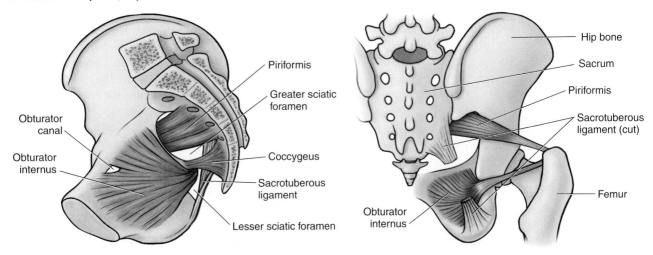

D Medial view

E Posterior view

Muscle	Proximal Attachment	Distal Attachment	Innervation	Main Action
Obturator internus	Pelvic surface of ilium and ischium; obturator membrane	Greater trochanter of femur	Nerve to obturator internus (L5, S1, S2)	Rotates thigh laterally; assists in holding head of femur in acetabulum
Piriformis	Pelvic surface of 2nd–4th sacral segments: superior margin of greater sciatic notch and sacrotuberous ligament		Anterior rami of S1 and S2	Rotates thigh laterally; abducts thigh; assists in holding head of femur in acetabulum

the tendinous arch and passes posteriorly in a nearly horizontal plane. The lateral fibers attach posteriorly to the coccyx, and the medial fibers merge with those of the contralateral side to form part of the **anococcygeal body** or **ligament.**

- The **iliococcygeus,** the posterolateral part of the levator ani, arising from the posterior part of the tendinous arch and ischial spine; it is thin and often poorly developed and blends with the anococcygeal body posteriorly.

The levator ani forms a dynamic floor for supporting the abdominopelvic viscera. Acting together, the parts of the levator ani raise the pelvic floor, following its descent when relaxed to allow defecation and urination, restoring its normal position. Further contraction occurs when the thoracic diaphragm and anterolateral abdominal wall muscles contract to compress the abdominal and pelvic contents. Therefore, it can resist the increased intra-abdominal pressure that would otherwise force the abdominopelvic contents (gas, solid and liquid wastes, and the viscera) through the pelvic outlet. This action occurs reflexively during forced expiration, coughing, sneezing, vomiting, and fixation of the trunk during strong movements of the upper limbs, as occurs when lifting a heavy object. The levator ani also has important functions in the voluntary control of urination, fecal continence (via the puborectalis), and support of the uterus.

Pelvic Fascia

The **pelvic fascia** is connective tissue that occupies the space between the membranous peritoneum and the muscular pelvic walls and floor not occupied by pelvic organs. This "layer" is a continuation of the comparatively thin endoabdominal fascia that lies between the muscular abdominal walls and the peritoneum superiorly.

MEMBRANOUS PELVIC FASCIA: PARIETAL AND VISCERAL

The **parietal pelvic fascia** is a membranous layer of variable thickness that lines the internal (deep or pelvic) aspect of the muscles forming the walls and floor of the pelvis. (Fig. 3.5). The parietal pelvic fascia covers the pelvic surfaces of the **obturator internus, piriformis, coccygeus, levator ani, and part of the urethral sphincter muscles** (Fig. 3.5 *B, E, & F*). The name given to the fascia is derived from the muscle it encloses (e.g., obturator fascia). This layer is continuous superiorly with the transversalis and iliopsoas fascias.

The **visceral pelvic fascia** includes the membranous fascia that directly ensheathes the pelvic organs, forming the adventitial layer of each. The membranous parietal and visceral layers become continuous where the organs penetrate the pelvic floor (Fig. 3.5 *A & C*). Here the parietal fascia thickens, forming the **tendinous arch of pelvic fascia,** a continuous bilateral band running from the pubis to the sacrum along the pelvic floor adjacent to the viscera (Fig. 3.5 *B, D, & E*).

The anteriormost part of this tendinous arch (**puboprostatic ligament** in males; **pubovesical ligament** in females) connects the prostate to the pubis in the male or the fundus (base) of the bladder to the pubis in the female. The posteriormost part of the band runs as the sacrogenital ligaments from the sacrum around the side of the rectum to attach to the prostate in the male or the vagina in the female.

ENDOPELVIC FASCIA: LOOSE AND CONDENSED

Usually, the abundant connective tissue remaining between the parietal and the visceral membranous layers is considered part of the visceral fascia, but various authors label parts of it as parietal. It is probably more realistic to consider this remaining fascia simply as extraperitoneal or **subperitoneal endopelvic fascia** (Fig. 3.5 *A & B*), which is continuous with both the parietal and the visceral membranous fascias.

Injury to Pelvic Floor

During childbirth, the pelvic floor supports the fetal head while the cervix of the uterus is dilating to permit delivery of the fetus. The perineum, levator ani, and pelvic fascia may be injured during childbirth. It is the pubococcygeus, the main and most medial part of the levator ani, that is usually torn (Fig. B3.1). This part of the muscle is important because it encircles and supports the urethra, vagina, and anal canal. Weakening of the levator ani and pelvic fascia resulting from stretching or tearing during childbirth may alter the position of the neck of the bladder and urethra. These changes cause *urinary stress incontinence,* characterized by dribbling of urine when intra-abdominal pressure is raised during coughing and lifting, for instance.

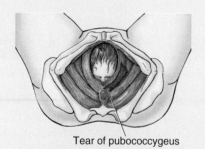

Tear of pubococcygeus

Figure B3.1.

Some of this fascia is extremely loose areolar (fatty) tissue, relatively devoid of all but minor lymphatics and nutrient vessels. The **retropubic** (or *prevesical*, extended posterolaterally as *paravesical*) and **retrorectal** (or *presacral*) **spaces** are *potential spaces* in the loose fatty tissue that accommodate the expansion of the urinary bladder and rectal ampulla as they fill. Other parts of the endopelvic fascia have fibrous consistency. These parts are often described as "fascial condensations" or pelvic "ligaments." The **hypogastric sheath** is a thick band of condensed pelvic fascia that gives passage to essentially all the vessels and nerves passing from the lateral wall of the pelvis to the pelvic viscera, along with the ureters and, in the male, the ductus deferens (Fig. 3.5 *B & E*). As it extends medially from the lateral wall, the hypogastric sheath divides into three laminae ("leaflets" or "wings") that pass to or between the pelvic organs, conveying neurovascular structures and providing support. The three laminae of the hypogastric sheath, from anterior to posterior, are (Fig. 3.5 *B & E*):

- The **lateral ligament of the bladder,** passing to the bladder, conveying the superior vesical arteries and veins.
- The middle lamina in the male, forming the **rectovesical septum** between the posterior surface of the bladder and the prostate anteriorly and the rectum posteriorly (Fig. 3.5 *B*). In the female, the middle lamina is substantial and passes medially to the uterine cervix and vagina as the **transverse cervical (cardinal) ligament,** also known clinically as the *lateral cervical* or *Mackenrodt ligament*. In its superiormost portion, at the base of the broad ligament, the uterine artery runs transversely toward the cervix while the ureters course immediately inferior to them as they pass on each side of the cervix toward the bladder.
- The posteriormost lamina passes to the rectum, conveying the middle rectal artery and vein.

The transverse cervical ligament, and the way in which the uterus normally "rests" on top of the bladder, provides the main passive support for the uterus. The perineal muscles provide dynamic support for the uterus by contracting during movements of increased intra-abdominal pressure (e.g., sneezing and coughing).

There is a surgically important potential **pelvirectal space** in the loose extraperitoneal connective tissue superior to the pelvic diaphragm. It is divided into anterior and posterior regions by the **lateral rectal ligaments** (rectal stalks), which are the posterior laminae of the hypogastric sheaths. These ligaments connect the rectum to the parietal pelvic fascia at the S2–S4 levels (Fig. 3.5 *B & D*).

Pelvic Nerves

Pelvic structures are innervated mainly by the **sacral** (S1–S4) and **coccygeal spinal nerves** and the pelvic part of the *autonomic nervous system*. The piriformis and coccygeus muscles form a bed for the sacral and coccygeal nerve plexuses (Table 3.4). The anterior rami of the S2 and S3 nerves emerge between the digitations of these muscles. The descending part of the anterior rumus of L4 nerve unites with the anterior ramus of the L5 nerve to form the thick, cord-like **lumbosacral trunk.** It passes inferiorly, anterior to the ala of the sacrum to join the sacral plexus.

SACRAL PLEXUS

The **sacral plexus** is located on the posterolateral wall of the lesser pelvis, where it is closely related to the anterior surface of the piriformis (Table 3.4). The two main nerves of the sacral plexus are the *sciatic* and *pudendal*. Most branches of the sacral plexus leave the pelvis through the *greater sciatic foramen*.

The **sciatic nerve,** the largest nerve in the body, is formed by the anterior rami of spinal nerves L4–S3. The anterior rami converge on the anterior surface of the piriformis. Most commonly, the sciatic nerve passes through the *greater sciatic foramen* inferior to the piriformis to enter the gluteal (buttock) region.

The **pudendal nerve** is the main nerve of the perineum and the chief sensory nerve of the external genitalia. It is derived from the anterior rami of spinal nerves S2–S4. It accompanies the internal pudendal artery and leaves the pelvis through the greater sciatic foramen between the piriformis and the coccygeus muscles. The pudendal nerve hooks around the ischial spine and sacrospinous ligament and enters the perineum through the lesser sciatic foramen. It supplies the skin and muscles of the perineum.

The **superior gluteal nerve** arises from the anterior rami of spinal nerves L4–S1 and leaves the pelvis through the greater sciatic foramen, superior to the piriformis (Table 3.4). It supplies three muscles in the gluteal region: the gluteus medius and minimus and the tensor of fascia lata (see Chapter 5).

The **inferior gluteal nerve** arises from the anterior rami of spinal nerves L5–S2 and leaves the pelvis through the greater sciatic foramen, inferior to the piriformis and superficial to the sciatic nerve. It accompanies the inferior gluteal artery and breaks up into several branches that supply the overlying gluteus maximus muscle (see Chapter 5).

OBTURATOR NERVE

The **obturator nerve** arises from the lumbar plexus (anterior rami of spinal nerves L2–L4) in the abdomen (greater pelvis) and enters the lesser pelvis (Table 3.4). It runs in the extraperitoneal fat along the lateral wall of the pelvis to the **obturator canal,** the opening in the obturator membrane, where it divides into anterior and posterior branches that leave the pelvis through this canal and supply the medial thigh muscles (see Chapter 5).

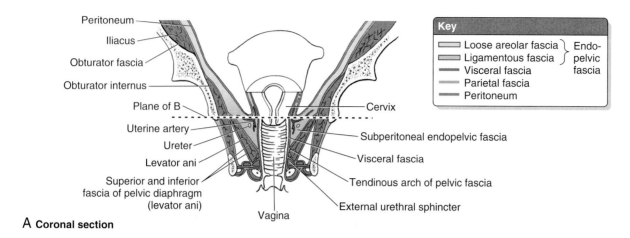

Peritoneum
Iliacus
Obturator fascia
Obturator internus
Plane of B
Uterine artery
Ureter
Levator ani
Superior and inferior fascia of pelvic diaphragm (levator ani)
Vagina
Cervix
Subperitoneal endopelvic fascia
Visceral fascia
Tendinous arch of pelvic fascia
External urethral sphincter

Key
Loose areolar fascia } Endo-
Ligamentous fascia } pelvic
Visceral fascia   fascia
Parietal fascia
Peritoneum

A Coronal section

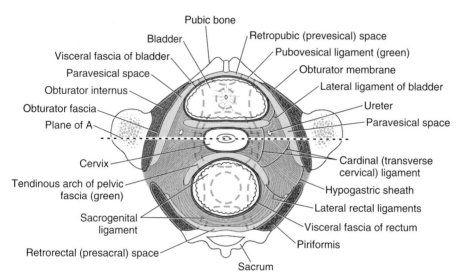

Pubic bone
Bladder
Visceral fascia of bladder
Paravesical space
Obturator internus
Obturator fascia
Plane of A
Cervix
Tendinous arch of pelvic fascia (green)
Sacrogenital ligament
Retrorectal (presacral) space
Sacrum

Retropubic (prevesical) space
Pubovesical ligament (green)
Obturator membrane
Lateral ligament of bladder
Ureter
Paravesical space
Cardinal (transverse cervical) ligament
Hypogastric sheath
Lateral rectal ligaments
Visceral fascia of rectum
Piriformis

B Female endopelvic fascia, transverse section

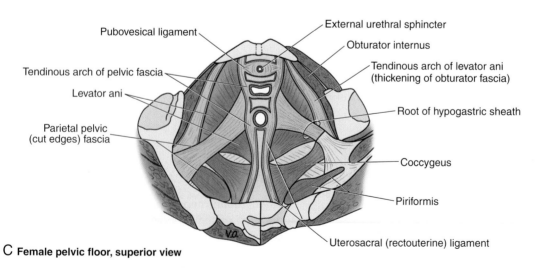

Pubovesical ligament
Tendinous arch of pelvic fascia
Levator ani
Parietal pelvic (cut edges) fascia

External urethral sphincter
Obturator internus
Tendinous arch of levator ani (thickening of obturator fascia)
Root of hypogastric sheath
Coccygeus
Piriformis
Uterosacral (rectouterine) ligament

C Female pelvic floor, superior view

Figure 3.5. Pelvic fascia: endopelvic fascia and fascial ligaments. A–C. The female pelvis is shown.

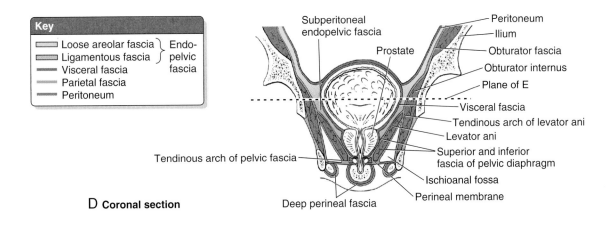

Key
- Loose areolar fascia ⎫ Endo-
- Ligamentous fascia ⎬ pelvic
- Visceral fascia ⎭ fascia
- Parietal fascia
- Peritoneum

Subperitoneal endopelvic fascia
Prostate
Peritoneum
Ilium
Obturator fascia
Obturator internus
Plane of E
Visceral fascia
Tendinous arch of levator ani
Levator ani
Superior and inferior fascia of pelvic diaphragm
Ischioanal fossa
Perineal membrane
Tendinous arch of pelvic fascia
Deep perineal fascia

D **Coronal section**

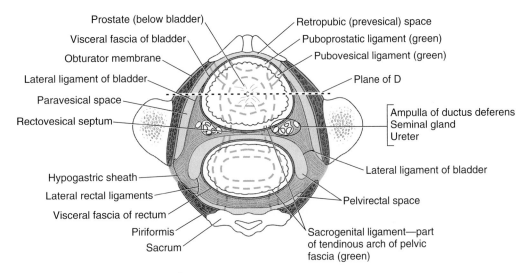

Prostate (below bladder)
Visceral fascia of bladder
Obturator membrane
Lateral ligament of bladder
Paravesical space
Rectovesical septum
Retropubic (prevesical) space
Puboprostatic ligament (green)
Pubovesical ligament (green)
Plane of D
Ampulla of ductus deferens
Seminal gland
Ureter
Lateral ligament of bladder
Hypogastric sheath
Lateral rectal ligaments
Visceral fascia of rectum
Piriformis
Sacrum
Pelvirectal space
Sacrogenital ligament—part of tendinous arch of pelvic fascia (green)

E **Male endopelvic fascia, transverse section**

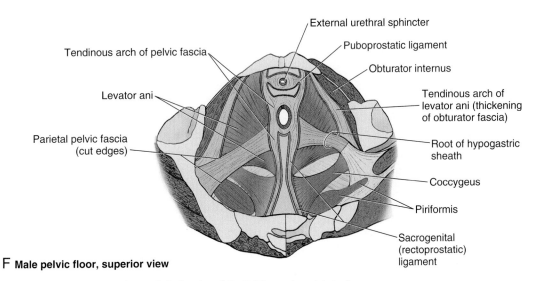

External urethral sphincter
Puboprostatic ligament
Obturator internus
Tendinous arch of pelvic fascia
Levator ani
Parietal pelvic fascia (cut edges)
Tendinous arch of levator ani (thickening of obturator fascia)
Root of hypogastric sheath
Coccygeus
Piriformis
Sacrogenital (rectoprostatic) ligament

F **Male pelvic floor, superior view**

Figure 3.5. *(continued)* **D–F.** The male pelvis is shown.

COCCYGEAL PLEXUS

The **coccygeal plexus** is a small network of nerve fibers formed by the anterior rami of spinal nerves S4 and S5 and the **coccygeal nerves.** It lies on the pelvic surface of the coccygeus and supplies this muscle, part of the levator ani, and the sacrococcygeal joint. The **anococcygeal nerves** arising from this plexus pierce the sacrotuberous ligament and supply a small area of skin between the tip of the coccyx and the anus.

PELVIC AUTONOMIC NERVES

Autonomic innervation of the pelvic cavity is via four routes: the *sacral sympathetic trunks, periarterial plexuses, hypogastric plexuses,* and *pelvic splanchnic nerves.*

Injury to Pelvic Nerves

During childbirth, the fetal head may compress the mother's sacral plexus, producing pain in her lower limbs. The obturator nerve is vulnerable to injury during surgery (e.g., during removal of cancerous lymph nodes from the lateral pelvic wall). *Injury to the obturator nerve* may cause painful spasms of the adductor muscles of the thigh and sensory deficits in the medial thigh region (see Chapter 5).

The **sacral sympathetic trunks** are the inferior continuation of the lumbar sympathetic trunks (Fig. 3.6). Each sacral trunk usually has four sympathetic ganglia. The sacral trunks descend on the pelvic surface of the sacrum just medial to the pelvic sacral foramina, and commonly converge to form the small median **ganglion impar** anterior to the coccyx. The sympathetic trunks descend posterior to the rectum in the extraperitoneal connective tissue and send communicating branches (gray rami communicantes) to each of the anterior rami of the sacral and coccygeal nerves. They also send branches to the median sacral artery and the inferior hypogastric plexus. The primary function of the sacral sympathetic trunks is to provide postsynaptic fibers to the sacral plexus for sympathetic innervation of the lower limb.

The **periarterial plexuses** of the superior rectal, ovarian, and internal iliac arteries provide postsynaptic, sympathetic, vasomotor fibers to each of the arteries and its derivative branches.

The **hypogastric plexuses** (superior and inferior) are networks of sympathetic and visceral afferent nerve fibers (Fig. 3.6). The main part of the **superior hypogastric plexus** lies just inferior to the bifurcation of the aorta and descends into the pelvis. This plexus is the inferior prolongation of the **intermesenteric plexus** (see Chapter 2), which also receives the L3 and L4 splanchnic nerves. The superior hypogastric plexus enter the pelvis, dividing into **left** and **right hypogastric nerves,** which descend anterior to the sacrum. These nerves descend lateral to the rectum within the *hypogastric sheaths* and then spread as they merge with pelvic splanchnic nerves (parasympathetic) to form the **right** and

Table 3.4 Nerves of the Sacral and Coccygeal Plexuses

Nerve[a]	Segmental Origin	Distribution
1 Sciatic	L4, L5, S1, S2, S3	Articular branches to hip joint and muscular branches to flexors of knee (hamstring muscles), and all muscles in leg and foot
2 Superior gluteal	L4, L5, S1	Gluteus medius gluteus minimus and tensor of fascia lata muscles
3 Inferior gluteal	L5, S1, S2	Gluteus maximus muscle
4 Nerve to piriformis	S1, S2	Piriformis muscle
5 Nerve to quadratus femoris and inferior gemellus	L4, L5, S1	Quadratus femoris and inferior gemellus muscles
6 Nerve to obturator internus and superior gemellus	L5, S1, S2	Obturator internus and superior gemellus muscles
7 Pudendal	S2, S3, S4	Structures in perineum: sensory to genitalia, muscular branches to perineal muscles, sphincter urethrae and external anal sphincter
8 Nerves to levator ani and coccygeus	S3, S4	Levator ani and coccygeus muscles
9 Posterior femoral cutaneous	S2, S3	Cutaneous branches to buttock and uppermost medial and posterior surfaces of thigh
10 Perforating cutaneous	S2, S3	Cutaneous branches to medial part of buttock
11 Pelvic splanchnic	S2, S3, S4	Pelvic viscera via inferior hypogastric and pelvic plexus

[a]Numbers refer to the figure on facing page.

Table 3.4 Nerves of the Sacral and Coccygeal Plexuses *(continued)*

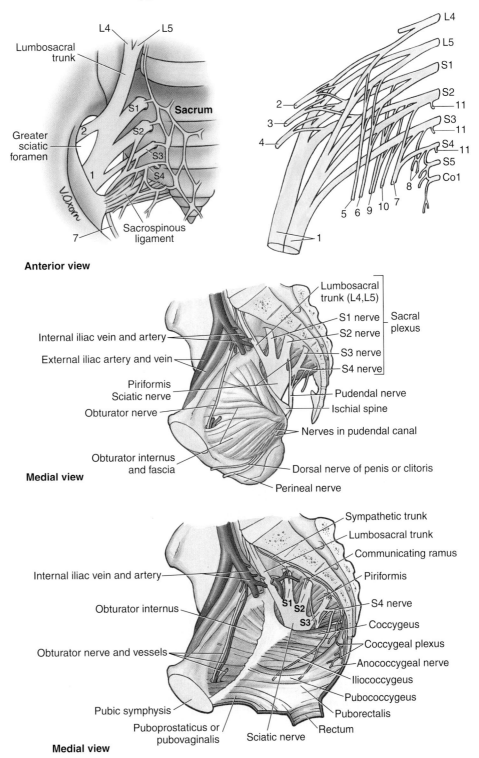

Anterior view

- Lumbosacral trunk
- L4
- L5
- Sacrum
- Greater sciatic foramen
- Sacrospinous ligament

Medial view

- Internal iliac vein and artery
- External iliac artery and vein
- Piriformis
- Sciatic nerve
- Obturator nerve
- Obturator internus and fascia
- Lumbosacral trunk (L4,L5)
- S1 nerve
- S2 nerve
- S3 nerve
- S4 nerve
- Sacral plexus
- Pudendal nerve
- Ischial spine
- Nerves in pudendal canal
- Dorsal nerve of penis or clitoris
- Perineal nerve

Medial view

- Internal iliac vein and artery
- Obturator internus
- Obturator nerve and vessels
- Pubic symphysis
- Puboprostaticus or pubovaginalis
- Sciatic nerve
- Sympathetic trunk
- Lumbosacral trunk
- Communicating ramus
- Piriformis
- S4 nerve
- Coccygeus
- Coccygeal plexus
- Anococcygeal nerve
- Iliococcygeus
- Pubococcygeus
- Puborectalis
- Rectum

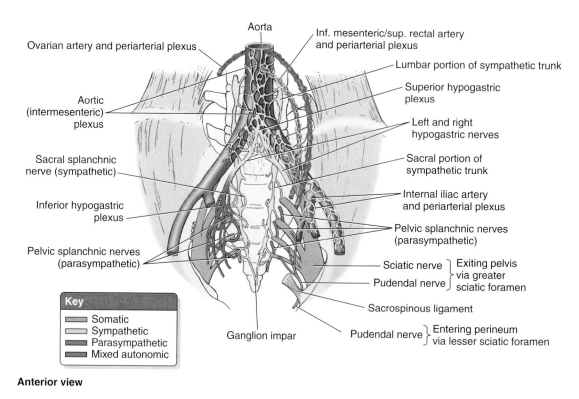

Anterior view

Figure 3.6. Autonomic nerves of pelvis.

left inferior hypogastric plexuses. Subplexuses of the inferior hypogastric plexuses, **pelvic plexuses**, in both sexes pass to the lateral surfaces of the rectum and to the inferolateral surfaces of the urinary bladder, and in males to the prostate and seminal glands (vesicles) and in females to the cervix of the uterus and lateral parts of the fornix of the vagina.

The **pelvic splanchnic nerves** contain presynaptic parasympathetic and visceral afferent fibers derived from the S2–S4 spinal cord segments and visceral afferent fibers from cell bodies in the spinal ganglia of the corresponding spinal nerves (Fig. 3.6; Table 3.4). The pelvic splanchnic nerves merge with the hypogastric nerves to form the inferior hypogastric (and pelvic) plexuses.

The **hypogastric/pelvic system of plexuses**, receiving sympathetic fibers via the lumbar splanchnic nerves and parasympathetic fibers via the pelvic splanchnic nerves, innervate the pelvic viscera. The **sympathetic component** produces vasomotion, inhibits peristaltic contraction of the rectum, and stimulates contraction of the genital organs during orgasm (producing ejaculation in the male). The **parasympathetic fibers** stimulate contraction of the rectum and bladder for defecation and urination, respectively. Parasympathetic fibers in the prostatic plexus penetrate the pelvic floor to supply the erectile bodies of the external genitalia, producing erection.

VISCERAL AFFERENT INNERVATION IN THE PELVIS

Visceral afferent fibers travel with the autonomic nerve fibers, although the sensory impulses are conducted centrally retrograde to the efferent impulses. Visceral afferent fibers in the pelvis conducting reflexive sensation (information that does not reach consciousness) travel with parasympathetic fibers to the spinal sensory ganglia of S2–S4, e.g., visceral afferent fibers that transmit pain sensations from the viscera inferior to the pelvic pain line (structures that do not contact the peritoneum, and the distal sigmoid colon and rectum). Visceral afferent fibers conducting pain from the viscera superior to the pelvic pain line (structures in contact with the peritoneum, except for the distal sigmoid colon and rectum) follow the sympathetic fibers retrogradely to inferior thoracic and superior lumbar spinal ganglia. The **pelvic pain line** corresponds to the inferior limit of peritoneum, except in the case of the large intestine, where the pain line occurs in the middle of the sigmoid colon.

Pelvic Arteries and Veins

Four main arteries enter the lesser pelvis in females, three in males:

- The paired **internal iliac arteries** deliver the most blood to the lesser pelvis (Fig. 3.8). They bifurcate into an anterior

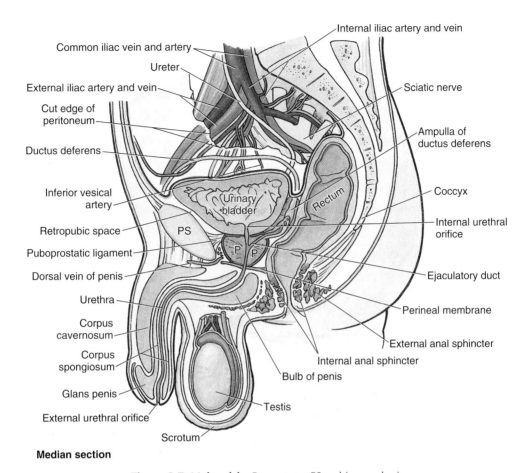

Internal iliac artery and vein

Common iliac vein and artery

Ureter

External iliac artery and vein

Cut edge of peritoneum

Ductus deferens

Inferior vesical artery

Retropubic space

Puboprostatic ligament

Dorsal vein of penis

Urethra

Corpus cavernosum

Corpus spongiosum

Glans penis

External urethral orifice

Scrotum

Sciatic nerve

Ampulla of ductus deferens

Coccyx

Internal urethral orifice

Ejaculatory duct

Perineal membrane

External anal sphincter

Internal anal sphincter

Bulb of penis

Testis

Urinary bladder

Rectum

PS

P P

Median section

Figure 3.7. Male pelvis. *P,* prostate; *PS,* pubic symphysis.

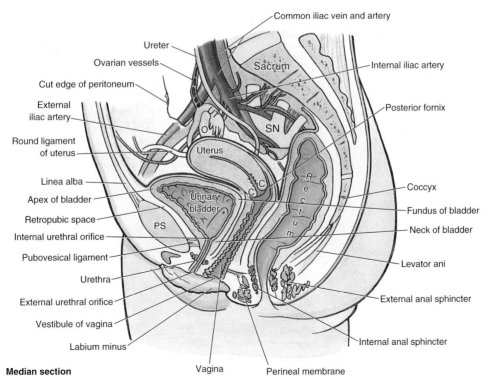

Common iliac vein and artery

Ureter

Ovarian vessels

Cut edge of peritoneum

External iliac artery

Round ligament of uterus

Linea alba

Apex of bladder

Retropubic space

Internal urethral orifice

Pubovesical ligament

Urethra

External urethral orifice

Vestibule of vagina

Labium minus

Sacrum

Internal iliac artery

Posterior fornix

Coccyx

Fundus of bladder

Neck of bladder

Levator ani

External anal sphincter

Internal anal sphincter

Uterus

Urinary bladder

PS

SN

O

UT

C

C

Rectum

Median section

Vagina

Perineal membrane

Figure 3.8. Female pelvis. *C,* cervix of uterus; *O,* ovary; *PS,* pubic symphysis; *SN,* sciatic nerve; *UT,* uterine tube.

Table 3.5 Arteries and Veins of the Pelvis

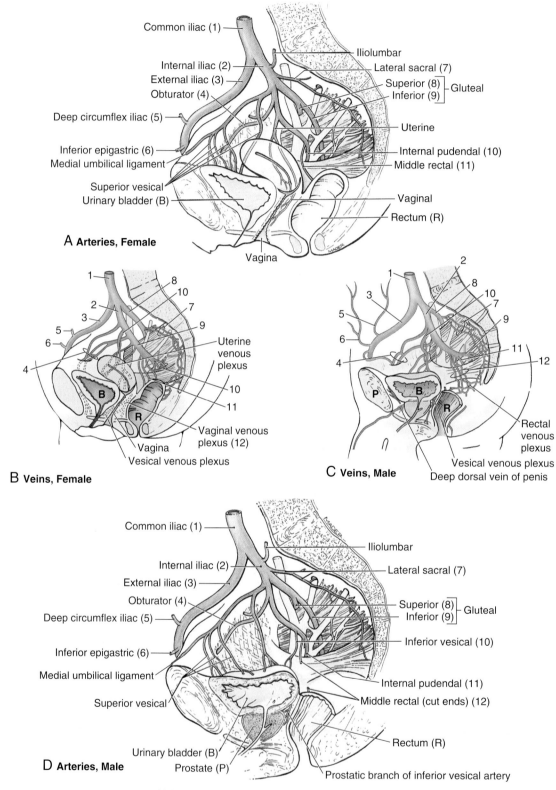

A **Arteries, Female**

- Common iliac (1)
- Internal iliac (2)
- External iliac (3)
- Obturator (4)
- Deep circumflex iliac (5)
- Inferior epigastric (6)
- Medial umbilical ligament
- Superior vesical
- Urinary bladder (B)
- Vagina
- Iliolumbar
- Lateral sacral (7)
- Superior (8) / Inferior (9) — Gluteal
- Uterine
- Internal pudendal (10)
- Middle rectal (11)
- Vaginal
- Rectum (R)

B **Veins, Female**

- Uterine venous plexus
- 10
- 11
- Vaginal venous plexus (12)
- Vagina
- Vesical venous plexus

C **Veins, Male**

- 11
- 12
- Rectal venous plexus
- Vesical venous plexus
- Deep dorsal vein of penis

D **Arteries, Male**

- Common iliac (1)
- Internal iliac (2)
- External iliac (3)
- Obturator (4)
- Deep circumflex iliac (5)
- Inferior epigastric (6)
- Medial umbilical ligament
- Superior vesical
- Urinary bladder (B)
- Prostate (P)
- Iliolumbar
- Lateral sacral (7)
- Superior (8) / Inferior (9) — Gluteal
- Inferior vesical (10)
- Internal pudendal (11)
- Middle rectal (cut ends) (12)
- Rectum (R)
- Prostatic branch of inferior vesical artery

Veins share names with arteries shown in A and D.

Median section

Table 3.5 Arteries and Veins of the Pelvis *(continued)*

Artery	Origin	Course	Distribution
Internal iliac	Common iliac artery	Passes over pelvic brim to reach pelvic cavity	Main blood supply to pelvic organs, gluteal muscles, and perineum
Anterior division of internal iliac artery	Internal iliac artery	Passes anteriorly and divides into visceral branches and obturator artery	Pelvic viscera and muscles in medial compartment of thigh
Umbilical	Anterior division of internal iliac artery	Short pelvic course and ends as superior vesical artery in females	Superior aspect of urinary bladder in females; ductus deferens in males
Obturator		Runs anteroinferiorly on lateral pelvic wall	Pelvic muscles, nutrient artery to ilium, and head of femur
Superior vesical artery	Patent part of umbilical artery	Passes to superior aspect of urinary bladder	Superior aspect of urinary bladder
Artery to ductus deferens	Superior or inferior vesical artery	Runs retroperitoneally to ductus deferens	Ductus deferens
Inferior vesical		Passes retroperitoneally to inferior aspect of male urinary bladder	Urinary bladder, pelvic part of ureter, seminal gland, and prostate
Middle rectal		Descends in pelvis to rectum	Seminal gland, prostate, and rectum
Internal pudendal	Anterior division of internal iliac artery	Leaves pelvis through greater sciatic foramen and enters perineum (ischioanal fossa) by passing through lesser sciatic foramen	Main artery to perineum, including muscles of anal canal and perineum; skin and urogenital triangle; erectile bodies
Inferior gluteal		Leaves pelvis through greater sciatic foramen	Piriformis, coccygeus, levator ani, and gluteal muscles
Uterine		Runs medially on levator ani; crosses ureter to reach base of broad ligament	Pelvic part of ureter, uterus, ligament of uterus, uterine tube, and vagina
Vaginal	Uterine artery	At junction of body and cervix of uterus, it descends to vagina	Vagina and branches to inferior part of urinary bladder
Gonadal (testicular and ovarian)	Abdominal aorta	Descends retroperitoneally; testicular artery passes into deep inguinal ring; ovarian artery crosses brim of pelvis and runs medially in suspensory ligament to ovary	Testis and ovary, respectively
Posterior division of internal iliac artery	Internal iliac artery	Passes posteriorly and gives rise to parietal branches	Pelvic wall and gluteal region
Iliolumbar	Posterior division of internal iliac artery	Ascends anterior to sacroiliac joint and posterior to common iliac vessels and psoas major	Iliacus, psoas major, quadratus lumborum muscles, and cauda equina in vertebral canal
Lateral sacral (superior and inferior)		Run on superficial aspect of piriformis	Piriformis and vertebral canal

division and a posterior division, providing the visceral branches and parietal branches, respectively.

- The paired **ovarian arteries.**
- The **median sacral artery.**
- The **superior rectal artery.**

The origin, course, and distribution of these arteries and their branches are summarized in Table 3.5.

The pelvis is drained:

- Mainly by the internal iliac veins and their tributaries.
- Superior rectal veins (see portal venous system, Chapter 2).
- Median sacral vein.
- Gonadal veins.
- Internal vertebral venous plexus (see Chapter 4).

Pelvic venous plexuses are formed by the interjoining of veins in the pelvis (Table 3.5). The various plexuses (rectal, vesical, prostatic, uterine, and vaginal) unite and drain mainly into the **internal iliac vein,** but some drain through the superior rectal vein into the inferior mesenteric vein or through lateral sacral veins into the internal vertebral venous plexus.

Pelvic Viscera

The pelvic viscera include the inferior part of the intestinal tract (rectum), the urinary bladder, and parts of the ureters and reproductive system (Figs. 3.7 and 3.8). Although the sigmoid colon and parts of the small bowel extend into the pelvic cavity, they are mobile at their abdominal attachments; therefore, they are abdominal rather than pelvic viscera.

Urinary Organs

The pelvic urinary organs are the (Fig. 3.9A & B):

- Ureters, which carry urine from the kidneys.
- Urinary bladder, which temporarily stores urine.
- Urethra, which conducts urine from the urinary bladder to the exterior.

URETERS

The **ureters** are retroperitoneal muscular tubes that connect the kidneys to the urinary bladder. Urine is transported down the ureters by peristaltic contractions. The ureters run inferiorly from the kidneys, passing over the pelvic brim at the bifurcation of the common iliac arteries (Figs. 3.7 and 3.8). The ureters then run posteroinferiorly on the lateral walls of the pelvis, and anterior to the internal iliac arteries. Opposite the ischial spine, they curve anteromedially, superior to the levator ani, to enter the urinary bladder. The ureters pass inferomedially through the muscular wall of the urinary bladder. This oblique passage through the bladder wall forms a one-way "flap valve"; the internal pressure of the filling bladder causes the intramural passage to collapse. In males, the only structure that passes between the ureter and the peritoneum is the *ductus deferens*. The ureter lies posterolateral to the ductus deferens and enters the posterosuperior angle of the bladder (Fig. 3.8). In females, the ureter passes medial to the origin of the uterine artery and continues to the level of the ischial spine, where it is crossed superiorly by the uterine artery. The ureter then passes close to the lateral part of the fornix of the vagina and enters the posterosuperior angle of the bladder.

Vasculature of Ureters. Branches of the common and internal iliac arteries supply the pelvic part of the ureters (Fig. 3.9D). The most constant arteries supplying this part of the ureters in females are branches of the **uterine arteries.** The sources of similar branches in males are the **inferior vesical arteries.** Veins from the ureters accompany the arteries and have corresponding names. **Lymph** drains into the lumbar (caval/aortic), common iliac, external iliac, and internal iliac lymph nodes (Fig. 3.12A).

Innervation of Ureters. The nerves to the ureters derive from adjacent autonomic plexuses (renal, aortic, superior and inferior hypogastric). The ureters are superior to the pelvic pain line; therefore, afferent (pain) fibers from the ureters follow sympathetic fibers retrogradely to reach the spinal ganglia and spinal cord segments T11–L1 or L2 (Fig. 3.9C).

URINARY BLADDER

The **urinary bladder,** a hollow viscus with strong muscular walls, is in the lesser pelvis when empty, posterior and slightly superior to the pubic bones. It is separated from these bones by the *retropubic space* and lies inferior to the peritoneum, where it rests on the pelvic floor (Figs. 3.7 and 3.8). The bladder is relatively free within the extraperitoneal subcutaneous fatty tissue, except for its neck, which is held firmly by the lateral ligaments of the bladder and the tendinous arch of pelvic fascia, especially the *puboprostatic ligament* in males and the *pubovesical ligament* in females. As the bladder fills, it ascends superiorly into the extraperitoneal fatty tissue of the anterior abdominal wall and enters the greater pelvis. A full bladder may ascend to the level of the umbilicus. When empty the bladder is somewhat tetrahedral and externally has an apex, body, fundus, and neck. The four surfaces are a superior surface, two inferolateral surfaces, and a posterior surface (Fig. 3.9).

The **apex of the bladder** (anterior end) points toward the superior edge of the pubic symphysis. The **fundus of the bladder** is opposite the apex, formed by the somewhat convex posterior wall. The **body of the bladder** is the part between the apex and the fundus. *In females,* the fundus is closely related to the anterior wall of the vagina; *in males,* it is related to the rectum. The **neck of the bladder** is where

Ureteric Calculi

Ureteric calculi (stones) may cause complete or intermittent *obstruction of urinary flow.* The obstruction may occur anywhere along the ureter; however, it occurs most often where the ureters are relatively constricted: (1) at the junction of the ureters and renal pelvis, (2) where they cross the external iliac artery and the pelvic brim, and (3) where they passes through the wall of the bladder. The severity of the pain associated with calculi can be extremely intense; it depends on the location, type, size, and texture of the calculus. Ureteric calculi can be removed by open surgery, endoscopy, or **lithotripsy** (shock waves are used to break the stones into small fragments that can be passed in the urine.

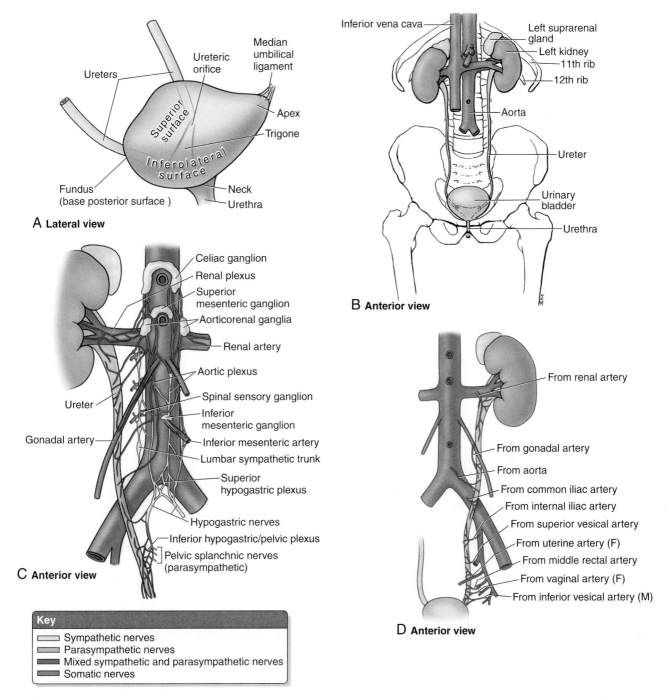

Figure 3.9. Urinary System. A. Parts of the urinary bladder are shown. **B.** An overview of the urinary organs is presented. **C.** The innervation of the ureter is detailed. **D.** Arterial supply of ureter is shown. F=Female, M=Male.

the fundus and inferolateral surfaces converge inferiorly. The **bladder bed** is formed on each side by the pubic bones and the fascia covering the obturator internus and levator ani muscles and posteriorly by the rectum or vagina (Fig. 3.10). The bladder is enveloped by loose connective tissue, the vesical fascia. Only the superior surface is covered by peritoneum.

The walls of the bladder are composed chiefly of the **detrusor muscle** (Fig. 3.10A). Toward the neck of the male bladder, its muscle fibers form the involuntary **internal urethral sphincter.** This sphincter contracts during ejaculation to prevent retrograde ejaculation of semen into the bladder. Some fibers run radially and assist in opening the **internal urethral orifice.** In males, the muscle fibers in the neck of

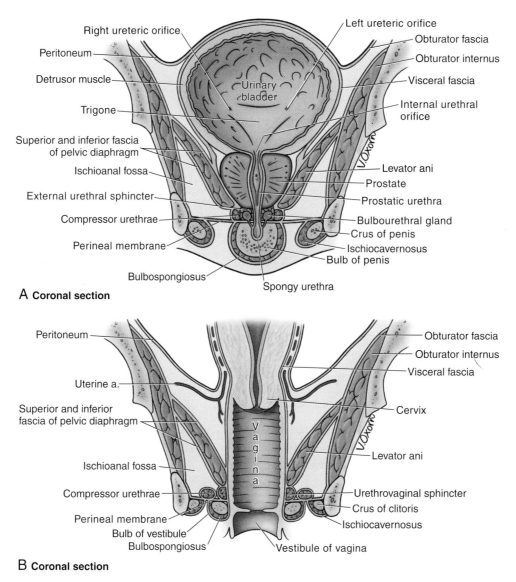

A Coronal section

Right ureteric orifice
Peritoneum
Detrusor muscle
Trigone
Superior and inferior fascia of pelvic diaphragm
Ischioanal fossa
External urethral sphincter
Compressor urethrae
Perineal membrane
Bulbospongiosus

Left ureteric orifice
Obturator fascia
Obturator internus
Visceral fascia
Internal urethral orifice
Urinary bladder
Levator ani
Prostate
Prostatic urethra
Bulbourethral gland
Crus of penis
Ischiocavernosus
Bulb of penis
Spongy urethra

B Coronal section

Peritoneum
Uterine a.
Superior and inferior fascia of pelvic diaphragm
Ischioanal fossa
Compressor urethrae
Perineal membrane
Bulb of vestibule
Bulbospongiosus

Obturator fascia
Obturator internus
Visceral fascia
Cervix
Vagina
Levator ani
Urethrovaginal sphincter
Crus of clitoris
Ischiocavernosus
Vestibule of vagina

Figure 3.10. Structures near urinary bladder. Both the male (**A**) and female (**B**) pelves are shown.

the bladder are continuous with the fibromuscular tissue of the prostate, whereas in females, these fibers are continuous with muscle fibers in the wall of the urethra. The **ureteric orifices** and the internal urethral orifice are at the angles of the **trigone of the bladder** (Figs. 3.10*A* and 3.11*A*). The ureteric orifices are encircled by loops of detrusor musculature that tighten when the bladder contracts to assist in preventing reflux of urine into the bladder. The **uvula of the bladder** is a slight elevation of the trigone.

Vasculature of Bladder. The main arteries supplying the bladder are branches of the internal iliac arteries (Table 3.5). The *superior vesical arteries* supply anterosuperior parts of the bladder. In males, the fundus and neck of the bladder are supplied by the *inferior vesical arteries*. In females, the inferior vesical arteries are replaced by the *vaginal arter-*

ies, which send small branches to the posteroinferior parts of the bladder. The obturator and inferior gluteal arteries also supply small branches to the bladder.

The names of the **veins draining the bladder** correspond to the arteries and are tributaries of the internal iliac veins. In males, the *vesical venous plexus* is continuous with the *prostatic venous plexus* (Fig. 3.11*B*), and the combined plexus envelops the fundus of the bladder and prostate, the seminal glands, the ductus deferentes (plural of ductus deferens), and the inferior ends of the ureters. The prostatic venous plexus also receives blood from the *deep dorsal vein of the penis*. The *vesical venous plexus* mainly drains through the inferior vesical veins into the internal iliac veins (Table 3.4); however, it may drain through the sacral veins into the *internal vertebral venous plexuses* (see

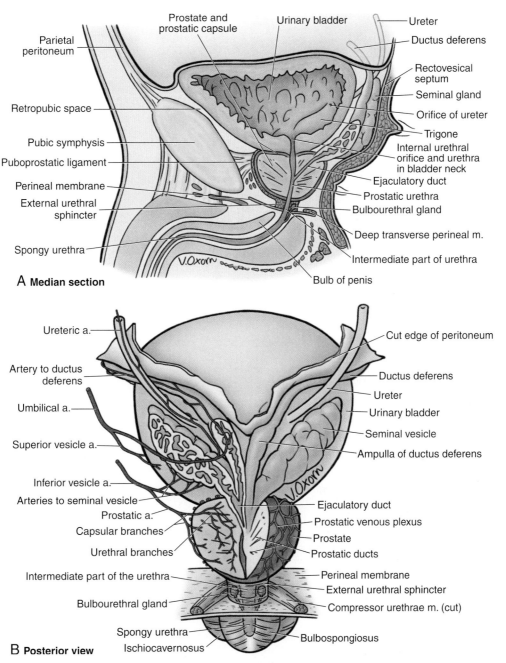

Figure 3.11. Urinary bladder, seminal glands, ductus deferentes, and prostate. A. Relationships of the bladder, prostate, ductus deferens, and ejaculatory duct are demonstrated. **B.** The left seminal gland and ampulla of ductus deferens have been opened and the prostate has been cut away to expose the ejaculatory duct.

Chapter 4). In females, the vesical venous plexus envelops the pelvic part of the urethra and the neck of the bladder, receives blood from the *dorsal vein of the clitoris,* and communicates with the *vaginal or uterovaginal venous plexus* (Table 3.5). In both sexes, **lymphatic vessels** leave the superior surface of the bladder and pass to the *external iliac lymph nodes* (Tables 3.6 and 3.7), whereas those from the fundus pass to the *internal iliac lymph nodes*. Some vessels from the neck of the bladder drain into the sacral or common iliac lymph nodes.

Innervation of Bladder. *Sympathetic fibers* to the bladder are conveyed from the T11–L2 or L3 spinal cord levels to the vesical (pelvic) plexuses, primarily through the hypogastric plexuses and nerves, whereas parasympathetic fibers from the sacral spinal cord levels are conveyed by the pelvic splanchnic nerves and the inferior hypogastric

Table 3.6 Lymphatic Drainage of the Female Pelvis and Perineum

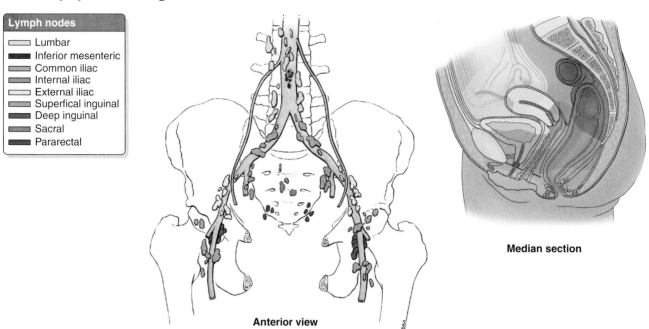

Lymph nodes
Lumbar
Inferior mesenteric
Common iliac
Internal iliac
External iliac
Superfical inguinal
Deep inguinal
Sacral
Pararectal

Anterior view

Median section

Lymph Node Group	Typically Drains
Lumbar (along ovarian vessels)	Gonads and associated structures, common iliac nodes (ovary, uterine tube except isthmus and intrauterine parts, fundus of uterus)
Inferior mesenteric	Superiormost rectum, sigmoid colon, descending colon, pararectal nodes
Internal iliac	Inferior pelvic structures, deep perineal structures, sacral nodes (base of bladder, inferior pelvic ureter, anal canal above pectinate line, inferior rectum, middle and upper vagina, cervix, body of uterus)
External iliac	Anterosuperior pelvic structures, deep inguinal nodes (superior bladder, superior pelvic ureter, upper vagina, cervix, lower body of uterus)
Superficial inguinal	Lower limb; superficial drainage of inferolateral quadrant of trunk, including anterior abdominal wall inferior to umbilicus, gluteal region, superficial perineal structures (superolateral uterus near attachment of round ligament, skin of perineum including vulva, ostium of vagina inferior to hymen, prepuce of clitoris, perianal skin, anal canal inferior to pectinate line)
Deep inguinal	Glans clitoris, superficial inguinal nodes
Sacral	Posteroinferior pelvic structures, inferior rectum, inferior vagina
Pararectal	Superior rectum

plexuses (Fig. 3.12). *Parasympathetic fibers* are motor to the detrusor muscle in the bladder wall and inhibitory to the internal sphincter of males. Hence, when the visceral afferent fibers are stimulated by stretching, the bladder contracts, the internal sphincter relaxes in males, and urine flows into the urethra. Adults suppress this reflex until it is convenient to void. The sympathetic innervation that stimulates ejaculation simultaneously causes contraction of the internal urethral sphincter, to prevent reflux of semen into the bladder.

Sensory fibers from the bladder are visceral; reflex afferents and pain (e.g., from overdistention) afferents from the inferior part of the bladder follow the course of the parasympathetic fibers. The superior surface of the bladder is cov-

ered with peritoneum and is, therefore, superior to the pain line; thus pain fibers from the superior part of the bladder follow the sympathetic fibers retrogradely.

MALE URETHRA

The **male urethra** is a muscular tube that conveys urine from the *internal urethral orifice* of the urinary bladder to the exterior through the *external urethral orifice* at the tip of the glans penis (Fig. 3.11*A*). The urethra also provides an exit for semen (sperms and glandular secretions). For descriptive purposes, the urethra is divided into four parts: intramural part of the urethra (preprostatic urethra), prostatic

Table 3.7 Lymphatic Drainage of the Male Pelvis and Perineum

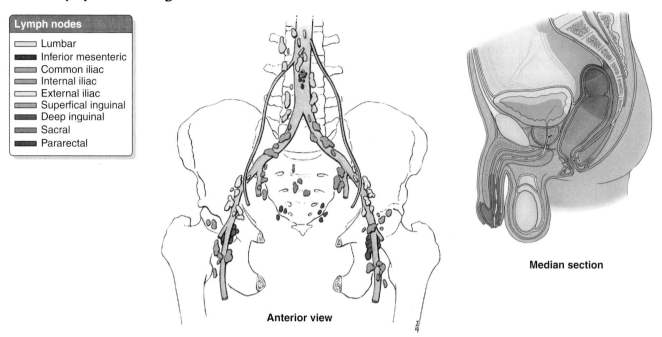

Lymph nodes
☐ Lumbar
◼ Inferior mesenteric
▨ Common iliac
▨ Internal iliac
☐ External iliac
▨ Superfical inguinal
◼ Deep inguinal
▨ Sacral
◼ Pararectal

Anterior view

Median section

Lymph Node Group	Typically Drains
Lumbar along testicular vessels	Urethra, testis, epididymis
Inferior mesenteric	Superiormost rectum, sigmoid colon, descending colon, pararectal nodes
Internal iliac	External and internal iliac lymph nodes
External iliac	Inferior pelvic structures, deep perineal structures, sacral nodes (prostatic urethra, prostate, base of bladder, inferior pelvic ureter, inferior seminal glands, cavernous bodies, anal canal above pectinate line, inferior rectum)
Superficial inguinal	Lower limb; superficial drainage of inferolateral quadrant of trunk, including anterior abdominal wall inferior to umbilicus, gluteal region, superficial perineal structures (skin of perineum including skin and prepuce of penis, scrotum, perianal skin, anal canal inferior to pectinate line)
Deep inguinal	Glans of penis, superficial inguinal nodes, distal spongy urethra
Sacral	Posteroinferior pelvic structures, inferior rectum
Pararectal	Superior rectum

urethra, intermediate (membranous) part of the urethra, and spongy (penile) part of the urethra (Figs. 3.11*A* and 3.13; Table 3.8).

Vasculature of Male Urethra. The urethra in the bladder neck and the prostatic urethra are supplied by the *prostatic branches of the inferior vesical and middle rectal arteries* (Table 3.5). The intermediate and spongy parts of the urethra are supplied by the *internal pudendal artery*. The **veins** accompany the arteries and have similar names. The **lymphatic vessels** drain mainly into the *internal iliac lymph nodes* (Table 3.7), but some lymph passes to the *external iliac lymph nodes*. Lymphatic vessels from the spongy urethra pass to the *deep inguinal lymph nodes*.

Innervation of Male Urethra. The nerves of the male urethra are derived from the **prostatic nerve plexus** (mixed

sympathetic, parasympathetic and visceral afferent fibers) (Fig. 3.12). This plexus is one of the pelvic plexuses (an inferior extension of the vesical plexus) arising as an organ-specific extension of the inferior hypogastric plexus.

FEMALE URETHRA

The short **female urethra** passes anteroinferiorly from the *internal urethral orifice* of the urinary bladder, posterior, and then inferior to the pubic symphysis to the *external urethral orifice* in the vestibule of the vagina (Fig. 3.8). The urethra lies anterior to the vagina; its axis is parallel with the vagina. The urethra passes with the vagina through the pelvic diaphragm, external urethral sphincter, and perineal membrane. Urethral glands are present, particularly in its supe-

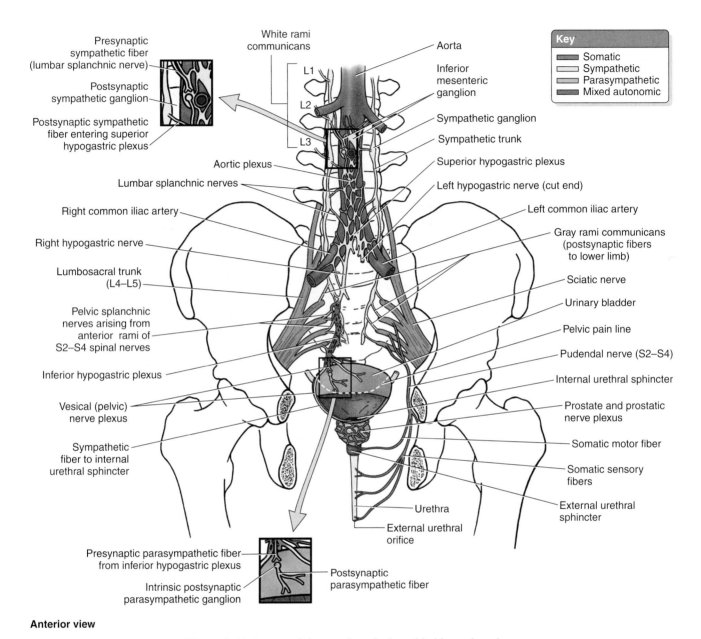

Key
- Somatic
- Sympathetic
- Parasympathetic
- Mixed autonomic

Presynaptic sympathetic fiber (lumbar splanchnic nerve)

Postsynaptic sympathetic ganglion

Postsynaptic sympathetic fiber entering superior hypogastric plexus

White rami communicans

L1

L2

L3

Aortic plexus

Lumbar splanchnic nerves

Right common iliac artery

Right hypogastric nerve

Lumbosacral trunk (L4–L5)

Pelvic splanchnic nerves arising from anterior rami of S2–S4 spinal nerves

Inferior hypogastric plexus

Vesical (pelvic) nerve plexus

Sympathetic fiber to internal urethral sphincter

Aorta

Inferior mesenteric ganglion

Sympathetic ganglion

Sympathetic trunk

Superior hypogastric plexus

Left hypogastric nerve (cut end)

Left common iliac artery

Gray rami communicans (postsynaptic fibers to lower limb)

Sciatic nerve

Urinary bladder

Pelvic pain line

Pudendal nerve (S2–S4)

Internal urethral sphincter

Prostate and prostatic nerve plexus

Somatic motor fiber

Somatic sensory fibers

External urethral sphincter

Urethra

External urethral orifice

Presynaptic parasympathetic fiber from inferior hypogastric plexus

Postsynaptic parasympathetic fiber

Intrinsic postsynaptic parasympathetic ganglion

Anterior view

Figure 3.12. Autonomic innervation of urinary bladder and urethra.

rior part; the **paraurethral glands** are homologues to the prostate. These glands have a common paraurethral duct, which opens (one on each side) near the external urethral orifice. The inferior half of the urethra is in the perineum and is discussed in that section.

Vasculature of Female Urethra. Blood is supplied by the *internal pudendal* and *vaginal arteries* (Table 3.5). The veins follow the arteries and have similar names. Most lymphatic vessels from the urethra pass to the *sacral* and *internal iliac lymph nodes* (Table 3.6). A few vessels drain into the *inguinal lymph nodes.*

Innervation of Female Urethra. The nerves to the urethra arise from the *vesical (nerve) plexus* and the *pudendal*

nerve (Fig. 3.12). The pattern is similar to that in the male, given the absence of a prostatic plexus and an internal urethral sphincter. Visceral afferents from most of the urethra run in *pelvic splanchnic nerves,* but the termination receives somatic afferents from the pudendal nerve.

Male Internal Genital Organs

The male internal genital organs include the testes, epididymides (plural of epididymis), ductus deferentes (plural of ductus deferens), seminal glands, ejaculatory ducts, prostate, and bulbourethral glands (Fig. 3.11). The testes and epididymides are described in Chapter 2.

Suprapubic Cystotomy

As the bladder fills, it extends superiorly in the extraperitoneal fatty tissue of the anterior abdominal wall. The bladder then lies adjacent to this wall without the intervention of peritoneum. Consequently, the distended bladder may be punctured (*suprapubic cystostomy*) or approached surgically for the introduction of indwelling catheters or instruments without traversing the peritoneum and entering the peritoneal cavity.

Rupture of Bladder

Because of the superior position of a distended bladder, it may be ruptured by injuries to the inferior part of the anterior abdominal wall or by fractures of the pelvis. The rupture of the superior part of the bladder frequently tears the peritoneum, resulting in passage (extravasation) of urine into the peritoneal cavity. Posterior rupture of the bladder usually results in passage of urine subperitoneally into the perineum.

Cystoscopy

The interior of the bladder and its three orifices can be examined with a *cystoscope*, a lighted tubular endoscope that is inserted through the urethra into the bladder. The cystoscope consists of a light; an observing lens; and various attachments for grasping, removing, cutting, and cauterizing (Fig. B3.2).

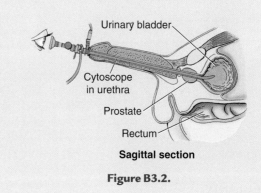

Sagittal section

Figure B3.2.

DUCTUS DEFERENS

The **ductus deferens** (deferent duct, vas deferens) is the continuation of the duct of the epididymis (see Chapter 2). The ductus deferens (Figs. 3.7 and 3.11):

- Begins in the tail of the epididymis at the inferior pole of the testis.
- Ascends in the spermatic cord.
- Passes through the inguinal canal.

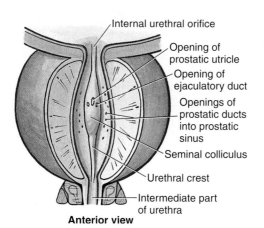

Figure 3.13. Posterior wall of prostatic urethra. Observe the openings of the ejaculatory and prostatic ducts.

- Crosses over the external iliac vessels and enters the pelvis.
- Passes along the lateral wall of the pelvis where it lies external to the parietal peritoneum.
- Ends by joining the duct of the seminal gland to form the *ejaculatory duct*.

During the course of the ductus deferens, no other structure intervenes between it and the peritoneum. The ductus crosses superior to the ureter near the posterolateral angle of the bladder, running between the ureter and the peritoneum to reach the fundus of the urinary bladder. Posterior to the bladder, the ductus deferens at first lies superior to the seminal gland, then it descends medial to the ureter and the gland. Here, the ductus deferens enlarges to form the **ampulla of the ductus deferens** before its termination. The ductus then narrows and joins the duct of the seminal gland to form the **ejaculatory duct**.

Vasculature of Ductus Deferens. The tiny *artery to the ductus deferens* usually arises from a superior (sometimes inferior) vesical artery and accompanies the ductus deferens as far as the testis (Table 3.5). It terminates by anastomosing with the testicular artery, posterior to the testis. The veins accompany the arteries and have similar names. The lymphatic vessels from the ductus deferens drain into the *external iliac lymph nodes* (Table 3.7).

Table 3.8 Parts of the Male Urethra

Part	Length (cm)	Location/Disposition	Features
Intramural (preprostatic) part	0.5–1.5	Extends almost vertically through neck of bladder	Surrounded by internal urethral sphincter; diameter and length vary, depending on whether bladder is filling or emptying
Prostatic urethra	3.0–4.0	Descends through anterior prostate, forming gentle, anteriorly concave curve; is bounded anteriorly by vertical, trough-like part (rhabdosphincter) of external urethral sphincter	Widest and most dilatable part; features urethral crest with seminal colliculus, flanked by prostatic sinuses into which the prostatic ducts open; ejaculatory ducts open onto colliculus; hence urinary and reproductive tracts merge in this part
Intermediate (membranous) part	1.0–1.5	Passes through deep perineal pouch, surrounded by circular fibers of external urethral sphincter; penetrates perineal membrane	Narrowest and least distensible part (except for external urethral orifice)
Spongy urethra	~ 15	Courses through corpus spongiosum; initial widening occurs in bulb of penis; widens again distally as navicular fossa (in the glans penis)	Longest and most mobile part; bulbourethral glands open into bulbous part; distally, urethral glands open into small urethral lacunae entering lumen of this part

SEMINAL GLANDS

Each **seminal gland** (vesicle) is an elongated structure that lies between the fundus of the bladder and the rectum (Fig. 3.11). The seminal glands are obliquely placed structures superior to the prostate and do not store sperms. They secrete a thick alkaline fluid that mixes with the sperms as they pass into the ejaculatory ducts and urethra. The superior ends of the seminal glands are covered with peritoneum and lie posterior to the ureters, where the peritoneum of the *rectovesical pouch* separates them from the rectum (Table 3.3). The inferior ends of the seminal glands are closely related to the rectum and are separated from it only by the rectovesical septum.

Sterilization of Males

The common method of sterilizing males is **deferentectomy,** popularly called a *vasectomy*. During this procedure, part of the ductus deferens is ligated and/or excised through an incision in the superior part of the scrotum. Hence the ejaculated fluid from the seminal glands, prostate, and bulbourethral glands contains no sperms. The unexpelled sperms degenerate in the epididymis and the proximal part of the ductus deferens.

Vasculature of Seminal Glands.   The arteries to the seminal glands derive from the *inferior vesical* and *middle rectal arteries* (Table 3.5). The veins accompany the arteries and have similar names. The iliac lymph nodes receive lymph from the seminal glands: the *external iliac nodes* from the superior part, and the *internal iliac lymph nodes* from the inferior part. (Table 3.7).

EJACULATORY DUCTS

Each **ejaculatory duct** is a slender tube that arises by the union of the duct of a seminal gland with the ductus deferens (Fig. 3.11). The ejaculatory ducts arise near the neck of the bladder and run close together as they pass anteroinferiorly through the posterior part of the prostate. The ducts converge to open by slit-like apertures on, or just within, the opening of the prostatic utricle (Fig. 3.13). Prostatic secretions join the seminal fluid in the prostatic urethra after the termination of the ejaculatory ducts.

Vasculature of Ejaculatory Ducts.   The *arteries to the ductus deferentes,* usually branches of the superior (but frequently inferior) vesical arteries, supply the ejaculatory ducts (Table 3.5). The veins join the *prostatic* and *vesical venous plexuses.* The lymphatic vessels drain into the *external iliac lymph nodes* (Table 3.7).

PROSTATE

The walnut-size **prostate** surrounds the *prostatic urethra* (Fig. 3.11). The glandular part makes up approximately two thirds of the prostate; the other third is fibromuscular. The structure has a dense **fibrous capsule of the prostate** that incorporates the prostatic plexuses of nerves and veins. This is surrounded by the visceral layer of the pelvic fascia, forming a fibrous *prostatic sheath* that is thin anteriorly, continuous anterolaterally with the *puboprostatic ligaments,* and dense posteriorly, continuous with the *rectovesical septum.*

The prostate has

- A **base** (superior aspect) that is closely related to the neck of the bladder.
- An **apex** (inferior aspect) that is in contact with fascia on the superior aspect of the urethral sphincter and deep perineal muscles.
- A muscular **anterior surface** that features mostly transversely oriented muscle fibers forming a vertical trough-like hemisphincter (rhabdosphincter), which is part the urethral sphincter, separated from the pubic symphysis by retroperitoneal fat in the **retropubic space** (Fig. 3.11*A*).
- A **posterior surface** that is related to the ampulla of the rectum.

- **Inferolateral surfaces** that are related to the levator ani.

Although not clearly distinct anatomically, the following **lobes of the prostate** are traditionally described.

- The **isthmus of the prostate** (historically, the anterior lobe) lies anterior to the urethra. It is primarily muscular and represents the superior continuation of the urethral sphincter muscle.
- The **inferoposterior** (posterior) **lobe** lies posterior to the urethra and inferior to the ejaculatory ducts; it is readily palpable by digital rectal examination.
- The **right** and **left** (lateral) **lobes** on either side of the urethra form the major part of the prostate.
- The **middle** (*median*) **lobe** lies between the urethra and the ejaculatory ducts and is closely related to the neck of the bladder. Enlargement of the middle lobe is believed to be partially responsible for the formation of the *uvula* that may project into the internal urethral orifice.

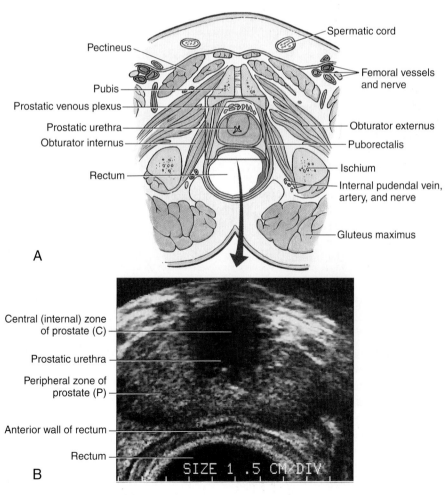

Figure 3.14. Relations of prostate. A. Details of the central and peripheral zones male pelvis are shown. **B.** The zones are seen in this transverse (transrectal) ultrasound scan.

Urologists and sonographers usually divide the prostate into peripheral and central (internal) zones (Fig. 3.14). The central zone is comparable to the middle lobe.

The **prostatic ducts** (20–30) open chiefly into the **prostatic sinuses** that lie on either side of the **seminal colliculus** on the posterior wall of the prostatic urethra (Fig. 3.13). Prostatic fluid provides about 20% of the volume of semen.

Vasculature of Prostate.   The prostatic **arteries** are mainly branches of the *internal iliac artery* (Table 3.5), especially the *inferior vesical arteries* but also the *internal pudendal* and *middle rectal arteries.* The **veins** join to form the **prostatic venous plexus** around the sides and base of the prostate (Fig. 3.11). This plexus, between the fibrous capsule of the prostate and the prostatic sheath, drains into the *internal iliac veins.* The plexus is continuous superiorly with the *vesical venous plexus* and communicates posteriorly with the *internal vertebral venous plexus* (see Chapter 4). The lymphatic vessels drain chiefly into the *internal iliac nodes,* but some pass to the *sacral lymph nodes* (Table 3.7).

BULBOURETHRAL GLANDS

The two pea-size **bulbourethral glands** (Cowper glands) lie posterolateral to the intermediate part of the urethra, largely embedded within the external urethral sphincter (Fig. 3.13).

The **ducts of the bulbourethral glands** pass through the perineal membrane with the intermediate urethra and open through minute apertures into the proximal part of the spongy urethra in the bulb of the penis. Their mucus-like secretion enters the urethra during sexual arousal.

INNERVATION OF THE INTERNAL GENITAL ORGANS OF THE MALE PELVIS

The ductus deferens, seminal glands, ejaculatory ducts, and prostate are richly innervated by *sympathetic nerve fibers* originating from cell bodies in the intermediolateral cell column. They traverse the paravertebral ganglia of the sympathetic trunk to become components of the lumbar (abdominopelvic) splanchnic nerves and the hypogastric and pelvic plexuses (Fig. 3.15). *Presynaptic parasympathetic fibers* from the S2–S3 spinal cord segments traverse the pelvic splanchnic nerves, which also join the inferior hypogastric–pelvic plexuses. Synapses with postsynaptic sympathetic and parasympathetic neurons occur with the plexuses, en route to or near the pelvic viscera. As part of an orgasm, the sympathetic system stimulates contractions of the ductus deferens, and the combined contraction of and secretion from the seminal and prostate glands provides the vehicle (semen) and the expulsive force to dis-

Prostatic Enlargement and Prostatic Cancer

The prostate is of medical interest because benign enlargement or **benign hypertrophy of the prostate** is common after middle age. An enlarged prostate projects into the urinary bladder and impedes urination by distorting the prostatic urethra. The middle lobe usually enlarges the most and obstructs the internal urethral orifice.

Prostatic cancer is common in men older than 55 years. In most cases, the cancer develops in the posterolateral region. This may be palpated during a digital rectal examination (Fig. B3.3). A malignant prostate feels hard and often irregular. In advanced stages, cancer cells metastasize (spread) to the iliac and sacral lymph nodes and later to distant nodes and bone. The prostatic plexus, closely associated with the prostatic sheath, gives passage to parasympathetic fibers, which give rise to the cavernous nerves that convey the fibers that cause penile erection. A major concern regarding **prostatectomy** is that impotency may

be a consequence. All or part of the prostate, or just the hypertrophied part, is removed (*transurethral resection of the prostate;* TURP).

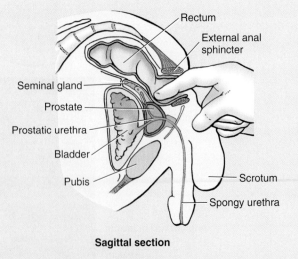

Sagittal section

Figure B3.3.

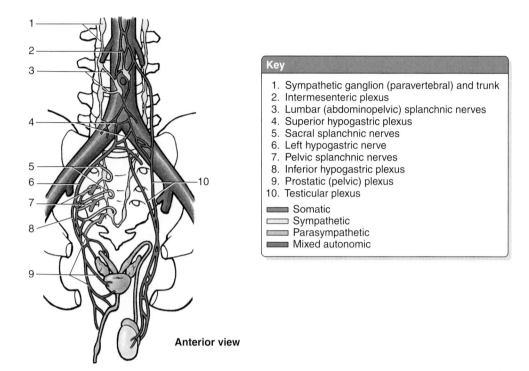

Key

1. Sympathetic ganglion (paravertebral) and trunk
2. Intermesenteric plexus
3. Lumbar (abdominopelvic) splanchnic nerves
4. Superior hypogastric plexus
5. Sacral splanchnic nerves
6. Left hypogastric nerve
7. Pelvic splanchnic nerves
8. Inferior hypogastric plexus
9. Prostatic (pelvic) plexus
10. Testicular plexus

Somatic
Sympathetic
Parasympathetic
Mixed autonomic

Anterior view

Figure 3.15. Autonomic innervation of testis, ductus deferens, prostate, and seminal glands.

charge the sperm during ejaculation. The function of the parasympathetic innervation is unclear. However, the parasympathetic fibers in the prostatic nerve plexus form the cavernous nerves that pass to the erectile bodies of the penis, which are responsible for producing penile erection.

Female Internal Genital Organs

The female internal genital organs include the vagina, uterus, uterine tubes, and ovaries.

VAGINA

The **vagina**, a musculomembranous tube, extends from the cervix of the uterus to the **vestibule**, the cleft between the labia minora into which the vagina and urethra open (Fig. 3.16). The vestibule contains the vaginal and external urethral orifices and the openings of the two greater vestibular glands. The superior end of the vagina surrounds the *cervix* of the uterus.

The vagina:

- Serves as a canal for menstrual fluid.
- Forms the inferior part of the pelvic (birth) canal.
- Receives the penis and ejaculate during sexual intercourse.
- Communicates superiorly with the **cervical canal**, and inferiorly with the vestibule (Fig. 3.16). The cervical

canal extends from the isthmus of the uterus to the external os (opening) of the uterus.

The vagina is usually collapsed so its anterior and posterior walls are in contact, except at its superior end, where the cervix holds them apart. The **vaginal fornix**, the recess around the protruding cervix, is usually described as having *anterior, posterior,* and *lateral parts*. The **posterior vaginal fornix** is the deepest part and is closely related to the rectouterine pouch (Fig. 3.16B). Four muscles compress the vagina and act like sphincters: **pubovaginalis, external urethral sphincter, urethrovaginal sphincter,** and **bulbospongiosus** (Table 3.9). The relations of the vagina are

- Anteriorly: the fundus of the urinary bladder and urethra.
- Laterally: the levator ani, visceral pelvic fascia, and ureters.
- Posteriorly (inferior to superior): the anal canal, rectum, and rectouterine pouch.

Vasculature of Vagina. The **arteries** supplying the superior part of the vagina derive from the *uterine arteries;* the arteries supplying the middle and inferior parts of the vagina derive from the *vaginal arteries* and *internal pudendal arteries* (Fig. 3.17A; Table 3.5). The **veins** form the **vaginal venous plexuses** along the sides of the vagina and within the vaginal

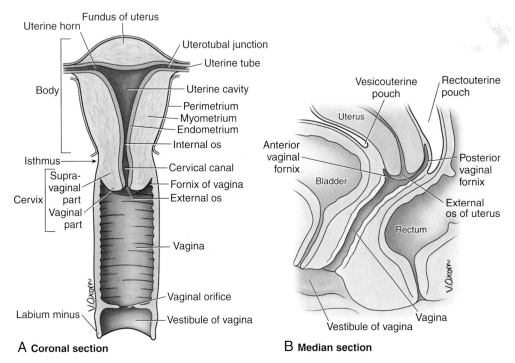

Figure 3.16. Uterus and vagina.

mucosa (Fig. 3.17*B*). These veins communicate with the *uterine venous plexus* as the **uterovaginal plexus** and drain into the internal iliac veins through the uterine vein.

The lymphatic vessels drain from the vagina as follows (Table 3.6):

- Superior part: to the internal and external iliac lymph nodes.
- Middle part: to the internal iliac lymph nodes.

- Inferior part: to the sacral and common iliac nodes.
- External orifice: to the superficial inguinal lymph nodes.

UTERUS

The uterus (womb) is a thick-walled, pear-shaped, hollow muscular organ. The non-gravid (not pregnant) uterus usually lies in the lesser pelvis, with its body lying on the urinary bladder and its cervix between the urinary bladder

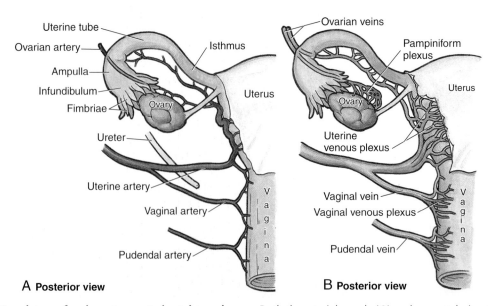

Figure 3.17. Vasculature of vagina, uterus, uterine tube, and ovary. Both the arterial supply (**A**) and venous drainage (**B**) are shown.

Table 3.9 Supporting and Compressor Muscles of the Pelvis

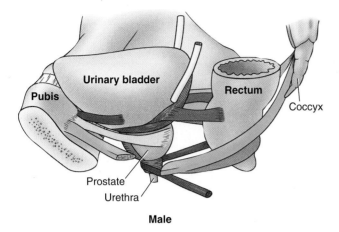

Male

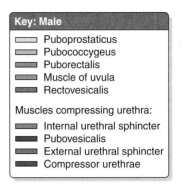

Key: Male
- Puboprostaticus
- Pubococcygeus
- Puborectalis
- Muscle of uvula
- Rectovesicalis

Muscles compressing urethra:
- Internal urethral sphincter
- Pubovesicalis
- External urethral sphincter
- Compressor urethrae

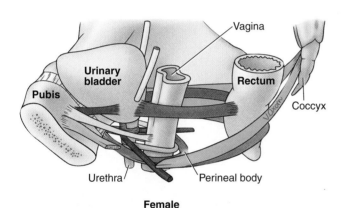

Female

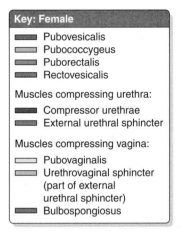

Key: Female
- Pubovesicalis
- Pubococcygeus
- Puborectalis
- Rectovesicalis

Muscles compressing urethra:
- Compressor urethrae
- External urethral sphincter

Muscles compressing vagina:
- Pubovaginalis
- Urethrovaginal sphincter (part of external urethral sphincter)
- Bulbospongiosus

and the rectum (Fig. 3.16*B*). The adult uterus is usually anteverted (tipped anterosuperiorly relative to the axis of the vagina) and *anteflexed* (uterine body is flexed or bent anteriorly relative to the cervix) so that its mass lies over the bladder (Fig. 3.8). The position of the uterus changes with the degree of fullness of the bladder and rectum. The uterus is divisible into two main parts (Fig. 3.16*A*):

- The **body of the uterus,** forming the superior two thirds of the structure, includes the **fundus of the uterus,** the rounded part of the body that lies superior to the orifices of the uterine tubes, and the **isthmus of the uterus,** the relatively constricted region of the body (about 1 cm long) just superior to the cervix. The **uterine horns** (L. *cornua*) are the superolateral regions where the uterine tubes enter. The body of the uterus lies between the layers of the broad ligament and is freely movable (Fig. 3.18*A*).
- The **cervix of the uterus,** the cylindrical, narrow inferior part of the uterus, which has a *supravaginal part* between the isthmus and the vagina and a *vaginal part* that protrudes into the vagina and surrounds the *external os of*

the uterus. The *supravaginal part of the cervix* is separated from the bladder anteriorly by loose connective tissue and from the rectum posteriorly by the rectouterine pouch (Fig. 3.16*B*). The cervix is mostly fibrous, with a small amount of smooth muscle and elastin.

The wall of the body of the uterus consists of three layers (Fig. 3.16*A*):

- **Perimetrium:** the outer serous coat, which consists of peritoneum supported by a thin layer of connective tissue.
- **Myometrium:** the middle muscular coat of smooth muscle, which becomes greatly distended during pregnancy; the main branches of the blood vessels and nerves of the uterus are located in this coat.
- **Endometrium:** the inner mucous coat, which firmly adheres to the myometrium and is actively involved in the menstrual cycle, differing in structure with each stage; if conception occurs, the blastocyst becomes implanted in this layer; if conception does not occur, the inner surface of the coat is shed through menstruation.

Distention and Examination of Vagina

The vagina can be markedly distended by the fetus during childbirth, particularly in an anteroposterior direction. Lateral distention of the vagina is limited by the ischial spines, which project posteromedially, and the sacrospinous ligaments extending from these spines to the lateral margins of the sacrum and coccyx. The interior of the vagina can be distended for examination using a *vaginal speculum* (Fig. B3.4). The cervix, ischial spines, and sacral promontory can be palpated with the digits in the vagina and/or rectum (*manual pelvic examination*).

Culdocentesis

An endoscopic instrument (*culdoscope*) can be inserted through an incision made in the posterior part of the vaginal fornix into the peritoneal cavity to drain a pelvic abscess (collection of pus) in the rectouterine pouch (*culdocentesis*). Similarly, fluid in this part of the perineal cavity (e.g., blood) can be aspirated at this site.

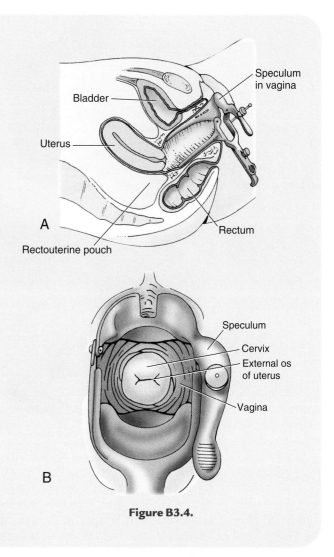

Figure B3.4.

Ligaments of the Uterus.   Externally, the **ligament of the ovary** attaches to the uterus posteroinferior to the uterotubal junction (Fig. 3.18*A*). The **round ligament of the uterus** attaches anteroinferiorly to this junction. These two ligaments are vestiges of the *ovarian gubernaculum,* related to the descent of the gonad from its developmental position on the posterior abdominal wall (see Chapter 2).

The **broad ligament of the uterus** is a double layer of peritoneum (mesentery) that extends from the sides of the uterus to the lateral walls and floor of the pelvis (Fig. 3.18*A*). This ligament assists in keeping the uterus relatively centered in the pelvis but mostly contains the ovaries, uterine tubes, and related structures as well as the vasculature that serves them. The two layers of the ligament are continuous with each other at a free edge, which surrounds the uterine tube. Laterally, the ligament is prolonged superiorly over the ovarian vessels as the **suspensory ligament of the ovary** (Fig. 3.18). Between the layers of the broad ligament on each side of the uterus, the **ligament of the ovary** lies posterosuperiorly and the *round ligament of the uterus,* anteroinferiorly. The part of the broad ligament by which the ovary is suspended is the **mesovarium** (Fig. 3.18*B*). The part of the broad ligament forming the mesentery of the uterine tube is the **mesosalpinx**. The major part of the broad ligament serves as a mesentery for the uterus and is the **mesometrium**, which lies inferior to the mesosalpinx and mesovarium.

The principal supports of the uterus are both dynamic and passive. Dynamic support is provided by the pelvic fascia. Passive support is provided by the way in which the uterus normally rests on top of the bladder. The cervix is the least mobile part of the uterus because of the passive support provided by attached condensations of endopelvic

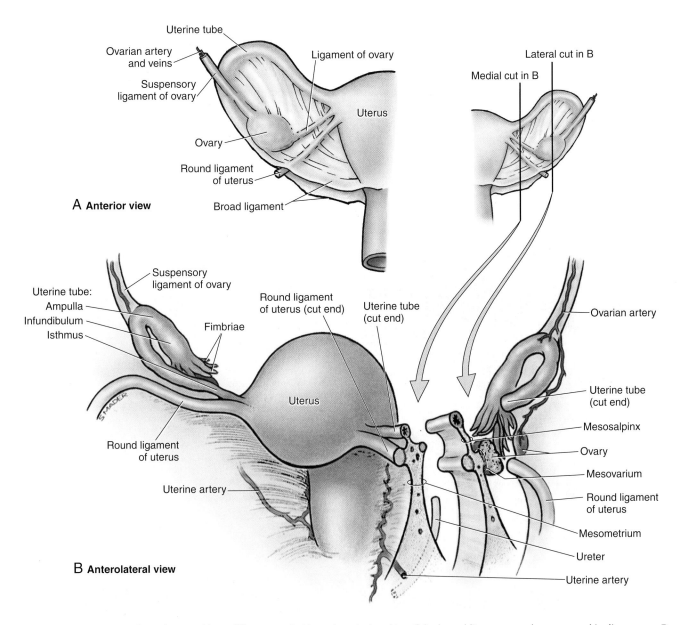

Figure 3.18. Uterus, uterine tubes, and broad ligament. A. Note the relationship of the broad ligament to the ovary and its ligaments. **B.** This sagittal sections shows the mesentery of the uterus (mesometrium), ovary (mesovarium), and uterine tube (mesosalpinx).

fascia (ligaments), which may also contain smooth muscle (Fig. 3.5 B & C):

- *Transverse cervical* (cardinal) *ligaments* extend from the cervix and lateral parts of the fornix of the vagina to the lateral walls of the pelvis.
- *Uterosacral ligaments* pass superiorly and slightly posteriorly from the sides of the cervix to the middle of the sacrum; they are palpable on rectal examination.

Relations of the Uterus. Peritoneum covers the uterus anteriorly and superiorly, except for the cervix (Fig. 3.18; Table 3.3). The peritoneum is reflected anteriorly from the uterus onto the bladder and posteriorly over the posterior part of the fornix of the vagina onto the rectum. Anteriorly, the uterine body is separated from the urinary bladder by the **vesicouterine pouch** where the peritoneum is reflected from the uterus onto the posterior margin of the superior surface of the bladder (Fig. 3.16B); the inferior uterine body (isthmus) and cervix lie in direct contact with the bladder without intervening peritoneum. This allows uterine/cervical cancer to invade the urinary bladder. Posteriorly, the uterine body and supravaginal part of the cervix are separated from the sigmoid colon by a layer of peritoneum and the peritoneal cavity and from the rectum by the *rectouterine pouch* (Fig. 3.16B). Laterally, the uterine artery crosses the ureter superiorly, near the cervix, in the root of the broad ligament (Fig. 3.18*B*).

Vasculature of Uterus. The *arteries* derive mainly from the **uterine arteries,** with potential collateral supply from the ovarian arteries (Fig. 3.17*A;* Table 3.5). The *uterine veins* run in the broad ligament, draining the **uterine venous plexus** formed on each side of the uterus and vagina (Fig. 3.17*B*). Veins from this plexus drain into the internal iliac veins.

The *uterine lymphatic vessels* follow three main routes (Table 3.6):

* Most vessels from the uterine fundus and superior uterine body pass along the ovarian vessels to the lumbar (caval/aortic) lymph nodes, but some vessels pass along the round ligament of the uterus to the *superficial inguinal lymph nodes.*

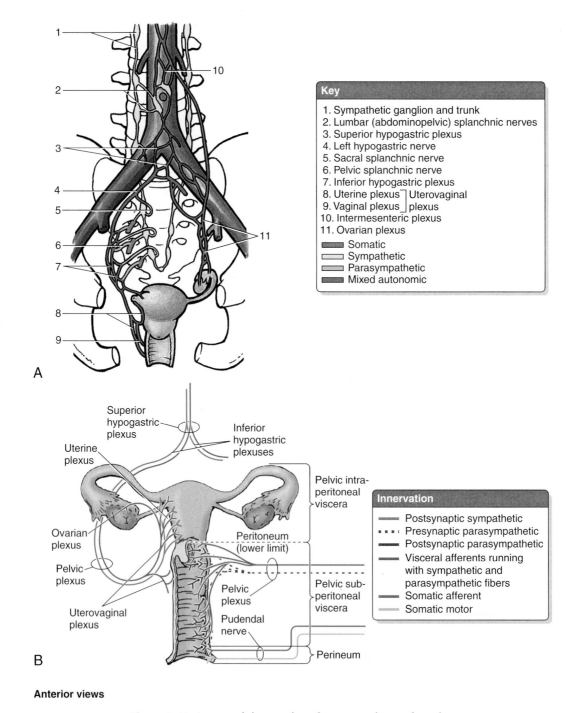

Key

1. Sympathetic ganglion and trunk
2. Lumbar (abdominopelvic) splanchnic nerves
3. Superior hypogastric plexus
4. Left hypogastric nerve
5. Sacral splanchnic nerve
6. Pelvic splanchnic nerve
7. Inferior hypogastric plexus
8. Uterine plexus ⎤ Uterovaginal
9. Vaginal plexus ⎦ plexus
10. Intermesenteric plexus
11. Ovarian plexus

▬ Somatic
▭ Sympathetic
▬ Parasympathetic
▬ Mixed autonomic

Innervation

▬ Postsynaptic sympathetic
•••• Presynaptic parasympathetic
▬ Postsynaptic parasympathetic
▬ Visceral afferents running with sympathetic and parasympathetic fibers
▬ Somatic afferent
▬ Somatic motor

Anterior views

Figure 3.19. Autonomic innervation of uterus, vagina, and ovaries.

- Vessels from most of the uterine body pass within the broad ligament to the *external iliac lymph nodes.*
- Vessels from the uterine cervix pass along the uterine vessels, within the transverse cervical ligaments, to the *internal iliac lymph nodes* and along the uterosacral ligaments to the *sacral lymph nodes.*

Innervation of the Vagina and Uterus.   The innervation of the inferior part of the vagina is somatic, from the *deep perineal nerve,* a branch of the *pudendal nerve.* The innervation of most of the vagina and the entire uterus, however, is visceral. The nerves are derived from the **uterovaginal nerve plexus,** which travels with the uterine artery at the junction of the base of the peritoneal broad ligament and the superior part of the transverse cervical ligament (Fig. 3.19). The uterovaginal plexus is one of the pelvic plexuses that extend to the pelvic viscera from the inferior hypogastric plexus.

Sympathetic, parasympathetic, and visceral afferent fibers pass through this plexus. Sympathetic innervation originates in the inferior thoracic spinal cord segments and passes through *lumbar splanchnic nerves* and the intermesenteric–hypogastric–pelvic series of plexuses. Parasympathetic innervation originates in the S2–S4 spinal cord segments and passes through the *pelvic splanchnic nerves* to the inferior hypogastric–uterovaginal plexus. Visceral afferent fibers, carrying pain sensation from the intraperitoneal uterine fundus and body, travel retrogradely with the sympathetic fibers to the lower thoracic–upper lumbar spinal ganglia; those from the subperitoneal uterine cervix and vagina (inferior to the pelvic pain line) travel with the parasympathetic fibers to the spinal sensory ganglia of S2–S4. All visceral afferent fibers from the uterus and vagina not concerned with pain (those conveying unconscious sensations) also follow the latter route.

Hysterectomy

Hysterectomy (excision of the uterus) is performed through the lower anterior abdominal wall or through the vagina (Fig. B3.5). Because the uterine artery crosses anterior to the ureter near the lateral fornix of the vagina, the ureter is in danger of being inadvertently clamped or severed when the uterine artery is tied off during a hysterectomy. The point of crossing of the artery and the ureter is approximately 2 cm superior to the ischial spine.

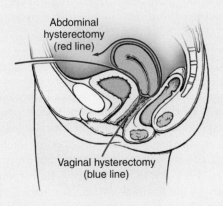

Abdominal hysterectomy (red line)

Vaginal hysterectomy (blue line)

Figure B3.5.

Cervical Examination and Pap Smear

The vagina can be distended with a vaginal speculum to enable inspection of the cervix and prepare a Pap smear. A spatula is placed on the external os of the uterus. The spatula is rotated to scrape cellular material from the vaginal cervix, followed by insertion of a cytobrush into the cervical canal that is used to gather cellular material from the supravaginal cervical mucosa. The cellular material is placed on glass slides for microscopic examination.

Laparoscopic Examination of Pelvic Viscera

Laparoscopy involves inserting a *laparoscope* into the peritoneal cavity through a small incision below the umbilicus (Fig. B3.6). Insufflation of inert gas creates a pneumoperitoneum to provide space to visualize the pelvic organs. Additional openings (ports) can be made to introduce other instruments for manipulation or to enable therapeutic procedures (e.g., ligation of the uterine tubes).

Caudal Epidural Block

A caudal epidural block is a popular choice for participatory childbirth. It must be administered in advance of childbirth, which is not possible with a precipitous

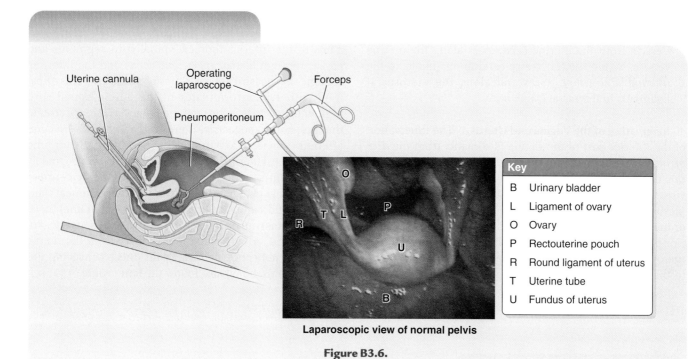

Laparoscopic view of normal pelvis

Figure B3.6.

Key

B	Urinary bladder
L	Ligament of ovary
O	Ovary
P	Rectouterine pouch
R	Round ligament of uterus
T	Uterine tube
U	Fundus of uterus

birth. The anesthetic agent is administered using an indwelling catheter in the *sacral canal* (see Chapter 4), enabling administration of more anesthetic agent for a deeper or more prolonged anesthesia if necessary. Within the sacral canal, the anesthesia bathes the S2–S4 spinal nerve roots, including the pain fibers from the uterine cervix and upper vagina, and the afferent fibers from the pudendal nerve. Thus the entire birth canal (pelvic floor and majority of the perineum) are anesthetized but the lower limbs are usually not affected. Because visceral afferent fibers from the uterine fundus ascend to the upper lumbar spinal ganglia, they are also not affected and sensations of uterine contraction are still perceived.

UTERINE TUBES

The **uterine tubes** (formerly called fallopian tubes) extend laterally from the *uterine horns* and open into the peritoneal cavity near the ovaries (Fig. 3.18). The uterine tubes lie in the *mesosalpinx* in the free edges of the broad ligament. In the "ideal" disposition, the tubes extend posterolaterally to the lateral pelvic walls, where they ascend and arch over the ovaries; but ultrasound studies demonstrate that the position of the tubes and ovaries is variable (dynamic) in life, and right and left sides are often asymmetrical.

Each uterine tube is divisible into four parts (Fig. 3.18*B*):

- The **infundibulum** is the funnel-shaped distal end that opens into the peritoneal cavity through the **abdominal ostium**. The finger-like processes of the infundibulum, the **fimbriae**, spread over the medial surface of the ovary; one large **ovarian fimbria** is attached to the superior pole of the ovary.
- The **ampulla**, the widest and longest part, begins at the medial end of the infundibulum.

- The **isthmus**, the thick-walled part, enters the uterine horn.
- The **uterine part** is the short intramural segment that passes through the wall of the uterus and opens through the **uterine ostium** into the uterine cavity at the uterine horn.

OVARIES

The almond-shaped **ovaries** are typically located near the attachment of the broad ligament to the lateral pelvic walls, suspended from both by peritoneal folds, the *mesovarium* from the posterosuperior aspect of the broad ligament and the *suspensory ligament of the ovary* from the pelvic wall (Figs. 3.18*A* and 3.20*B*). The suspensory ligament conveys the ovarian vessels, lymphatics, and nerves to and from the ovary and constitutes the lateral part of the mesovarium. The ovary also attaches to the uterus by the *ligament of ovary*, which runs within the mesovarium. This ligament is a remnant of the superior part of the ovarian

Infections of Female Genital Tract

Because the female genital tract communicates with the peritoneal cavity through the abdominal ostia of the uterine tubes, infections of the vagina, uterus, and uterine tubes may result in *peritonitis*. Conversely, inflammation of the tube (*salpingitis*) may result from infections that spread from the peritoneal cavity. A major cause of infertility in women is blockage of the uterine tubes, often the result of infection that causes salpingitis.

Patency of the Uterine Tubes

Patency of the uterine tubes may be determined by a radiographic procedure involving injection of a water-soluble radiopaque material into the uterus, **hysterosalpingography.** The material enters the uterine tubes and, if the tubes are patent, passes from the abdominal ostium into the peritoneal cavity. Patency can also be determined by **hysteroscopy,** examination of the interior of the tubes using an endoscopic instrument (*hysteroscope*) introduced through the vagina and uterus.

Ligation of Uterine Tubes

Ligation of the uterine tubes is a surgical method of birth control. **Abdominal tubal ligation** is usually performed through a short suprapubic incision made just at the pubic hairline. **Laparoscopic tubal ligation** is done with a laparoscope, which is similar to a small telescope with a powerful light. It is inserted through a small incision, usually near the umbilicus.

Ectopic Tubal Pregnancy

Occasionally, a blastocyst fails to reach the uterus and may implant in the mucosa of the uterine tube (most commonly the ampulla), producing an **ectopic tubal pregnancy.** On the right side, the appendix often lies close to the ovary and uterine tube. This close relationship explains why a *ruptured tubal pregnancy* and the resulting peritonitis may be misdiagnosed as acute appendicitis. In both cases, the parietal peritoneum is inflamed in the same general area and the pain is referred to the right lower quadrant of the abdomen. Tubal rupture and the severe hemorrhage constitute a threat to the mother's life and result in death of the embryo.

---

gubernaculum of the fetus and connects the proximal (uterine) end of the ovary to the lateral angle of the uterus, just inferior to the entrance of the uterine tube. Because the ovary is suspended in the peritoneal cavity and its surface is not covered by peritoneum, the oocyte expelled at ovulation passes into the peritoneal cavity but is usually trapped by the fimbriae of the uterine tube and carried to the ampulla.

Vasculature of Ovaries and Uterine Tubes. The *ovarian arteries* arise from the abdominal aorta and descend along the posterior abdominal wall. At the pelvic brim, they cross over the external iliac vessels and enter the suspensory ligaments (Figs. 3.17*A* and 3.18*B*). The ovarian artery sends branches through the mesovarium to the ovary and through the mesosalpinx to supply the uterine tube. The ascending branches of the uterine arteries (branches of the internal iliac arteries) course along the lateral aspects of the uterus to approach the medial aspects of the ovaries and tubes. The ovarian and ascending uterine artery terminate by bifurcating into ovarian and tubal branches and anastomose with each other, providing a collateral circulation from abdominal and pelvic sources.

Ovarian veins draining the ovary form a **pampiniform plexus of veins** in the broad ligament near the ovary and uterine tube (Fig. 3.17*B*). The veins of the plexus merge to form a singular **ovarian vein,** which leaves the lesser pelvis with the ovarian artery. The right ovarian vein ascends to enter the *inferior vena cava;* the left ovarian vein drains into the *left renal vein.* The tubal veins drain into the *ovarian veins* and *uterine (uterovaginal) venous plexus* (Fig. 3.17*B*). The lymphatic vessels from the ovary join those from the uterine tubes and fundus of the uterus as they ascend to the *right* and *left* (caval/aortic) *lumbar lymph nodes* (Table 3.6).

Innervation of the Ovaries and Uterine Tubes. The nerves descend along the ovarian vessels from the *ovarian plexus,* and from the *uterine (pelvic) plexus* (Fig. 3.19). Because the ovaries and uterine tubes are superior to the *pelvic pain line,* the visceral afferent pain fibers ascend retrogradely with the sympathetic fibers of the ovarian plexus and lumbar splanchnic nerves to the cell bodies in the T11–L1 spinal sensory ganglia. Visceral afferent reflex fibers follow parasympathetic fibers retrogradely through the uterine (pelvic) and inferior hypogastric plexuses and pelvic splanchnic nerves to cell bodies in the S2–S4 spinal sensory ganglia.

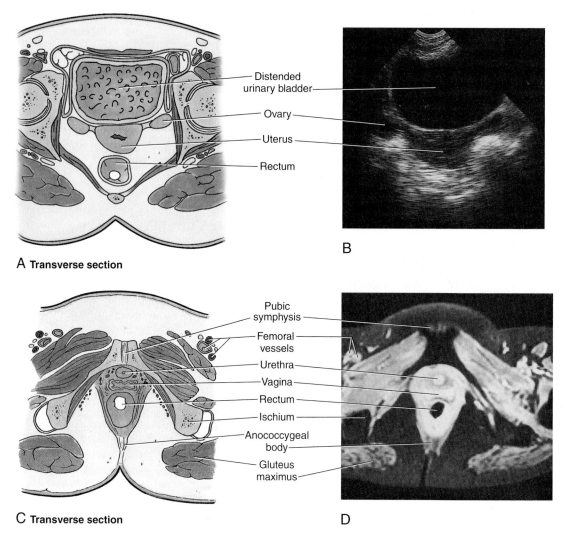

Distended urinary bladder

Ovary

Uterus

Rectum

A **Transverse section**

B

Pubic symphysis

Femoral vessels

Urethra

Vagina

Rectum

Ischium

Anococcygeal body

Gluteus maximus

C **Transverse section**

D

Figure 3.20. Imaging of female pelvis. A and B. Structures seen on an ultrasound scan are identified. **C and D.** Structures seen via MRI are identified.

Rectum

The **rectum** is the pelvic part of the alimentary tract that is continuous proximally with the sigmoid colon and distally with the anal canal (Fig. 3.21A). The **rectosigmoid junction** lies at the level of the S3 vertebra. The rectum follows the curve of the sacrum and coccyx, forming the **sacral flexure of the rectum.** The rectum ends anteroinferior to the tip of the coccyx where the rectum turns posteroinferiorly and becomes the **anal canal.** The dilated terminal part, the **ampulla of the rectum,** supports and retains the fecal mass before it is expelled during defecation. The rectum is S-shaped and has three flexures as it follows the sacrococcygeal curve (Fig. 3.21B). Its terminal part bends sharply in a posterior direction, **anorectal flexure,** as it perforates the pelvic diaphragm to become the anal canal.

The roughly 80° anorectal flexure (angle) is an important mechanism for fecal continence and is maintained during the resting state by the tonus of the puborectalis muscle and by its active contraction during peristaltic contractions if defecation is not to occur (Fig. 3.21B). The relation of puborectalis during defecation results in straightening of the anorectal junction. Three sharp **lateral flexures of the rectum (superior, intermediate,** and **inferior)** are apparent when the rectum is viewed anteriorly. The flexures are formed in relation to three internal infoldings (**transverse rectal folds**): two on the left and one on the right side. The folds overlie thickened parts of the circular muscle layer of the rectal wall (Fig. 3.21A & C).

Peritoneum covers the anterior and lateral surfaces of the superior third of the rectum (Table 3.3), only the anterior surface of the middle third, and no surface of the inferior third because it is subperitoneal. In males, the peritoneum reflects from the rectum to the posterior wall of the bladder, where it forms the floor of the *rectovesical pouch*. In females, the peritoneum reflects from the rectum to the posterior

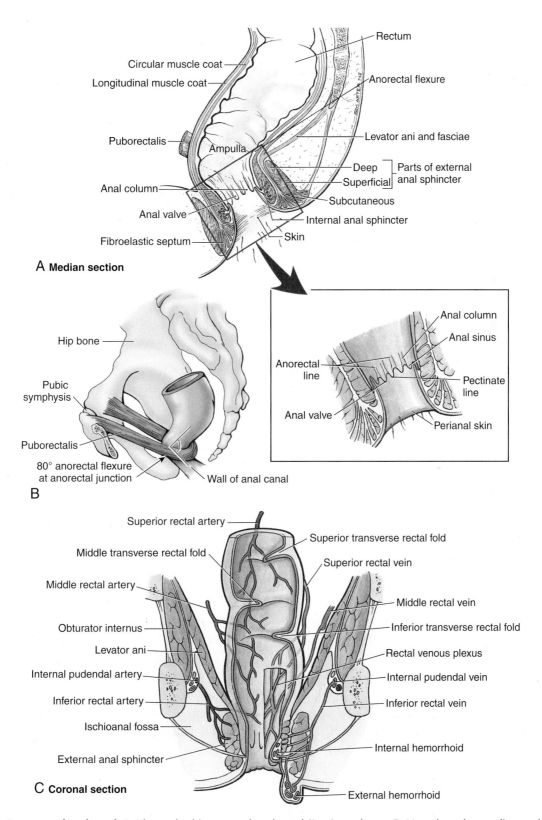

Figure 3.21. Rectum and anal canal. A. The anal sphincters and anal canal (*inset*) are shown. **B.** Note the puborectalis muscle. **C.** The arterial supply (right side) and venous drainage (left side) with hemorrhoids are shown.

fornix of the vagina, where it forms the floor of the *rectouterine pouch*. In both sexes, lateral reflections of peritoneum from the upper third of the rectum form *pararectal fossae,* which permit the rectum to distend as it fills with feces.

The rectum rests posteriorly on the inferior three sacral vertebrae and the coccyx, anococcygeal ligament, median sacral vessels, and inferior ends of the sympathetic trunks and sacral plexuses. In males, the rectum is related anteriorly to the fundus of the urinary bladder, terminal parts of the ureters, ductus deferentes, seminal glands, and prostate (Figs. 3.16 and 3.17). The *rectovesical septum* lies between the fundus of the bladder and the ampulla of the rectum and is closely associated with the seminal glands and prostate. In females, the rectum is related anteriorly to the vagina and is separated from the posterior part of the fornix and cervix by the *rectouterine pouch* (Figs. 3.8, 3.11*B,* and 3.20*C*). Inferior to this pouch, the weak rectovaginal septum separates the superior half of the posterior wall of the vagina from the rectum.

VASCULATURE OF RECTUM

The continuation of the inferior mesenteric artery, the *superior rectal artery,* supplies the proximal part of the rectum. The right and left *middle rectal arteries,* usually arising from the inferior vesical (male) or uterine (female) arteries, supply the middle and inferior parts of the rectum. The *inferior rectal arteries,* arising from the internal pudendal arteries, supply the anorectal junction and anal canal (Fig.

3.21*C*). Blood from the rectum drains via superior, middle, and inferior rectal veins. Because the superior rectal vein drains into the portal venous system and the middle and inferior rectal veins drain into the systemic system, this communication is an important area of *portacaval anastomosis* (see Chapter 2). The submucosal rectal venous plexus surrounds the rectum and communicates with the vesical venous plexus in males and the uterovaginal venous plexus in females. The **rectal venous plexus** consists of two parts, the **internal rectal venous plexus** just deep to the epithelium of the rectum and the external **rectal venous plexus** external to the muscular wall of the rectum.

Lymphatic vessels from the superior half of the rectum pass to the **pararectal lymph nodes,** located directly on the muscle layer of the rectum (Fig. 3.22), and then ascend to the *inferior mesenteric lymph nodes* either via the *sacral lymph nodes* or by passing through the nodes along the superior rectal vessels. Lymphatic vessels from the inferior half of the rectum drain into the *sacral lymph nodes* or, especially from the distal ampulla, follow the middle rectal vessels to drain into the *internal iliac lymph nodes.*

INNERVATION OF RECTUM

The nerve supply to the rectum is from the sympathetic and parasympathetic systems (Fig. 3.23). The *sympathetic supply* is from the lumbar spinal cord, conveyed via the lumbar splanchnic nerves and the hypogastric (pelvic) plexuses and through periarterial plexuses on the branches of the in-

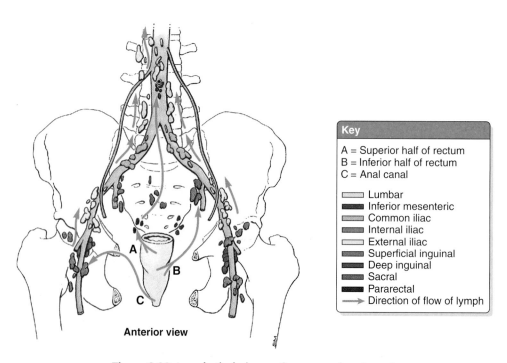

Key

A = Superior half of rectum
B = Inferior half of rectum
C = Anal canal

Lumbar
Inferior mesenteric
Common iliac
Internal iliac
External iliac
Superficial inguinal
Deep inguinal
Sacral
Pararectal
→ Direction of flow of lymph

Anterior view

Figure 3.22. Lymphatic drainage of rectum and anal canal.

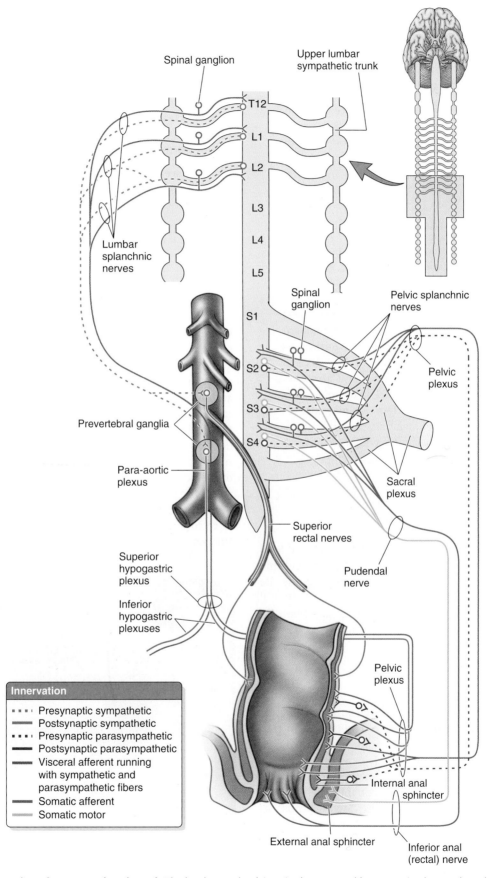

Figure 3.23. Innervation of rectum and anal canal. The lumbar and pelvic spinal nerves and hypogastric plexuses have been retracted laterally for clarity.

Resection of Rectum

When resecting the rectum in males (e.g., during cancer treatment), the plane of the rectovesical septum (a fascial septum extending superiorly from the perineal body) is located so that the prostate and urethra can be separated from the rectum. In this way, these organs are not often damaged during surgery.

Rectal Examination

Many structures related to the anteroinferior part of the rectum may be palpated through its walls (e.g., the prostate and seminal glands in males and the cervix in females). In both sexes, the pelvic surfaces of the sacrum and coccyx may be palpated. The ischial spines and tuberosities may also be palpated. Enlarged internal iliac lymph nodes, pathologic thickening of the ureters, swellings in the ischioanal fossae (e.g., ischioanal abscesses and abnormal contents in the rectovesical pouch in the male or the rectouterine pouch in the female) may also be palpated. Tenderness of an inflamed appendix may also be detected rectally if it descends into the lesser pelvis (pararectal fossa).

ferior mesenteric artery and superior rectal arteries. The *parasympathetic supply* is from the S2–S4 spinal cord level, passing via the pelvic splanchnic nerves (S2–S4) and inferior hypogastric plexuses to the rectal (pelvic) plexus. Because the rectum is inferior (distal) to the pelvic pain line, all visceral afferent fibers follow the parasympathetic fibers retrogradely to the S2–S4 spinal sensory ganglia.

Perineum

The **perineum** refers to both an external surface area and a shallow "compartment" of the body. The perineum (perineal compartment) lies inferior to the inferior pelvic aperture and is separated from the pelvic cavity by the pelvic diaphragm. In the anatomical position, the perineum (perineal area) is the narrow region between the proximal parts of the thighs. However, when the lower limbs are abducted, the perineum is a diamond-shaped area extending from the mons pubis anteriorly, the medial surfaces (insides) of the thighs laterally, and the gluteal folds and superior end of the intergluteal (natal) cleft posteriorly.

The osseofibrous structures marking the boundaries of the perineum (perineal compartment) are the (Fig. 3.24):

- *Pubic symphysis,* anteriorly.
- *Inferior pubic rami* and *ischial rami,* anterolaterally.
- *Ischial tuberosities,* laterally.
- *Sacrotuberous ligaments,* posterolaterally.
- Inferiormost *sacrum* and *coccyx,* posteriorly.

A transverse line joining the anterior ends of the ischial tuberosities divides the perineum into two triangles (Fig. 3.24):

- The **anal triangle** lies posterior to this line and contains the anal canal and its orifice, the anus.
- The **urogenital (UG) triangle**, containing the root of the scrotum and penis in males and the vulva of females, is anterior to this line.

The urogenital triangle is "closed" by the **perineal membrane** (Table 3.10), a thin sheet of tough deep fascia, which stretches between the right and the left sides of the pubic arch. The perineal membrane covers the anterior part of the pelvic outlet and is perforated by the urethra in both sexes and by the vagina of the female. The **perineal body** is an irregular fibromuscular mass located in the median plane between the anal canal and the perineal membrane. It lies deep to the skin, with relatively little overlying subcutaneous tissue, posterior to the vestibule of the vagina or bulb of the penis and anterior to the anus and anal canal. Anteriorly, the perineal body blends with the posterior border of the perineal membrane and superiorly with the rectovesical or rectovaginal septum. It contains collagenous and elastic fibers and both skeletal and smooth muscle.

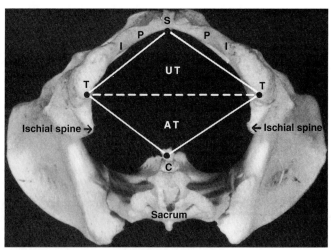

Inferior view

Figure 3.24. Urogenital and anal triangles of perineum. *AT,* anal triangle; *C,* coccyx; *I,* ischial rami; *P,* inferior pubic rami; *S,* pubic symphysis; *T,* ischial tuberosities; *UT,* urogenital triangle.

Disruption of Perineal Body

The perineal body is an especially important structure in women because it is the final support of the pelvic viscera. Stretching or tearing of this attachment of the perineal muscles from the perineal body can occur during childbirth, removing support. As a result, *prolapse of pelvic viscera*, including prolapse of the bladder (through the urethra) and prolapse of the uterus and/or vagina (through the vaginal orifice) may occur.

Episiotomy

During vaginal surgery and labor, an *episiotomy* (surgical incision of the perineum and inferoposterior vaginal wall) is often made to enlarge the vaginal orifice and to prevent a jagged tear of the perineal muscles.

The perineal body is the site of convergence of several muscles (Table 3.10):

- Bulbospongiosus.
- External anal sphincter.
- Superficial and deep transverse perineal muscles.
- Smooth and voluntary slips of muscle from the external urethral sphincter, levator ani, and muscular coats of the rectum.

Fasciae and Pouches of Urogenital Triangle

PERINEAL FASCIAE

The **perineal fascia** consists of superficial and deep layers (Fig. 3.25). The **subcutaneous tissue of the perineum**, or *superficial perineal fascia,* consists of a fatty superficial layer and a deep membranous layer (Colles fascia). In females, the fatty layer makes up the substance of the labia majora and mons pubis and is continuous anteriorly and superiorly with the fatty layer of subcutaneous tissue of the abdomen (Camper fascia). In males, the fatty layer is greatly diminished in the urogenital triangle and is replaced altogether in the penis and scrotum with smooth (dartos) muscle. It is continuous between the penis or scrotum and the thighs with the fatty layer of subcutaneous tissue of the abdomen. In both sexes, it is continuous posteriorly with the ischioanal fat-pad in the anal region.

The **membranous layer of subcutaneous tissue of the perineum** is attached posteriorly to the posterior margin of the perineal membrane and the perineal body. Laterally, it is attached to the fascia lata (deep fascia) of the superiormost medial aspect of the thigh. Anteriorly, in the male, the membranous layer of subcutaneous tissue is continuous with the dartos fascia of the penis and scrotum; however, on each side of and anterior to the scrotum, the membranous layer becomes continuous with the membranous layer of subcutaneous tissue of the abdomen (Scarpa fascia). In females, the membranous layer passes superior to the fatty layer forming the labia majora and becomes continuous with the membranous layer of the subcutaneous tissue of the abdomen.

The **(deep) perineal fascia** (investing or Gallaudet fascia) intimately invests the ischiocavernosus, bulbospongiosus, and superficial transverse perineal muscles. It is also attached laterally to the ischiopubic rami. Anteriorly, it is fused to the suspensory ligament of the penis and is continuous with the deep fascia covering the external oblique muscle of the abdomen and the rectus sheath. The deep perineal fascia is fused with the suspensory ligament of the clitoris in females and with the deep fascia of the abdomen in males.

SUPERFICIAL PERINEAL POUCH

The **superficial perineal pouch** (compartment) is a potential space between the membranous layer of subcutaneous tissue and the perineal membrane, bounded laterally by the ischiopubic rami (Fig. 3.25; Table 3.10).

In males, the superficial perineal pouch contains the:

- *Root* (bulb and crura) *of the penis* and associated muscles (*ischiocavernosus* and *bulbospongiosus*).
- Proximal (bulbous) part of the *spongy urethra.*
- *Superficial transverse perineal muscles.*
- *Deep perineal branches* of the internal pudendal vessels and pudendal nerves.

In females, the superficial perineal pouch contains the:

- *Clitoris* and associated muscle (ischiocavernosus).
- *Bulbs of the vestibule* and the surrounding muscle (bulbospongiosus).
- *Greater vestibular glands.*
- *Deep perineal branches* of the internal pudendal vessels and pudendal nerves.
- *Superficial transverse perineal muscles.*

DEEP PERINEAL POUCH

The **deep perineal pouch** (space) is bounded inferiorly by the perineal membrane, superiorly by the inferior fascia of the pelvic diaphragm, and laterally by the inferior portion of the obturator fascia (covering obturator internus muscle). It includes the fat-filled anterior recesses of the ischioanal fossa

Table 3.10 Muscles of the Perineum

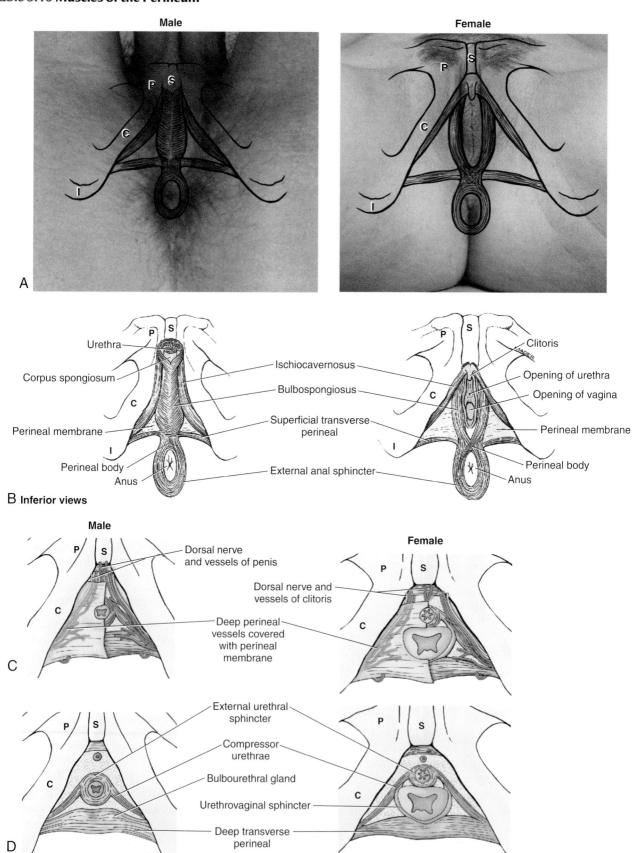

Male

Female

A

B **Inferior views**

Urethra

Corpus spongiosum

Perineal membrane

Perineal body

Anus

Ischiocavernosus

Bulbospongiosus

Superficial transverse
perineal

External anal sphincter

Clitoris

Opening of urethra

Opening of vagina

Perineal membrane

Perineal body

Anus

Male

Female

Dorsal nerve
and vessels of penis

Dorsal nerve and
vessels of clitoris

Deep perineal
vessels covered
with perineal
membrane

C

External urethral
sphincter

Compressor
urethrae

Bulbourethral gland

Urethrovaginal sphincter

Deep transverse
perineal

D

Table 3.10 Muscles of the Perineum (continued)

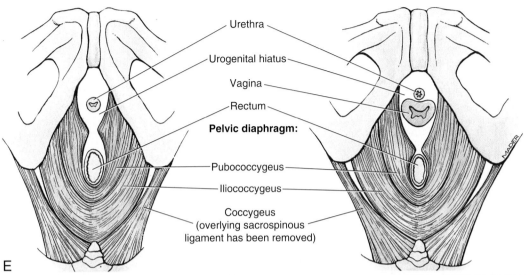

E

Muscle	Origin	Course and Insertion	Innervation	Main Action(s)
External anal sphincter	Skin and fascia surrounding anus and coccyx via anococcygeal ligament	Passes around lateral aspects of anal canal, inserting into perineal body	Inferior anal nerve, branch of pudendal nerve (S2–S4)	Constricts anal canal during peristalsis, resisting defecation; supports and fixes perineal body/pelvic floor
Bulbospongiosus	*Male:* median raphe on ventral surface of bulb of penis and perineal body *Female:* perineal body	*Male:* surrounds lateral aspects of bulb of penis and most proximal part of body of penis, inserting into perineal membrane, dorsal aspect of corpora spongiosum and cavernosa, and fascia of bulb of penis *Female:* passes on each side of lower vagina, enclosing bulb and greater vestibular gland; inserts onto pubic arch and fascia of corpora cavernosa of clitoris	Muscular (deep) branch of perineal nerve, branch of pudendal nerve (S2–S4)	Supports and fixes perineal body/ pelvic floor *Male:* compresses bulb of penis to expel last drops of urine/semen; assists erection by compressing outflow via deep perineal vein and by pushing blood from bulb into body of penis *Female:* "sphincter" of vagina; assists in erection of clitoris (and bulb of vestibule[?]); compresses greater vestibular gland
Ischiocavernosus	Internal surface of ischiopubic ramus and ischial tuberosity	Embraces crus of penis or clitoris, inserting onto inferior and medial aspects of crus and to perineal membrane medial to crus	Muscular (deep) branch of perineal nerve, branch of pudendal nerve (S2–S4)	Maintains erection of penis or clitoris by compressing outflow veins and pushing blood from root of penis or clitoris into body of penis or clitoris
Superficial transverse perineal	Internal surface of ischiopubic ramus and ischial tuberosity; compressor urethrae portion only	Passes along superior posterior border of perineal membrane to perineal body	Muscular (deep) branch of perineal nerve, branch of pudendal nerve (S2–S4); dorsal nerve of penis or clitoris, terminal branch of pudendal nerve (S2–S4)	Support and fix perineal body (pelvic floor) to support abdominopelvic viscera and resist increased intra-abdominal pressure
Deep transverse perineal		Passes along superior posterior border of perineal membrane to perineal body, and external anal sphincter		
External urethral sphincter		Surrounds urethra superior to perineal membrane *Males:* also ascends anterior aspect of prostate *Females:* some fibers also enclose vagina (urethrovaginal sphincter)		Compresses urethra to maintain urinary continence *Females:* urethrovaginal sphincter portion also compresses vagina

C, conjoint ramus formed by inferior rami of ischium and pubis; *I,* ischial tuberosity; *P,* body of pubis; *S,* pubic symphysis.

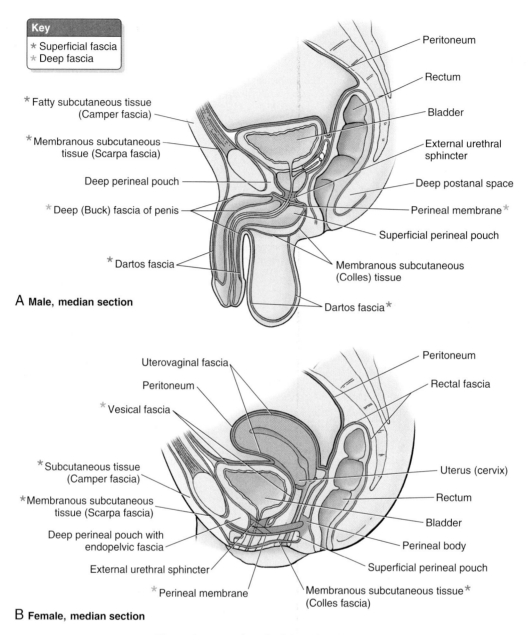

Key
* Superficial fascia
* Deep fascia

* Fatty subcutaneous tissue (Camper fascia)

* Membranous subcutaneous tissue (Scarpa fascia)

Deep perineal pouch

* Deep (Buck) fascia of penis

* Dartos fascia

Peritoneum

Rectum

Bladder

External urethral sphincter

Deep postanal space

Perineal membrane *

Superficial perineal pouch

Membranous subcutaneous (Colles) tissue

Dartos fascia *

A **Male, median section**

Uterovaginal fascia

Peritoneum

* Vesical fascia

* Subcutaneous tissue (Camper fascia)

* Membranous subcutaneous tissue (Scarpa fascia)

Deep perineal pouch with endopelvic fascia

External urethral sphincter

* Perineal membrane

Peritoneum

Rectal fascia

Uterus (cervix)

Rectum

Bladder

Perineal body

Superficial perineal pouch

Membranous subcutaneous tissue * (Colles fascia)

B **Female, median section**

Figure 3.25. Fasciae of pelvis and perineum.

(Figs. 3.25 and Fig. 3.27). In *both sexes,* the deep perineal pouch contains part of the urethra centrally, the inferior part of the external urethral sphincter muscle, and the anterior extensions of the ischioanal fat-pads. In *males,* the deep perineal pouch contains the *intermediate part of the urethra, deep transverse perineal muscles, bulbourethral glands,* and dorsal neurovascular structures of the penis. In *females,* it contains the proximal part of the *urethra,* a mass of smooth muscle in place of deep transverse perineal muscles, and the dorsal neurovasculature of the clitoris.

Traditionally, a trilaminar UG diaphragm was described as making up the deep perineal pouch. The long-held

concept of a flat, essentially two-dimensional UG diaphragm is erroneous (Wendell-Smith, 1995). According to this concept, the UG diaphragm consisted of the perineal membrane (inferior fascia of UG diaphragm) inferiorly and a superior fascia of the UG diaphragm superiorly, between which was a flat muscular sheet composed of a disc-like sphincter urethra and the transversely oriented deep transverse perineal muscle. The descriptions of only the perineal membrane and of the deep transverse perineal muscles of the male appear to be supported by evidence (Myers et al., 1998a, 1998b).

In the female, deep transverse perineal muscles are mainly smooth muscle. Immediately superior to the posterior half of the perineal membrane, the flat, sheet-like deep transverse perineal muscle, when developed (typically only in males), offers dynamic support for the pelvic viscera. As described by Oelrich (1980), however, the urethral sphincter muscle is not a flat, planar structure, and the only "superior fascia" is the fascia of the external urethral sphincter muscle. In both views, the strong perineal membrane is the inferior boundary (floor) of the deep pouch. The perineal membrane, with the perineal body, is the final passive support of the pelvic viscera.

The **external urethral sphincter** is more tube- and trough-like than disc-like, and in the male, only a part of the muscle forms a circular investment (a true sphincter) for the intermediate part of the urethra inferior to the prostate (Fig. 3.26A). Its larger, trough-like part extends vertically to the neck of the bladder, displacing the prostate and investing the prostatic urethra anteriorly and anterolaterally only. As the prostate develops from urethral glands, the posterior and posterolateral muscle atrophies or is displaced by the prostate. Whether this part of the muscle compresses or dilates the prostatic urethra is a matter of some controversy.

In the female, the external urethral sphincter is more properly a "urogenital sphincter," according to Oelrich (1983). Here, too, he described a part forming a true anular sphincter around the urethra, with several additional parts extending from it (Fig. 3.26B): a superior part, extending to the neck of the bladder; a subdivision described as extending inferolaterally to the ischial ramus on each side (the **compressor urethrae muscle**); and another band-like part, which encircles both the vagina and the urethra (**urethrovaginal sphincter**). In both males and females, the musculature described is oriented perpendicular to the perineal membrane rather than lying in the plane parallel to it. Some dispute the encircling of the urethra in the female, stating that the muscle is not capable of sphincteric action.

Features of Anal Triangle

ISCHIOANAL FOSSAE

The **ischioanal fossae** (formerly ischiorectal fossae) around the wall of the anal canal are large fascia-lined, wedge-shaped spaces between the skin of the anal region and the pelvic diaphragm (Fig. 3.27). The apex of each fossa lies superiorly where the levator ani muscle arises from the obturator fascia. The ischioanal fossae, wide inferiorly and narrow superiorly, are filled with fat and loose connective tissue. The two ischioanal fossae communicate by means of

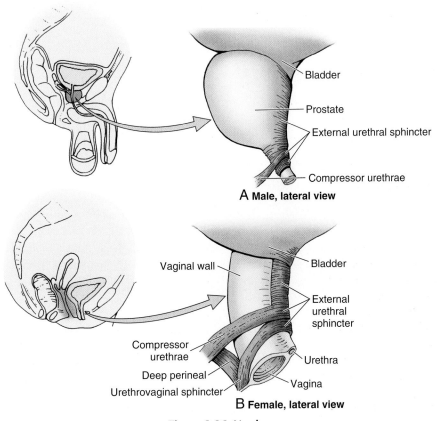

A **Male, lateral view**

- Bladder
- Prostate
- External urethral sphincter
- Compressor urethrae

B **Female, lateral view**

- Vaginal wall
- Bladder
- External urethral sphincter
- Compressor urethrae
- Deep perineal
- Urethrovaginal sphincter
- Urethra
- Vagina

Figure 3.26. Urethra.

Rupture of Urethra in Males and Extravasation of Urine

Rupture of the intermediate part of the urethra results in extravasation of urine and blood into the deep perineal pouch (Fig. B3.7A). The fluid may pass superiorly through the urogenital hiatus and distribute extraperitoneally around the prostate and bladder.

Rupture of the spongy urethra in the bulb of the penis results in urine passing (extravasating) into the superficial perineal space (Fig. B3.7B). The attachments of the perineal fascia determine the direction of flow of the extravasated urine. Urine and blood may pass into the loose connective tissue in the scrotum, around the penis, and superiorly, deep to the membranous layer of subcutaneous connective tissue of the inferior anterior abdominal wall. The urine cannot pass far into the thighs because the membranous layer of superficial perineal fascia blends with the fascia lata (deep fascia) enveloping the thigh muscles, just distal to the inguinal ligament. In addition, urine cannot pass posteriorly into the anal triangle because the superficial and deep layers of perineal fascia are continuous with each other around the superficial perineal muscles and with the posterior edge of the perineal membrane between them.

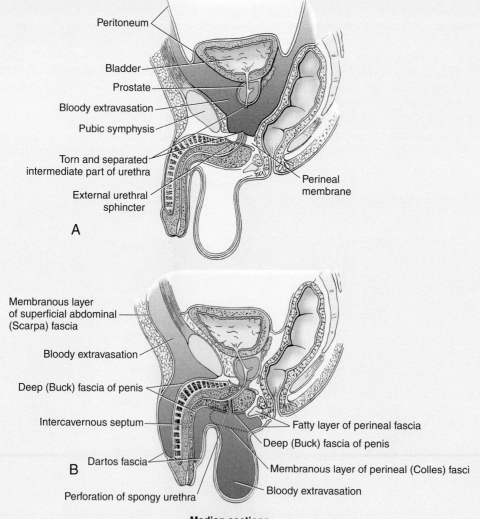

Median sections

Figure B3.7.

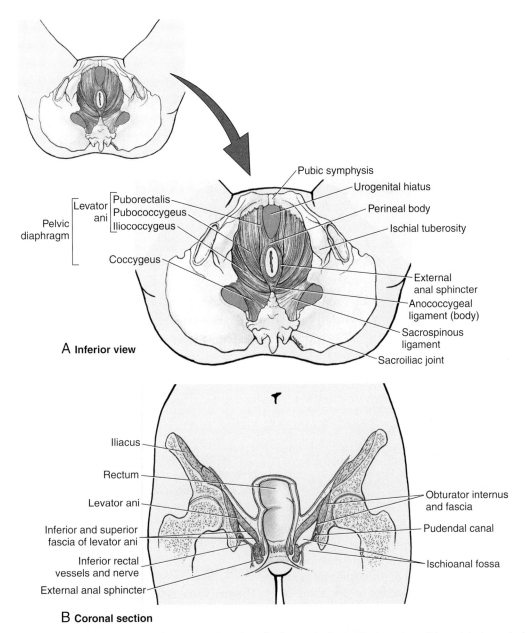

Figure 3.27. Pelvic diaphragm and ischioanal fossae. A. The pelvic diaphragm is shown. **B.** A section of the pelvis through the rectum, anal canal, and ischioanal fossae is shown.

the *deep postanal space* over the *anococcygeal ligament* (body), a fibrous mass located between the anal canal and the tip of the coccyx (Fig. 3.27B).

Each ischioanal fossa is bounded

- Laterally by the ischium and the inferior part of the obturator internus, covered with obturator fascia.
- Medially by the external anal sphincter, with a sloping superior medial wall or roof formed by the levator ani as it descends to blend with the sphincter; both structures surround the anal canal.
- Posteriorly by the sacrotuberous ligament and gluteus maximus.

- Anteriorly by the bodies of the pubic bones, inferior to the origin of the puborectalis; these parts of the fossae, extending into the UG triangle superior to the perineal membrane, are known as the **anterior recesses of the ischioanal fossae.**

The ischioanal fossae are traversed by tough, fibrous bands and filled with fat, forming the **fat bodies of the ischioanal fossae.** These fat bodies support the anal canal but are readily displaced to permit expansion of the anal canal during the passage of feces. The fat bodies are traversed by several neurovascular structures, including the inferior anal/rectal vessels and nerves and two other cuta-

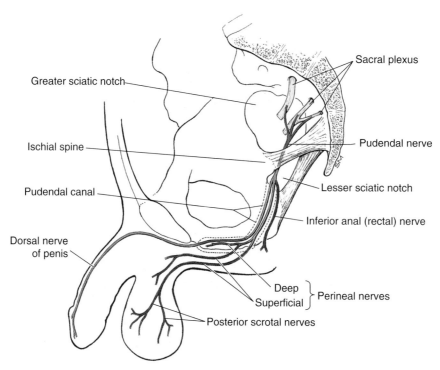

Figure 3.28. Pudendal nerve. The five regions in which the nerve runs are shown in color. The perineal nerves in the female give rise to labial branches and the dorsal nerve of the clitoris.

neous nerves: the perforating branch of S2 and S3 and the perineal branch of the S4 nerve.

PUDENDAL CANAL

The **pudendal canal** (Alcock canal) is essentially a horizontal passageway within the obturator fascia (Figs. 3.27 *B* and 3.28), which covers the medial aspect of the obturator internus muscle and lines the lateral wall of the ischioanal fossa. The pudendal canal begins at the posterior border of the ischioanal fossa and runs from the *lesser sciatic notch* adjacent to the ischial spine to the posterior edge of the perineal membrane. The internal pudendal artery and vein, the pudendal nerve, and the nerve to the obturator internus enter this canal at the lesser sciatic notch, inferior to the ischial spine. The internal pudendal vessels supply and drain blood from the perineum; the pudendal nerve innervates most of the same area. As the artery and nerve enter the canal, they give rise to the **inferior rectal artery** and then pass medially to supply the external anal sphincter and perianal skin. Toward the distal (anterior) end of the pudendal canal, the artery and nerve both bifurcate, giving rise to the *perineal nerve and artery*, which are distributed mostly to the superficial pouch (inferior to the perineal membrane) and to the **dorsal artery and nerve of penis** or **clitoris**, which run in the deep pouch (superior to the membrane). The perineal nerve has two branches: The **superficial perineal nerves** give rise to poste-

rior scrotal or labial (cutaneous) branches, and the **deep perineal nerve** supplies the muscles of the deep and superficial perineal pouches, the skin of the vestibule of the vagina, and the mucosa of the inferiormost part of the vagina. The **dorsal nerve of the penis or clitoris**, is the primary sensory nerve serving the male or female organ, especially the glans.

ANAL CANAL

The **anal canal** is the terminal part of the large intestine that extends from the superior aspect of the pelvic diaphragm to the **anus**. The canal begins where the rectal ampulla abruptly narrows at the level of the U-shaped sling formed by the puborectalis muscle (Fig. 3.21*A* & *B*). The canal ends at the anus, the external outlet of the alimentary tract. The anal canal, surrounded by internal and external anal sphincters, descends posteroinferiorly between the **anococcygeal ligament** and the **perineal body**. The anal canal is normally collapsed except during passage of feces. Both sphincters must relax before defecation can occur. The **external anal sphincter** is a large voluntary sphincter that forms a broad band on each side of the inferior two thirds of the anal canal (Fig. 3.21). This sphincter blends superiorly with the puborectalis muscle and is described as having subcutaneous, superficial, and deep parts. The external anal sphincter is supplied mainly by S4 through the inferior rectal nerve (Fig. 3.23).

Ischioanal Abscesses

The ischioanal fossae are occasionally the sites of infection, which may result in the formation of *ischioanal abscesses* (Fig. B3.8). These collections of pus are quite painful. Diagnostic signs of an ischioanal abscess are fullness and tenderness between the anus and the ischial tuberosity. A perianal abscess may rupture spontaneously, opening into the anal canal, rectum, or perianal skin.

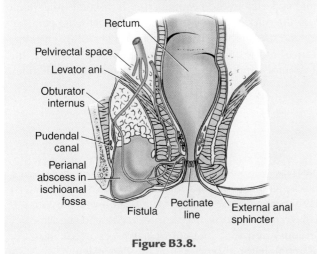

Figure B3.8.

The **internal anal sphincter** is an involuntary sphincter surrounding the superior two thirds of the anal canal. It is a thickening of the circular muscle layer. Its contraction (tonus) is stimulated and maintained by the sympathetic fibers from the superior rectal (periarterial) and hypogastric plexuses. It is inhibited (loses its tonic contraction and is allowed to expand passively) by the parasympathetic fibers. This sphincter is tonically contracted most of time to prevent leakage of fluid or flatus; however, it relaxes temporarily in response to distension of the rectal ampulla by feces or gas, requiring voluntary contraction of the puborectalis and the external anal sphincter if defecation or flatulence is not to occur.

Interior of Anal Canal. The superior half of the mucous membrane of the anal canal is characterized by a series of longitudinal ridges called **anal columns** (Fig. 3.21*A*). These columns contain the terminal branches of the superior rectal artery and vein. The **anorectal junction**, indicated by the superior ends of the anal columns, is where the rectum joins the anal canal. The inferior ends of these columns are joined by **anal valves**. Superior to the valves are small recesses called **anal sinuses**. When compressed by feces, the anal sinuses exude mucus that aids in evacuation of feces from the anal canal. The inferior comb-shaped limit of the anal valves forms an irregular line, the **pectinate line** (Fig. 3.29), which indicates the junction of the superior part of the anal canal (visceral; derived from the hindgut) and the inferior part (somatic; derived from the embryonic proctodeum). The anal canal superior to the pectinate line differs from the part inferior to the pectinate line in its

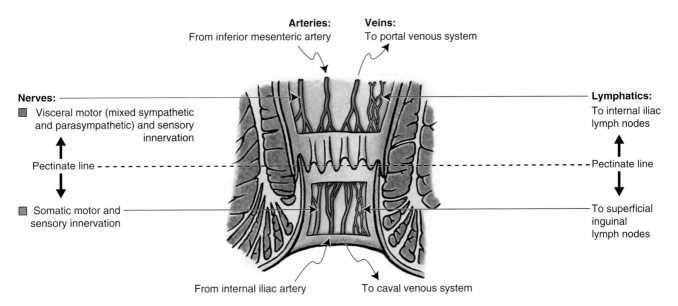

Figure 3.29. Innervation and vascular supply of anal canal superior and inferior to pectinate line. The vessels and nerves superior to the pectinate line are visceral; those inferior to the pectinate line are somatic.

arterial supply, innervation, and venous and lymphatic drainage. These differences result from their different embryological origins (Moore and Persaud, 2003).

Vasculature and Lymphatic Drainage of Anal Canal. The *superior rectal artery* supplies the anal canal superior to the pectinate line (Fig. 3.21*C*). The two *inferior rectal arteries* supply the inferior part of the anal canal as well as the surrounding muscles and perianal skin. The *middle rectal arteries* assist with the blood supply to the anal canal by forming anastomoses with the superior and inferior rectal arteries.

The *internal rectal venous plexus* drains in both directions from the level of the pectinate line. Superior to the pectinate line, the internal rectal venous plexus drains chiefly into the *superior rectal vein* (a tributary of the inferior mesenteric vein) and the portal system (Fig. 3.21*C*). Inferior to the pectinate line, the internal rectal venous plexus drains into the *inferior rectal veins* (tributaries of the

caval venous system) around the margin of the external anal sphincter. The *middle rectal veins* (tributaries of the internal iliac veins) mainly drain the muscularis externa of the rectal ampulla and form anastomoses with the superior and inferior rectal veins. The rectal venous plexuses receive multiple arteriovenous anastomoses from the superior and middle rectal arteries.

Superior to the pectinate line, the lymphatic vessels drain into the *internal iliac lymph nodes* and through them into the common iliac and lumbar lymph nodes (Fig. 3.22). Inferior to the pectinate line, the lymphatic vessels drain into the *superficial inguinal lymph nodes*.

Innervation of Anal Canal. The nerve supply to the anal canal superior to the pectinate line is visceral innervation from the *inferior hypogastric plexus* (sympathetic, parasympathetic, and visceral afferent fibers) (Fig. 3.23). The superior part of the anal canal is inferior to the pelvic pain line; all visceral afferents travel with the parasympathetic fibers

Hemorrhoids

Internal hemorrhoids ("piles") are prolapses of the rectal mucosa containing the normally dilated veins of the *internal rectal venous plexus* (Fig B3.9). They are thought to result from a breakdown of the muscularis mucosae, a smooth muscle layer deep to the mucosa. Internal hemorrhoids that prolapse through the anal canal are often compressed by the contracted sphincters, impeding blood flow. As a result, they tend to strangulate and ulcerate. Owing to the presence of abundant arteriovenous anastomoses, bleeding from internal hemorrhoids is usually bright red. *External hemorrhoids* are thromboses (blood clots) in the veins of the *external rectal venous plexus* and are covered by skin (Fig. B3.9). Predisposing factors for hemorrhoids include pregnancy, chronic constipation, and any disorder that impedes venous return, including increased intra-abdominal pressure.

The anastomoses among the superior, middle, and inferior rectal veins form clinically important communications between the portal and the systemic venous systems (Fig. 3.29). The superior rectal vein drains into the inferior mesenteric vein, whereas the middle and inferior rectal veins drain through the systemic system into the inferior vena cava. Any abnormal increase in pressure in the valveless portal system or veins of the trunk may cause enlargement of the superior rectal veins, resulting in increase in blood flow or stasis in the internal rectal venous plexus. In *portal hypertension*, as in *hepatic cirrhosis*, the portocaval

anastomosis among the superior, middle, and inferior rectal veins, along with portocaval anastomoses elsewhere, may become varicose. It is important to note that the veins of the rectal plexuses *normally* appear varicose (dilated and tortuous) and that internal hemorrhoids occur most commonly in the absence of portal hypertension.

Because visceral afferent nerves supply the anal canal superior to the pectinate line, an incision or a needle insertion in this region is painless. However, the anal canal inferior to the pectinate line is quite sensitive (e.g., to the prick of a hypodermic needle) because it is supplied by the *inferior rectal nerves*, containing somatic sensory fibers.

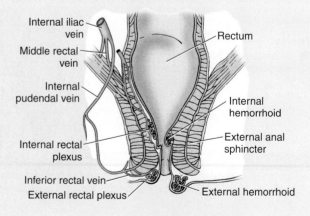

Internal iliac vein

Rectum

Middle rectal vein

Internal pudendal vein

Internal hemorrhoid

Internal rectal plexus

External anal sphincter

Inferior rectal vein

External rectal plexus

External hemorrhoid

Anterior view of coronal sections

Figure B3.9.

Urethral Catheterization

Urethral catheterization is done to remove urine from a person who is unable to micturate. It is also performed to irrigate the bladder and to obtain an uncontaminated sample of urine. When inserting the catheters and urethral sounds (slightly conical instruments for exploring and dilating a constricted urethra) the curves of the male urethra must be considered.

to spinal sensory ganglia S2–S4. Superior to the pectinate line, the anal canal is sensitive only to stretching. The nerve supply of the anal canal inferior to the pectinate line is somatic, derived from the *inferior anal (rectal) nerves*, branches of the pudendal nerve. Therefore, this part of the anal canal is sensitive to pain, touch, and temperature. Somatic efferent fibers stimulate the contraction of the voluntary external anal sphincter.

Male Perineum

The male perineum includes the external genitalia (urethra, scrotum, and penis), perineal muscles, and anal canal.

DISTAL MALE URETHRA

The urethra in the bladder neck (intramural part) and the prostatic urethra, the first two parts of the male urethra, are described with the pelvis (Table 3.8). The **intermediate (membranous) part of the urethra** begins at the apex of the prostate and traverses the deep perineal pouch, surrounded by the external urethral sphincter. It then penetrates the perineal membrane, ending as the urethra enters the bulb of the penis (Fig. 3.11*A*). Posterolateral to this part of the urethra are the small *bulbourethral glands* (Fig. 3.11) and their slender ducts, which open into the proximal part of the spongy urethra.

The **spongy urethra** begins at the distal end of the intermediate part of the urethra and ends at the *external urethral orifice* (Figs. 3.30*D* and 3.31). The lumen of the spongy urethra is expanded in the bulb of the penis to form the **intrabulbar fossa** and in the glans of the penis to form the **navicular fossa**. On each side, the ducts of the bulbourethral glands open into the proximal part of the spongy urethra. There are also many minute openings of the ducts of mucus-secreting **urethral glands** (Littré glands) into the spongy urethra.

The *arterial supply* of the intermediate and spongy parts of the urethra is from branches of the *dorsal artery of the penis*. The *veins* accompany the arteries and have similar

names. *Lymphatic vessels* from the intermediate part of the urethra drain mainly into the *internal iliac lymph nodes* (Fig. 3.32*A*), *whereas most vessels from the spongy urethra pass to the* deep inguinal lymph nodes, but some vessels pass to the external iliac lymph nodes. The *innervation* of the intermediate part of the urethra is the same as that of the prostatic part (Fig. 3.32*B*). The dorsal nerve of the penis, a branch of the *pudendal nerve*, provides somatic innervation of the spongy part of the urethra.

SCROTUM

The **scrotum** is a cutaneous fibromuscular sac for the testes and associated structures (Fig. 3.31*A*). It is situated posteroinferior to the penis and inferior to the pubic symphysis. The bilateral embryonic formation of the scrotum is indicated by the midline **scrotal raphe** (Fig. 3.30*C*), which is continuous on the ventral surface of the penis with the **penile raphe** and posteriorly along the median line of the perineum as the **perineal raphe**. Internally deep to the scrotal raphe, the scrotum is divided into two compartments, one for each testis, by a prolongation of dartos fascia, the **septum of the scrotum**. The contents of the scrotum (testes and epididymides) are described with the abdomen (see Chapter 2).

Vasculature of Scrotum. The anterior aspect of the scrotum is supplied by the **anterior scrotal arteries**, terminal branches of the **external pudendal arteries** (Table 3.6), and the posterior aspect is supplied by the **posterior scrotal arteries**, terminal branches of the *internal pudendal arteries*. The scrotum also receives branches from the cremasteric arteries, branches of inferior epigastric arteries. The *scrotal veins* accompany the arteries and drain primarily to the *external pudendal veins*. *Lymphatic vessels* from the scrotum drain into the *superficial inguinal lymph nodes* (Fig. 3.32*A*).

Innervation of Scrotum. The anterior aspect of the scrotum is supplied by the **anterior scrotal nerves** derived from the *ilioinguinal nerve*, and by the *genital branch of the genitofemoral nerve*. The posterior aspect of the scrotum is supplied by **posterior scrotal nerves**, branches of the superficial perineal branches of the pudendal nerve (Fig. 3.32*B*), and by the *perineal branch of the posterior femoral cutaneous nerve*.

PENIS

The penis is the male organ of copulation and the outlet for urine and semen. The penis consists of a *root, body*, and *glans penis* (Fig. 3.30*D*). It is composed of three cylindrical bodies of erectile cavernous tissue: the paired **corpora cavernosa** and the single **corpus spongiosum** ventrally. (Note that in the anatomical position, the penis is erect; when the penis is flaccid, its dorsum is directed anteriorly. Each *cavernous body* has a fibrous outer covering or capsule, the **tunica albuginea** (Fig. 3.30*B*). Superficial to the outer covering is the **deep fascia of the penis** (Buck fascia), the

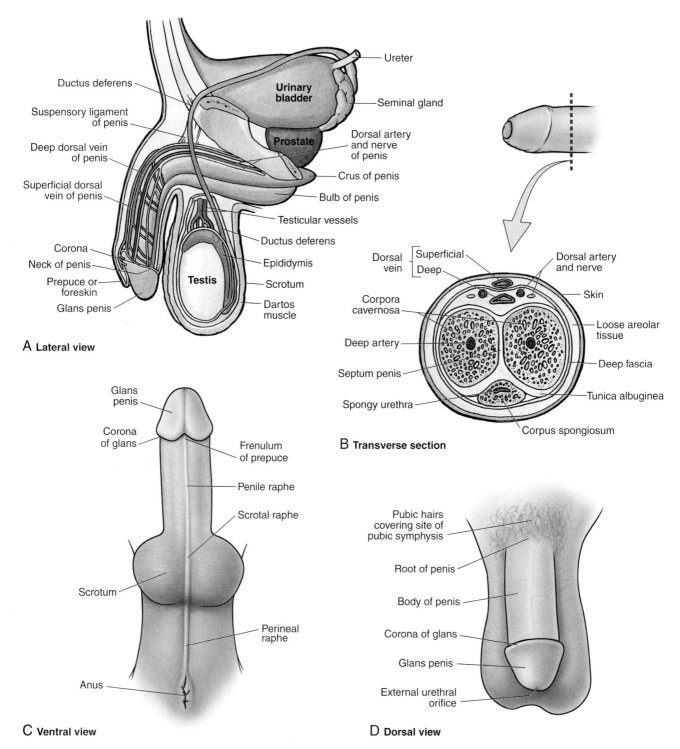

A Lateral view

B Transverse section

C Ventral view

D Dorsal view

Figure 3.30. Male urogenital organs. A. The urinary bladder, prostate, seminal gland, and male genital organs are identified. **B.** This section through the body of the penis reveals the internal structures. **C.** Note that the spongy urethra is deep to the penile raphe. **D.** The surface anatomy of the penis is shown.

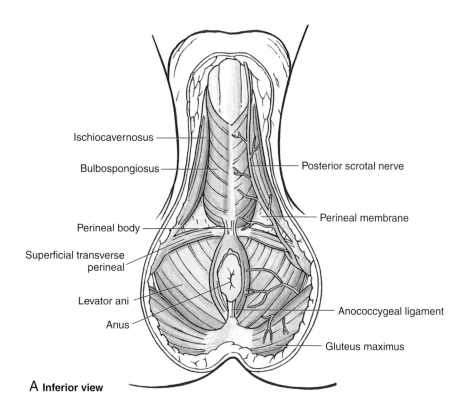

Ischiocavernosus

Bulbospongiosus

Posterior scrotal nerve

Perineal membrane

Perineal body

Superficial transverse perineal

Levator ani

Anus

Anococcygeal ligament

Gluteus maximus

A Inferior view

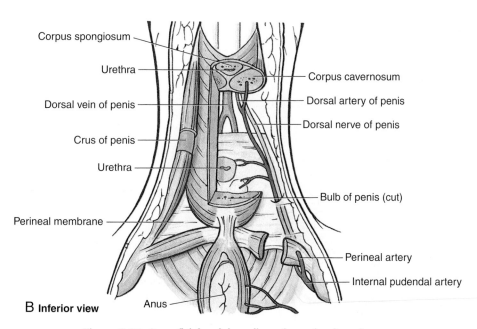

Corpus spongiosum

Urethra

Dorsal vein of penis

Crus of penis

Urethra

Perineal membrane

Corpus cavernosum

Dorsal artery of penis

Dorsal nerve of penis

Bulb of penis (cut)

Perineal artery

Internal pudendal artery

Anus

B Inferior view

Figure 3.31. Superficial and deep dissections of male perineum.

continuation of the deep perineal fascia that forms a membranous covering for the corpora, binding them together. The corpus spongiosum contains the spongy urethra. The corpora cavernosa are fused with each other in the median plane, except posteriorly where they separate to form the **crura of the penis** (Figs. 3.30A and 3.31B).

The **root of the penis** consists of the crura, bulb, and **ischiocavernosus** and **bulbospongiosus muscles** (Fig. 3.31; Table 3.10). The root is located in the superficial perineal pouch (Fig. 3.25A). The **crura** and **bulb of the penis** contain masses of erectile tissue. Each crus is attached to the inferior part of the internal surface of the corresponding ischial

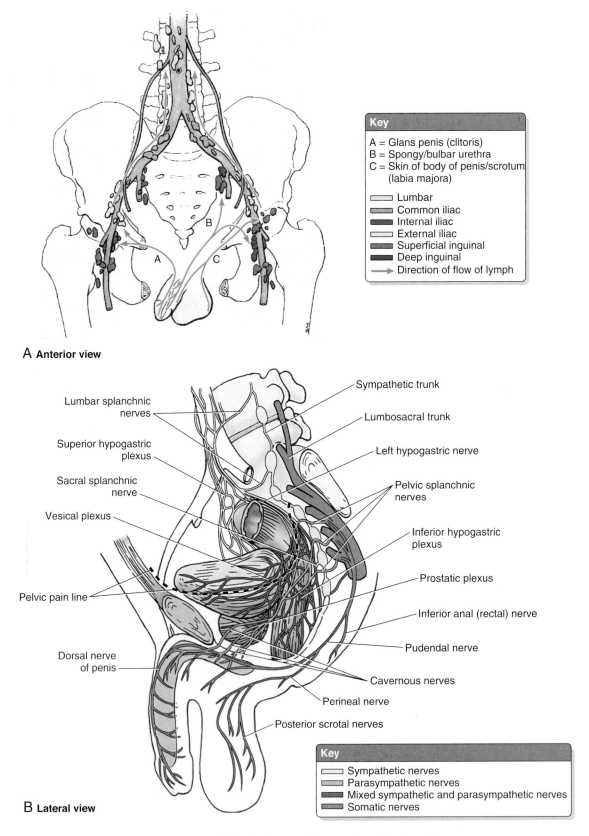

A Anterior view

Key

A = Glans penis (clitoris)
B = Spongy/bulbar urethra
C = Skin of body of penis/scrotum
    (labia majora)

▢ Lumbar
▢ Common iliac
▢ Internal iliac
▢ External iliac
▢ Superficial inguinal
▢ Deep inguinal
→ Direction of flow of lymph

Lumbar splanchnic nerves
Superior hypogastric plexus
Sacral splanchnic nerve
Vesical plexus
Pelvic pain line
Dorsal nerve of penis

Sympathetic trunk
Lumbosacral trunk
Left hypogastric nerve
Pelvic splanchnic nerves
Inferior hypogastric plexus
Prostatic plexus
Inferior anal (rectal) nerve
Pudendal nerve
Cavernous nerves
Perineal nerve
Posterior scrotal nerves

B Lateral view

Key

▢ Sympathetic nerves
▢ Parasympathetic nerves
▢ Mixed sympathetic and parasympathetic nerves
▢ Somatic nerves

Figure 3.32. Lymphatic drainage and innervation of male perineum.

ramus, anterior to the ischial tuberosity. The bulb of the penis is penetrated by the urethra, continuing from its intermediate part.

The **body of the penis** (usually pendulous) is the free part that is suspended from the pubic symphysis. Except for a few fibers of the bulbospongiosus near the root of the penis and the ischiocavernosus that embrace the crura, the penis has no muscles. Distally, the corpus spongiosum of the penis expands to form the **glans** (Fig. 3.30). The margin of the glans (head) projects beyond the ends of the corpora cavernosa to form the **corona of the gland.** The corona overhangs the neck of the glans. The **neck of the glans** separates the glans from the body of the penis. The slit-like opening of the spongy urethra, the *external urethral orifice,* is located near the tip of the glans (Fig. 3.30). The thin skin and fascia of the penis are prolonged as a double layer of skin, the **prepuce** (foreskin), which covers the glans to a variable extent (Fig. 3.30*A*). The **frenulum of the prepuce** is a median fold that passes from the prepuce to the urethral surface of the glans.

The **suspensory ligament of the penis** is a condensation of the deep fascia that arises from the anterior surface of the pubic symphysis and splits to form a sling that is attached to the deep fascia of the penis at the junction of its root and body (Fig. 3.30*A*). The fibers of the suspensory ligament are short and taut. The **fundiform ligament of the penis** is a band of the subcutaneous tissue that descends in the midline from the linea alba superior to the pubic symphysis. It passes inferiorly and splits to surround the penis and then unites and blends with the dartos fascia forming the scrotal septum.

The **superficial perineal muscles** are the superficial transverse perineal, bulbospongiosus, and ischiocavernosus (Table 3.10). These muscles are in the superficial perineal pouch and are supplied by the perineal nerves. Because of their function during erection and the activity of the bulbospongiosus subsequent to urination and ejaculation, to expel the last drops of urine and semen, the perineal muscles are generally more developed in males than in females.

Vasculature of Penis. The penis is supplied by *branches of the internal pudendal arteries* (Table 3.11).

- **Dorsal arteries of the penis** run in the interval between the corpora cavernosa on each side of the deep dorsal vein, supplying the fibrous tissue around the corpora cavernosa and the penile skin.
- **Deep arteries of the penis** pierce the crura and run distally near the center of the corpora cavernosa, supplying the erectile tissue in these structures.
- **Arteries of the bulb of the penis** supply the posterior (bulbous) part of the corpus spongiosum and the bulbourethral gland. They give off numerous branches (**helicine arteries of penis**) that open directly into the cavernous spaces. When the penis is flaccid, these arteries are coiled, restricting blood flow.

- **Superficial** and **deep branches of the external pudendal arteries** supply the penile skin, anastomosing with branches of the internal pudendal arteries.

Blood from the cavernous spaces of the corpora is drained by a venous plexus that becomes the **deep dorsal vein of the penis** in the deep fascia (Fig. 3.30*A* & *B*). This vein passes deep between the laminae of the suspensory ligament of the penis, anterior to the perineal membrane, to enter the prostatic venous plexus. Blood from the superficial coverings of the penis drains into the **superficial dorsal vein(s)**, which ends in the *superficial external pudendal vein.* Some blood also passes to the internal pudendal vein.

Lymph from the skin of the penis drains initially to the *superficial inguinal lymph nodes,* that from the glans and distal spongy urethra drain to the *deep inguinal* and *external iliac nodes.* The cavernous bodies and proximal spongy urethra drain to the *internal iliac nodes* (Fig. 3.32*A*).

Innervation of Penis. The nerves derive from the S2–S4 segments of the spinal cord. Sensory and sympathetic innervation is primarily from the *dorsal nerve of the penis,* a terminal branch of the **pudendal nerve** (Fig. 3.32*B*), which arises in the pudendal canal and passes anteriorly into the deep perineal pouch. It then runs along the dorsum of the penis lateral to the dorsal artery and supplies the skin and glans. The penis is supplied with a variety of sensory nerve endings, especially the glans penis. Branches of the *ilioinguinal nerve* supply the skin at the root of the penis. Cavernous nerves, conveying parasympathetic fibers independently from the prostatic nerve plexus, innervate the helicine arteries.

PERINEAL MUSCLES OF THE MALE

The *superficial perineal muscles* include the *superficial transverse perineal, ischiocavernosus,* and *bulbospongiosus* (Fig. 3.31). Details of their attachments, innervation, and actions are provided in Table 3.10. The ischiocavernosus and bulbospongiosus muscles both constrict venous outflow from the erectile bodies to assist erection, simultaneously pushing blood from the penile root into the body. The bulbospongiosus muscle constricts around the bulb of the penis to express the final drops of urine or semen.

Female Perineum

The female perineum includes the female external genitalia, perineal muscles, and anal canal.

FEMALE EXTERNAL GENITALIA

The **female external genitalia** include the mons pubis and labia majora (enclosing the pudendal cleft), labia minora (enclosing the vestibule), clitoris, bulbs of the vestibule, and

Table 3.11 Arterial Supply of the Perineum

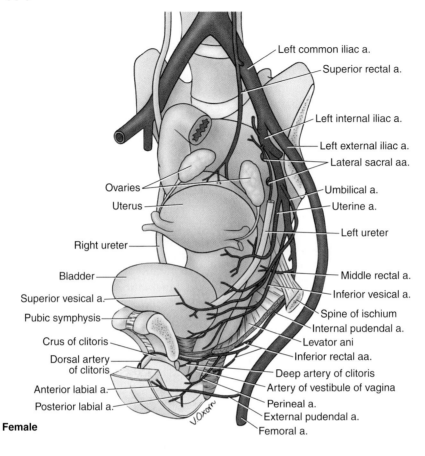

Left common iliac a.
Superior rectal a.
Left internal iliac a.
Left external iliac a.
Lateral sacral aa.
Ovaries
Uterus
Umbilical a.
Uterine a.
Left ureter
Right ureter
Bladder
Middle rectal a.
Superior vesical a.
Inferior vesical a.
Pubic symphysis
Spine of ischium
Internal pudendal a.
Crus of clitoris
Levator ani
Dorsal artery
of clitoris
Inferior rectal aa.
Deep artery of clitoris
Anterior labial a.
Artery of vestibule of vagina
Posterior labial a.
Perineal a.
External pudendal a.
Female
Femoral a.

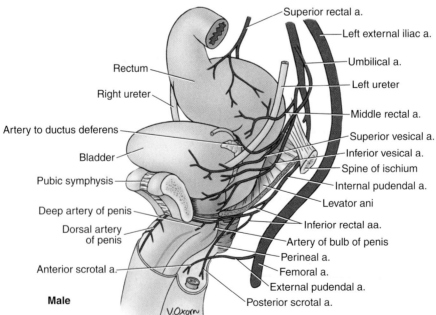

Superior rectal a.
Left external iliac a.
Umbilical a.
Rectum
Left ureter
Right ureter
Middle rectal a.
Artery to ductus deferens
Superior vesical a.
Inferior vesical a.
Bladder
Spine of ischium
Pubic symphysis
Internal pudendal a.
Deep artery of penis
Levator ani
Dorsal artery
of penis
Inferior rectal aa.
Artery of bulb of penis
Perineal a.
Anterior scrotal a.
Femoral a.
External pudendal a.
Male
Posterior scrotal a.

Table 3.11 Arterial Supply of the Perineum *(continued)*

Artery	Origin	Course	Distribution
Internal pudendal	Internal iliac artery	Leaves pelvis through greater sciatic foramen; hooks around ischial spine to enter perineum via lesser sciatic foramen; enters pudendal canal	Primary artery of perineum and external genital organs
Inferior rectal	Internal pudendal artery	Arises at entrance to pudendal canal; crosses ischioanal fossa to anal canal	Anal canal inferior to pectinate line; anal sphincters; perianal skin
Perineal		Arises within pudendal canal; passes to superficial perineal pouch (space) on exit	Supplies superficial perineal muscles and scrotum in male; vestibule in female
Posterior scrotal or labial	Terminal branch of perineal artery	Runs in subcutaneous tissue of posterior scrotum or labia majora	Skin of scrotum or labia majora and minora
Artery of bulb of penis or vestibule		Pierces perineal membrane to reach bulb of penis or vestibule of vagina	Supplies bulb of penis and bulbourethral gland in male; bulb of vestibule and greater vestibular gland in female
Deep artery of penis or clitoris	Terminal branch of internal pudendal artery	Pierces perineal membrane to reach corpora cavernosa of penis or clitoris	Supplies most erectile tissue of penis or clitoris via helicine arteries
Dorsal artery of penis or clitoris		Pierces perineal membrane and passes through suspensory ligament of penis or clitoris to run on dorsum of penis or clitoris	Deep perineal pouch; skin of penis; erectile tissue of penis or clitoris; distal corpus spongiosum of penis, including spongy urethra
External pudendal, superficial and deep branches	Femoral artery	Pass medially across thigh to reach scrotum or labia majora (anterior aspect of urogenital triangle)	Anterior aspect of scrotum and skin at root of penis in male; mons pubis and anterior aspect of labia in female

Erection, Emission, and Ejaculation

When a male is stimulated erotically, arteriovenous anastomoses, by which blood is normally able to bypass the "empty" potential spaces or sinuses of the corpora cavernosa are closed. The smooth muscle in the fibrous trabeculae and coiled arteries relaxes as a result of *parasympathetic stimulation* (S2–S4 through the cavernous nerves from the *prostatic nerve plexus*). As a result, the arteries straighten, enlarging their lumina and allowing blood to flow into and dilate the cavernous spaces in the corpora of the penis. The bulbospongiosus and ischiocavernosus muscles compress the veins of the corpora cavernosa, impeding the return of venous blood. As a result, the corpora cavernosa and corpus spongiosum become engorged with blood, causing the erectile bodies to become turgid (enlarged and rigid), and an **erection** occurs.

During **emission,** semen (sperms and glandular secretions) is delivered to the prostatic urethra through the ejaculatory ducts after peristalsis of the ductus deferentes and seminal glands. Prostatic fluid is added to the seminal fluid as the smooth muscle in the prostate contracts. Emission is a sympathetic response (L1–L2 nerves).

During **ejaculation,** semen is expelled from the urethra through the external urethral orifice. Ejaculation results from:

- Closure of the internal urethral sphincter at the neck of the urinary bladder, a sympathetic response (L1–L2 nerves).
- Contraction of the urethral muscle, a parasympathetic response (S2–S4 nerves).
- Contraction of the bulbospongiosus muscles, from the pudendal nerves (S2–S4).

After ejaculation, the penis gradually returns to a flaccid state (**remission**), resulting from sympathetic stimulation that causes constriction of the smooth muscle in the coiled arteries. The bulbospongiosus and ischiocavernosus muscles relax, allowing more blood to be drained from the cavernous spaces into the deep dorsal vein.

greater and lesser vestibular glands. The synonymous terms **pudendum** and **vulva** include all these parts. The term *pudendum* is commonly used clinically (Fig. 3.33). The vulva serves as sensory and erectile tissue for sexual arousal and intercourse, directs the flow of urine, and prevents entry of foreign material into the urogenital tract.

Mons Pubis. The **mons pubis** is the rounded fatty eminence anterior to the pubic symphysis, pubic tubercle, and superior pubic rami (Fig. 3.33). The amount of fat in the mons increases at puberty and decreases after menopause. After puberty, the mons pubis is covered with coarse pubic hairs.

Labia Majora. The **labia majora** are prominent folds of skin that bound the **pudendal cleft**, the slit between the labia majora and indirectly provide protection for the urethral and vaginal orifices (Fig. 3.33). Each labium majus—largely filled with subcutaneous fat containing smooth muscle and the termination of the round ligament of the uterus—passes inferoposteriorly from the mons pubis toward the anus. The external aspects of the labia in the adult are covered with pigmented skin containing many sebaceous glands and are covered with crisp pubic hair. The internal aspects of the labia are smooth, pink, and hairless. The labia are thicker anteriorly where they join to form the **anterior commissure**. Posteriorly, they merge to form the **posterior commissure**, which usually disappears after the first vaginal birth.

Labia Minora. The **labia minora** are folds of fat-free, hairless skin. They have a core of spongy connective tissue containing erectile tissue and many small blood vessels. Although the internal surface of each labium minus consists of thin moist skin, it has the typical pink color of a mucous membrane and contains many sensory nerve endings. The labia minora are enclosed in the pudendal cleft within the labia majora and surround the vestibule into which the external urethral and vaginal orifices open. Anteriorly, the labia minora form two laminae: the medial laminae unite as the **frenulum of the clitoris** (Fig. 3.33), and the lateral laminae unite to form the **prepuce** (foreskin) **of the clitoris**. In young women, especially virgins, the labia minora are connected posteriorly by a small transverse fold, the **frenulum of the labia minora** (fourchette).

Clitoris. The **clitoris** is an erectile organ located where the labia minora meet anteriorly. The clitoris consists of a **root** and a **body**, which are composed of two crura, two corpora cavernosa, and the **glans of the clitoris**. The glans is covered by the prepuce of the clitoris (Figs. 3.33 and 3.34A). The clitoris is highly sensitive and enlarges on tactile stimulation. The glans is the most highly innervated part of the clitoris.

Vestibule. The **vestibule** is the space surrounded by the labia minora, which contains the openings of the urethra, vagina, and ducts of the greater and lesser vestibular glands (Figs. 3.3 and 3.34A). The *external urethral orifice* is located posteroinferior to the glans clitoris and anterior to the vaginal orifice. On each side of the external urethral orifice are the openings of the ducts of the **paraurethral glands**. The size and appearance of the **vaginal orifice** vary with the condition of the **hymen**, a thin fold of mucous membrane within the vaginal orifice surrounding the lumen. After its rupture, only remnants of the hymen, **hymenal caruncles** (tags) are visible (Fig. 3.33A).

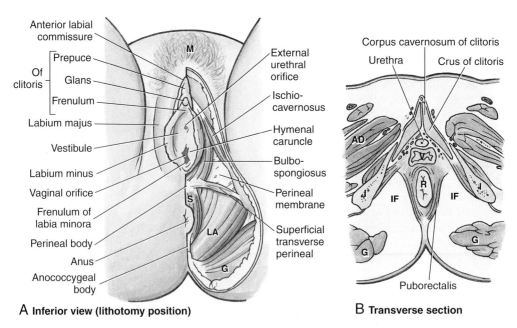

Anterior labial commissure
Of clitoris
— Prepuce
— Glans
— Frenulum
Labium majus
Vestibule
Labium minus
Vaginal orifice
Frenulum of labia minora
Perineal body
Anus
Anococcygeal body

External urethral orifice
Ischio-cavernosus
Hymenal caruncle
Bulbo-spongiosus
Perineal membrane
Superficial transverse perineal

Corpus cavernosum of clitoris
Urethra
Crus of clitoris

A Inferior view (lithotomy position)   **B** Transverse section

Figure 3.33. Female perineum. A. The left side has been dissected to show the muscles. **B.** The structures of the perineum are shown. *AD,* adductor muscles of thigh; *G,* gluteus maximus; *I,* ischium; *IF,* ischioanal fossa; *LA,* levator ani; *M,* mons pubis; *S,* external anal sphincter; *R,* rectum; *V,* vagina.

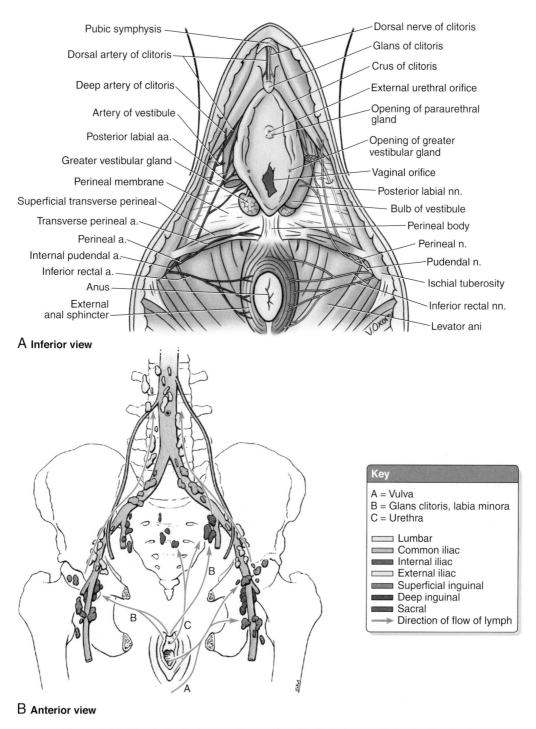

Pubic symphysis

Dorsal artery of clitoris

Deep artery of clitoris

Artery of vestibule

Posterior labial aa.

Greater vestibular gland

Perineal membrane

Superficial transverse perineal

Transverse perineal a.

Perineal a.

Internal pudendal a.

Inferior rectal a.

Anus

External anal sphincter

Dorsal nerve of clitoris

Glans of clitoris

Crus of clitoris

External urethral orifice

Opening of paraurethral gland

Opening of greater vestibular gland

Vaginal orifice

Posterior labial nn.

Bulb of vestibule

Perineal body

Perineal n.

Pudendal n.

Ischial tuberosity

Inferior rectal nn.

Levator ani

A Inferior view

Key

A = Vulva
B = Glans clitoris, labia minora
C = Urethra

☐ Lumbar
☐ Common iliac
☐ Internal iliac
☐ External iliac
☐ Superficial inguinal
☐ Deep inguinal
☐ Sacral
→ Direction of flow of lymph

B Anterior view

Figure 3.34. Blood supply, innervation and lymphatic drainage of vulva (pudendum).

Bulbs of Vestibule. The **bulbs of the vestibule** are paired masses of elongated erectile tissue that lie along the sides of the vaginal orifice under cover of the bulbospongiosus muscles (Fig. 3.34A). The bulbs are homologous with the bulb of the penis and the corpus spongiosum.

Vestibular Glands. The **greater vestibular glands** (Bartholin glands) are located on each side of the vestibule,

posterolateral to the vaginal orifice (Fig. 3.34A). These glands are round or oval and are partly overlapped posteriorly by the bulbs of the vestibule, and both are partially surrounded by the bulbospongiosus muscles. The slender ducts of these glands pass deep to the bulbs and open into the vestibule on each side of the vaginal orifice. These glands secrete mucus into the vestibule during sexual arousal. The **lesser vestibular glands** are smaller glands on each side of the vestibule that open into it between the urethral and the vaginal orifices. These glands secrete mucus into the vestibule, which moistens the labia and vestibule.

Vasculature of Vulva. The *arterial supply* to the vulva is from the *external and internal pudendal arteries* (Table 3.11). The *internal pudendal artery* supplies most of the skin, external genitalia, and perineal muscles. The labial arteries are branches of the internal pudendal artery, as are those of the clitoris (Fig. 3.34*A*). The *labial veins* are tributaries of the *internal pudendal veins* and accompanying veins (L. *venae comitantes*). Venous engorgement during the excitement phase of the sexual response causes an increase in the size and consistency of the clitoris and the bulbs of the vestibule. As a result the clitoris becomes turgid.

The vulva contains a rich network of *lymphatic vessels* that pass laterally to the *superficial inguinal lymph nodes* (Fig. 3.34*B*). The glans of the clitoris and anterior labia minora may also drain to the deep inguinal nodes or internal iliac nodes.

Innervation of Vulva. The anterior aspect of the vulva is supplied by **anterior labial nerves**, derived from the *ilioinguinal nerve* and the *genital branch of the genitofemoral nerve*. The posterior aspect is supplied by the *perineal branch of the posterior cutaneous nerve of the thigh* laterally and the *pudendal nerve* centrally. The pudendal nerve is the main nerve of the perineum. Its **posterior labial nerves** supply the labia; *deep and muscular branches* supply the orifice of the vagina and superficial perineal muscles; and the *dorsal nerve of the clitoris* supplies deep perineal muscles and sensation to the clitoris (Fig. 3.34*A*). The bulb of the vestibule and erectile bodies of the clitoris receive parasympathetic fibers via cavernous nerves from the uterovaginal plexus. Parasympathetic stimulation produces increased vaginal secretion, erection of the clitoris, and engorgement of erectile tissue in the bulbs of the vestibule.

PERINEAL MUSCLES OF THE FEMALE

The *superficial perineal muscles* include the *superficial transverse perineal, ischiocavernosus,* and *bulbospongiosus* (Fig. 3.33*A*). Details of their attachments, innervation and actions are provided in Table 3.10.

Dilation of Urethra

The female urethra is distensible because it contains considerable elastic tissue, as well as smooth muscle. It can easily dilate without injury to it. Consequently, the passage of catheters or cystoscopes in females is much easier than it is in males.

Inflammation of Greater Vestibular Glands

The greater vestibular glands (Bartholin glands) are usually not palpable, except when infected. *Bartholinitis,* inflammation of the greater vestibular glands, may result from a number of pathogenic organisms. Infected glands may enlarge to a diameter of 4–5 cm and impinge on the wall of the rectum.

Pudendal and Ilioinguinal Nerve Blocks

To relieve the pain experienced during childbirth, *pudendal nerve block anesthesia* may be performed by injecting a local anesthetic agent into the tissues surrounding the pudendal nerve. The injection may be made where the pudendal nerve crosses the lateral aspect of the sacrospinous ligament, near its attachment to the ischial spine. Although a pudendal nerve block anesthetizes most of the perineum, it does not abolish sensation from the anterior part of the perineum that is innervated by the ilioinguinal nerve. To abolish pain from the anterior part of the perineum, an *ilioinguinal nerve block* is performed (Fig. B3.10).

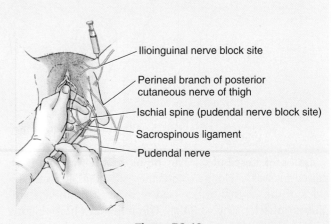

Ilioinguinal nerve block site

Perineal branch of posterior cutaneous nerve of thigh

Ischial spine (pudendal nerve block site)

Sacrospinous ligament

Pudendal nerve

Figure B3.10.

MRI provides excellent evaluation of pelvic structures and permits delineation of the uterus and ovaries (Figs. 3.35 and 3.36). It also permits the identification of tumors and congenital anomalies.

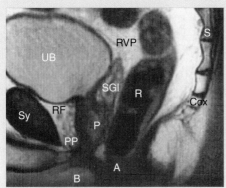

A **Median section**

Key

A	Anus
Ad	Adductor muscles
B	Bulb of penis
C	Conjoint ramus
Cav	Corpus cavernosum of penis
Cox	Coccyx
Cr	Crus of penis
IAF	Ischioanal fossa
IL	Iliacus
IT	Ischial tuberosity
LA	Levator ani
Max	Gluteus maximus
OE	Obturator externus
OI	Obturator internus
P	Prostate
PP	Prostatic venous plexus
R	Rectum
RP	Root of penis
RVP	Rectovesical pouch
S	Sacrum
SGI	Seminal gland
Sy	Pubic symphysis
U	Urethra
UB	Urinary bladder

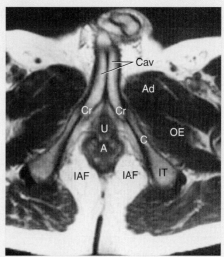

B **Transverse section**

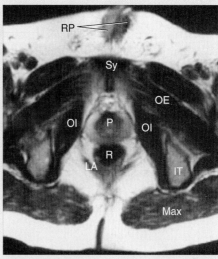

C **Transverse section**

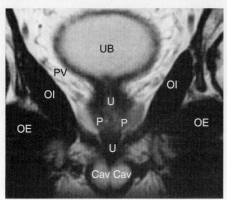

D **Coronal section**

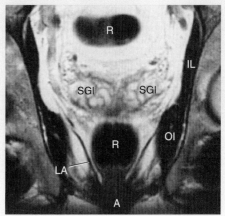

E **Coronal section**

Figure 3.35. MRI studies of male pelvis and perineum.

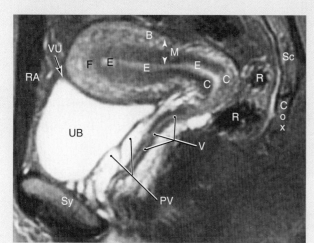

A **Median section**

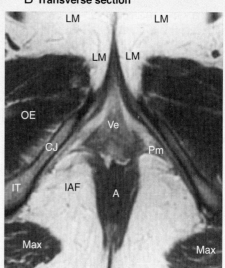

B **Transverse section**

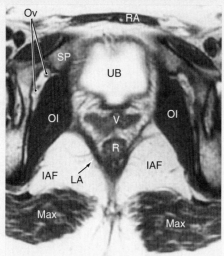

C **Transverse section**

D **Transverse section**

Key							
A	Anus	LM	Labium majus	RA	Rectus abdominis
B	Body of uterus	M	Myometrium	Sc	Sacrum
C	Cervix of uterus	Max	Gluteus maximus	SP	Superior ramus of pubis
Cox	Coccyx	OE	Obturator externus	Sy	Pubic symphysis
CJ	Conjoint ramus	OI	Obturator internus	U	Uterus
E	Endometrium	Ov	Ovary	UB	Urinary bladder
F	Fundus of uterus	Pm	Perineal membrane	V	Vagina
IAF	Ischioanal fossa	PV	Perivaginal veins	Ve	Vestibule of vagina
IT	Ischial tuberosity	R	Rectum	VU	Vesicouterine pouch
LA	Levator ani				

Figure 3.36. MRI studies of female pelvis and perineum.

4 Back

The back, the posterior aspect of the trunk inferior to the neck and superior to the gluteal region (buttocks), is the region of the body to which the head, neck, and limbs are attached. Because of their close association with the trunk, the back of the neck and the posterior and deep cervical muscles and vertebrae are described in this chapter. The back consists of skin, subcutaneous tissue (a layer of loose irregular connective tissue consisting of fatty tissue containing cutaneous nerves and vessels), deep fascia, muscles, ligaments, vertebral column, ribs (in the thoracic region), spinal cord and meninges (membranes covering spinal cord), and various segmental nerves and vessels.

Vertebral Column

The vertebral column (spine), extending from the cranium (skull) to the apex of the coccyx, forms the skeleton of the neck and back and is the main part of the axial skeleton (articulated bones of the cranium, vertebral column, ribs, and sternum). The vertebral column protects the spinal cord and spinal nerves, supports the weight of the body superior to the level of the pelvis, provides a partly rigid and flexible axis for the body and a pivot for the head, and plays an important role in posture and locomotion.

The adult vertebral column typically consists of 33 vertebrae arranged in five regions: 7 cervical, 12 thoracic, 5 lumbar, 5 sacral, and 4 coccygeal (Fig. 4.1). The **lumbosacral angle** occurs at the junction of the lumbar region of the vertebral column and sacrum. Significant motion occurs between only the superior 25 vertebrae. The 5 sacral vertebrae are fused in adults to form the **sacrum**, and the 4 coccygeal vertebrae are fused to form the **coccyx**. The vertebrae gradually become larger as the vertebral column descends to the sacrum and then become progressively smaller toward the apex of the coccyx. These structural differences are related to the fact that the successive vertebrae bear increasing amounts of the body's weight. The vertebral column is flexible because it consists of small bones, the **vertebrae**, that are separated by **intervertebral (IV) discs.** The 25 cervical, thoracic, lumbar, and first sacral vertebrae articulate at synovial *zygapophysial joints,* which facilitate and control the vertebral column's flexibility. The vertebral bodies contribute approximately three quarters of the height of the vertebral column, and the fibrocartilage of IV discs contribute approximately one quarter. The shape and strength of the vertebrae and IV discs, ligaments, and muscles provide stability to the vertebral column.

Curvatures of Vertebral Column

The vertebral column in adults has four curvatures: cervical, thoracic, lumbar, and sacral (Fig. 4.1C). The curvatures provide a flexible support (shock-absorbing resilience) for the body. The **thoracic** and **sacral (pelvic) curvatures (kyphoses)** are concave anteriorly, whereas the **cervical** and **lumbar curvatures (lordoses)** are concave posteriorly. The thoracic and sacral curvatures are **primary curvatures**, developing during the fetal period. Primary curvatures are retained throughout life as a consequence of differences in height between the anterior and the posterior parts of the vertebrae. The cervical and lumbar curvatures are **secondary curvatures**, which begin to appear in the cervical region during the fetal period but do not become obvious until infancy. Secondary curvatures are maintained primarily by differences in thickness between the anterior and the posterior parts of the IV discs. The **cervical curvature** becomes prominent when an infant

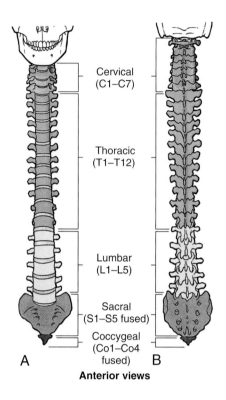

Cervical (C1–C7)

Thoracic (T1–T12)

Lumbar (L1–L5)

Sacral (S1–S5 fused)

Coccygeal (Co1–Co4 fused)

A   B

Anterior views

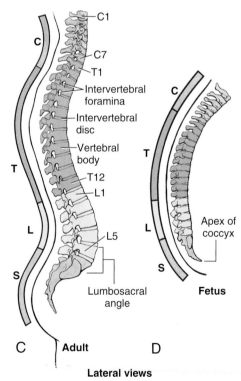

C

C1

C7

T1

Intervertebral foramina

Intervertebral disc

Vertebral body

T

T12

L1

L

L5

S

Lumbosacral angle

Apex of coccyx

C

T

L

S

Fetus

C   **Adult**   D

Lateral views

Figure 4.1. Vertebral column and curvatures. A and B. The composition of the adult vertebral column is shown. **C** and **D.** Note the curvatures of the vertebral column of the adult and fetus.

begins to hold his or her head erect. The **lumbar curvature** becomes obvious when an infant begins to walk and assumes the upright posture. This curvature, generally more pronounced in females, ends at the **lumbosacral angle**, formed at the junction of the L5 vertebra with the sacrum. The **sacral curvature** of females is reduced so that the coccyx protrudes less into the pelvic outlet.

The curvatures provide additional flexibility (shock-absorbing resilience) to the vertebral column, augmenting that provided by the IV discs. Although the flexibility provided by the IV disc is passive and limited primarily by the zygapophysial (facet) joints and longitudinal ligaments, that provided by the curvatures is actively resisted by the contraction of muscle groups antagonistic to the movement.

Abnormal Curvatures of Vertebral Column

Abnormal curvatures in some people result from developmental anomalies; in others, the curvatures result from pathological processes such as *osteoporosis*. This process is characterized by demineralization of the bones caused by a disruption of the normal balance of calcium deposition and resorption. The bones become weakened and brittle, and are subject to fracture.

Excess thoracic kyphosis (clinically shortened to **kyphosis** and colloquially called "humpback") is characterized by an abnormal increase in the thoracic curvature; the vertebral column curves posteriorly (Fig. B4.1*A* & *B*). This abnormality can result from erosion of the anterior part of one or more vertebrae. Progressive erosion and collapse of vertebrae results in an overall loss of height. *Dowager('s) hump* is a colloquial name for excess thoracic kyphosis in older women resulting from osteoporosis; however, kyphosis occurs in geriatric people of both sexes.

Excess lumbar lordosis (clinically shortened to **lordosis** and colloquially called "hollow back") is characterized by an anterior rotation of the pelvis (the upper sacrum tilts anteroinferiorly) at the hip joints, producing an abnormal increase in the lumbar curvature; the vertebral column becomes more convex anteriorly (Fig. B4.1*A* & *C*). This *abnormal extension deformity* may be associated with weakened trunk musculature, especially of the anterolateral abdominal wall. To compensate for alterations to their normal line of gravity, women develop a temporary lordosis during late pregnancy.

Scoliosis (crooked or curved back) is characterized by an abnormal lateral curvature that is accompanied by rotation of the vertebrae (Fig. 4.1*D* & *E*). The spinous processes turn toward the cavity of the abnormal curvature. Scoliosis is the most common deformity of the vertebral column in pubertal girls (aged 12–15 years). Asymmetric weakness of the intrinsic back muscles (*myopathic scoliosis*), failure of half of a vertebra to develop (*hemivertebra*), and a difference in the length of the lower limbs are causes of scoliosis.

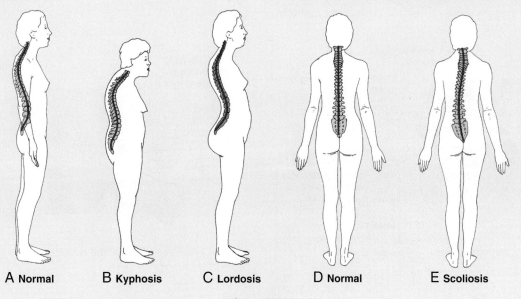

A Normal   B Kyphosis   C Lordosis   D Normal   E Scoliosis

Figure B4.1.

Structure and Function of Vertebrae

Vertebrae vary in size and other characteristics from one region of the vertebral column to another and to a lesser degree within each region. A *typical vertebra* consists of a vertebral body, vertebral arch, and seven processes (Fig. 4.2A). The **vertebral body** (the anterior, more massive part of the vertebra) gives strength to the vertebral column and supports body weight. The size of vertebral bodies, especially from T4 inferiorly, increase to bear the progressively greater body weight. In life, most of the superior and inferior surfaces of vertebral bodies are covered with hyaline cartilage, which are remnants of the cartilaginous model from which the bone develops, except at the periphery where there is a ring of smooth bone, the **epiphysial rim** (Fig. 4.2A). The cartilaginous remnants permit some diffusion of fluid between the IV disc and capillaries in the vertebral body.

The **vertebral arch** lies posterior to the vertebral body and is formed by right and left pedicles and laminae. The **pedi-** cles are short, stout processes that join the vertebral arch to the vertebral body. The pedicles project posteriorly to meet two broad, flat plates of bone, called **laminae,** which unite in the midline. The vertebral arch and the posterior surface of the vertebral body form the walls of the **vertebral foramen.** The succession of vertebral foramina in the articulated column forms the **vertebral canal,** which contains the spinal cord, meninges (protective membranes), fat, spinal nerve roots, and vessels. The indentations formed by the projection of the body and articular processes superior and inferior of the pedicles are **vertebral notches** (Fig. 4.2C). The superior and inferior vertebral notches of adjacent vertebrae contribute to the formation of the **IV foramina,** which give passage to spinal nerve roots and accompanying vessels and contain the spinal ganglia (Fig. 4.2D).

Seven processes arise from the vertebral arch of a typical vertebra:

- One median **spinous process** projects posteriorly (and usually inferiorly) from the vertebral arch at the junc-

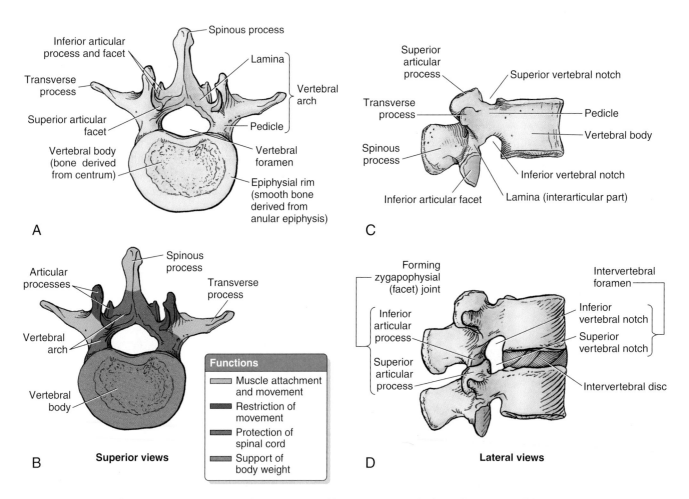

Figure 4.2. Parts and functions of a typical vertebra, represented by L2. A and **C.** The bony formations of the vertebrae are identified. **B.** Functional components include the vertebral body (*purple*), a vertebral arch (*red*), and seven processes: three for muscle attachment and leverage (*green*) and four that participate in synovial joints with adjacent vertebrae (*blue*). **D.** The intervertebral foramen is shown.

tion of the laminae and typically overlaps the vertebra below.

- Two **transverse processes** project posterolaterally from the junctions of the pedicles and laminae.
- Four **articular processes**—two **superior** and two **inferior**—also arise from the junctions of the pedicles and laminae, each bearing an **articular surface (facet)**.

The spinous process and two transverse processes project from the vertebral arch and afford attachments for deep back muscles and serve as levers that help the muscles move the vertebrae. The four articular processes are in apposition with corresponding processes of vertebrae superior and inferior to them, forming *zygapophysial (facet) joints*. The direction of the articular facets on the articular processes determine the types of movements permitted and restricted between the adjacent vertebrae of each region. The interlocking of the articular processes also assists in keeping adjacent vertebrae aligned, particularly preventing one vertebrae from slipping anteriorly on the vertebra below.

Laminectomy

A laminectomy is the surgical excision of one or more spinous processes and their supporting laminae in a particular region of the vertebral column (Fig. B4.2, *1*) and also commonly denotes the removal of most of the vertebral arch by transecting the pedicles (Fig. B4.2, *2*). Laminectomies provide access to the vertebral canal to relieve pressure on the spinal cord or nerve roots, commonly caused by a tumor, herniated IV disc, or bony hypertrophy (excess growth).

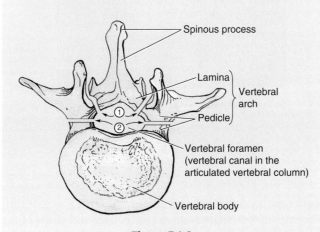

Figure B4.2.

Regional Characteristics of Vertebrae

Each of the 33 vertebrae is unique. However, most of the vertebrae demonstrate characteristic features identifying them as belonging to one of the five regions of the

Dislocation of Vertebrae

The bodies of the cervical vertebrae can be dislocated in neck injuries with less force than is required to fracture them. Because of the large vertebral canal in the cervical region, slight dislocation can occur without damaging the spinal cord. When a cervical vertebra is severely dislocated, it injures the spinal cord. If the dislocation does not result in "facet jumping" with locking of the displaced articular processes, the cervical vertebrae may self-reduce ("slip back into place") so that a radiograph may not indicate that the cord has been injured. MRI may reveal the resulting soft tissue damage.

Dislocation of vertebrae in the thoracic and lumbar regions is uncommon because of the interlocking of their articular processes; however, owing to the abrupt transition from the relatively inflexible thoracic region to the much more mobile lumbar region, T11 or T12 are the most commonly fractured non-cervical vertebrae (i.e., a "broken back" versus a "broken neck").

Fractures of the interarticular parts of the vertebral laminae of L5 (*spondylolysis of L5*) may result in forward displacement of the L5 vertebral body relative to the sacrum (the S1 vertebra)—*spondylolisthesis*). Spondylolysis of L5, or susceptibility to it, probably results from a failure of the centrum of L5 to unite adequately with the neural arches during development. Spondylolisthesis at the L5–S1 articulation may (but does not necessarily) result in pressure on the spinal nerves of the cauda equina as they pass into the superior part of the sacrum, causing back and lower limb pain. The intrusion of the L5 body into the pelvic inlet reduces the AP diameter of the pelvic inlet, which may interfere with parturition (childbearing) (Fig. B4.3).

Fractures of Vertebrae

Fractures and fracture-dislocations of the vertebral column usually result from sudden forceful flexion, as in an automobile accident. Typically,

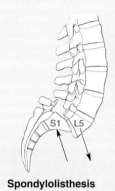

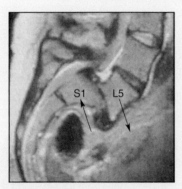

Spondylolisthesis

Figure B4.3.

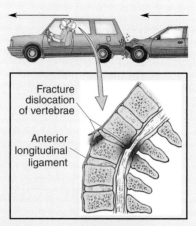

Hyperextension injury

Figure B4.4.

the injury is a crush or compression fracture of the body of one or more vertebrae. If violent anterior movement of the vertebra occurs in addition to compression, a vertebra may be displaced anteriorly on the vertebra inferior to it, such as dislocation of C6 or C7 vertebrae. Usually this dislocates and fractures the articular facets between the two vertebrae and ruptures the interspinous ligaments. Irreparable injuries to the spinal cord accompany most severe flexion injuries of the vertebral column. Severe hyperextension is most likely to injure the posterior parts of the vertebrae—the vertebral arches and their processes. Severe hyperextension of the neck (e.g., as occurs in diving injuries) may pinch the posterior arch of C1 vertebra between the occipital bone and the C2 vertebra. In these cases, the C1 vertebra usually breaks at one or both grooves for the vertebral arteries. The anterior longitudinal ligament and adjacent anulus fibrosus of the C2–C3 IV disc may also rupture. If this occurs, the cranium, C1, and C2 are separated from the rest of the axial skeleton, and the spinal cord is usually severed. Individuals with this injury seldom survive (Fig. B4.4).

Spina Bifida

The common congenital anomaly of the vertebral column is **spina bifida occulta,** in which the laminae (embryonic neural arches) of L5 and/or S1 fail to develop normally and fuse. This bony defect, present in up to 24% of people, is concealed by skin but its location is often in-

dicated by a tuft of hair. Most people with spina bifida occulta have no back problems. In severe types of the anomaly, such as **spina bifida cystica,** one or more vertebral arches may almost completely fail to develop (Moore and Persaud, 2003) (Fig. B4.5). Spina bifida cystica is associated with herniation of the meninges (*meningocele*) and/or the spinal cord (*meningomyelocele*). Usually, neurological symptoms are present in severe cases of meningomyelocele (e.g., paralysis of limbs and disturbances in bladder and bowel control).

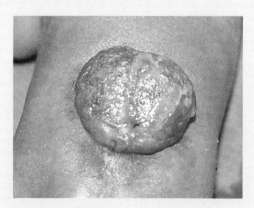

Spina bifida cystica

Figure B4.5.

vertebral column (e.g., cervical vertebrae are characterized by the presence of foramina in their transverse processes). In each region, the articular facets are oriented on the articular processes of the vertebrae in a characteristic direction that determines the type of movement permitted

between the adjacent vertebrae and, in aggregate, for the region. Regional variations in the size and shape of the vertebral canal accommodate the varying thickness of the spinal cord. The main regional characteristics of vertebrae are summarized in Tables 4.1–4.4.

Table 4.1 Cervical Vertebrae

Cervical vertebrae (C1–C7) form the skeleton of the neck; the atlas (C1) and the axis (C2) are atypical cervical vertebrae.

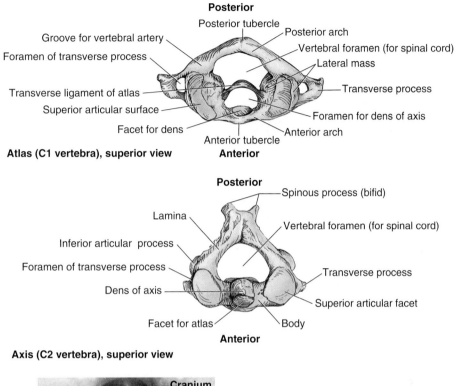

Atlas (C1 vertebra), superior view

Axis (C2 vertebra), superior view

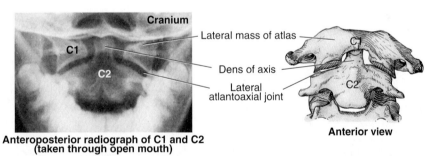

Anteroposterior radiograph of C1 and C2
(taken through open mouth)

Anterior view

Part	Distinctive Characteristics
Body	Small and wider from side to side than anteroposteriorly; superior surface is concave with uncus of body (uncinate process); inferior surface is convex
Vertebral foramen	Large and triangular
Transverse processes	Transverse foramina (L. *foramina transversarium*); small or absent in C7; vertebral arteries and accompanying venous and sympathetic plexuses pass through foramina (except C7, which transmits only small accessory vertebral veins); anterior and posterior tubercles
Articular processes	Superior facets directed superoposteriorly; inferior facets directed inferoanteriorly
Spinous process	C3–C5 short and bifid (split in two parts); process of C6 is long but that of C7 is longer (C7 is called *vertebra prominens*)

The ring-like C1 vertebra (atlas) is somewhat kidney-shaped when viewed from above or below. Its concave superior articular facets create a joint with the occipital condyles, and the flat inferior facets meet with the C2 vertebra. C1 has no spinous process or body and consists of two lateral masses connected by anterior and posterior arches. The C2 vertebra (axis) is the strongest cervical vertebra. Its distinguishing feature is the dens, which projects superiorly from its body and provides a pivot around which the atlas turns and carries the cranium. The dens articulates anteriorly with the anterior arch of the atlas and posteriorly with the transverse ligament of the atlas.

Table 4.1 Cervical Vertebrae *(continued)*

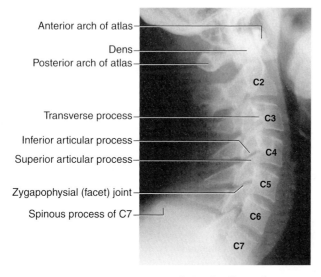

Lateral radiograph

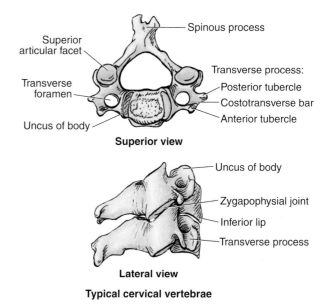

Superior view

Lateral view

Typical cervical vertebrae

Table 4.2 Thoracic Vertebrae

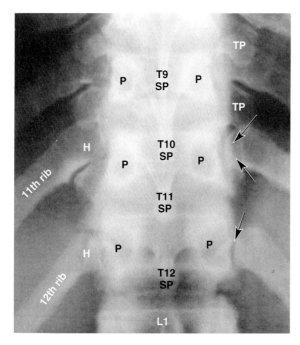

Posteroanterior radiograph

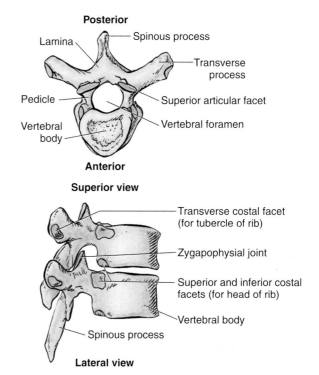

Superior view

Lateral view

Thoracic vertebrae (T1–T12) form the posterior part of the skeleton of the thorax and articulate with the ribs. The space between the vertebral bodies is the site of intervertebral disc. *P*, pedicle; *arrows*, costovertebral joints.

Table 4.2 Thoracic Vertebrae (continued)

Part	Distinctive Characteristics
Body	Heart-shaped; has one or two facets for articulation with head of rib (H)
Vertebral foramen	Circular and smaller than those in cervical and lumbar regions
Transverse process (TP)	Long and strong; extends posterolaterally; length diminishes from T1 to T12 (T1–T10 have facets for articulation with tubercle of rib)
Articular processes	Superior facets directed posteriorly and slightly laterally; inferior facets directed anteriorly and slightly medially
Spinous process (SP)	Long; slopes posteroinferiorly; tip extends to level of vertebral body below

Table 4.3 Lumbar Vertebrae

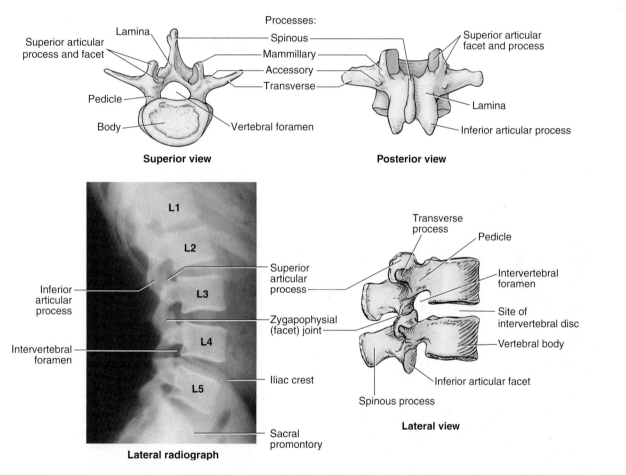

Superior view

Posterior view

Lateral radiograph

Lateral view

Lumbar vertebrae (L1–L5) are larger and heavier than the vertebrae in other regions. The space between vertebral bodies is the site of the intervertebral disc.

Part	Distinctive Characteristics
Body	Massive; kidney-shaped when viewed superiorly
Vertebral foramen	Triangular; larger than in thoracic vertebrae and smaller than in cervical vertebrae
Transverse processes	Long and slender; accessory process on posterior surface of base of each process
Articular processes	Superior facets directed posteromedially (or medially); inferior facets directed anterolaterally (or laterally); mammillary process on posterior surface of each superior articular process
Spinous process	Short and sturdy; hatchet shaped

Table 4.4 Sacrum and Coccyx

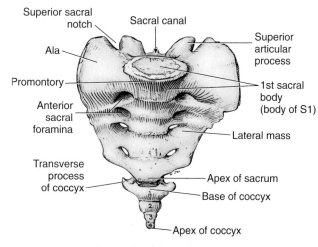

Base and pelvic surface, anteroinferior view

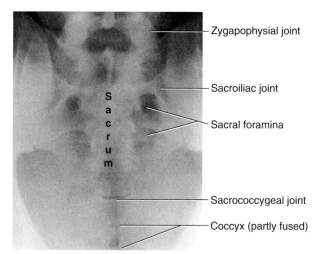

Posteroanterior radiograph

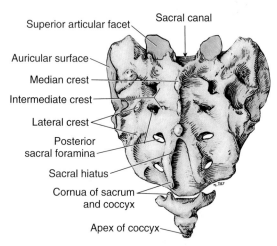

Dorsal surface, posterosuperior view

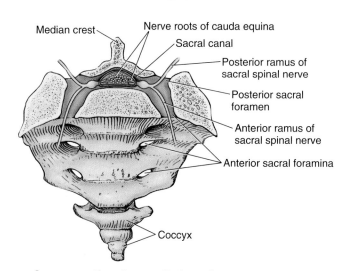

Sacrum, sectioned coronally through 1st sacral foramina, anterior view

The large, wedge-shaped **sacrum** in adults is composed of five fused sacral vertebrae. The sacrum provides strength and stability to the pelvis and transmits body weight to the pelvic girdle through the **sacroiliac joints.** The base of the sacrum is formed by the superior surface of the S1 vertebra. Its superior articular processes articulate with the inferior articular processes of the L5 vertebra. The projecting anterior edge of the body of the first sacral vertebra is the **sacral promontory.** On the pelvic and dorsal surfaces are four pairs of sacral foramina for the exit of the rami of the first four sacral nerves and the accompanying vessels. The pelvic surface of the sacrum is smooth and concave. The four transverse lines indicate where fusion of the sacral vertebrae occurred. The posterior surface of the sacrum is rough and convex. The fused spinous processes form the **median sacral crest.** The fused articular processes form the **intermediate sacral crests,** and the fused tips of the transverse processes form the **lateral sacral crests.** The inverted U-shaped **sacral hiatus** results from the absence of the laminae and spinous processes of the S4 and S5 vertebrae. The hiatus leads into the sacral canal, the inferior end of the vertebral canal. The **sacral cornua** (L. *horns*), representing the inferior articular processes of the S5 vertebra, project inferiorly on each side of the sacral hiatus and are a helpful guide to its location. The lateral surface of the sacrum has an ear-shaped (auricular) articular surface that participates in the sacroiliac joint.

The four vertebrae of the tapering **coccyx** are remnants of the skeleton of the embryonic tail-like caudal eminence. The distal three vertebrae fuse during middle life to form the coccyx, a beak-like bone that articulates with the sacrum.

Surface Anatomy of Vertebral Column

When the posterior surface of the trunk is observed, especially in a lateral view, the normal curvatures of the vertebral column are apparent (Fig. SA4.1*A*). The spinous processes from C7 vertebra inferiorly can be observed when the back is flexed (Fig. SA4.1*B*), but most of the spinous processes can be palpated, even in an obese individual, because the fat does not normally accumulate in the midline. Although C7 is the most superior process that is visible (vertebra prominens), the spinous process of T1 may be the most prominent. The spinous processes of C2–C6 may be palpated in the nuchal groove between the neck muscles; the C3–C5 spinous processes are separated from the surface by the nuchal ligament, making them harder to palpate. C1 has no spinous process. The transverse processes of the C1, C6, and C7 vertebrae are also palpable. Those of C1 can be palpated by deep pressure posteroinferior to the tips of the mastoid processes of the temporal bones (bony prominences posterior to the ears).

The spinous processes of thoracic vertebrae may be observed in thin people and can be palpated from superior to inferior starting at the C7 spinous process. The tips of the thoracic spinous processes do not indicate the level of the corresponding vertebral bodies because they overlap (lie at the level of) the vertebra below. The transverse processes of the thoracic vertebrae can usually be palpated on each side of the spinous processes in the thoracic region; and in thin individuals, the ribs can be palpated from tubercle to angle, at least in the lower back (inferior to the scapula).

The spinous processes of lumbar vertebrae are large and easy to observe when the trunk is flexed and can be palpated in the posterior median furrow (Fig. SA4.1*B*). A horizontal line joining the highest points of the iliac crests passes through the tip of the L4 spinous process and the L4–L5 IV disc. This is a useful landmark when performing lumbar puncture to obtain a sample of cerebrospinal fluid (see clinical correlation [blue] box "Lumbar Spinal Puncture," in this chapter). The transverse processes are covered with thick muscles and may or may not be palpable.

The S2 spinous process lies at the middle of a line drawn between the posterior superior iliac spines, in-

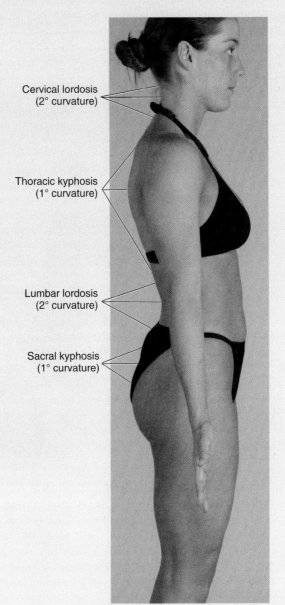

Cervical lordosis
(2° curvature)

Thoracic kyphosis
(1° curvature)

Lumbar lordosis
(2° curvature)

Sacral kyphosis
(1° curvature)

A **Lateral view of normal curvatures of back**

Figure SA4.1.

dicated by the skin dimples formed by the attachment of skin and deep fascia to these spines (Fig. SA4.1*C*). This level indicates the inferior extent of the subarachnoid space (lumbar cistern). The median crest of the sacrum can be palpated in the midline inferior to the

L5 spinous process. The sacral hiatus can be palpated at the inferior end of the sacrum in the superior part of the intergluteal (natal) cleft between the buttocks. Clinically the coccyx is examined with a gloved finger in the anal canal and its apex can be palpated approximately 2.5 cm posterosuperior to the anus. The sacral triangle is formed by the lines joining the posterior superior iliac spines and the superior part of the intergluteal cleft. The sacral triangle outlining the sacrum is a common area of pain resulting from low back sprains.

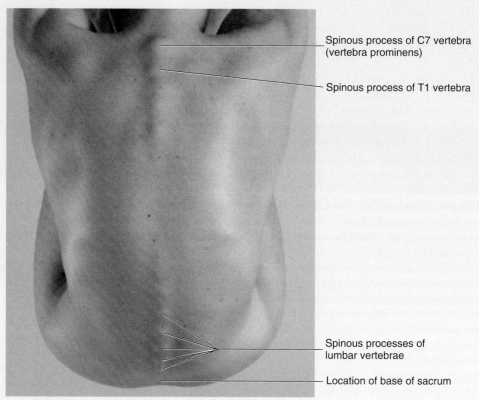

Spinous process of C7 vertebra (vertebra prominens)

Spinous process of T1 vertebra

Spinous processes of lumbar vertebrae

Location of base of sacrum

B **Posterior view during flexion of vertebral column**

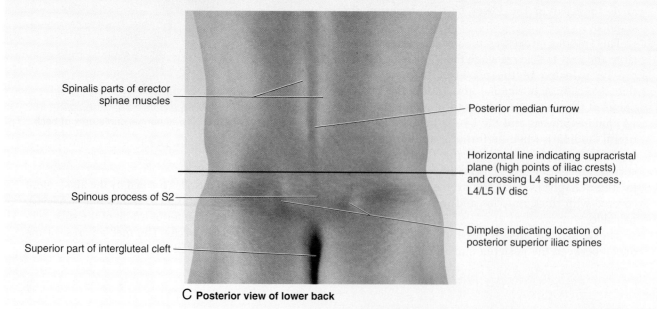

Spinalis parts of erector spinae muscles

Posterior median furrow

Horizontal line indicating supracristal plane (high points of iliac crests) and crossing L4 spinous process, L4/L5 IV disc

Spinous process of S2

Superior part of intergluteal cleft

Dimples indicating location of posterior superior iliac spines

C **Posterior view of lower back**

Figure SA4.1. (continued)

Joints of Vertebral Column

The joints of the vertebral column include the joints of vertebral bodies, joints of the vertebral arches, craniovertebral joints, costovertebral joints (Chapter 1), and sacroiliac joints (Chapter 3).

JOINTS OF THE VERTEBRAL BODIES

The joints of the vertebral bodies are *symphyses* (*secondary cartilaginous joints*) designed for weight bearing and strength. The articulating surfaces of adjacent vertebrae are connected by **IV discs** and ligaments (Fig. 4.3). The **IV discs**, interposed between the bodies of adjacent vertebrae, provide strong attachments between the vertebral bodies.

As well as permitting movement between adjacent vertebrae, the discs have resilient deformability, which allows them to serve as shock absorbers. Each IV disc consists of an *anulus fibrosus,* an outer fibrous part, composed of concentric lamellae of fibrocartilage and a gelatinous central mass, the *nucleus pulposus.*

The **anulus fibrosus** is a ring consisting of concentric lamellae of fibrocartilage forming the circumference of the IV disc. The anuli insert into the smooth, rounded *epiphysial rims* on the articular surfaces of the vertebral bodies (Fig. 4.3*C*). The fibers forming each lamella run obliquely from one vertebra to another; the fibers of one lamella typically run at right angles to those of adjacent ones.

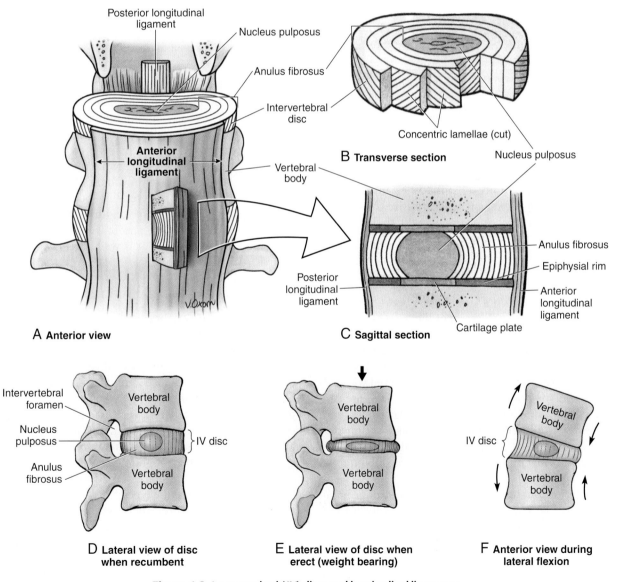

Figure 4.3. Intervertebral (*IV*) discs and longitudinal ligaments.

The **nucleus pulposus** is the central core of the IV disc (Fig. 4.3). At birth, the nuclei are about 88% water and are initially more cartilaginous than fibrous. The pulpy nuclei become broader when compressed and thinner when tensed or stretched. Compression and tension occur simultaneously in the same disc during movement of the vertebral column (e.g., anterior and lateral flexion, extension, rotation); the turgid nucleus acts as a semifluid fulcrum (Fig. 4.3D–F). With age, the nuclei pulposi dehydrate and lose elastin and proteoglycans while gaining collagen, eventually becoming dry and granular. As a result, the IV discs lose their turgor, becoming stiffer and more resistant to deformation. As this occurs, the anulus assumes a greater share of the vertical load and the associated stresses and strains. The lamellae of the anulus thicken with age and often develop fissures and cavities. Because the lamellae of the anulus fibrosus are thinner and less numerous posteriorly than they are anteriorly or laterally, the nucleus pulposus is not centered in the disc but is more posteriorly placed (Fig. 4.3C). The nucleus pulposus is avascular. It receives its nourishment by diffusion from blood vessels at the periphery of the anulus fibrosus and vertebral body.

There is no IV disc between the C1 (atlas) and C2 (axis) vertebrae. The most inferior functional disc is between the L5 and S1 vertebrae. The discs vary in thickness in different regions; they are thickest relative to the size of the vertebral bodies they connect in the cervical and lumbar regions (and absolutely thickest in the latter) and thinnest in the superior thoracic region. Their relative thickness is related to the range of movement, and their varying shapes produce the secondary curvatures of the vertebral column. The discs are thicker anteriorly in the cervical and lumbar regions, and their thickness is most uniform in the thoracic region.

Uncovertebral "joints" (of Luschka) are between the unci of the bodies (uncinate processes) of the C3–C6 vertebrae and the bevelled inferolateral surfaces of the vertebral bodies superior to them (Fig. 4.4). The joints are at the lateral and posterolateral margins of the IV discs. The articulating surfaces of these joint-like structures are covered with cartilage and contain a capsule filled with fluid. They are considered to be synovial joints by some; others consider them to be degenerative spaces (fissures) in the discs occupied by extracellular fluid. The uncovertebral "joints" are frequent sites of spur formation (projecting processes of bone) that may cause neck pain.

The **anterior longitudinal ligament** is a strong, broad fibrous band that covers and connects the anterolateral aspects of the vertebral bodies and IV discs (Figs. 4.3A and 4.5A). The ligament extends from the pelvic surface of the sacrum to the anterior tubercle of the C1 vertebra (atlas) and the occipital bone anterior to the foramen magnum.

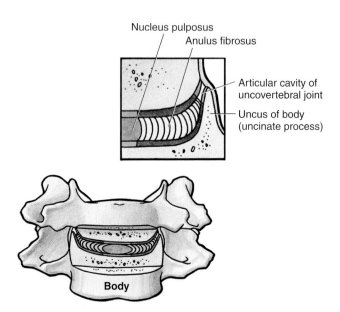

Figure 4.4. Uncovertebral joints. These joints are at the posterolateral margin of the cervical IV discs.

The anterior longitudinal ligament maintains stability of the intervertebral joints and limits extension of the vertebral column. The **posterior longitudinal ligament** is a much narrower, somewhat weaker band than the anterior longitudinal ligament. The ligament runs within the vertebral canal along the posterior aspect of the vertebral bodies (Fig. 4.3A & C). It is attached mainly to the IV discs and less so to the posterior edges of the vertebral bodies from C2 (axis) to the sacrum. The posterior longitudinal ligament helps prevent hyperflexion of the vertebral column and posterior herniation of the IV discs. It is well innervated with nociceptive (pain) nerve endings.

JOINTS OF THE VERTEBRAL ARCHES

The joints of the vertebral arches are the **zygapophysial joints** (facet joints). These articulations are synovial, plane joints between the superior and the inferior articular processes (G. *zygapophyses*) of adjacent vertebrae. Each joint is surrounded by a thin, loose **joint (articular) capsule**, which is attached to the margins of the articular surfaces of the articular processes of adjacent vertebrae (Fig. 4.5B & C). Accessory ligaments unite the laminae, transverse processes, and spinous processes and help stabilize the joints. The zygapophysial joints permit gliding movements between the articular processes; the shape and disposition of the articular surfaces determine the type of movement possible. The zygapophysial joints are innervated by articular branches that arise from the medial branches of the posterior rami of spinal nerves (Fig. 4.6). Each articular branch supplies two adjacent joints; therefore, each joint is supplied by two nerves.

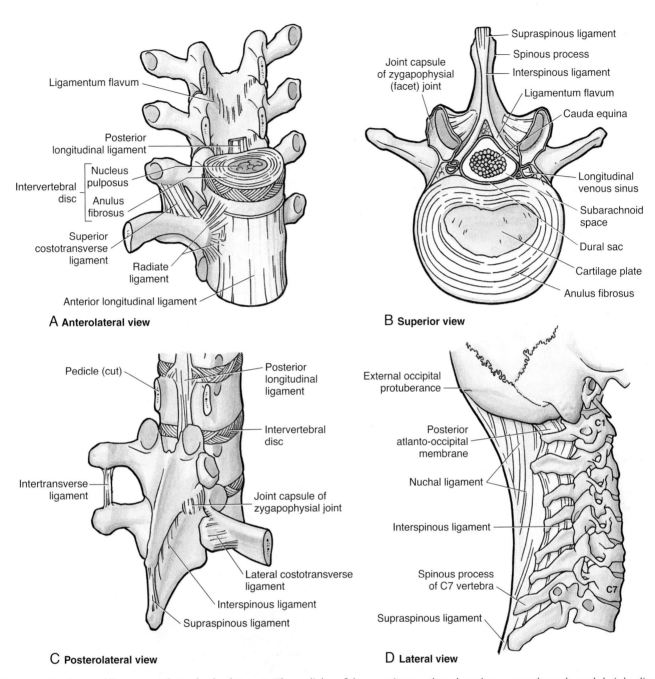

Figure 4.5. Joints and ligaments of vertebral column. A. The pedicles of the superior vertebrae have been sawn through, and their bodies have been removed. A rib and its costovertebral joint and associated ligaments are also shown. **B.** In this transverse section of an IV disc and associated ligaments, the nucleus pulposus has been removed to show the hyaline cartilage plate covering the superior surface of the vertebral body. **C.** The vertebral arch of the superior vertebra has been removed to show the posterior longitudinal ligament. **D.** The ligaments of the cervical region are identified.

ACCESSORY LIGAMENTS OF INTERVERTEBRAL JOINTS

The laminae of adjacent vertebral arches are joined by broad, pale, yellow elastic fibrous tissue called the **ligamenta flava** (L. *flavus,* yellow), which extend almost vertically from the lamina above to the lamina below (Fig. 4.5*A*). The ligaments bind the laminae of the adjoining vertebrae together, forming alternating sections of the posterior wall of the vertebral canal. The ligamenta flava resist separation of the vertebral laminae by arresting abrupt flexion of the vertebral column and thereby preventing injury to the IV discs.

Herniation of IV Discs

Herniation or protrusion of the gelatinous nucleus pulposus into or through the anulus fibrosus is a well-recognized cause of low back and lower limb pain. If degeneration of the posterior longitudinal ligament and wearing of the anulus fibrosus has occurred, the nucleus pulposus may herniate into the vertebral canal and compress the spinal cord or nerve roots of spinal nerves in the cauda equina (Fig. B4.6A). Herniations usually occur posterolaterally, where the anulus is relatively thin and does not receive support from the posterior or anterior longitudinal ligaments. A posterolateral herniation is more likely to be symptomatic because of the proximity of the spinal nerve roots.

The *localized back pain* of a herniated disc results from pressure on the longitudinal ligaments and periphery of the anulus fibrosus and from local inflammation, resulting from chemical irritation by substances from the ruptured nucleus pulposus. *Chronic pain* resulting from the spinal nerve roots being compressed by the herniated disc is referred to the area (dermatome) supplied by that nerve. Posterolateral herniation is most common in the lumbar region; approximately 95% of protrusions occur at the L4–L5 or L5–S1 levels. In patients of advanced years, the nerve roots are more likely being compressed by increased ossification (osteophytes) of the IV foramen as they exit. *Sciatica*, pain in the lower back and hip and radiating down the back of the thigh into the leg, is often caused by herniated lumbar IV discs or osteophytes that compress the L5 or S1 component of the sciatic nerve. The spinal nerve roots descend to the IV foramen from which the spinal nerve formed by their merging will exit. The nerve that exits a given IV foramen passes through the superior bony half of the foramen and thus lies above and is not affected by a herniating disc at that level. However, the nerve roots passing to the IV foramen immediately and farther below pass directly across the area of herniation. (i.e., herniation of the L4–L5 disc affects the L5 nerve root) (Fig. B4.6B).

Symptom-producing IV disc protrusions occur in the cervical region almost as often as in the lumbar region. In the cervical region, the IV discs are centrally placed in the anterior border of the IV foramen, and a herniating disc compresses the nerve actually exiting at that level. Recall, however, that cervical spinal nerves exit superior to the vertebra of the same number. Cervical disc protrusions result in pain in the neck, shoulder, arm, and hand.

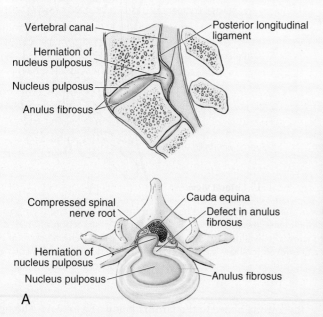

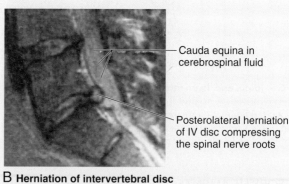

B **Herniation of intervertebral disc**

A

Figure B4.6.

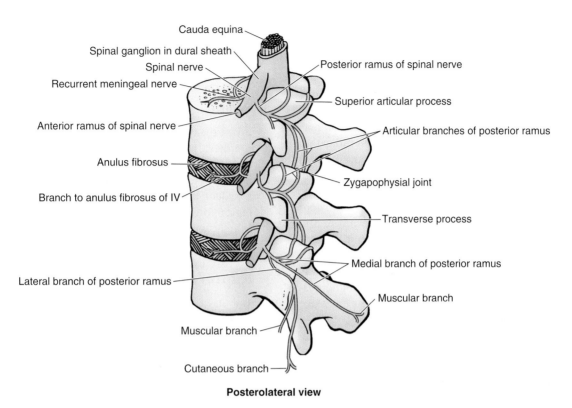

Cauda equina

Spinal ganglion in dural sheath

Spinal nerve

Recurrent meningeal nerve

Posterior ramus of spinal nerve

Superior articular process

Anterior ramus of spinal nerve

Articular branches of posterior ramus

Anulus fibrosus

Zygapophysial joint

Branch to anulus fibrosus of IV

Transverse process

Medial branch of posterior ramus

Lateral branch of posterior ramus

Muscular branch

Muscular branch

Cutaneous branch

Posterolateral view

Figure 4.6. Nerves of the vertebral joints. The posterior ramus arises from the spinal nerve outside the IV foramen and divides into medial and lateral branches, which supply the zygapophysial joints.

Injury and Disease of Zygapophysial Joints

When the zygapophyseal joints are injured or develop osteophytes during aging (osteoarthritis), the related spinal nerves are affected. This causes pain along the distribution pattern of the dermatomes and spasm in the muscles derived from the associated myotomes (a myotome consists of all the muscles or parts of muscles receiving innervation from one spinal nerve). *Denervation of lumbar zygapophysial joints* is a procedure that may be used for treatment of back pain caused by disease of these joints. The nerves are sectioned near the joints or are destroyed by radiofrequency *percutaneous rhizolysis* (root dissolution). The denervation process is directed at the articular branches of two adjacent posterior rami of the spinal nerves because each joint receives innervation from both the nerve exiting that level and the superjacent nerve (Fig. 4.6).

The strong elastic ligamenta flava help preserve the normal curvatures of the vertebral column and assist with straightening the column after flexing. Adjacent spinous processes are united by weak, almost membranous **interspinous ligaments** and strong fibrous **supraspinous ligaments** (Fig. 4.5 B & C). The latter ligament merges superiorly with the **nuchal ligament** (L. *ligamentum nuchae*), the strong median ligament of the neck (*nucha* refers to the back of neck). The nuchal ligament is composed of thickened fibroelastic tissue extending from the external occipital protuberance and posterior border of the foramen magnum to the spinous processes of the cervical vertebrae. Because of the shortness of the C3–C5 spinous processes, the nuchal ligament substitutes for bone in providing muscular attachments. The **intertransverse ligaments** (Fig. 4.5C), connecting adjacent transverse processes, consist of scattered fibers in the cervical region and fibrous cords in the thoracic region. In the lumbar region, they are thin and membranous.

CRANIOVERTEBRAL JOINTS

The craniovertebral joints include the atlanto-occipital joints, between the atlas (C1 vertebra) and the occipital bone of the cranium, and the atlantoaxial joints, between the C1 and the C2 vertebrae. *Atlanto,* a Greek prefix, refers to the atlas. These craniovertebral articulations are synovial joints that have no IV discs. Their design allows a wider range of movement than in the rest of the vertebral column.

Atlanto-Occipital Joints.   The atlanto-occipital joints, between the lateral masses of C1 (atlas) and the occipital condyles (Fig. 4.7C), permit nodding of the head, such as the neck flexion and extension that occurs when indicating approval (the "yes" movement). The main movement is flexion, with a little lateral flexion (bending) and rotation. These joints also permit sideways tilting of the head. The atlanto-occipital joints are synovial joints of the condyloid type and have thin, loose joint capsules. The cranium and C1 are also connected by **anterior** and **posterior atlanto-occipital membranes**, which extend from the anterior and posterior arches of C1 to the anterior and posterior margins of the foramen magnum (Fig. 4.7B). The anterior and posterior atlanto-occipital membranes help prevent excessive movement of these joints.

Atlantoaxial Joints.   There are three atlantoaxial articulations (Fig. 4.7A): two (right and left) **lateral atlantoaxial joints** between the lateral masses of C1 and the superior facets of C2, and one **median atlantoaxial joint** between the dens of C2 and the anterior arch and transverse ligament of the atlas. The median atlantoaxial joint is a pivot joint, whereas the lateral atlantoaxial joints are gliding-type synovial joints. Movement at all three atlantoaxial joints permits the head to be turned from side to side, as occurs when rotating the head to indicate disapproval (the "no" movement). During this movement, the cranium and C1 vertebra rotate on the C2 vertebra as a unit. During rotation of the head, the dens of C2 is the pivot, which is held in a socket formed anteriorly by the anterior arch of the atlas and posteriorly by the transverse ligament of the atlas. The **transverse ligament of the atlas** is a strong band extending between the tubercles on the medial aspects of the lateral masses of the C1 vertebrae. Vertically oriented but much weaker superior and inferior **longitudinal bands** pass from the transverse ligament to the occipital bone superiorly and to the body of C2 inferiorly. Together, the transverse ligament and the longitudinal bands form the **cruciate ligament** (formerly the cruciform ligament), so named because of its resemblance to a cross (Fig. 4.7C).

The **alar ligaments** extend from the sides of the dens to the lateral margins of the foramen magnum. These short, rounded cords attach the cranium to the C1 vertebra and serve as check ligaments, preventing excessive rotation at the joints.

The **tectorial membrane** is the strong superior continuation of the posterior longitudinal ligament across the median atlantoaxial joint through the foramen magnum to the central floor of the cranial cavity. It runs from the body of C2 to the internal surface of the occipital bone and covers the alar and transverse ligaments (Fig. 4.7B & C).

Rupture of Transverse Ligament of Atlas

When the transverse ligament of the atlas ruptures, the dens is set free, resulting in *atlantoaxial subluxation* or incomplete dislocation of the median atlantoaxial joint. When complete dislocation occurs, the dens may be driven into the upper cervical region of the spinal cord, causing *quadriplegia* (paralysis of all four limbs), or into the medulla of the brainstem, causing death.

Rupture of Alar Ligaments

The alar ligaments are weaker than the transverse ligament of the atlas. Consequently, combined flexion and rotation of the head may tear one or both alar ligaments. Rupture of an alar ligament results in an increase of approximately 30% in the range of movement to the opposite side.

Movements of Vertebral Column

The following movements of the vertebral column are possible (Fig. 4.8): flexion, extension, lateral flexion (bending), and rotation (torsion). The range of movement of the vertebral column varies according to the region and the individual. The normal range of movement possible in healthy young adults is typically reduced by 50% or more as they age. The mobility of the column results primarily from the compressibility and elasticity of the IV discs. The range of movement of the vertebral column is limited by the:

- Thickness, elasticity, and compressibility of the IV discs.
- Shape and orientation of the zygapophysial joints.
- Tension of the joint capsules of the above joints.
- Resistance of the back muscles and ligaments (such as the ligamenta flava and the posterior longitudinal ligament).
- Attachment to the thoracic (rib) cage.
- Bulk of the surrounding tissues.

The back muscles producing movements of the vertebral column are discussed subsequently; however, the movements are not produced exclusively by the back muscles. They are assisted by gravity and the action of the anterolateral abdominal muscles (see Chapter 2). Movements between adjacent vertebrae occur at the resilient nuclei pulposi of the IV

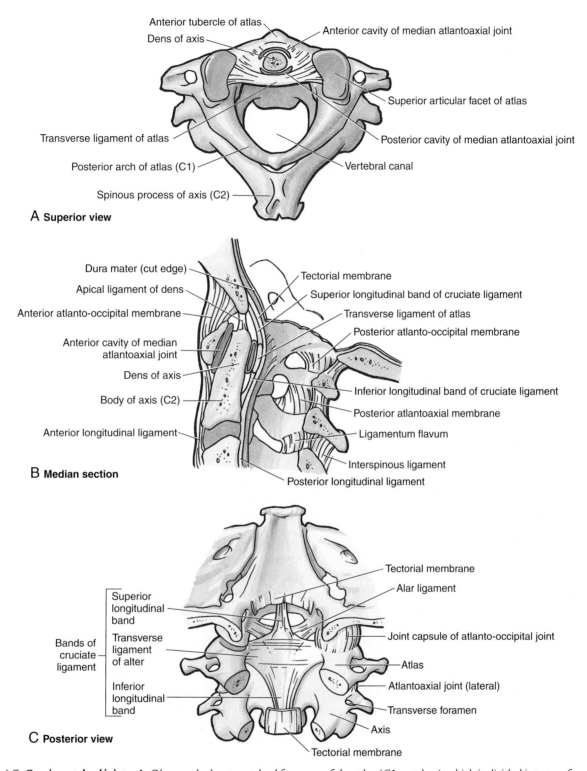

A Superior view

- Anterior tubercle of atlas
- Dens of axis
- Anterior cavity of median atlantoaxial joint
- Superior articular facet of atlas
- Transverse ligament of atlas
- Posterior cavity of median atlantoaxial joint
- Posterior arch of atlas (C1)
- Vertebral canal
- Spinous process of axis (C2)

B Median section

- Dura mater (cut edge)
- Apical ligament of dens
- Anterior atlanto-occipital membrane
- Anterior cavity of median atlantoaxial joint
- Dens of axis
- Body of axis (C2)
- Anterior longitudinal ligament
- Tectorial membrane
- Superior longitudinal band of cruciate ligament
- Transverse ligament of atlas
- Posterior atlanto-occipital membrane
- Inferior longitudinal band of cruciate ligament
- Posterior atlantoaxial membrane
- Ligamentum flavum
- Interspinous ligament
- Posterior longitudinal ligament

C Posterior view

- Bands of cruciate ligament
  - Superior longitudinal band
  - Transverse ligament of alter
  - Inferior longitudinal band
- Tectorial membrane
- Alar ligament
- Joint capsule of atlanto-occipital joint
- Atlas
- Atlantoaxial joint (lateral)
- Transverse foramen
- Axis
- Tectorial membrane

Figure 4.7. Craniovertebral joints. A. Observe the large vertebral foramen of the atlas (C1 vertebra), which is divided into two foramina by the transverse ligament. The larger posterior foramen is for the spinal cord, and the smaller anterior foramen is for the dens of the axis (C2 vertebra). **B.** The ligaments and joints are shown. **C.** The parts of the cruciate ligament are identified.

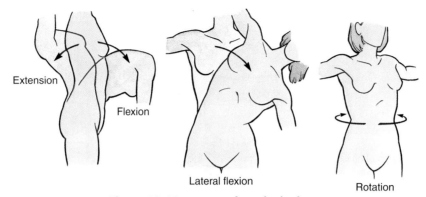

Figure 4.8. Movements of vertebral column.

discs and at the zygapophysial joints. The orientation of the latter joints permits some movements and restricts others. Although movements between adjacent vertebrae are relatively small, especially in the thoracic region, the summation of all of the small movements produces a considerable range of movement of the vertebral column as a whole (e.g., when flexing to touch the toes). Movements of the vertebral column are freer in the cervical and lumbar regions than elsewhere. Flexion, extension, lateral flexion, and rotation of the neck are especially free because the:

- IV discs, although thin relative to most other discs, are thick relative to the small size of the vertebral bodies at this level.
- Articular surfaces of the zygapophysial joints are relatively large and the joint planes are almost horizontal.
- Joint capsules of the zygapophysial joints are loose.
- Neck is relatively slender (with less surrounding soft tissue bulk).

Flexion of the vertebral column is greatest in the cervical region. The sagittally oriented joint planes of the lumbar region are conducive to flexion and extension. Extension of the vertebral column is most marked in the lumbar region and usually is more extensive than flexion; however, the interlocking articular processes here prevent rotation. The lumbar region, like the cervical region, has large IV discs (the largest ones occur here) relative to the size of the vertebral bodies. Lateral flexion of the vertebral column is greatest in the cervical and lumbar regions.

The thoracic region, in contrast, has IV discs that are thin relative to the size of the vertebral bodies. Relative stability is also conferred on this part of the vertebral column through its connection to the sternum by the ribs and costal cartilages. The joint planes here lie on an arc that is centered on the vertebral body, permitting rotation in the thoracic region. This rotation of the upper trunk, in combination with the rotation permitted in the cervical region and that at the atlantoaxial joints, enables the torsion of the axial skeleton that occurs as one looks back over the shoulder.

However, flexion is limited in the thoracic region, including lateral flexion.

Vasculature of Vertebral Column

Vertebrae are supplied by *periosteal* and *equatorial branches* of the major cervical and segmental arteries and their spinal branches. *Spinal branches* supplying the vertebrae are branches of the (Fig. 4.9A):

- Vertebral and ascending cervical arteries in the neck.
- Posterior intercostal arteries in the thoracic region.
- Subcostal and lumbar arteries in the abdomen.
- Iliolumbar and lateral and medial sacral arteries in the pelvis.

Spinal branches enter the IV foramina and divide into **anterior** and **posterior vertebral canal branches** that pass to the vertebral body and vertebral arch, respectively. The larger branches of the spinal branches continue as terminal *radicular* or *segmental medullary arteries* distributed to the posterior and anterior roots of the spinal nerves and their coverings and to the spinal cord.

Spinal veins form venous plexuses along the vertebral column both inside (**internal vertebral venous plexus**) and outside (**external vertebral venous plexus**) the vertebral canal (Fig. 4.9B & C). The large, tortuous **basivertebral veins** form within the vertebral bodies and emerge from foramina on the surfaces of the vertebral bodies (mostly the posterior aspect) and drain into the external and especially the internal vertebral venous plexuses. The **intervertebral veins** receive veins from the spinal cord and vertebral venous plexuses as they accompany the spinal nerves through the IV foramina to drain into the *vertebral veins* of the neck and *segmental veins* of the trunk.

Nerves of Vertebral Column

Other than the zygapophysial joints (innervated by articular branches of the medial branches of the posterior

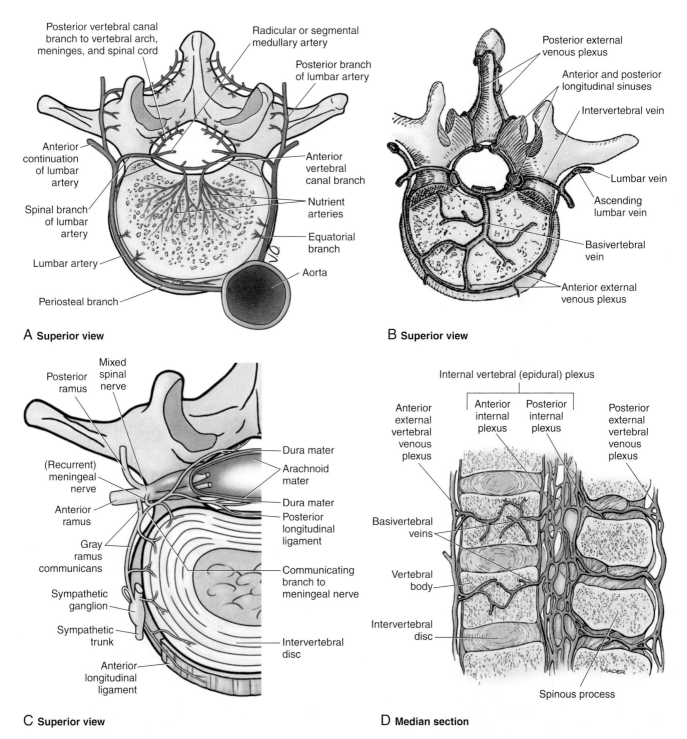

Figure 4.9. Blood, lymph, and nerve supply of vertebrae. The arterial supply (**A**), venous drainage (**B**), innervation (**C**), and vertebral venous plexuses (**D**) are shown.

rami), the vertebral column is innervated by (**recurrent**) **meningeal branches of the spinal nerves** (Fig.4.9C). Most of the meningeal branches run back through the IV foramen, but some branches remain outside the canal. The branches outside the canal supply the anuli fibrosi

and anterior longitudinal ligament; those inside the canal supply the periosteum, ligamenta flava, annuli fibrosi posteriorly, posterior longitudinal ligament, spinal dura mater, and blood vessels within the vertebral canal.

Spinal Cord and Meninges

The spinal cord, spinal meninges, spinal nerve roots, and neurovascular structures that supply them are in the **vertebral canal** (Fig. 4.10). The **spinal cord**, the major reflex center and conduction pathway between the body and the brain, is a cylindrical structure that is slightly flattened anteriorly and posteriorly. It is protected by the vertebrae and their associated ligaments and muscles, the spinal meninges, and the cerebrospinal fluid (CSF). The spinal cord begins as a continuation of the **medulla oblongata** (commonly called

the medulla), the caudal part of the brainstem. In the newborn, the inferior end of the spinal cord usually is opposite the IV disc between the L2 and the L3 vertebrae. In adults, the spinal cord usually ends opposite the IV disc between the L1 and the L2 vertebrae; however, its tapering end, the **medullary cone**, may terminate as high as T12 or as low as L3. Thus the spinal cord occupies only the superior two thirds of the vertebral canal. The spinal cord is enlarged in two regions for innervation of the limbs:

- The **cervical enlargement** extends from the C4 through the T1 segments of the spinal cord, and most of the an-

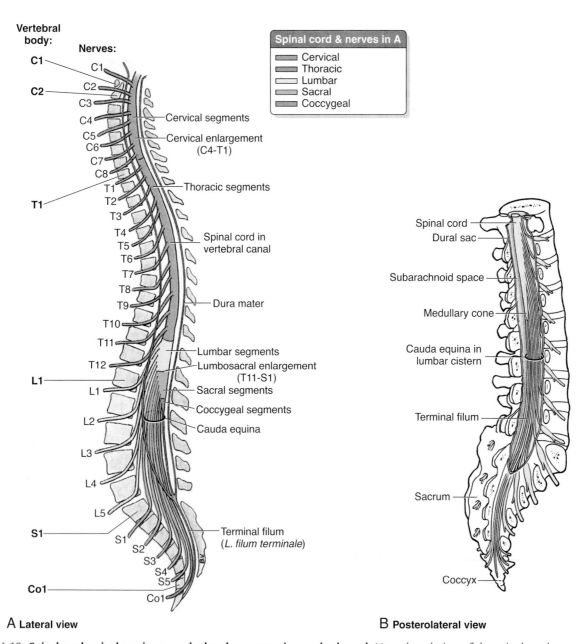

A Lateral view

B Posterolateral view

Figure 4.10. Spinal cord, spinal meninges, and related structures in vertebral canal. Note the relation of the spinal cord segments and spinal nerves to the adult vertebral column.

terior rami of the spinal nerves arising from it form the *brachial plexus of nerves,* which innervates the upper limbs (Chapter 6).

- The **lumbosacral (lumbar) enlargement** extends from the L1 through the S3 segments of the spinal cord, and the anterior rami of the spinal nerves arising from it contribute to the *lumbar* and *sacral plexuses of nerves,* which innervate the lower limbs (Chapter 5). The spinal nerve roots arising from the lumbosacral enlargement and medullary cone form the **cauda equina**, the bundle of spinal nerve roots running through the *lumbar cistern* (subarachnoid space).

Structure of Spinal Nerves

A total of 31 pairs of spinal nerves are attached to the spinal cord: 8 cervical, 12 thoracic, 5 lumbar, 5 sacral, and 1 coccygeal (Fig. 4.10*A*). Multiple rootlets emerge from the posterior and anterior surfaces of the spinal cord and converge to form **posterior** and **anterior roots of the spinal nerves** (Fig. 4.11*A & B*). The part of the spinal cord from which the rootlets of one pair of roots emerge is a **segment of the spinal cord.** The posterior roots of the spinal nerves contain afferent (or sensory) fibers from skin; subcutaneous and deep tissues; and, often, viscera. The anterior roots of spinal nerves contain efferent (or motor) fibers to skeletal muscle and many contain presynaptic autonomic fibers. The cell bodies of somatic axons contributing to the anterior roots are in the **anterior horns of gray matter** of the spinal cord (Fig. 4.11*C*), whereas the cell bodies of axons making up the posterior roots are outside the spinal cord in the **spinal ganglia** (posterior root ganglia) at the distal ends of the posterior roots. The posterior and anterior nerve roots unite at their points of exit from the vertebral canal to form a **spinal nerve.** The C1 nerves lack posterior roots in 50% of people, and the coccygeal nerve (Co1) may be absent. Each spinal nerve divides almost immediately into a **posterior ramus** and **anterior ramus** (Fig. 4.11*A*). The posterior rami supply the skin and deep muscles of the back; the anterior rami supply the limbs and the rest of the trunk.

In adults, the spinal cord is shorter than the vertebral column; hence there is a progressive obliquity of the spinal nerve roots as the cord descends (Fig. 4.10). Because of the increasing distance between the spinal cord segments and the corresponding vertebrae, the length of the nerve roots increases progressively as the inferior end of the vertebral column is approached. The lumbar and sacral nerve rootlets are the longest. They descend until they reach the IV foramina of exit in the lumbar and sacral regions of the vertebral column, respectively. The bundle of spinal nerve roots in the **lumbar cistern** (subarachnoid space) within the vertebral canal caudal to the termination of the spinal cord resembles a horse's tail, hence its name, *cauda equina* (L. horse tail) (Figs. 4.10*B* and 4.11*D*).

The inferior end of the spinal cord has a conical shape and tapers into the *medullary cone* (L. *conus medullaris*). From its inferior end, the **terminal filum** (L. *filum terminale*) descends among the spinal nerve roots in the cauda equina. It consists primarily of pia mater but its proximal end also includes vestiges of neural tissue, connective tissue, and neuroglial tissue. The terminal filum takes on layers of arachnoid and dura mater as it penetrates the inferior end of the dural sac and passes through the **sacral hiatus** to attach ultimately to the coccyx posteriorly. The terminal filum serves as an anchor for the end of the **dural sac**, the continuation of the dura inferior to the medullary cone.

Spinal Meninges and Cerebrospinal Fluid

Collectively, the dura mater, arachnoid mater, and pia mater surrounding the spinal cord form the **spinal meninges.** These membranes and CSF surround, support, and protect the spinal cord and the spinal nerve roots, including those in the cauda equina.

The **spinal dura mater**, composed of tough, fibrous, and some elastic tissue, is the outermost covering membrane of the spinal cord (Fig. 4.11). The spinal dura mater is separated from the vertebrae by the **epidural space** (Table 4.5). The dura forms the **spinal dural sac**, a long tubular sheath within the vertebral canal. The spinal dural sac adheres to the margin of the foramen magnum of the cranium, where it is continuous with the cranial dura mater. The spinal dural sac is pierced by the spinal nerves and is anchored inferiorly to the coccyx by the *terminal filum.* The spinal dura extends into the IV foramina and along the posterior and anterior nerve roots distal to the spinal ganglia to form **dural root sheaths,** or sleeves (Fig. 4.11*A*). These sheaths blend with the epineurium (outer connective tissue covering of spinal nerves) that adheres to the periosteum lining the IV foramina.

Table 4.5 Spaces Associated with Spinal Meninges

Space	Location	Contents
Extradural (epidural)	Between wall of vertebral canal and dura mater	Fat (loose connective tissue); internal vertebral venous plexuses; inferior to L2 vertebra, the roots of spinal nerves
Subarachnoid	Between arachnoid and pia mater	CSF; arachnoid trabeculae; radicular, segmental, medullary, and spinal arteries; veins

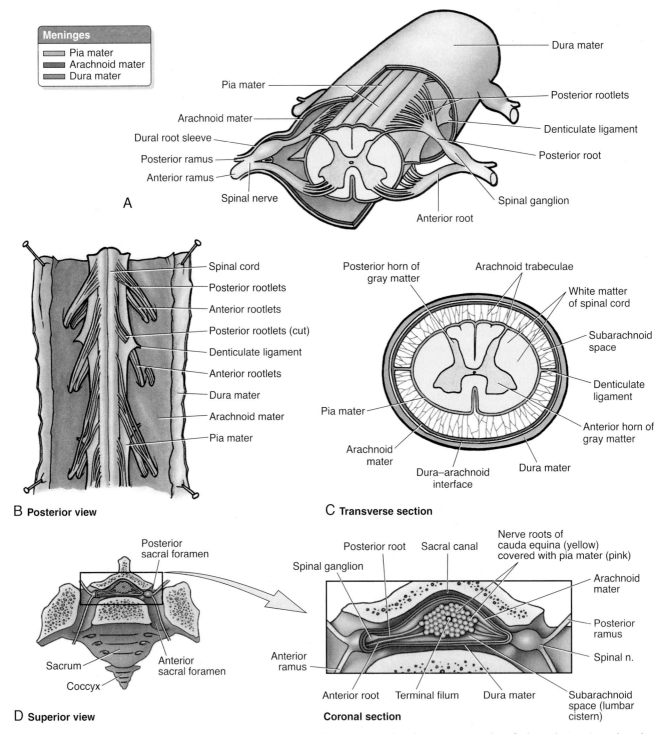

Meninges
- Pia mater
- Arachnoid mater
- Dura mater

Dura mater

Pia mater

Posterior rootlets

Arachnoid mater

Denticulate ligament

Dural root sleeve

Posterior root

Posterior ramus

Anterior ramus

Spinal nerve

Spinal ganglion

Anterior root

A

Spinal cord

Posterior rootlets

Anterior rootlets

Posterior rootlets (cut)

Denticulate ligament

Anterior rootlets

Dura mater

Arachnoid mater

Pia mater

B **Posterior view**

Posterior horn of gray matter

Arachnoid trabeculae

White matter of spinal cord

Subarachnoid space

Denticulate ligament

Pia mater

Anterior horn of gray matter

Arachnoid mater

Dura–arachnoid interface

Dura mater

C **Transverse section**

Posterior sacral foramen

Nerve roots of cauda equina (yellow) covered with pia mater (pink)

Spinal ganglion

Posterior root   Sacral canal

Arachnoid mater

Posterior ramus

Spinal n.

Anterior ramus

Sacrum

Anterior sacral foramen

Coccyx

Anterior root   Terminal filum   Dura mater

Subarachnoid space (lumbar cistern)

D **Superior view**

Coronal section

Figure 4.11. Spinal cord and spinal meninges. A. The structures of the spinal cord and meninges are identified. **B.** The meninges have been cut and spread out. The pia mater covers the spinal cord and projects laterally as the denticulate ligament. **C.** The parts of the spinal cord and meninges are shown. **D.** The first sacral foramina is shown in detail.

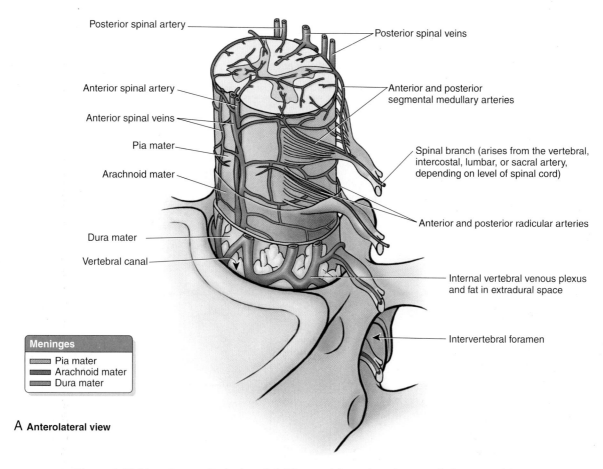

Figure 4.12. **Vasculature of spinal cord. A.** The arterial supply and venous drainage are shown.

The **spinal arachnoid mater** is a delicate, avascular membrane composed of fibrous and elastic tissue that lines the dural sac and the dural root sheaths. It encloses the CSF-filled subarachnoid space containing the spinal cord, spinal nerve roots, and spinal ganglia (Fig. 4.11*B* & *C*). The arachnoid mater is not attached to the dura but is held against the inner surface of the dura by the pressure of the CSF. In a *lumbar spinal puncture,* the needle traverses the dura and arachnoid mater simultaneously. Their apposition is the **dura–arachnoid interface,** often erroneously referred to as the "subdural space." No actual space occurs naturally at this site; it is rather, a weak cell layer (Haines, 2002). Bleeding into this layer creates a pathological space at the dura–arachnoid junction in which a *subdural hematoma* is formed. In the cadaver, because of the absence of CSF, the arachnoid falls away from the internal surface of the dura and lies loosely on the spinal cord. The arachnoid mater is separated from the pia mater on the surface of the spinal cord by the *subarachnoid space* containing CSF (Table 4.5). Delicate

strands of connective tissue, the **arachnoid trabeculae,** span the subarachnoid space connecting the arachnoid and pia (Fig. 4.11*B*).

The **spinal pia mater,** the innermost covering membrane of the spinal cord, consists of flattened cells with long, equally flattened processes that closely follow all the surface features of the spinal cord (Fig. 4.11*B* & *C*). The pia mater also directly covers the roots of the spinal nerves and spinal blood vessels. Inferior to the medullary cone, the pia continues as the terminal filum.

The spinal cord is suspended in the dural sac by the terminal filum and especially by the right and left sawtooth **denticulate ligaments** (L. *denticulus,* a small tooth), which run longitudinally along each side of the spinal cord. These ligaments consists of a fibrous sheet of pia mater extending midway between the posterior and the anterior nerve roots. Between 20 and 22 of these processes, shaped much like sharks' teeth, attach to the internal surface of the arachnoid-lined dural sac. The superior processes (uppermost part) of the right and left denticulate ligament attach to the cranial

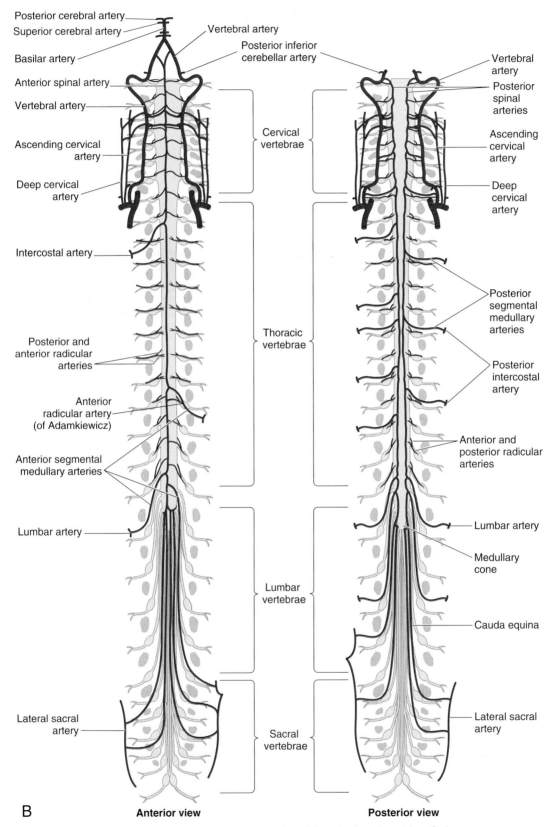

Figure 4.12. *(continued)* **B.** The arteries of the spinal cord are identified.

Lumbar Spinal Puncture

To obtain a sample of CSF from the lumbar cistern, a *lumbar puncture needle,* fitted with a stylet, is inserted into the subarachnoid space. Lumbar spinal puncture (spinal tap) is performed with the patient leaning forward or lying on the side with the back flexed. Flexion of the vertebral column facilitates insertion of the needle by stretching the ligamenta flava and spreading the laminae and spinous processes apart (Fig. B4.7). Under aseptic conditions, the needle is inserted in the midline between the spinous processes of the L3 and L4 (or the L4 and L5) vertebrae. At these levels in adults, there is little danger of damaging the spinal cord.

Epidural Block

An anesthetic agent can be injected into the extradural (epidural) space using the position described in clinical correlation "Lumbar Spinal Puncture." The anesthetic has a direct effect on the spinal nerve roots of the cauda equina after they exit from the dural sac (Fig. B4.8). The patient loses sensation inferior to the level of the block. An anesthetic agent can also be injected through the sacral hiatus into the extradural space in the sacral canal—a *caudal epidural block.* The agent spreads superiorly and acts on the spinal nerves (*caudal analgesia*). The distance the agent ascends (and hence the number of nerves affected) depends on the amount injected and on the position assumed by the patient.

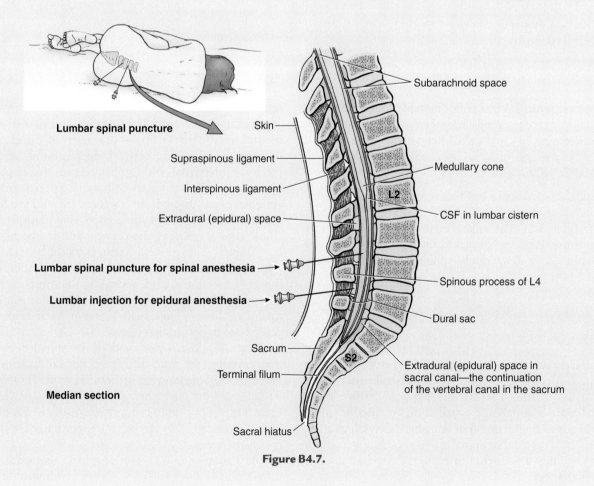

Lumbar spinal puncture

Skin

Supraspinous ligament

Interspinous ligament

Extradural (epidural) space

Lumbar spinal puncture for spinal anesthesia →

Lumbar injection for epidural anesthesia →

Sacrum

Terminal filum

Median section

Sacral hiatus

Subarachnoid space

Medullary cone

L2

CSF in lumbar cistern

Spinous process of L4

Dural sac

S2

Extradural (epidural) space in sacral canal—the continuation of the vertebral canal in the sacrum

Figure B4.7.

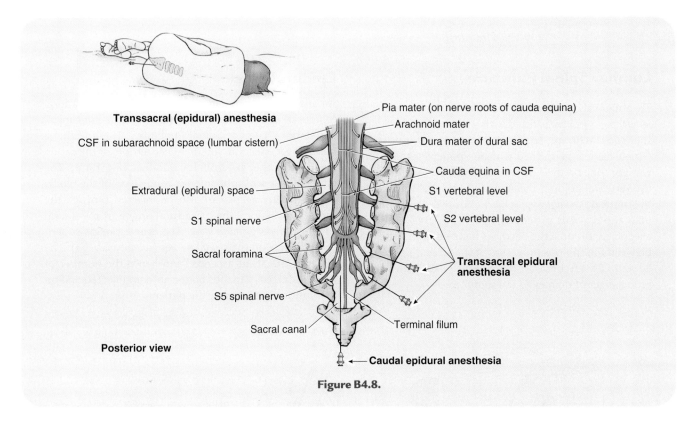

Transsacral (epidural) anesthesia

Pia mater (on nerve roots of cauda equina)

CSF in subarachnoid space (lumbar cistern)

Arachnoid mater

Dura mater of dural sac

Cauda equina in CSF

Extradural (epidural) space

S1 vertebral level

S1 spinal nerve

S2 vertebral level

Sacral foramina

Transsacral epidural anesthesia

S5 spinal nerve

Sacral canal

Terminal filum

Posterior view

← **Caudal epidural anesthesia**

Figure B4.8.

dura mater immediately superior to the foramen magnum. The inferior process extends from the medullary cone, passing between the T12 and the L1 nerve roots.

SUBARACHNOID SPACE

The subarachnoid space lies between the arachnoid mater and the pia mater and is filled with CSF (Figs. 4.10*B* and 4.11*B*; Table 4.5). The enlargement of the subarachnoid space in the dural sac, caudal to the medullary cone and containing CSF and the cauda equine is the **lumbar cistern** (Fig. 4.11*D*).

Vasculature of Spinal Cord and Spinal Nerve Roots

The arteries supplying the spinal cord are branches of the vertebral, ascending cervical, deep cervical, intercostal, lumbar, and lateral sacral arteries (Fig. 4.12). Three longitudinal arteries supply the spinal cord: an **anterior spinal artery**, formed by the union of branches of vertebral arteries, and paired **posterior spinal arteries**, each of which is a branch of either the vertebral artery or the posterior inferior cerebellar artery.

The spinal arteries run longitudinally from the medulla of the brainstem to the medullary cone of the spinal cord. By themselves, the anterior and posterior spinal arteries supply only the short superior part of the spinal cord. The circulation to much of the spinal cord depends on seg-

mental medullary and radicular arteries running along the spinal nerve roots. The **anterior** and **posterior segmental medullary arteries** are derived from spinal branches of ascending cervical, deep cervical, vertebral, posterior intercostal, and lumbar arteries that supply the spinal cord. The medullary segmental arteries enter the vertebral canal through the IV foramina and are located chiefly where the need for a good blood supply to the spinal cord is greatest: the cervical and lumbosacral enlargements. The **great anterior segmental medullary artery** (of Adamkiewicz) reinforces the circulation to two thirds of the spinal cord, including the lumbosacral enlargement. It is much larger than the other segmental medullary arteries and usually arises on the left side at low thoracic or upper lumbar levels.

Posterior and anterior roots of the spinal nerves and their coverings are supplied by **posterior** and **anterior radicular arteries,** which run along the nerve roots. These vessels do not reach the posterior or anterior spinal arteries. Segmental medullary arteries occur irregularly in the place of radicular arteries; they are larger vessels that make it to the spinal arteries.

The 3 **anterior** and 3 **posterior spinal veins** are arranged longitudinally (Fig. 4.9*B* & *C*); they communicate freely with each other and are drained by up to 12 **anterior** and **posterior medullary** and **radicular veins.** The veins draining the spinal cord join the **internal vertebral venous plexus** in the epidural space. The internal vertebral venous plexus passes superiorly through the foramen magnum to com-

Ischemia of the Spinal Cord

The segmental reinforcements of blood supply from the segmental medullary arteries are important in supplying blood to the anterior and posterior spinal arteries. Fractures, dislocations, and fracture–dislocations may interfere with the blood supply to the spinal cord from the spinal and medullary arteries. Deficiency of blood supply (ischemia) of the spinal cord affects its function and can lead to muscle weakness and paralysis. The spinal cord may also suffer circulatory impairment if the segmental medullary arteries, particularly the great anterior segmental medullary artery (of Adamkiewicz), are narrowed by *obstructive arterial disease*. Sometimes the aorta is purposely occluded ("cross-clamped") during surgery. Patients undergoing such surgeries, and those with ruptured aneurysms of the aorta or occlusion of the great anterior segmental medullary artery, may lose all sensation and voluntary movement inferior to the level of impaired blood sup-

ply to the spinal cord (*paraplegia*). This is secondary to death of neurons in the part of the spinal cord supplied by the anterior spinal artery.

When systemic blood pressure drops severely for 3–6 min., blood flow from the segmental medullary arteries to the anterior spinal artery supplying the midthoracic region of the spinal cord may be reduced or stopped. These patients may also lose sensation and voluntary movement in the areas supplied by the affected level of the spinal cord.

Alternative Circulation Pathways

The *vertebral venous plexuses* are important because blood may return from the pelvis or abdomen through these plexuses and reach the heart via the superior vena cava when the inferior vena cava is obstructed. These veins also can provide a route for metastasis of cancer cells to the vertebrae or the brain from an abdominal or pelvic tumor (e.g., prostate cancer).

---

municate with the dural venous sinuses and vertebral veins in the cranium (see Chapter 7). The internal vertebral plexus also communicates with the **external vertebral venous plexus** on the external surface of the vertebrae.

Muscles of Back

Most body weight is anterior to the vertebral column, especially in obese people. For this reason, the many strong muscles attached to the spinous and transverse processes of vertebrae are necessary to support and move the vertebral column. There are two major groups of muscles in the back. The **extrinsic back muscles** include *superficial* and *intermediate muscles* that produce and control limb and respiratory movements, respectively. The **intrinsic back muscles** include muscles that specifically act on the vertebral column, producing its movements and maintaining posture.

Extrinsic Back Muscles

The **superficial extrinsic back muscles** (trapezius, latissimus dorsi, levator scapulae, and rhomboids) connect the upper limbs to the trunk (see Chapter 6). These muscles, although located in the back region, for the most part, receive their nerve supply from the anterior rami of cervical nerves and act on the upper limb. The trapezius receives its motor fibers from a cranial nerve, the spinal accessory nerve (CN XI). The

intermediate extrinsic back muscles (serratus posterior superior and inferior) are thin muscles, commonly designated superficial respiratory muscles but are more likely proprioceptive rather than motor in function. They are described with muscles of the thoracic wall (see Chapter 1).

Intrinsic Back Muscles

The intrinsic back muscles (*muscles of back proper,* deep back muscles) are innervated by the posterior rami of spinal nerves and act to maintain posture and control movements of the vertebral column (Fig. 4.10). These muscles, extending from the pelvis to the cranium, are enclosed by deep fascia that attaches medially to the nuchal ligament, the tips of the spinous processes of the vertebrae, the supraspinous ligament, and the median crest of the sacrum. The fascia attaches laterally to the cervical and lumbar transverse processes and to the angles of the ribs. The thoracic and lumbar parts of the deep fascia constitute the **thoracolumbar fascia** (Fig. 4.13). The deep back muscles are grouped according to superficial, intermediate, and deep layers according to their relationship to the surface (Table 4.6).

SUPERFICIAL LAYER OF THE INTRINSIC BACK MUSCLES

The **splenius muscles** (L. *musculi splenii*) are thick and flat and lie on the lateral and posterior aspects of the neck,

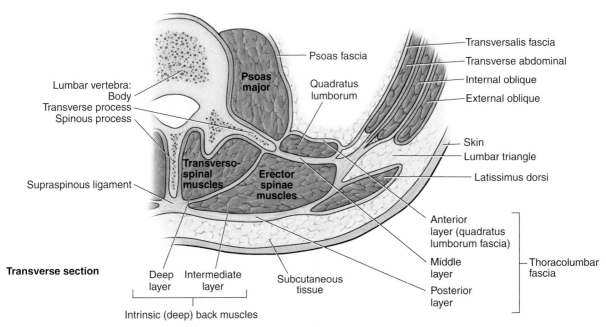

Lumbar vertebra:
Body
Transverse process
Spinous process

Supraspinous ligament

Transversospinal muscles

Erector spinae muscles

Psoas fascia

Psoas major

Quadratus lumborum

Transversalis fascia
Transverse abdominal
Internal oblique
External oblique

Skin
Lumbar triangle
Latissimus dorsi

Anterior layer (quadratus lumborum fascia)
Middle layer
Posterior layer
} Thoracolumbar fascia

Transverse section

Deep layer   Intermediate layer

Subcutaneous tissue

Intrinsic (deep) back muscles

Figure 4.13. Muscles of back and layers of thoracolumbar fascia.

covering the vertical muscles somewhat like a bandage, which explains their name (L. *splenion,* bandage). The splenii arise from the midline and extend superolaterally to the cervical vertebrae (**splenius cervicis**) and cranium (**splenius capitis**). These muscles cover and hold the deep neck muscles in position (Fig. 4.14; Table 4.6).

INTERMEDIATE LAYER OF INTRINSIC BACK MUSCLES

The **erector spinae muscles** (sacrospinalis) lie in a "groove" on each side of the vertebral column between the spinous processes and the angles of the ribs (Fig. 4.14). The mas-

Table 4.6A Superficial and Intermediate Layers of Intrinsic Back Muscles

Muscle	Origin	Insertion	Nerve Supply	Main Action(s)
Superficial layer of intrinsic back muscles				
Splenius	Arises from nuchal ligament and spinous processes of C7–T3 or T4 vertebrae	*Splenius capitis:* fibers run superolaterally to mastoid process of temporal bone and lateral third of superior nuchal line of occipital bone *Splenius cervicis:* tubercles of transverse processes of C1–C3 or C4 vertebrae	Posterior rami of spinal nerves	*Acting alone:* laterally flex neck and rotate head to side of active muscles *Acting together:* extend head and neck
Intermediate layer of intrinsic back muscles (Erector spinae)				
Iliocostalis Longissimus Spinalis	Arises by broad tendon from posterior part of iliac crest, posterior surface of sacrum, sacroiliac ligaments, sacral and inferior lumbar spinous processes, and supraspinous ligament	*Iliocostalis* (lumborum, thoracis, and cervicis): fibers run superiorly to angles of lower ribs and cervical transverse processes *Longissimus* (thoracis, cervicis, and capitis): fibers run superiorly to ribs between tubercles and angles to transverse processes in thoracic and cervical regions and to mastoid process of temporal bone *Spinalis* (thoracis, cervicis, and capitis): fibers run superiorly to spinous processes in upper thoracic region and to cranium	Posterior rami of spinal nerves	*Acting bilaterally:* extend vertebral column and head; as back is flexed, control movement by gradually lengthening their fibers *Acting unilaterally:* laterally flex vertebral column

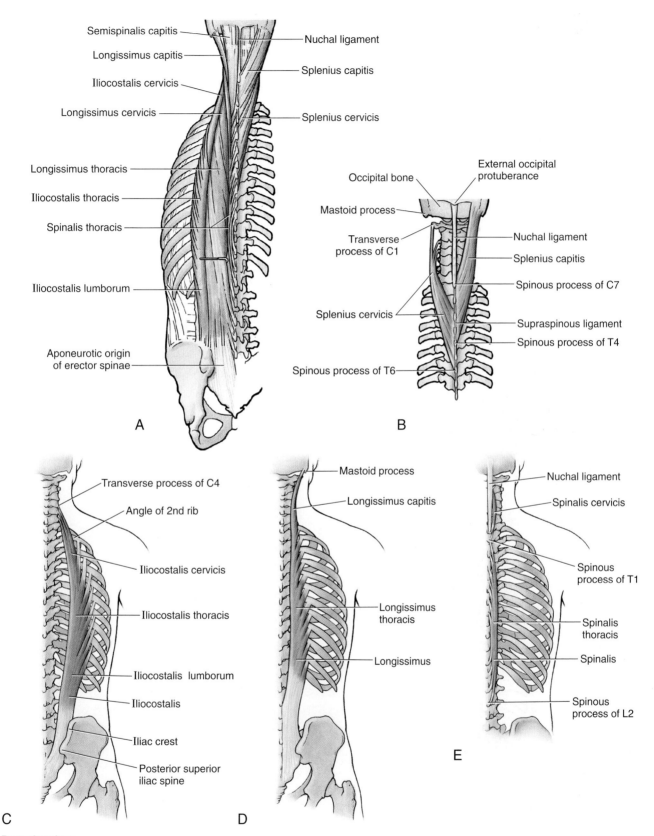

Posterior views

Figure 4.14. Superficial and intermediate layers of intrinsic back muscles. A. An overview is presented. Details of the splenius capitis and splenius cervicis (**B**), iliocostalis (**C**), longissimus (**D**), and spinalis (**E**) muscles are shown.

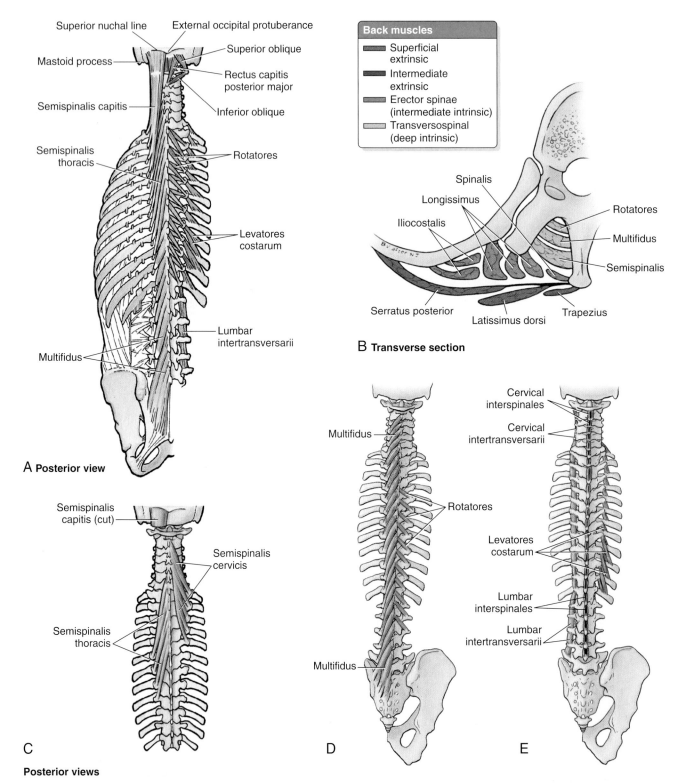

Back muscles
- Superficial extrinsic
- Intermediate extrinsic
- Erector spinae (intermediate intrinsic)
- Transversospinal (deep intrinsic)

A Posterior view

Superior nuchal line
External occipital protuberance
Superior oblique
Mastoid process
Rectus capitis posterior major
Semispinalis capitis
Inferior oblique
Semispinalis thoracis
Rotatores
Levatores costarum
Lumbar intertransversarii
Multifidus

B Transverse section

Spinalis
Longissimus
Iliocostalis
Rotatores
Multifidus
Semispinalis
Serratus posterior
Latissimus dorsi
Trapezius

C

Semispinalis capitis (cut)
Semispinalis cervicis
Semispinalis thoracis

D

Multifidus
Rotatores
Multifidus

E

Cervical interspinales
Cervical intertransversarii
Levatores costarum
Lumbar interspinales
Lumbar intertransversarii

Posterior views

Figure 4.15. Deep layer of intrinsic back muscles. A. An overview is presented. **B.** Note that the erector spinae muscle is in three columns and that the transversospinal muscle is in three layers. The semispinalis (**C**); multifidus and rotatores (**D**); and interspinales, intertransversarii, and levatores costarum (**E**) muscles are shown.

Table 4.6B Deep Layers of Intrinsic Back Muscles

Muscle	Origin	Insertion	Nerve Supply	Main Action(s)
Deep layer of intrinsic back muscles (Transverso spinal)				
Semispinalis (thoracis, cervicis, and capitis)	Arises from transverse processes of C4–T12 vertebrae	Fibers run superomedially to occipital bone and spinous processes in thoracic and cervical regions, spanning 4–6 segments	Posterior rami of spinal nerves	Extends head and thoracic and and cervical regions of vertebral column and rotates them contralaterally
Multifidus	Arises from posterior sacrum, posterior superior iliac spine of ilium, aponeurosis of erector spinae, sacroiliac ligaments, mammillary processes of lumbar vertebrae, transverse processes of T1–T3, and articular processes of C4–C7	Thickest in lumbar region, fibers pass obliquely supero-medially to entire length of spinous processes of vertebrae located 2–4 segments superior to origin		Stabilizes vertebrae during local movements of vertebral column
Rotatores (brevis and longus)	Arise from transverse processes of vertebrae; are best developed in thoracic region	Fibers pass superomedially to attach to junction of lamina and transverse process or spinous process of vertebra immediately (brevis) or 2 segments (longus) superior to vertebra of origin		Stabilize vertebrae and assist with local extension and rotatory movements of vertebral column; may function as organs of proprioception
Minor deep layer of intrinsic back muscles				
Interspinales	Superior surfaces of spinous processes of cervical and lumbar vertebrae	Inferior surfaces of spinous processes of vertebrae superior to vertebrae of origin	Posterior rami of spinal nerves	Aid in extension and rotation of vertebral column
Intertransversarii	Transverse processes of cervical and lumbar vertebrae	Transverse processes of adjacent vertebrae	Posterior and anterior rami of spinal nerves[a]	Aid in lateral flexion of vertebral column; acting bilaterally, stabilize vertebral column
Levatores costarum	Tips of transverse processes of C7 and T1–T11 vertebrae	Pass inferolaterally and insert on rib between its tubercle and angle	Posterior rami of C8–T11 spinal nerves	Elevate ribs, assisting respiration; assist with lateral flexion of vertebral column

[a]Most back muscles are innervated by posterior rami of the spinal nerves, but a few are innervated by anterior rami. Anterior intertransversarii muscles of the cervical region lateral intertransversarii of the lumbar region are supplied by anterior rami.

sive **erector spinae,** the chief extensor of the vertebral column divides into three muscle columns:

- Iliocostalis: lateral column.
- Longissimus: intermediate column.
- Spinalis: medial column.

Each column is divided regionally into three parts according to its superior attachments (e.g., iliocostalis lumborum, iliocostalis thoracis, and iliocostalis cervicis). The common origin of the three erector spinae columns is through a broad tendon that attaches inferiorly to the posterior part of the iliac crest, the posterior aspect of the sacrum, the sacroiliac ligaments, and the sacral and inferior lumbar spinous processes. Although the muscle columns are generally identified as isolated muscles, each column is actually composed of many overlapping shorter fibers—a design that provides

stability, localized action, and segmental vascular and neural supply. The attachments, nerve supply, and actions of the erector spinae are described in Table 4.6B.

DEEP LAYER OF INTRINSIC BACK MUSCLES

Deep to the erector spinae muscles is an obliquely disposed group of muscles—the **transversospinal muscle group** (L. *transversospinalis*)—composed of the semispinalis, multifidus, and rotatores. These muscles originate from transverse processes of vertebrae and pass to spinous processes of more superior vertebrae. They occupy the "gutter" between the collective transverse and spinous processes (Fig. 4.15; Table 4.6B).

- The semispinalis is superficial, spanning four to six segments.

- The multifidus is deeper, spanning two to four segments.
- The rotatores are deepest; spanning one to two segments.

The **semispinalis**, as its name indicates, arises from approximately half of the vertebral column (spine). It is divided into three parts according to the vertebral level of their superior attachments: semispinalis capitis, semispinalis cervicis, and semispinalis thoracis.

The **semispinalis capitis** is responsible for the longitudinal bulge on each side in the back of the neck near the median plane. It ascends from the cervical and thoracic transverse processes to the occipital bone. The **semispinalis thoracis and cervicis** pass superomedially from the transverse processes to the thoracic and cervical spinous processes of more superior vertebrae.

The **multifidus** consists of short, triangular muscular bundles that are thickest in the lumbar region. Each bundle passes obliquely superiorly and medially and attaches along the whole length of the spinous process of the adjacent superior vertebra.

The **rotatores** or rotator muscles—best developed in the thoracic region—are the deepest of the three layers of transversospinal muscles. They arise from the transverse process of one vertebra and insert into the root of the spinous processes of the next one or two vertebrae superiorly.

The **interspinales**, **intertransversarii**, and **levatores costarum** are the smallest of the deep back muscles. The interspinales and intertransversarii muscles connect spinous and transverse processes, respectively.

MUSCLES PRODUCING MOVEMENTS OF THE INTERVERTEBRAL JOINTS

The principal muscles producing movements of the cervical, thoracic, and lumbar IV joints and structures limiting these movements are summarized in Tables 4.7 and 4.8. Smaller muscles generally have higher densities of *muscle spindles* (sensors of proprioception—the sense of one's position—that are interdigitated among the muscle's fibers) than do large muscles. It has been presumed that this is because small muscles are used for the most precise movements, such as fine postural movements or manipulation, and therefore require more proprioceptive feedback. The movements described for small muscles are assumed from the location of their attachments, the direction of the muscle fibers, and from activity measured by *electromyography*. Muscles such as the rotatores, however, are so small and are placed in positions of such relatively poor mechanical advantage that their ability to produce the movements described is somewhat questionable. Furthermore, such small muscles often are redundant to other larger muscles having superior

Back Strain

Back strain is a common back problem that usually results from extreme movements of the vertebral column, such as extension or rotation. *Back strain refers to some stretching or microscopic tearing of muscle fibers and/or ligaments of the back.* The muscles usually involved are those producing movements of the lumbar IV joints, especially the erector spinae. If the weight is not properly balanced on the vertebral column, strain is exerted on the muscles. This is undoubtedly a common cause of low back pain. As a protective mechanism, the back muscles go into *spasm* after an injury or in response to inflammation of structures such as ligaments.

mechanical advantage. Hence it has been proposed that the smaller muscles of small–large muscle pairs function more as "kinesiological monitors" (organs of proprioception) and that the larger muscles are the producers of motion.

Suboccipital and Deep Neck Muscles

The **suboccipital region**—superior part of the back of the neck—is the triangular area (*suboccipital triangle*) inferior to the occipital region of the head, including the posterior aspects of the C1 and C2 vertebrae. The **suboccipital triangle** lies deep to the trapezius and semispinalis capitis muscles (Fig. 4.16). The four small muscles in the suboccipital region—rectus capitis posterior major and minor and superior and inferior oblique—are innervated by the posterior ramus of C1, the **suboccipital nerve**. These muscles are mainly postural muscles, but they act on the head—directly or indirectly—as indicated by *capitis* in their name.

- **Rectus capitis posterior major** arises from the spinous process of the C2 vertebra and inserts into the lateral part of the inferior nuchal line of the occipital bone.
- **Rectus capitis posterior minor** arises from the posterior tubercle on the posterior arch of the C1 vertebra and inserts into the medial third of the inferior nuchal line.
- **Inferior oblique of head** (L. *obliquus capitis inferior*) arises from the spinous process of the C2 vertebra and inserts into the transverse process of the C1 vertebra. The name of this muscle is somewhat misleading because it is the only "capitis" muscle that has no attachment to the cranium.
- **Superior oblique of head** (L. *obliquus capitis superior*) arises from the transverse process of C1 and inserts into

Table 4.7 Principal Muscles Producing Movement of the Cervical Intervertebral Joints

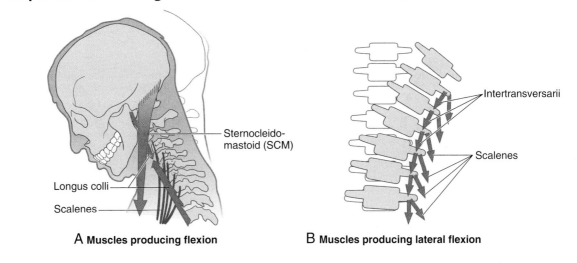

A **Muscles producing flexion**

B **Muscles producing lateral flexion**

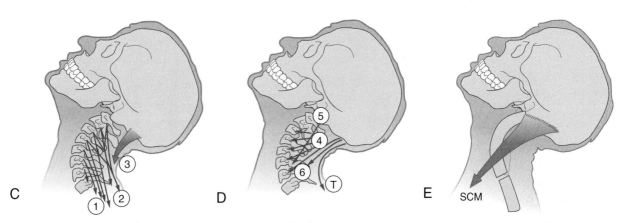

C–E, **Muscles producing extension**

Flexion	Extension	Lateral Bending	Rotation
Bilateral action of • Longus colli • Scalene • Sternocleidomastoid	Deep neck muscles, bilateral action of: • Semispinalis cervicis and iliocostalis cervicis (1) • Splenius cervicis and levator scapulae (2) • Splenius capitis (3) • Multifidus (4) • Longissimus capitis (5) • Semispinalis capitis (6) • Trapezius (T)	Unilateral action of • Iliocostalis cervicis • Longissimus capitis and cervicis • Splenius capitis and cervicis • Intertransversarii and scalenes	Unilateral action of • Rotatores • Semispinalis capitis and cervicis • Multifidus • Splenius cervicis
Limiting structures • Ligaments: posterior atlantoaxial, posterior longitudinal, flavum, tectorial membrane • Posterior neck muscles • Anulus fibrosus (tension posteriorly)	• Ligaments: anterior longitudinal, anterior atlantoaxial • Anterior neck muscles • Anulus fibrosus (tension anteriorly) • Spinous processes (contact between adjacent processes)	• Ligaments: alar ligament tension limits movement to contralateral side • Anulus fibrosus (tension anteriorly) • Zygapophysial (facet) joints	• Ligaments: alar ligament tension limits movement to ipsilateral side • Anulus fibrosus

Numbers and letters in parentheses refer to the figure.

Table 4.8 Principal Muscles Producing Movements of the Thoracic and Lumbar Intervertebral Joints

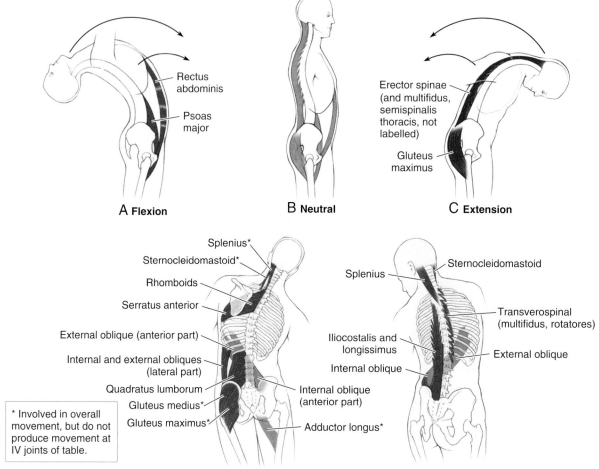

* Involved in overall movement, but do not produce movement at IV joints of table.

A Flexion

B Neutral

C Extension

D Lateral flexion (bending)
(Muscles shown contract to bend to opposite [left] side)

E Rotation
(Muscles shown contract to rotate to the left)

Flexion	Extension	Lateral bending	Rotation
Bilateral action of • Rectus abdominis • Psoas major • Gravity	Bilateral action of • Erector spinae • Multifidus • Semispinalis thoracis	Unilateral action of • Iliocostalis thoracis and lumborum • Longissimus thoracis • Multifidus • External and internal oblique • Quadratus lumborum • Rhomboids • Serratus anterior	Unilateral action of • Rotatores • Multifidus • Iliocostalis • Longissimus • External oblique acting synchronously with opposite internal oblique • Splenius thoracis
Limiting structures • Ligaments: supraspinous, interspinous, flavum • Capsules of zygapophysial (facet) joints • Extensor muscles • Vertebral bodies (apposition anteriorly) • IV disc (compression anteriorly • Anulus fibrosus (tension posteriorly)	• Ligaments: anterior longitudinal • Capsules of zygapophysial joints • Abdominal muscles • Spinous processes (contact between adjacent processes) • Anulus fibrosus (tension anteriorly) • IV discs (compression posteriorly)	• Ligaments: contralateral side • Contralateral muscles that laterally bend trunk • Contact between iliac crest and thorax • Anulus fibrosus (tension of contralateral fibers) • IV disc (compression ipsilaterally)	• Ligaments: costovertebral • Ipsilateral external oblique, contralateral internal oblique • Articular facets (apposition) • Anulus fibrosus

IV, intervertebral.

Surface Anatomy of Back Muscles

In the midline of the back there is a posterior median furrow that overlies the tips of the spinous processes of the vertebrae (Fig.SA4.2). The furrow is continuous superiorly with the nuchal groove in the neck. The erector spinae produce prominent vertical bulges on each side of the furrow. The superficially located trapezius and latissimus dorsi muscles connecting the upper limbs to the vertebral column are also clearly visible.

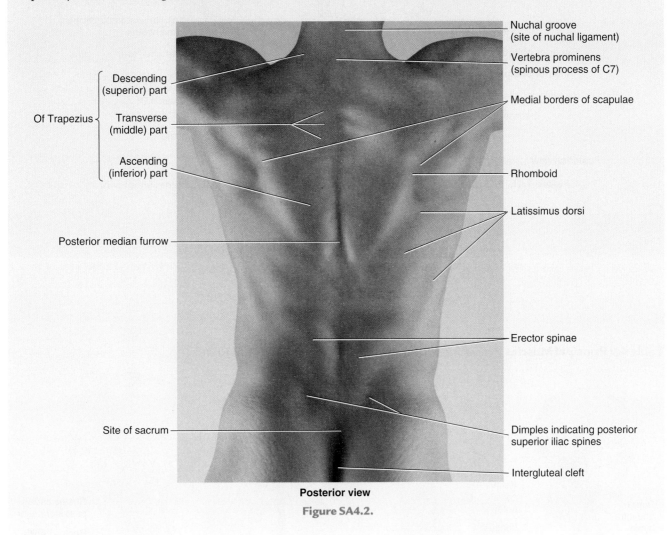

Posterior view

Figure SA4.2.

the occipital bone between the superior and the inferior nuchal lines.

The boundaries and contents of the suboccipital triangle are

- Superomedially, rectus capitis posterior major.
- Superolaterally, superior oblique.
- Inferolaterally, inferior oblique.
- Floor, posterior atlanto-occipital membrane and posterior arch of C1.

- Roof, semispinalis capitis.
- Contents, *vertebral artery* and *suboccipital nerve* (C1).

The actions of the suboccipital group of muscles is to extend the head on C1 and rotate the head and the C1 on C2 vertebrae. The principal muscles producing movements of the craniovertebral joints are summarized in Tables 4.9 and 4.10, and the nerve supply of the muscles in the suboccipital triangle, back of the neck, and back are summarized in Table 4.11.

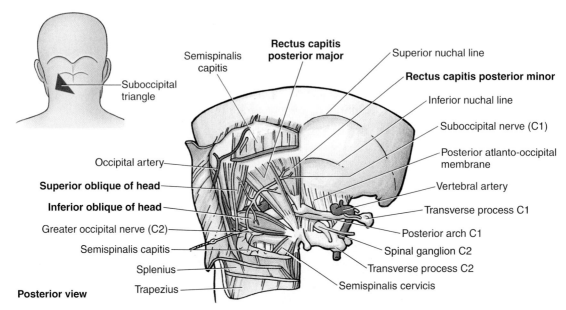

Suboccipital triangle

Semispinalis capitis

Rectus capitis posterior major

Superior nuchal line

Rectus capitis posterior minor

Inferior nuchal line

Suboccipital nerve (C1)

Posterior atlanto-occipital membrane

Vertebral artery

Transverse process C1

Posterior arch C1

Spinal ganglion C2

Transverse process C2

Semispinalis cervicis

Occipital artery

Superior oblique of head

Inferior oblique of head

Greater occipital nerve (C2)

Semispinalis capitis

Splenius

Trapezius

Posterior view

Figure 4.16. Suboccipital region and deep neck muscles. Muscles, nerves, and arteries are shown.

Table 4.9 Principal Muscles Producing Movement of the Atlanto-Occipital Joints

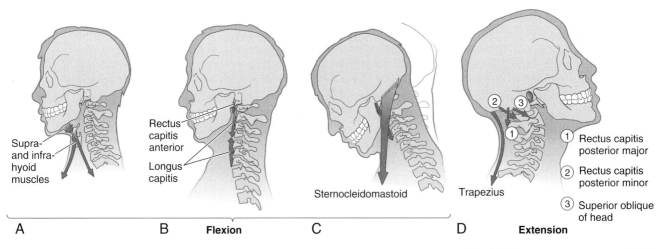

Supra- and infra-hyoid muscles

Rectus capitis anterior

Longus capitis

Sternocleidomastoid

Trapezius

① Rectus capitis posterior major
② Rectus capitis posterior minor
③ Superior oblique of head

A   B   **Flexion**   C   D   **Extension**

Flexion	Extension	Lateral bending (not shown)
Longus capitis	Rectus capitis posterior major and minor	Sternocleidomastoid
Rectus capitis anterior	Superior oblique of head	Superior oblique of head
Anterior fibers of sternocleidomastoid	Splenius capitis	Rectus capitis lateralis
Suprahyoid and infrahyoid muscles	Longissimus capitis	Longissimus capitis
	Trapezius	Splenius capitis

Table 4.10 Principal Muscles Producing Movement of the Atlantoaxial Joints[a]

Ipsilateral[b]		Contralateral
Inferior oblique of head	Head rotates to **left** by contraction of:	Sternocleidomastoid
Rectus capitis posterior, major and minor		Semispinalis capitis
Longissimus capitis	**Right:** Sternocleidomastoid Semispinalis capitis	
Splenius capitis		
	Left: Inferior oblique of head Rectus capitis posterior, major and minor Longissimus capitis Splenius capitis	

[a]Rotation is the specialized movement at these joints. Movement of one joint involves the other.
[b]Same side to which head is rotated.

Table 4.11 Nerve Supply of the Suboccipital Triangle, Back, and Back of Neck

Nerve	Origin	Course	Distribution
Suboccipital	Posterior ramus of C1 spinal nerve	Runs between cranium and C1 vertebra to reach suboccipital triangle	Muscles of suboccipital triangle
Greater occipital	Posterior ramus of C2 spinal nerve	Emerges inferior to inferior oblique of head and ascends to posterior scalp	Skin over neck and occipital bone
Lesser occipital	Anterior rami of spinal nerves C2–C3	Pass directly to skin	Skin of superior posterolateral neck and scalp posterior to ear
Posterior rami, nerves C3–C7	Posterior rami of spinal nerves C3–C7	Pass segmentally to muscles and skin	Intrinsic muscles of back and overlying skin adjacent to vertebral column

Ischemia of the Brainstem

The winding course of the vertebral arteries through the suboccipital triangle becomes clinically significant when blood flow through them is reduced, as occurs with *arteriosclerosis*. Under these conditions, prolonged turning of the head—as occurs when backing up a motor vehicle—may cause light-headedness, dizziness, and other symptoms resulting from interference with the blood supply to the brainstem.

Medical Imaging of Back

Conventional radiographs are excellent for high-contrast structures such as bone (Fig. 4.17A). The advent of digital radiography allows improved contrast resolution. **Myelography** is a radiopaque contrast study that allows visualization of the spinal cord and spinal nerve roots (Fig. 4.17B). In this procedure, CSF is withdrawn by lumbar puncture and replaced with contrast material injected into the spinal subarachnoid space. This technique shows the extent of the subarachnoid space and its extensions around the spinal nerve roots within the dural sheaths.

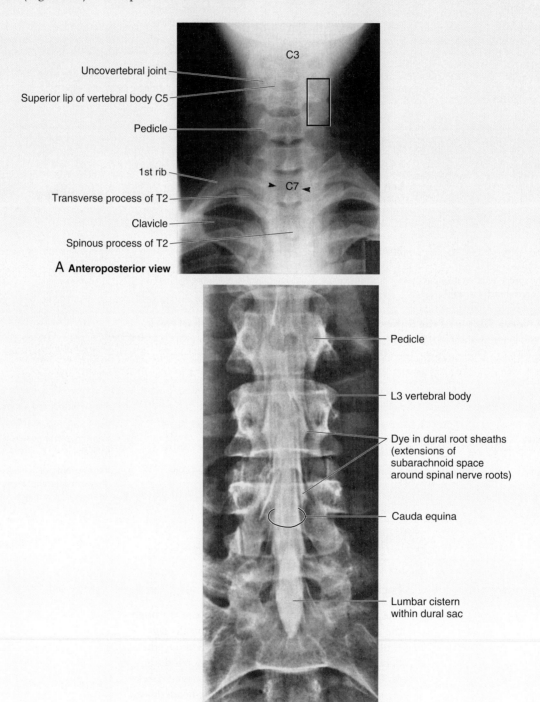

A Anteroposterior view

B Anteroposterior view

Figure 4.17. Imaging of the vertebral column. A. A radiograph of the cervical region of the vertebral column is shown. *Arrowheads,* margins of the column of air (*black*) in the trachea; *boxed area,* column of articular processes and the overlapping transverse processes. **B.** A Myelogram of the lumbar region of the vertebral column.

CT differentiates between the white and the gray matter of the brain and spinal cord. It has also improved the radiological assessment of fractures of the vertebral column, particularly in determining the degree of compression of the spinal cord. The dense vertebrae attenuate much of the X-ray beam and, therefore, appear white on the scans (Fig. 4.18C). The IV discs have a higher density than the surrounding adipose tissue in the extradural space and the CSF in the subarachnoid space. Herniations of the IV discs are thus recognizable in CT images.

MRI, like CT, is a computer-assisted imaging procedure, but X-rays are not used as with CT. MRI produces extremely good images of the vertebral column, spinal cord, and CSF (Fig. 4.18A & B). MRI clearly demonstrates the components of IV discs and shows their relationship to the vertebral bodies and longitudinal ligaments. Herniations of the nucleus pulposus and its relationship to the spinal nerve roots also are well defined. MRI is the imaging procedure of choice for evaluating IV disc disorders and is gradually replacing myelography and CT for the study of these disorders.

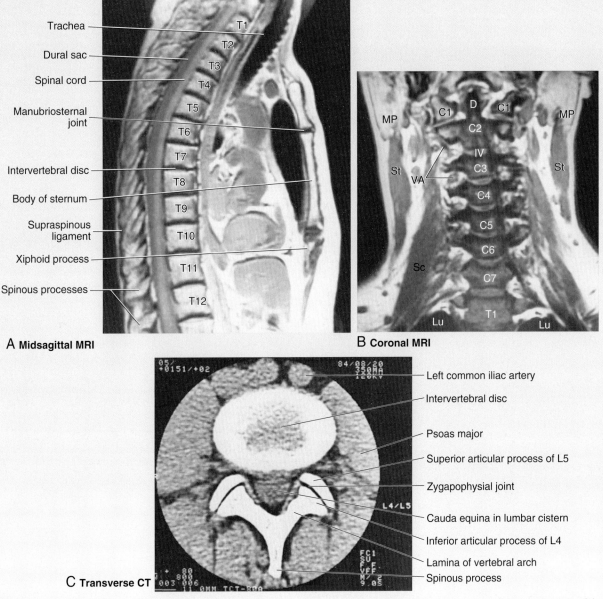

Figure 4.18. **MRI studies and CT scan of vertebral column.** **A.** An MRI study of the thoracic region is shown. **B.** An MRI study of the cervical region is shown. *D,* dens of axis; *IV,* intervertebral; *Lu,* lung; *MP,* mastoid process; *Sc,* scalenes; *St,* sternocleidomastoid; *Va,* vertebral arteries. **C.** In this CT scan of the L4–L5 IV disc, observe the cauda equina, zygapophysial joints, and vertebral arch.

5 Lower Limb

The lower limbs (extremities) are specialized for locomotion, supporting body weight, and maintaining balance. The lower limbs are connected to the trunk by the **pelvic girdle**, a bony ring composed of the sacrum and right and left hip bones joined anteriorly at the **pubic symphysis** (L. *symphysis pubis*). The lower limb has six major parts or regions (Fig. 5.1):

- **Gluteal region** (L. *regio glutealis*), including the **buttocks** (L. *nates, clunes*) and the **hip** (L. *coxa*) or **hip region** (L. *regio coxae*), which overlies the hip joint and greater trochanter of the femur.
- **Thigh** or **femoral region** (L. *regio femoris*), containing the **femur,** which connects the hip and knee.
- **Knee** (L. *crus*) or **knee region** (L. *regio genus*), containing the distal femur, proximal tibia and fibula, and the *patella* (knee cap) as well as the joints between these

bony structures; the fat-filled hollow posterior to the knee (L. *poples*) is called the *popliteal fossa*.
- **Leg** (L. *crus*) or leg region (L. *regio cruris*), connecting the knee and ankle and containing the **tibia** (shin bone) and **fibula** (calf bone); the **calf** (L. *sura*) of the leg is the posterior prominence.
- **Ankle** (L. *tarsus*) or **talocrural region** (L. *regio talocruralis*), including the narrow distal part of the leg and ankle (talocrural) joint.
- **Foot** (L. *pes*) or **foot region** (L. *regio pedis*), the distal part of the lower limb, containing the *tarsus* (which connects the ankle and foot), *metatarsus,* and *phalanges* (toe bones); the superior surface is the **dorsum of the foot**, and the inferior, ground-contacting surface is the **sole** or **plantar region.** The **toes** are the **digits of the foot;** the **great toe** (L. *hallux*) has only two phalanges (digital bones), and the other digits have three.

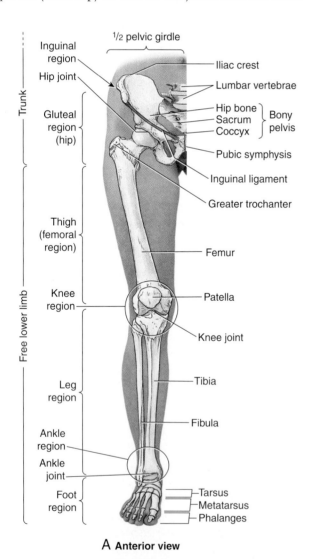

A Anterior view

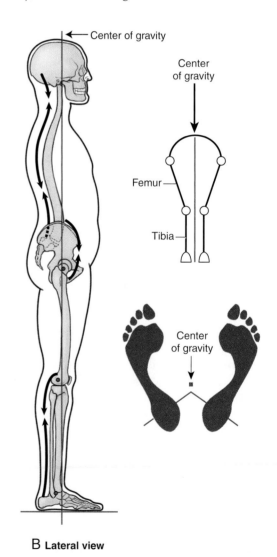

B Lateral view

Figure 5.1. Lower limb. A. The regions and bones of the lower limb are shown. **B.** The center of gravity in a relaxed standing position is demonstrated.

Bones of Lower Limb

Body weight is transferred from the vertebral column through the *sacroiliac joints* to the pelvic girdle and from the pelvic girdle through the hip joints to the femurs (L. *femora*). Weight is then transferred from the knee joint to the ankle joint by the tibia. The fibula does not articulate with the femur and does not bear weight. At the ankle, the weight is transferred to the talus. The talus is the keystone of a longitudinal arch formed by the tarsal and metatarsal bones of each foot, which distribute the weight evenly between the heel and the forefoot when standing. To support the erect bipedal posture better, the femurs are oblique (directed inferomedially) within the thighs so that when standing the knees are adjacent and are placed directly inferior to the trunk, returning the center of gravity to the vertical lines of the supporting legs and feet (Fig. 5.1*B*). The femurs of females are slightly more oblique than those of males, reflecting the greater width of their pelves.

Hip Bone

Each mature **hip bone** is formed by the fusion of three primary bones: *ilium, ischium,* and *pubis* (Figs. 5.2 and 5.3). At puberty, these bones are still separated by a **triradiate cartilage.** The cartilage disappears and the bones begin to fuse at 15–17 years of age; fusion is complete between 20 and 25 years of age.

The **ilium,** the superior and largest part of the hip bone, contributes to the superior part of the **acetabulum** (Fig. 5.3), the cup-like cavity (socket) on the lateral aspect of the hip bone for articulation with the head of the femur. The ilium consists of a **body,** which joins the pubis and ischium to the acetabulum, and an **ala** (wing), which is bordered superiorly by the **iliac crest.**

The **ischium** forms the posteroinferior part of the acetabulum and hip bone. The ischium consists of a **body,** where it joins the ilium and superior ramus of the pubis to form the acetabulum. The **ramus of the ischium** joins the inferior ramus of the pubis to form the **ischiopubic ramus** (Fig. 5.3*B*). The **pubis** forms the anterior part of the acetabulum and the anteromedial part of the hip bone. The right pubis has a **body** that articulates with the left pubis at the pubic symphysis. It also has two **rami,** superior and inferior.

To place the hip bone in the anatomical position, manipulate it so that the acetabulum faces laterally and slightly anteriorly (Fig. 5.3*B*). When the hip bone is in the anatomical position, the:

- Anterior superior iliac spine (ASIS) and anterosuperior aspect of the pubis lie in the same vertical plane.
- Symphysial surface of the pubis is vertical, parallel to the median plane.

Fractures of Hip Bone

Fractures of the hip bone are commonly referred to as "pelvic fractures." The term *hip fracture* is most commonly applied (unfortunately) to fractures of the femoral heads, neck, or trochanters. Avulsion fractures of the hip bone may occur during sports that require sudden acceleration or deceleration forces. A small part of the bone with a piece of tendon or ligament attached is "avulsed" (torn away)—for example, the anterior superior and inferior iliac spines, the ischiopubic rami, and the ischial tuberosities.

- Internal aspect of the body of the pubis faces almost directly superiorly.
- Acetabulum faces inferolaterally, with the acetabular notch directed inferiorly.
- Obturator foramen lies inferomedial to the acetabulum.

Femur

The femur is the longest and heaviest bone in the body. The femur consists of a **shaft** (body) and superior (or proximal) and inferior (or distal) ends (Fig. 5.2). Most of the shaft is smoothly rounded, except for a prominent double-edge ridge on its posterior aspect—the **linea aspera**—which diverges inferiorly. The proximal end of the femur consists of a head, neck, and two trochanters (greater and lesser). The **head of the femur** is covered with articular cartilage, except for a medially placed depression or pit, the **fovea for the ligament of the head.** The **neck of the femur** is trapezoidal; the narrow end supports the head and its broader base is continuous with the shaft.

Where the neck joins the shaft are two large, blunt elevations—the trochanters. The conical **lesser trochanter,** with its rounded tip, extends medially from the posteromedial part of the junction of the femoral neck and shaft (Fig. 5.2*A*). The **greater trochanter** is a large, laterally placed mass that projects superomedially where the neck joins the shaft. The **intertrochanteric line** is a roughened ridge running from the greater to the lesser trochanter. A similar but smoother ridge, the **intertrochanteric crest,** joins the trochanters posteriorly (Fig. 5.2*B*).

The distal end of the femur ends in two spirally curved **femoral condyles (medial and lateral).** The femoral

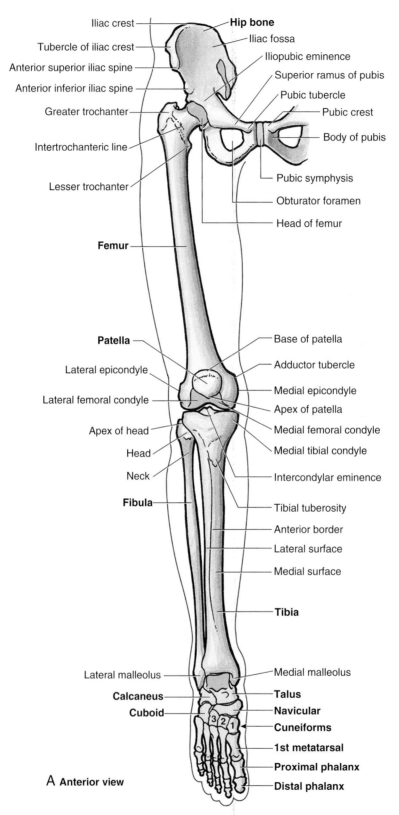

Iliac crest — **Hip bone**
Tubercle of iliac crest — Iliac fossa
Anterior superior iliac spine — Iliopubic eminence
Anterior inferior iliac spine — Superior ramus of pubis
Greater trochanter — Pubic tubercle
Intertrochanteric line — Pubic crest
Lesser trochanter — Body of pubis
Pubic symphysis
Obturator foramen
Head of femur
Femur
Patella — Base of patella
Adductor tubercle
Lateral epicondyle — Medial epicondyle
Lateral femoral condyle — Apex of patella
Apex of head — Medial femoral condyle
Head — Medial tibial condyle
Neck — Intercondylar eminence
Fibula — Tibial tuberosity
Anterior border
Lateral surface
Medial surface
Tibia
Lateral malleolus — Medial malleolus
Calcaneus — **Talus**
Cuboid — **Navicular**
Cuneiforms
1st metatarsal
Proximal phalanx
A **Anterior view** — **Distal phalanx**

Figure 5.2. Bones of lower limb.

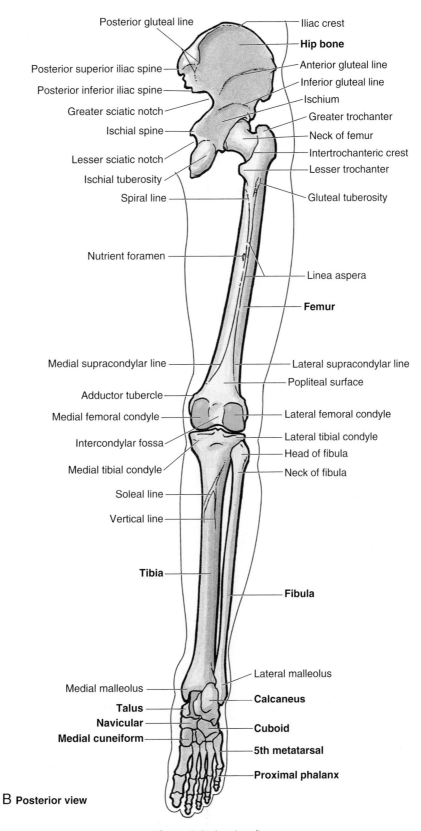

Posterior gluteal line

Posterior superior iliac spine

Posterior inferior iliac spine

Greater sciatic notch

Ischial spine

Lesser sciatic notch

Ischial tuberosity

Spiral line

Nutrient foramen

Medial supracondylar line

Adductor tubercle

Medial femoral condyle

Intercondylar fossa

Medial tibial condyle

Soleal line

Vertical line

Tibia

Medial malleolus

Talus

Navicular

Medial cuneiform

Iliac crest

Hip bone

Anterior gluteal line

Inferior gluteal line

Ischium

Greater trochanter

Neck of femur

Intertrochanteric crest

Lesser trochanter

Gluteal tuberosity

Linea aspera

Femur

Lateral supracondylar line

Popliteal surface

Lateral femoral condyle

Lateral tibial condyle

Head of fibula

Neck of fibula

Fibula

Lateral malleolus

Calcaneus

Cuboid

5th metatarsal

Proximal phalanx

B **Posterior view**

Figure 5.2. *(continued)*

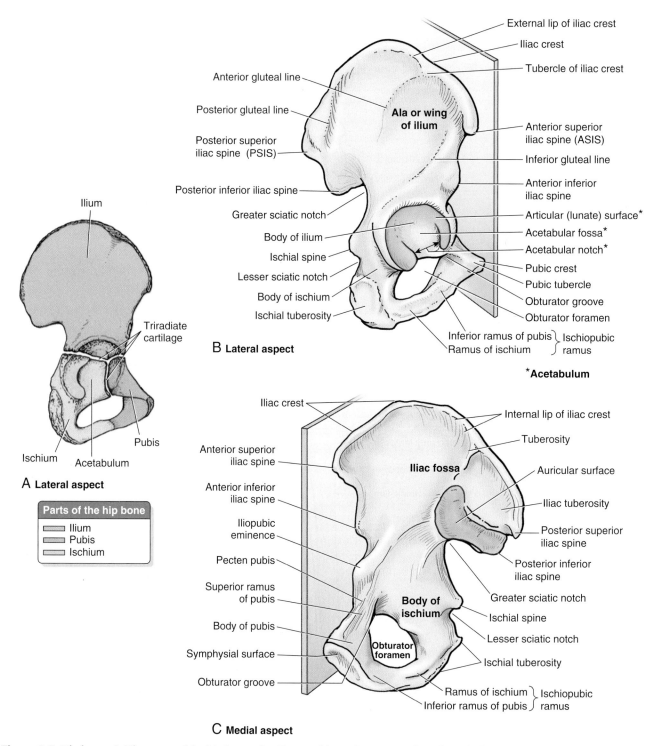

External lip of iliac crest
Iliac crest
Tubercle of iliac crest
Anterior gluteal line
Posterior gluteal line
Ala or wing of ilium
Anterior superior iliac spine (ASIS)
Posterior superior iliac spine (PSIS)
Inferior gluteal line
Posterior inferior iliac spine
Anterior inferior iliac spine
Greater sciatic notch
Articular (lunate) surface*
Body of ilium
Acetabular fossa*
Ischial spine
Acetabular notch*
Lesser sciatic notch
Pubic crest
Body of ischium
Pubic tubercle
Ischial tuberosity
Obturator groove
Obturator foramen
Inferior ramus of pubis ⎱ Ischiopubic
Ramus of ischium ⎰ ramus
B Lateral aspect

*Acetabulum

Ilium
Triradiate cartilage
Pubis
Ischium
Acetabulum
A Lateral aspect

Parts of the hip bone
Ilium
Pubis
Ischium

Iliac crest
Internal lip of iliac crest
Anterior superior iliac spine
Tuberosity
Iliac fossa
Auricular surface
Anterior inferior iliac spine
Iliac tuberosity
Iliopubic eminence
Posterior superior iliac spine
Pecten pubis
Posterior inferior iliac spine
Superior ramus of pubis
Greater sciatic notch
Body of ischium
Body of pubis
Ischial spine
Lesser sciatic notch
Symphysial surface
Obturator foramen
Ischial tuberosity
Obturator groove
Ramus of ischium ⎱ Ischiopubic
Inferior ramus of pubis ⎰ ramus

C Medial aspect

Figure 5.3. Hip bone. A. The parts of the hip bone of a 13-year-old are shown. **B and C.** The right hip bone of an adult is shown in the anatomical position. In this position, the anterior superior iliac spine and the anterior aspect of the pubis lie in the same vertical plane.

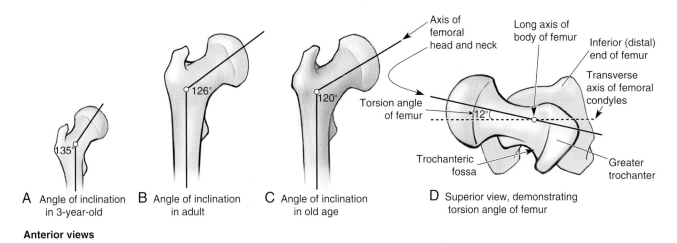

A Angle of inclination
in 3-year-old

B Angle of inclination
in adult

C Angle of inclination
in old age

D Superior view, demonstrating
torsion angle of femur

Anterior views

Figure 5.4. **Angle of inclination and torsion angle of femur.**

condyles articulate with the tibial condyles to form the knee joint.

The proximal femur is bent (L-shaped) so that the long axis of the head and neck project superomedially at an angle to that of the obliquely oriented shaft (Fig. 5.4). This obtuse **angle of inclination** in the adult is 115–140°, averaging 126°. The angle is less in females because of the increased width between the acetabula and the greater obliquity of the shaft. The angle of inclination allows greater mobility of the femur at the hip joint because it places the head and neck more perpendicular to the acetabulum. This is advantageous for bipedal walking; however, it imposes considerable strain on the neck of the femur. Fractures of the neck may occur in older people as a result of a slight stumble if the neck has been weakened by osteoporosis. In addition, when the femur is viewed superiorly (so that one is looking along the long axis of the shaft), it is apparent that the two axes lie at an angle (the **torsion angle,** or **angle of declination**), the mean of which is 7° in males and 12° in females (Fig. 5.4D). The torsion angle, combined with the angle of inclination, allows rotatory movements of the femoral head within the obliquely placed acetabulum to convert into flexion and extension, abduction and adduction, and rotational movements of the thigh.

Patella

The patella (knee cap) is a large sesamoid bone, formed intratendinously after birth, located anterior to the knee joint (Fig. 5.2A). This triangular-shaped bone articulates with the patellar surface of the femur. The subcutaneous **anterior surface** of the patella is convex; the thick **base** (superior border) slopes inferoanteriorly; the two lateral and medial **borders** converge inferiorly to form the pointed **apex,** and the **articular surface** (posterior surface) has a smooth, oval articular area that is divided into articular facets by a vertical ridge.

Tibia

The large, weight-bearing **tibia** (shin bone) articulates with the femoral condyles superiorly, the talus inferiorly, and the fibula laterally at its proximal and distal ends (Figs. 5.2 and 5.5). The large **nutrient foramen** of the tibia is located on the posterior aspect of the proximal third of the bone. From it, the **nutrient canal** runs inferiorly in the tibia before it opens into the medullary (marrow) cavity. The distal end of the tibia is smaller than the proximal end and has facets for articulation with the fibula and talus. The **medial malleolus** is an inferiorly directed projection from the medial side of the distal end of the tibia.

Fibula

The slender **fibula** lies posterolateral to the tibia and serves mainly for muscle attachment (Figs. 5.2 and 5.5). At its distal end, the fibula enlarges to form the **lateral malleolus,** which is more prominent and more posteriorly placed than the medial malleolus and extends approximately 1 cm farther distally. The fibula is not directly involved in weight bearing; however, its lateral malleolus helps hold the talus in its socket. The shafts of the tibia and fibula are connected by an **interosseous membrane** throughout most of their lengths.

Femoral Fractures

The neck of the femur is most frequently fractured, especially in females secondary to osteoporosis. Fractures of the proximal femur can occur at several locations—for example, transcervical and intertrochanteric (Fig. B5.1A & B). The femoral shaft is large and strong; however, a violent direct injury, such as may be sustained in an automobile accident, may fracture it, causing, for example, a spiral fracture (Fig. B5.1C). Fractures of the distal femur may be complicated by separation of the condyles, resulting in misalignment of the knee joint.

Coxa Vara and Coxa Valga

The angle of inclination varies with age, sex, and development of the femur (e.g., consequent to a congenital defect in ossification of the femoral neck). It also may change with any pathological process that weakens the neck of the femur (e.g., rickets). When the angle of inclination is decreased, the condition is **coxa vara** (Fig. B5.1D); when it is increased, the condition is **coxa valga** (Fig. B5.1E). Coxa vara causes a mild passive abduction of the hip.

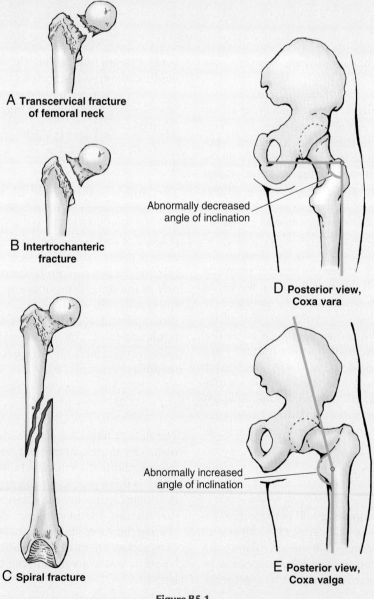

A **Transcervical fracture of femoral neck**

B **Intertrochanteric fracture**

C **Spiral fracture**

Abnormally decreased angle of inclination

D **Posterior view, Coxa vara**

Abnormally increased angle of inclination

E **Posterior view, Coxa valga**

Figure B5.1

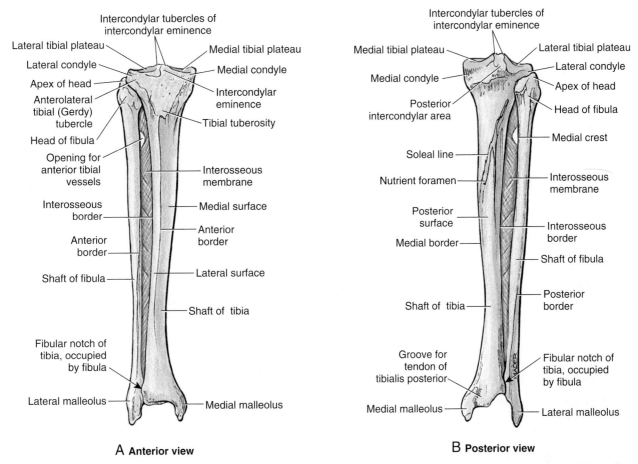

A Anterior view

B Posterior view

Figure 5.5. Right tibia and fibula. The shafts are connected by the dense interosseous membrane composed of strong oblique fibers.

Tarsus, Metatarsus, and Phalanges

The **bones of the foot** include the tarsus, metatarsus, and phalanges (Figs. 5.2 and 5.6).

TARSUS

The tarsus consists of seven bones: calcaneus, talus, cuboid, navicular, and three cuneiforms. Only the talus articulates with the leg bones. The **calcaneus** (heel bone) is the largest and strongest bone in the foot. It articulates with the talus superiorly and the cuboid anteriorly (Fig. 5.6A). The calcaneus transmits most of the body weight from the talus to the ground. The **talar shelf** (L. *sustentaculum tali*), projecting from the superior border of the medial surface of the calcaneus, supports the head of the talus (Fig. 5.6B). The lateral surface of the calcaneus has an oblique ridge (Fig. 5.6C), the **fibular trochlea**. The posterior part of the calcaneus has a prominence, the **calcaneal tuberosity** (L. *tuber calcanei*), which has medial, lateral, and anterior tubercles (Fig. 5.6B).

The **talus** (ankle bone) has a **head, neck,** and **body** (Fig. 5.6C). The talus rests on the anterior two thirds of the calcaneus. The superior surface, the **trochlea of the talus,** bears the weight of the body transmitted from the tibia and articulates with the two malleoli. The head of the talus articulates anteriorly with the navicular. The rounded **head of talus** rests partially on the **talar shelf** of the calcaneus (Fig. 5.6B & E).

The **navicular** (L. little ship), a flattened, boat-shaped bone, is located between the talar head and the cuneiforms. The medial surface of the navicular projects inferiorly as the **tuberosity of navicular.** If the tuberosity is too prominent, it may press against the medial part of the shoe and cause foot pain.

The **cuboid** is the most lateral bone in the distal row of the tarsus. Anterior to the **tuberosity of cuboid** (Fig. 5.6B), on the lateral and plantar surfaces of the bone, is a groove for the tendon of the fibularis longus muscle (Fig. 5.6B & C).

There are three cuneiforms: **medial** (1st), **intermediate** (2nd), and **lateral** (3rd). Each cuneiform (L. *cuneus,* wedge-shaped) articulates with the navicular posteriorly and the base of the appropriate metatarsal anteriorly. In addition, the lateral cuneiform articulates with the cuboid.

Tibial and Fibular Fractures

The tibial shaft is narrowest at the junction of its inferior and middle thirds, which is the most frequent site of fracture. Because its anterior surface is subcutaneous, the tibial shaft is the most frequent site of a *compound fracture*, one in which the skin is perforated and blood vessels are torn (Fig. B5.2*A*), or diagonal fracture (Fig. B5.2*B*). Fracture of the tibia through the nutrient canal predisposes to non-union of the bone fragments, resulting from damage to the nutrient artery. *Fibular fractures* commonly occur just proximal to the lateral malleolus and often are associated with fracture–dislocations of the ankle joint (Fig. B5.2*C*). When a person slips, forcing the foot into an excessively inverted position, the ankle ligaments tear, forcibly tilting the talus against the lateral malleolus and shearing it off.

Bone Grafts

The fibula is a common source of bone for grafting. Even after a segment of the fibular shaft has been removed, walking, running, and jumping can be normal. Free vascularized fibulas have been used to restore skeletal integrity to limbs in which congenital bone defects exist and to replace segments of bone after trauma or excision of a malignant tumor. The periosteum and nutrient artery are generally removed with the piece of bone so that the graft will remain alive and grow when transplanted to another site. The transplanted piece of fibula, secured in its new site, eventually restores the blood supply of the bone to which it has been attached.

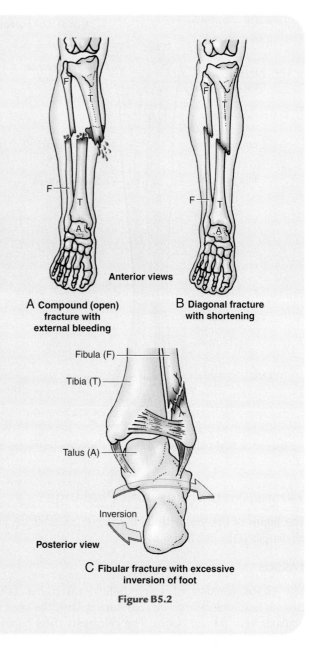

Anterior views

A **Compound (open) fracture with external bleeding**

B **Diagonal fracture with shortening**

Fibula (F)

Tibia (T)

Talus (A)

Inversion

Posterior view

C **Fibular fracture with excessive inversion of foot**

Figure B5.2

METATARSUS

The **metatarsus** consists of five metatarsals, which connect the tarsus and phalanges. They are numbered from the medial side of the foot (Fig. 5.6*B* & *C*). The **1st metatarsal** is shorter and stouter than the others. The **2nd metatarsal** is the longest. Each metatarsal has a **base** (proximally), a **shaft**, and a **head** (distally). The bases of the metatarsals articulate with the cuneiform and cuboid bones, and the heads articulate with the proximal phalanges. The bases of the 1st and 5th metatarsals have large tuberosities; the **tuberosity of the 5th metatarsal** projects over the lateral margin of the cuboid (Fig. 5.6*C*).

PHALANGES

There are 14 **phalanges**. The 1st digit (great toe) has two phalanges (proximal and distal); the other four digits have three each: proximal, middle, and distal (Fig. 5.6*A* & *B*). Each **phalanx** has a **base** (proximally), a **shaft**, and a **head** (distally).

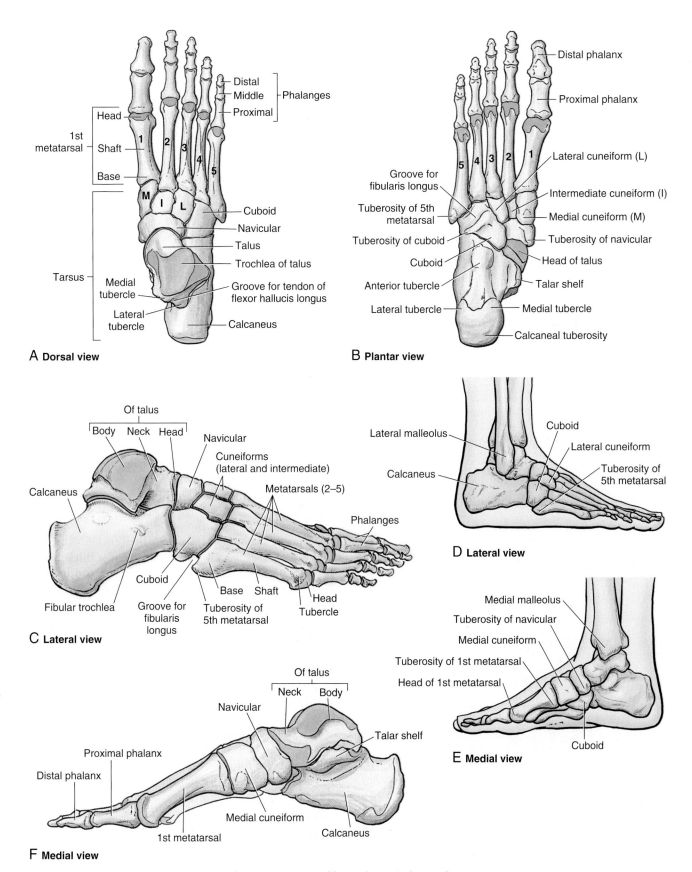

Figure 5.6. Bones of foot. *Blue,* articular cartilages.

Fractures of Foot Bones

Calcaneal fractures occur in people who fall on their heels (e.g., from a ladder). Usually the bone breaks into several fragments (*comminuted fracture*) that disrupt the subtalar joint, where the talus articulates with the calcaneus (Fig. B5.3A). *Fractures of the talar neck* may occur during severe dorsiflexion of the ankle (e.g., when a person is pressing extremely hard on the brake pedal of a car during a head-on collision). Metatarsal and phalangeal fractures usually occur when a heavy object falls on the foot or when the foot is run over by a wheel bearing a heavy weight. Metatarsal fractures are also common in dancers, especially female ballet dancers using the *demipointe* technique. The "dancer's fracture" usually occurs when the dancer loses balance, putting the full body weight on the metatarsal and fracturing the bone (Fig. B5.3B).

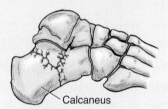

A Lateral view, comminuted fracture of calcaneus

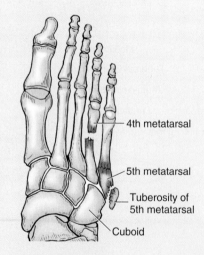

4th metatarsal

5th metatarsal

Tuberosity of 5th metatarsal

Cuboid

B Dorsum of foot, fractures of metatarsals

Figure B5.3

Fascia, Vessels, and Cutaneous Nerves of Lower Limb

The **subcutaneous tissue (superficial fascia)** lies deep to the skin and consists of loose connective tissue that contains a variable amount of fat, cutaneous nerves, superficial veins, lymphatic vessels, and lymph nodes (Fig. 5.7). The subcutaneous tissue of the hip and thigh is continuous with that of the inferior part of the anterolateral abdominal wall and buttock. At the knee, the subcutaneous tissue loses its fat and blends with the deep fascia; but fat is present in the subcutaneous tissue of the leg.

The **deep fascia** is especially strong, investing the limb like an elastic stocking. The deep fascia limits outward extension of contracting muscles, making muscular contraction more efficient in compressing veins to push blood toward the heart (Fig. 5.7A). The *deep fascia of the thigh* is called **fascia lata** (L. *lata,* broad). The fascia lata attaches to and is continuous with:

- The inguinal ligament, pubic arch, body of pubis, and pubic tubercle superiorly. The membranous layer of subcutaneous tissue (Scarpa fascia) of the inferior abdominal wall also attaches to the fascia lata just inferior to the inguinal ligament.
- The iliac crest laterally and posteriorly.
- The sacrum, coccyx, sacrotuberous ligament, and ischial tuberosity posteriorly.
- The exposed parts of the bones around the knee and the deep fascia of the leg distally.

The fascia lata is substantial because it encloses the large thigh muscles, especially laterally where it is thickened to form the **iliotibial tract** (Fig. 5.7B). This broad band of fibers is also the aponeurosis of the *tensor of fascia lata* and *gluteus maximus* muscles. The iliotibial tract extends from the iliac tubercle to the anterolateral tibial tubercle (Gerdy tubercle) on the lateral condyle of the tibia.

The thigh muscles are separated into three **fascial compartments:** anterior, medial, and posterior. The walls of these compartments are formed by the fascia lata and three fascial intermuscular septa that arise from the deep aspect of the fascia lata and attach to the linea aspera of the femur (Fig. 5.7C). The **lateral intermuscular septum** is strong; the other two septa are relatively weak. The lateral intermuscular septum extends from the iliotibial tract to the lateral lip of the linea aspera and lateral supracondylar line of the femur.

The **saphenous opening** in the fascia lata is a gap or hiatus in the fascia lata inferior to the medial part of the inguinal ligament, about 4 cm inferolateral to the pubic tubercle (Fig. 5.7A). Its medial margin is smooth; but its superior, lateral, and inferior margins form a sharp edge, the **falciform margin.** The sieve-like **cribriform fascia** (L. *cribrum,* a sieve)

text continues on page 328.

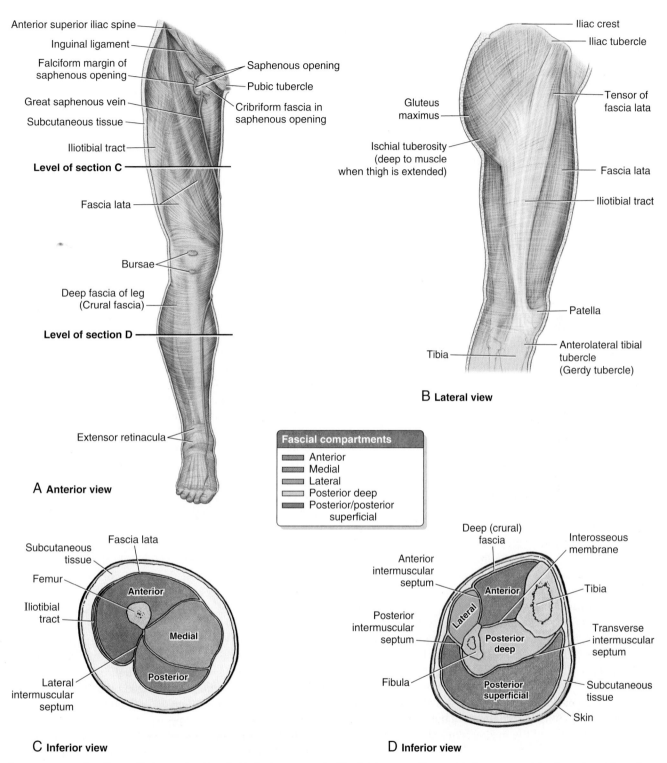

Fascial compartments
- Anterior
- Medial
- Lateral
- Posterior deep
- Posterior/posterior superficial

A **Anterior view**

B **Lateral view**

C **Inferior view**

D **Inferior view**

Figure 5.7. Fascia of lower limb. A. The deep fascia is shown. **B.** The iliotibial tract, a fibrous reinforcement of the fascia lata (deep fascia of thigh), is shown. **C.** This transverse section of the thigh shows the fascial compartments. **D.** This transverse section of the leg shows the fascial compartments.

Surface Anatomy of Lower Limb Bones

Pelvic Girdle and Femur

When your hands are on your hips, they rest on the **iliac crests**, the curved superior borders of the alae (wings) of the ilium. The anterior third of the crest is easily palpated because it is subcutaneous. The highest point of the crest is at the level of the intervertebral (IV) disc between the L4 and the L5 vertebrae The iliac crest ends anteriorly at the rounded **anterior superior iliac spine,** which is easy to palpate, especially in thin persons, because it is subcutaneous and often visible (Fig. SA5.1A & B). The iliac crest ends posteriorly at the **posterior superior iliac spine** (PSIS), which may be difficult to palpate (Fig. SA5.1C). Its position is easy to locate because it lies at the bottom of a skin dimple, approximately 4 cm lateral to the midline demarcating the sacroiliac joints. The dimple exists because the skin and fascia attach to the PSIS.

The **ischial tuberosity** is easily palpated in the inferior part of the buttock when the thigh is flexed. It bears body weight when sitting. The thick gluteus maximus and fat obscure the tuberosity when the thigh is extended. The **gluteal fold**, a prominent skin fold containing fat, coincides with the inferior border of the gluteus maximus muscle.

The **greater trochanter of the femur** is easily palpable on the lateral side of the hip approximately 10 cm inferior to the iliac crest (Fig. SA5.1B & C). Because it lies close to the skin, the greater trochanter causes discomfort when you lie on your side on a hard surface. In the anatomical position, a line joining the tips of the greater trochanters normally passes through the centers of the femoral heads and pubic tubercles. The **shaft of the femur** usually is not palpable because it is covered with large muscles. The **femoral condyles** are subcutaneous and easily palpated when the knee is flexed or extended. The patellar surface of the femur is where the **patella** slides during flexion and extension of the leg. The lateral and medial margins of the patellar surface can be palpated when the leg is flexed. The **adductor tubercle**, a small prominence of bone, may be felt at the superior part of the medial femoral condyle.

Tibia and Fibula

The **tibial tuberosity**, an oval elevation on the anterior surface of the tibia, is palpable approximately 5 cm distal (inferior) to the apex of the patella (Fig. SA5.1B).

The subcutaneous **anterior border and medial surface of the tibia** is also easy to palpate. The skin covering it is freely movable. The prominence at the ankle, the **medial malleolus,** is also subcutaneous, and its inferior end is blunt. The **medial** and **lateral tibial condyles** can be palpated anteriorly at the sides of the patellar ligament, especially when the knee is flexed. The **head of the fibula** can be palpated easily at the level of the superior part of the tibial tuberosity because its knob-like head is subcutaneous at the posterolateral aspect of the knee. The **neck of fibula** can be palpated just distal to the fibular head. Only the distal quarter of the shaft of the fibula is palpable. Feel your **lateral malleolus,** noting that it is subcutaneous and that its inferior end is sharp. Note that the tip of the lateral malleolus extends farther distally and more posteriorly than does the tip of the **medial malleolus.**

Bones of the Foot

The **talar head** is palpable anteromedial to the proximal part of the lateral malleolus when the foot is inverted and anterior to the medial malleolus when the foot is everted. Eversion of the foot makes the talar head more prominent as it moves away from the navicular. The talar head occupies the space between the talar shelf and the navicular tuberosity. When the foot is plantarflexed, the superior surface of the **body of the talus** can be palpated on the anterior aspect of the ankle, anterior to the inferior end of the tibia (Fig. SA5.1D).

The weight-bearing **medial tubercle of the calcaneus** on the plantar surface of the foot is broad and large but is not palpable because of the thick overlying skin and subcutaneous tissue (Fig. SA5.1E). The **fibular trochlea**, a lateral extension of the calcaneus, may be detectable as a small tubercle on the lateral subcutaneous aspect of the calcaneus, anteroinferior to the tip of the lateral malleolus. The **talar shelf** is the only part of the medial aspect of the calcaneus that may be palpated as a small prominence just distal to the tip of the medial malleolus.

The **tuberosity of the navicular** is easily seen and palpated on the medial aspect of the foot, inferoanterior to the tip of the medial malleolus. Usually, palpation of bony prominences on the plantar surface of the foot is difficult because of the thick skin, fascia, and pads of fat. The cuboid and cuneiforms are difficult to identify individually by palpation. The **cuboid** can be felt on the

continued >

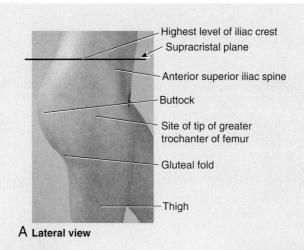

Highest level of iliac crest

Supracristal plane

Anterior superior iliac spine

Buttock

Site of tip of greater trochanter of femur

Gluteal fold

Thigh

A **Lateral view**

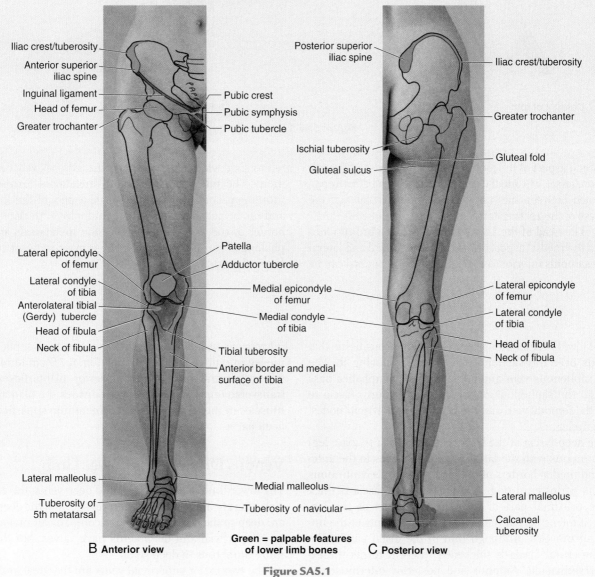

Iliac crest/tuberosity

Anterior superior iliac spine

Inguinal ligament

Head of femur

Greater trochanter

Pubic crest

Pubic symphysis

Pubic tubercle

Posterior superior iliac spine

Iliac crest/tuberosity

Greater trochanter

Ischial tuberosity

Gluteal fold

Gluteal sulcus

Lateral epicondyle of femur

Lateral condyle of tibia

Anterolateral tibial (Gerdy) tubercle

Head of fibula

Neck of fibula

Patella

Adductor tubercle

Medial epicondyle of femur

Medial condyle of tibia

Tibial tuberosity

Anterior border and medial surface of tibia

Lateral epicondyle of femur

Lateral condyle of tibia

Head of fibula

Neck of fibula

Lateral malleolus

Tuberosity of 5th metatarsal

Medial malleolus

Tuberosity of navicular

Lateral malleolus

Calcaneal tuberosity

B **Anterior view**

Green = palpable features of lower limb bones

C **Posterior view**

Figure SA5.1

continued >

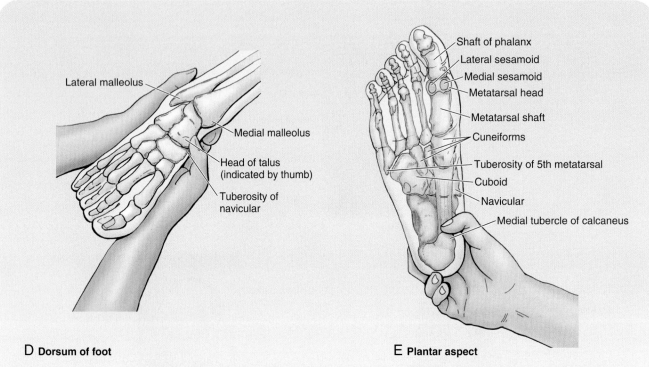

Lateral malleolus

Medial malleolus

Head of talus
(indicated by thumb)

Tuberosity of
navicular

Shaft of phalanx
Lateral sesamoid
Medial sesamoid
Metatarsal head
Metatarsal shaft
Cuneiforms
Tuberosity of 5th metatarsal
Cuboid
Navicular
Medial tubercle of calcaneus

D Dorsum of foot

E Plantar aspect

Figure SA5.1 *(continued)*

lateral aspect of the foot, posterior to the base of the 5th metatarsal. The **medial cuneiform** can be indistinctly palpated between the tuberosity of the navicular and the base of the 1st metatarsal.

The **head of the 1st metatarsal** forms a prominence on the medial aspect of the foot. The medial and lateral **sesamoids** inferior to the head of this metatarsal can be felt to slide when the 1st digit is moved passively over them. The **tuberosity of the 5th metatarsal** forms a prominent landmark on the lateral aspect of the foot and can be palpated easily at the midpoint of the lateral border of the foot. The shafts of the **metatarsals** and **phalanges** can be felt on the dorsum of the foot between the extensor tendons. ●

is a localized membranous layer of subcutaneous tissue that spreads over the saphenous opening, enclosing it. The **great saphenous vein** and some efferent lymphatics pass through the saphenous opening and cribriform fascia to enter the femoral vein and the deep inguinal lymph nodes, respectively.

The **deep fascia of the leg**, the **crural fascia** (L. *crus,* leg) is continuous with the fascia lata and attaches to the anterior and medial borders of the tibia, where it is continuous with its periosteum (Fig. 5.7A). The crural fascia is thick in the proximal part of the anterior aspect of the leg, where it forms part of the proximal attachments of the underlying muscles. Although thin in the distal part of the leg, the crural fascia is thickened where it forms the **extensor retinacula. Anterior** and **posterior intermuscular septa** pass from the deep surface of the crural fascia and attach to the corresponding margins of the fibula. The

interosseous membrane and the intermuscular septa divide the leg into three compartments (Fig. 5.7D): anterior (dorsiflexor), lateral (fibular), and posterior (plantarflexor). The **transverse intermuscular septum** divides the plantarflexor muscles in the posterior compartment into superficial and deep parts.

Venous Drainage of Lower Limb

The lower limb has superficial and deep veins; the superficial veins are in the subcutaneous tissue, and the deep veins are deep to the deep fascia and accompany all major arteries. Superficial and deep veins have valves, but they are more numerous in deep veins.

The two major **superficial veins** are the great and small saphenous veins (Fig. 5.8). The **great saphenous vein** is formed by the union of the **dorsal digital vein of the great** toe and the **dorsal venous arch** of the foot. The great saphenous vein (Fig. 5.8*A*):

- Ascends anterior to the medial malleolus.
- Passes posterior to the medial condyle of the femur (about a hand's breath posterior to the medial border of the patella).
- Anastomoses freely with the small saphenous vein.
- Traverses the saphenous opening in the fascia lata.
- Empties into the *femoral vein.*

The **small saphenous vein** arises on the lateral side of the foot from the union of the dorsal digital vein of the fifth digit with the *dorsal venous arch.* The small saphenous vein (Fig. 5.8*C*):

- Ascends posterior to the lateral malleolus as a continuation of the lateral marginal vein.
- Passes along the lateral border of the calcaneal tendon.
- Inclines to the midline of the fibula and penetrates the deep fascia.
- Ascends between the heads of the gastrocnemius muscle.
- Empties into the popliteal vein in the popliteal fossa.

Perforating veins penetrate the deep fascia close to their origin from the superficial veins (Fig. 5.8*C*). They contain

valves that allow blood to flow only from the superficial veins to the deep veins. The perforating veins pass through the deep fascia at an oblique angle so that when muscles contract and pressure increases inside the deep fascia, the perforating veins are compressed. Compression of the perforating veins also prevents blood from flowing from the deep to the superficial veins. This pattern of venous blood flow—from superficial to deep—is important for proper venous return from the limb because it enables muscular contractions to propel blood toward the heart against the pull of gravity (*musculovenous pump;* see Introduction).

The **deep veins** in the lower limb accompany all the major arteries (L. *venae comitantes*) and their branches. Instead of occurring as a single vein in the limbs, the deep veins are usually paired, frequently interconnecting veins that flank the artery they accompany. They are contained within a vascular sheath with the artery, whose pulsations also help compress and move blood in the veins (Fig. 5.8*D* & *E*). The deep veins from the leg flow into the popliteal vein posterior to the knee, which becomes the femoral vein in the thigh. The deep vein of the thigh joins the terminal portion of the femoral vein. The femoral vein passes deep to the inguinal ligament to become the external iliac vein in the pelvis.

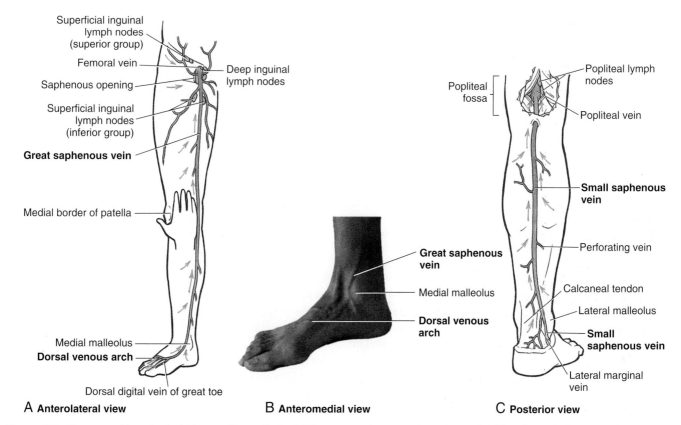

A Anterolateral view   **B Anteromedial view**   **C Posterior view**

Figure 5.8. Venous and lymphatic drainage of lower limb. A. The great saphenous vein and superficial lymphatic drainage are shown. *Arrows,* superficial lymphatic drainage to the inguinal nodes. **B.** The course of the great saphenous vein in the ankle region is shown. **C.** The small saphenous vein and superficial lymphatic drainage (*arrows*) to the popliteal lymph nodes are demonstrated.

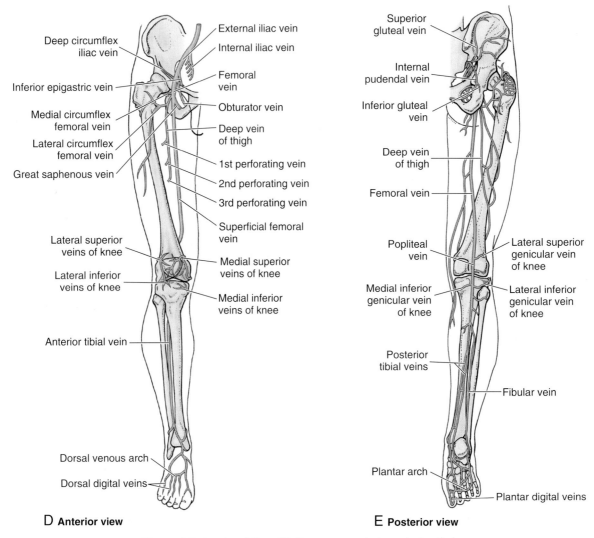

D Anterior view

E Posterior view

Figure 5.8. *(continued)* **D and E.** Deep venous drainage is detailed.

Lymphatic Drainage of Lower Limb

The lower limb has superficial and deep lymphatic vessels. The **superficial lymphatic vessels** converge on and accompany the saphenous veins and their tributaries. The lymphatic vessels accompanying the great saphenous vein end in the **superficial inguinal lymph nodes** (Fig. 5.8A). Most lymph from these nodes passes to the **external iliac lymph nodes**, located along the external iliac vein; but some lymph may also pass to the **deep inguinal lymph nodes**, located on the medial aspect of the femoral vein. The lymphatic vessels accompanying the small saphenous vein enter the **popliteal lymph nodes**, which surround the popliteal vein in the fat of the popliteal fossa (Fig. 5.8C). The **deep lymphatic vessels** of the leg accompany deep veins and enter the popliteal lymph nodes. Most lymph from these nodes ascends through deep lymphatic vessels to the deep inguinal lymph nodes. Lymph from the deep nodes passes to the external iliac lymph nodes.

Cutaneous Innervation of Lower Limb

Cutaneous nerves in the subcutaneous tissue supply the skin of the lower limb (Fig. 5.9). These nerves, except for some in the proximal part of the limb, are branches of the lumbar and sacral plexuses (see Chapters 3 and 4). The area of skin supplied by cutaneous branches from a single spinal nerve is a **dermatome** (Fig. 5.9A & B). Dermatomes L1–L5 extend as a series of bands from the posterior midline of the trunk into the limbs, passing laterally and inferiorly around the limb to its anterior and medial aspects, reflecting the medial rotation that occurs developmentally. Dermatomes S1 and S2 pass inferiorly down the posterior aspect of the limb, separating near the ankle to pass to the

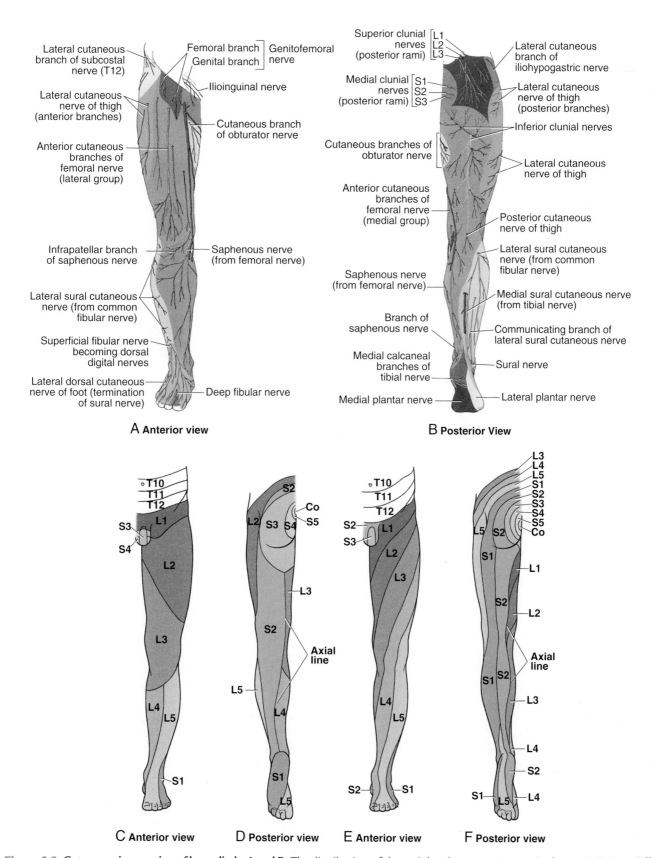

Figure 5.9. Cutaneous innervation of lower limb. A and B. The distribution of the peripheral cutaneous nerves is shown. **C–F.** Two different dermatome maps are frequently used (C and D, Foerster, 1933; E and F, Keegan and Garrett, 1948).

Varicose Veins, Thrombosis, and Thromboembolism

Varicose veins form when the valves that usually prevent blood flow from the deep veins through the perforating veins to the superficial veins are incompetent. As a result, the superficial veins become **varicose** (dilated so that their cusps do not close) and tortuous—*varicose veins* (Fig. B5.4).

The veins of the lower limb are subject to **venous thrombosis** (blood clotting)—for example, after a bone fracture, muscular inactivity, and external pressure on the veins (tight cast). **Venous stasis** (stagnation) is an important cause of thrombus formation. A thrombus that breaks free from a lower limb vein and travels to the lungs results in a **pulmonary thromboembolism** (obstruction of the pulmonary artery).

Saphenous Vein Grafts

Vein grafts obtained by surgically harvesting parts of the great saphenous vein are used to bypass obstructions in blood vessels (e.g., an occlusion of a coronary artery or its branches). When part of the vein is used as a bypass,

it is reversed so that the valves do not obstruct blood flow. Because there are so many other leg veins, removal of the great saphenous vein rarely affects circulation seriously, provided the deep veins are intact.

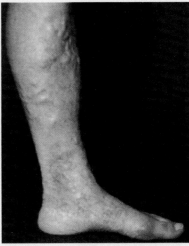

Medial view

Figure B5.4 Varicose veins.

Enlarged Inguinal Lymph Nodes

Lymph nodes enlarge when diseased. **Abrasions** and **minor sepsis,** caused by pathogenic microorganisms or their toxins in the blood or other tissues, may produce slight enlargement of the superficial inguinal nodes (**lymphadenopathy**) in otherwise healthy people. Malignancies (e.g., of the external genitalia and uterus) and perineal abscesses also result in enlargement of these nodes.

lateral and medial margins of the foot. Although simplified into distinct zones in dermatome maps, adjacent dermatomes overlap, except at the **axial line**, the line of junction of dermatomes supplied from discontinuous spinal levels.

Thigh and Gluteal Region

In evolution, the development of a prominent gluteal region is closely associated with the assumption of bipedalism and an erect posture. Modification of the shape of the femur necessary for bipedal walking allows the superior placement of the abductors of the thigh into the gluteal region. The remaining thigh muscles are organized into three compartments: *anterior* or *extensor, medial* or *adductor,* and *posterior* or *flexor* by intermuscular septa (Fig. 5.7C). Generally, the anterior group is innervated by the femoral nerve, the medial group by the obturator nerve, and the posterior group by the tibial portion of the sciatic nerve.

Anterior Thigh Muscles

The large **anterior compartment of the thigh** contains the **anterior thigh muscles,** *flexors of the hip* and *extensors of the* knee. The attachments, nerve supply, and main actions of these muscles are shown in Figure 5.10 and Table 5.1. The anterior thigh muscles are:

- **Pectineus:** a flat quadrangular muscle, located in the anterior part of the superomedial aspect of the thigh, that adducts and flexes the thigh and assists with medial rotation of the thigh.

- **Iliopsoas** (the chief flexor of the thigh): formed by the merger of two muscles, the psoas major and iliacus. The fleshy parts of the two muscles lie in the posterior wall of the abdomen and greater pelvis, merging as they enter the thigh by passing deep to the inguinal ligament and attaching to the lesser trochanter of the femur. It is in a unique position not only to produce movement but to stabilize (fixate). This muscle is also a postural muscle, active during standing in maintaining normal lumbar lordosis and, indirectly, the compensatory thoracic kyphosis.

- **Sartorius**, the tailor's muscle (L. *sartus,* patched or repaired): a long, ribbon-like muscle that is the most superficial muscle in the anterior thigh; it passes obliquely (lateral to medial) across the superoanterior part of the thigh. It acts across both the hip and the knee joints; and when acting bilaterally, the muscles bring the lower limbs into the cross-legged sitting position. None of the actions is strong; therefore, it is mainly a synergist, acting with other thigh muscles that produce these movements.

- **Quadriceps femoris** (L. four-headed femoral muscle): the great extensor of the leg that forms the main bulk of the anterior thigh muscles. It covers almost all the anterior aspect and sides of the femur. This muscle has four parts:

  - **Rectus femoris,** the "kicking muscle" (L. *rectus,* straight): this straight muscle is located on the anterior aspect of the thigh; it also crosses the hip joint and helps the iliopsoas flex this joint. Its ability to extend the knee is compromised during hip flexion.
  - **Vastus lateralis:** the largest component of the quadriceps, located on the lateral aspect of the thigh.
  - **Vastus intermedius:** lies deep to the rectus femoris between the vastus medialis and the vastus lateralis.
  - **Vastus medialis:** covers the medial aspect of the thigh.

A small, flat muscle, the **articular muscle of the knee** (L. *articularis genus*), a derivative of the vastus intermedius

Hip and Thigh Contusions

Sports broadcasters and trainers refer to a *hip pointer,* which is a *contusion of the iliac crest* that usually occurs at its anterior part (i.e., where the sartorius attaches to the ASIS), commonly seen in association with collision sports. **Contusions** cause bleeding from ruptured capillaries and infiltration of blood into the muscles, tendons, and other soft tissues.

Another term commonly used is *charley horse,* which may refer either to the cramping of an individual thigh muscle because of ischemia or to contusion and rupture of blood vessels sufficient enough to form a *hematoma.* This is associated with localized pain and/or muscle stiffness and commonly follows direct trauma (e.g., a stick slash in hockey).

Paralysis of the Quadriceps

The quadriceps is tested with the person in the supine position with the knee partly flexed. The person extends the knee against resistance. If the quadriceps is functioning normally, it should be observable and palpable. If the quadriceps is paralyzed, the person cannot extend the leg against resistance and usually presses on the distal end of the thigh during walking to prevent inadvertent flexion of the knee joint. Weakness of the vastus medialis and lateralis, resulting from arthritis or trauma to the knee joint for example, can result in abnormal patellar movement and loss of joint stability.

Patellar Tendon Reflex

Tapping the patellar ligament with a reflex hammer normally elicits the **patellar tendon reflex** (knee jerk). This reflex is tested by having the person sit with the legs dangling. A firm strike on the patellar ligament with a reflex hammer usually causes the leg to extend. If the reflex is normal, a hand on the patient's quadriceps should feel the muscle contract. This reflex tests the L2–L4 nerves. *Diminution or absence of the patellar tendon reflex* may result from any lesion that interrupts the innervation of the quadriceps muscle (e.g., peripheral nerve disease).

Chondromalacia Patellae

Chondromalacia patellae ("runner's knee") is a common knee problem in running sports and is seen in marathon runners and basketball players, for example. The soreness and aching around or deep to the patella results from *quadriceps imbalance.* This condition may result from a blow to the patella or from extreme flexion of the knee (e.g., during squatting when power lifting).

Table 5.1 Anterior Thigh Muscles

Muscle	Proximal Attachment	Distal Attachment	Innervation[a]	Main Action(s)
Pectineus	Superior ramus of pubis	Pectineal line of femur, just inferior to lesser trochanter	Femoral nerve (**L2**, L3); may receive branch from obturator nerve	Adducts and flexes thigh; assists with medial rotation of thigh
Sartorius	Anterior superior iliac spine and superior part of notch inferior to it	Superior part of medial surface of tibia	Femoral nerve (L2, L3)	Flexes, abducts, and laterally rotates thigh at hip joint; flexes leg at knee joint[c]
Iliopsoas				
Psoas major[b]	Sides of T12–L5 vertebrae and discs between them; transverse processes of all lumbar vertebrae	Lesser trochanter of femur	Anterior rami of lumbar nerves (**L1, L2**, L3)	Acting conjointly in flexing thigh at hip joint and in stabilizing this joint; psoas major is also a postural muscle that helps control deviation of the trunk and is active during standing
Iliacus	Iliac crest, iliac fossa, ala of sacrum, and anterior sacroiliac ligaments	Tendon of psoas major, lesser trochanter, and femur distal to it	Femoral nerve (**L2**, L3)	
Quadriceps femoris				
Rectus femoris	Anterior inferior iliac spine and ilium superior to acetabulum	Via common tendinous (quadriceps tendon) and independent attachments to base of patella; indirectly via patellar ligament to tibial tuberosity; medial and lateral vasti also attach to tibia and patella via aponeuroses (medial and lateral patellar retinacula)	Femoral nerve (L2, **L3, L4**)	Extends leg at knee joint; rectus femoris also steadies hip joint and helps iliopsoas flex thigh
Vastus lateralis	Greater trochanter and lateral lip of linea aspera			
Vastus medialis	Intertrochanteric line and medial lip of linea aspera of femur			
Vastus intermedius	Anterior and lateral surfaces of shaft of femur			

[a] The spinal cord segmental innervation is indicated (e.g., "**L1, L2,** L3" means that the nerves supplying the psoas major are derived from the first three lumbar segments of the spinal cord). Numbers in boldface (**L1, L2**) indicate the main segmental innervation. Damage to one or more of the listed spinal cord segments or to the motor nerve roots arising from them results in paralysis of the muscles concerned.

[b] The psoas minor is a small muscle that attaches proximally to the T12–L1 vertebrae and disc and distally to the pectineal line and iliopectineal eminence.

[c] The four actions of the sartorius (L. *sartor*, tailor) produce the once common cross-legged sitting position used by tailors; hence the name.

(Fig. 5.10*E*), attaches superiorly to the inferior part of the anterior aspect of the femur and inferiorly to the synovial membrane of the knee joint and the wall of the *suprapatellar bursa*. The muscle pulls the synovial membrane superiorly during extension of the leg, thereby preventing folds of the membrane from being compressed between the femur and the patella within the knee joint.

The tendons of the four parts of the quadriceps unite in the distal part of the thigh to form the **quadriceps tendon** (Fig. 5.10*B*). The **patellar ligament** (L. *ligamentum patellae*), attached to the **tibial tuberosity**, is the continuation of the quadriceps tendon in which the patella is embedded. The vastus medialis and lateralis also attach independently to the patella and form aponeuroses, the **medial** and **lateral patellar retinacula**, which reinforce the joint capsule of the knee on

each side of the patella en route to attachment to the anterior border of the tibial plateau. The patella provides additional leverage for the quadriceps in placing the tendon more anteriorly, farther from the joint's axis, causing it to approach the tibia from a position of greater mechanical advantage.

Medial Thigh Muscles

The medial thigh muscles—collectively called the **adductor group**—are in the medial compartment of the thigh and are innervated primarily by the obturator nerve (Fig. 5.11; Table 5.2). The adductor group consists of:

- **Adductor longus:** the most anterior muscle in the group.
- **Adductor brevis:** deep to the pectineus and adductor longus muscles.

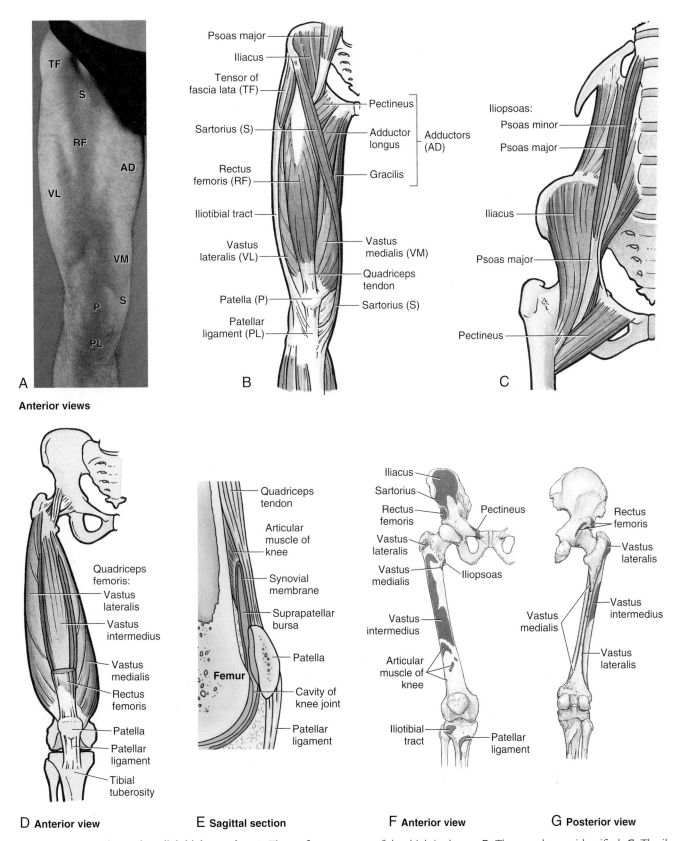

A

Anterior views

Psoas major
Iliacus
Tensor of fascia lata (TF)
Sartorius (S)
Rectus femoris (RF)
Iliotibial tract
Vastus lateralis (VL)
Patella (P)
Patellar ligament (PL)
Pectineus
Adductor longus
Gracilis
} Adductors (AD)
Vastus medialis (VM)
Quadriceps tendon
Sartorius (S)

B

Iliopsoas:
Psoas minor
Psoas major
Iliacus
Psoas major
Pectineus

C

Quadriceps femoris:
Vastus lateralis
Vastus intermedius
Vastus medialis
Rectus femoris
Patella
Patellar ligament
Tibial tuberosity

D Anterior view

Quadriceps tendon
Articular muscle of knee
Synovial membrane
Suprapatellar bursa
Patella
Cavity of knee joint
Patellar ligament
Femur

E Sagittal section

Iliacus
Sartorius
Rectus femoris
Vastus lateralis
Vastus medialis
Pectineus
Iliopsoas
Vastus intermedius
Articular muscle of knee
Iliotibial tract
Patellar ligament

F Anterior view

Rectus femoris
Vastus lateralis
Vastus intermedius
Vastus medialis
Vastus lateralis

G Posterior view

Figure 5.10. Anterior and medial thigh muscles. A. The surface anatomy of the thigh is shown. **B.** The muscles are identified. **C.** The iliopsoas (psoas major and iliacus) and pectineus are shown. **D.** The quadriceps femoris is demonstrated. Note that most of the rectus femoris has been removed to show the vastus intermedius. **E.** The articular muscle of the knee is detailed. **F and G.** The attachments of the muscles are identified.

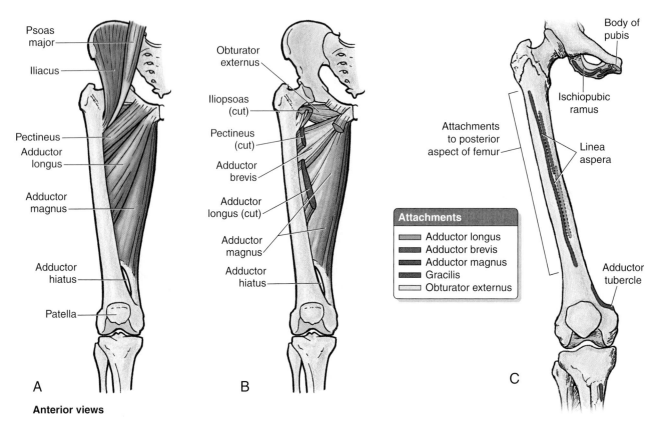

Anterior views

Figure 5.11. Medial thigh muscles. The muscles are exposed by superficial (**A**) and deep (**B**) dissections. **C.** The muscle attachments are shown.

Table 5.2 Medial Thigh Muscles

Muscle[a]	Proximal Attachment[b]	Distal Attachment[b]	Innervation[c]	Main Action(s)
Adductor longus	Body of pubis inferior to pubic crest	Middle third of linea aspera of femur	Obturator nerve (L2, **L3**, L4)	Adducts thigh
Adductor brevis	Body and inferior ramus of pubis	Pectineal line and proximal part of linea aspera of femur		Adducts thigh and to some extent flexes it
Adductor magnus	*Adductor part:* inferior ramus of pubis, ramus of ischium *Hamstring part:* ischial tuberosity	*Adductor part:* gluteal tuberosity, linea aspera, medial supracondylar line *Hamstring part:* adductor tubercle of femur	*Adductor part:* obturator nerve (L2, **L3, L4**) *Hamstring part:* tibial part of sciatic nerve (**L4**)	Adducts thigh; its adductor part also flexes thigh, and its hamstring part extends it
Gracilis	Body and inferior ramus of pubis	Superior part of medial surface of tibia	Obturator nerve (**L2**, L3)	Adducts thigh, flexes leg, and helps rotate it medially
Obturator externus	Margins of obturator foramen and obturator membrane	Trochanteric fossa of femur	Obturator nerve (L3, **L4**)	Laterally rotates thigh; steadies head of femur in acetabulum

[a]Collectively, the first four muscles listed are the adductors of the thigh, but their actions are more complex (e.g., they act as flexors of the hip joint during flexion of the knee joint and are active during walking).
[b]See Figure 5.11C for muscle attachments.
[c]The spinal cord segmental innervation is indicated (e.g., "L2, **L3, L4**" means that the nerves supplying the adductor magnus are derived from the second to fourth lumbar segments of the spinal cord). Numbers in boldface (**L3, L4**) indicate the main segmental innervation. Damage to one or more of the listed spinal cord segments or to the motor nerve roots arising from them results in paralysis of the muscles concerned.

- **Adductor magnus:** the largest adductor muscle, composed of adductor and "hamstring" parts; the parts differ in their attachments, nerve supply, and main actions.
- **Gracilis:** a long, strap-like muscle lying along the medial side of the thigh and knee; it is the only adductor muscle to cross and act at the knee joint as well as the hip joint.
- **Obturator externus:** a deeply placed fan-shaped muscle in the superomedial part of the thigh.

The **adductor hiatus** is an opening or gap between the distal aponeurotic attachment of the adductor part of the adductor magnus and the tendon of the "hamstring" part leading from the anterior compartment of the thigh into the popliteal fossa (Fig. 5.11 B). The adductor hiatus transmits the femoral artery and vein from the adductor canal in the thigh to the popliteal fossa posterior to the knee. The main action of the adductor group of muscles is to adduct the thigh (e.g., when pressed together while riding a horse). They are used to stabilize the stance when standing on both feet, to correct lateral sway of the trunk, and when there is a side-to-side shift. The adductors contribute to flexion of the extended thigh and to extension of the flexed thigh when running or against resistance

Groin Pull

The terms *pulled groin* and *groin injury* refer to a strain, stretching, and probably some tearing of the proximal attachments of the anteromedial thigh muscles. The injury usually involves the flexor and adductor thigh muscles. Groin pulls usually occur in sports that require quick starts, such as hockey, baseball, basketball, and short-distance racing.

Transplantation of Gracilis

Because the gracilis is a relatively weak member of the adductor group, it can be removed without noticeable loss of its actions on the leg. Hence surgeons often transplant the gracilis, or part of it, with its nerve and blood vessels to replace a damaged muscle in the hand, for example. Once transplanted, the muscle soon produces good digital flexion and extension. The gracilis may also be used to create a replacement for a non-functional external anal sphincter.

Neurovascular Structures and Relationships in Anteromedial Thigh

Femoral Triangle and Adductor Canal

The femoral triangle is a subfascial space in the anterosuperior third of the thigh (Fig. 5.12). It appears as a triangular depression inferior to the inguinal ligament when the thigh is flexed, abducted, and laterally rotated. The femoral triangle is bounded

- Superiorly by the inguinal ligament, which forms the *base of the femoral triangle.*
- Medially by the adductor longus.
- Laterally by the sartorius; the *apex* is where the lateral border of the sartorius crosses the medial border of the adductor longus.

The muscular *floor of the femoral triangle* is formed by the iliopsoas laterally and pectineus medially. The *roof of the femoral triangle* is formed by fascia lata, cribriform fascia, subcutaneous tissue, and skin. Deep to the inguinal ligament, the **subinguinal space** is an important passageway connecting the trunk/abdominopelvic cavity to the lower limb. It is created as the inguinal ligament spans the gap between the ASIS and the pubic tubercle. The space is divided into two compartments, or lacunae, by the iliopsoas fascia. The lateral compartment is the *muscular lacuna,* through which the iliopsoas muscle and femoral nerve pass; the *vascular lacuna* allows the passage of the veins, arteries, and lymphatics between the greater pelvis and the femoral triangle.

The contents of the femoral triangle, from lateral to medial, are the (Fig. 5.12):

- Femoral nerve and its (terminal) branches.
- Femoral sheath and its contents.
- Femoral artery and several of its branches.
- Femoral vein and its proximal tributaries (e.g., the great saphenous vein and deep femoral veins).
- Deep inguinal lymph nodes and associated lymphatic vessels.

The femoral triangle is bisected by the femoral artery and vein, which pass to and from the adductor canal at its apex (Fig. 5.12 B). The **adductor canal** (subsartorial canal, Hunter canal) extends from the apex of the femoral triangle, where the sartorius crosses over the adductor longus, to the adductor hiatus in the tendon of adductor magnus. It provides an intermuscular passage for the femoral artery and vein, the saphenous nerve, and the nerve to vastus medialis, delivering the femoral vessels to the popliteal fossa where they become popliteal vessels. The adductor canal is bounded anteriorly and laterally by the vastus medialis;

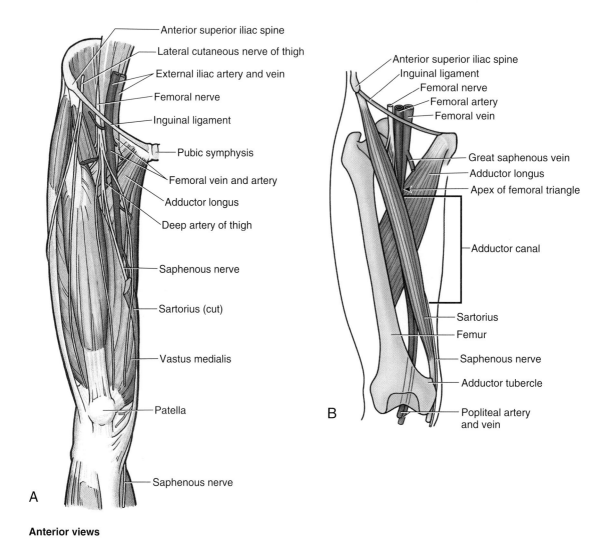

Anterior views

Figure 5.12. **Nerves and vessels of anterior thigh. A.** The femoral nerve and thigh vessels are defined. **B.** The adductor canal is shown.

posteriorly by the adductor longus and adductor magnus; and medially by the sartorius, which overlies the groove between the above muscles, forming the roof of the canal.

Femoral Nerve

The **femoral nerve** (L2–L4) is the largest branch of the lumbar plexus. The nerve originates in the abdomen within the psoas major and descends posterolaterally through the pelvis to the midpoint of the inguinal ligament. It then passes deep to this ligament and enters the femoral triangle, lateral to the femoral vessels (Fig. 5.12). After entering the triangle, the femoral nerve divides into several terminal branches to the anterior thigh muscles. It also sends articular branches to the hip and knee joints and provides cutaneous branches to the anteromedial thigh (Fig. 5.9*C*). The terminal cutaneous branch of the femoral nerve, the **saphenous nerve**, descends through the femoral triangle, lateral to the femoral sheath containing the femoral vessels. The saphenous nerve ac-

companies the femoral artery and vein through the adductor canal and becomes superficial by passing between the sartorius and the gracilis when the femoral vessels transverse the adductor hiatus (Fig. 5.11). The saphenous nerve runs anteroinferiorly to supply the skin and fascia on the anteromedial aspects of the knee, leg, and foot.

Femoral Sheath

The **femoral sheath** is a funnel-shaped, fascial tube of varying length (usually 3–4 cm) that passes deep to the inguinal ligament and encloses proximal parts of the femoral vessels and creates the femoral canal medial to them (Fig. 5.13). The sheath is formed by an inferior prolongation of the transversalis and iliopsoas fascia from the abdomen/greater pelvis. The sheath femoral does not enclose the femoral nerve. The sheath terminates inferiorly by becoming continuous with the tunica adventitia, the loose connective tissue covering of the femoral vessels. When a long femoral sheath occurs, its medial wall is pierced by the great saphenous vein and lymphatic vessels. The femoral sheath allows the femoral artery and vein to glide deep to the inguinal ligament during movements of the hip joint. The femoral sheath is subdivided into three compartments by vertical septa of extraperitoneal connective tissue that extend from the abdomen along the femoral vessels. The compartments of the femoral sheath are the *lateral compartment* for the femoral artery; *intermediate com-*

partment for the femoral vein; and *medial compartment,* which constitutes the femoral canal.

The **femoral canal**, is the smallest of the three compartments. It is short and conical and lies between the medial edge of the femoral sheath and the femoral vein. The femoral canal:

- Extends distally to the level of the proximal edge of the saphenous opening.

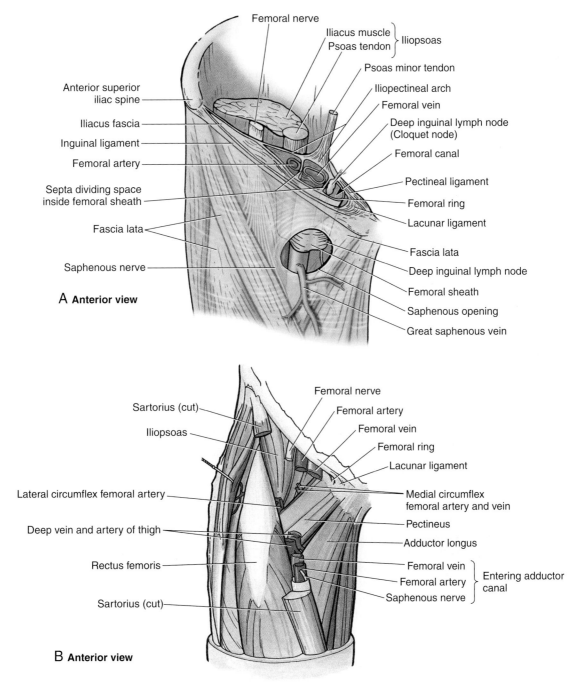

A Anterior view

B Anterior view

Figure 5.13. Femoral triangle. A. The femoral sheath and its contents at the superior end of the anterior aspect of the thigh are shown. Note that the femoral nerve is external and lateral to the sheath. **B.** This deep dissection shows the floor of the femoral triangle.

- Allows the femoral vein to expand when venous return from the lower limb is increased or when increased intra-abdominal pressure causes a temporary stasis in the vein (i.e., taking a breath and holding it, while bearing down).
- Contains loose connective tissue, fat, a few lymphatic vessels and sometimes a deep inguinal lymph node (Cloquet node).

The base of the femoral canal, formed by the small (approximately 1 cm wide) proximal opening at its abdominal end, is the oval **femoral ring** (Fig. 5.13). This opening is closed by extraperitoneal fatty tissue that forms the femoral septum. The **femoral septum** is pierced by lymphatic vessels connecting the inguinal and external iliac nodes. The boundaries of the femoral ring are *laterally,* a septum between the femoral canal and the femoral vein; *posteriorly,* the superior ramus of the pubis covered by the pectineus and its fascia; *medially,* the lacunar ligament; and *anteriorly,* the medial part of the inguinal ligament.

Femoral Artery

The **femoral artery**, the chief artery to the lower limb, is the continuation of the external iliac artery distal to the inguinal ligament (Fig. 5.12; Table 5.3). The femoral artery:

- Enters the femoral triangle deep to the midpoint of the inguinal ligament (midway between the ASIS and the pubic tubercle), lateral to the femoral vein.
- Lies posterior to the fascia lata and descends on the adjacent borders of the iliopsoas and pectineus, which make up the floor of the femoral triangle.
- Bisects the femoral triangle and exits at its apex to enter the adductor canal, deep to the sartorius.
- Exits the adductor canal by passing through the adductor hiatus and becoming the *popliteal artery.*

The **deep artery of the thigh** (L. *arteria profunda femoris*) is the largest branch of the femoral artery and the chief artery to the thigh. It arises from the femoral artery in the femoral triangle (Fig. 5.12A; Table 5.3); in the middle third of the thigh, it is separated from the femoral artery and vein by the adductor longus. The deep artery of the thigh gives off **perforating arteries** that wrap around the posterior aspect of the femur and supply the adductor magnus, hamstring, and vastus lateralis muscles.

The *circumflex femoral arteries* are usually branches of the deep artery of the thigh, but they may arise directly from the femoral artery. They encircle the thigh, anastomose with each other and other arteries, and supply the thigh muscles and the proximal end of the femur. The **medial circumflex femoral artery** supplies most of the blood to the head and neck of the femur via its branches, the **posterior retinacular arteries**. It passes deeply between the iliopsoas and pectineus to reach the posterior part of the thigh. The

lateral circumflex femoral artery passes laterally across the joint capsule, mainly supplying muscles on the lateral side of the thigh (Table 5.3).

Femoral Vein

The *femoral vein* is the continuation of the popliteal vein proximal to the adductor hiatus (Fig. 5.12A). As it ascends through the adductor canal, the femoral vein lies postero-lateral and then posterior to the femoral artery (Fig. 5.12B). The femoral vein enters the femoral sheath lateral to the femoral canal and ends posterior to the inguinal ligament, where it becomes the external iliac vein. In the inferior part of the femoral triangle, the femoral vein receives the deep vein of the thigh, the great saphenous vein, and other tributaries. The *deep vein of the thigh,* formed by the union of three or four perforating veins, enters the femoral vein inferior to the inguinal ligament and inferior to the termination of the great saphenous vein.

Obturator Artery and Nerve

The **obturator artery** usually arises from the internal iliac artery (Table 5.3). In approximately 20% of people, an enlarged pubic branch of the inferior epigastric artery either takes the place of the obturator artery (*replaced obturator artery*) or joins it as an *accessory obturator artery.* The obturator artery passes through the obturator foramen, enters the medial compartment of the thigh, and divides into anterior and posterior branches, which straddle the adductor brevis muscle. The obturator artery supplies the obturator externus, pectineus, adductors of thigh, and gracilis. Its posterior branch gives off an acetabular branch that supplies the head of the femur.

The **obturator nerve** (L2–L4) descends along the medial border of the psoas muscle and enters the thigh through the obturator foramen. It divides into anterior and posterior branches, which, like the arteries, straddle the adductor brevis. The anterior branch supplies the adductor longus, adductor brevis, gracilis, and pectineus; the posterior branch supplies the obturator externus and adductor magnus.

Gluteal Region and Posterior Thigh

The gluteal region (hip and buttocks) is the prominent area posterior to the pelvis. It is bounded superiorly by the iliac crest, greater trochanter and ASIS and inferiorly by the *gluteal fold.* The gluteal fold also demarcates the superior boundary of the thigh (Fig. 5.15). The *intergluteal cleft* separates the buttocks from each other.

The parts of the bony pelvis—hip bones, sacrum, and coccyx—are bound together by *gluteal ligaments* (Fig. 5.14). The **sacrotuberous** and **sacrospinous ligaments** convert the

Table 5.3 Arteries of the Anterior and Medial Thigh

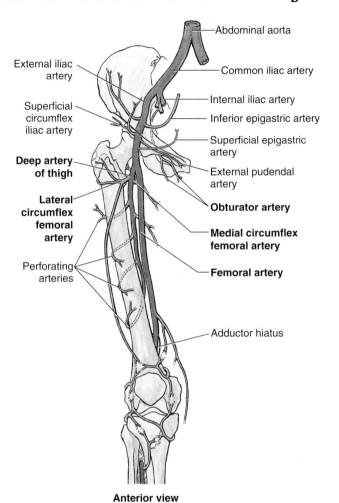

Anterior view

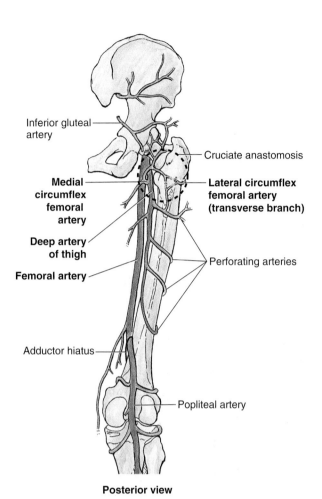

Posterior view

Artery	Origin	Course	Distribution
Femoral	Continuation of external iliac artery distal to inguinal ligament	Descends through femoral triangle; enters adductor canal; terminates as it traverses adductor hiatus; becomes popliteal artery	Anterior and anteromedial aspects of thigh
Deep artery of thigh	Femoral artery 1–5 cm inferior to inguinal ligament	Passes inferiorly, deep to adductor longus	Perforating branches pass through adductor magnus to supply muscles in medial, posterior, and lateral part of anterior compartments
Lateral circumflex femoral	Deep artery of thigh; may arise from femoral artery	Passes laterally deep to sartorius and rectus femoris and dividing into ascending, transverse and descending arteries	Ascending branch supplies anterior part of gluteal region; transverse branch winds around femur; descending branch joins genicular periarticular anastomosis
Medial circumflex femoral	Deep artery of thigh; may arise from femoral artery	Passes medially and posteriorly between pectineus and iliopsoas; enters gluteal region and divides into two branches	Supplies most blood to head and neck of femur; transverse branch takes part in cruciate anastomosis of thigh; ascending branch joins inferior gluteal artery
Obturator	Internal iliac artery or (in ~20%) as an accessory or replaced obturator artery from the inferior epigastric artery	Passes through obturator foramen; enters medial compartment of thigh; and divides into anterior and posterior branches	Anterior branch supplies obturator externus, pectineus, adductors of thigh, and gracilis; posterior branch supplies muscles attached to ischial tuberosity

Femoral Pulse and Cannulation of the Femoral Artery

The pulse of the femoral artery is usually palpable just inferior to the midpoint of the inguinal ligament. Normally, the pulse is strong; however, if the common or external iliac arteries are partially occluded, the pulse may be diminished. The femoral artery may be compressed here to control arterial bleeding after lower limb trauma. The femoral artery may be cannulated just inferior to the midpoint of the inguinal ligament (e.g., for cardioangiography—radiography of the heart and great vessels after the introduction of contrast material). For *left cardiac angiography,* a long slender catheter is inserted percutaneously into the femoral artery and passed superiorly in the aorta to the openings of the coronary arteries (see Chapter 1).

Cannulation of the Femoral Vein

The femoral vein usually is not palpable, but its position can be located by feeling the pulsations of the femoral artery, which lies just lateral to it. In thin people, the femoral vein may be close to the surface and may be mistaken for the great saphenous vein. It is thus important to know that the femoral vein has no tributaries at this level, except for the great saphenous vein that joins it approximately 3 cm inferior to the inguinal ligament. To secure blood samples and take pressure recordings from the chambers of the right side of the heart and/or from the pulmonary artery and to perform *right cardiac angiography,* a long slender catheter is inserted into the femoral vein as it passes through the femoral triangle. Under fluoroscopic control, the catheter is passed superiorly through the external and common iliac veins into the inferior vena cava and right atrium of the heart.

Femoral Hernia

The femoral ring is a weak area in the lower anterior abdominal wall that is the site of a *femoral hernia,* a protrusion of abdominal viscera (often a loop of small intestine) through the femoral ring into the femoral canal (Fig. 5.13A). A femoral hernia is more common in women than in men. The hernial sac compresses the contents of the femoral canal and distends its wall. Initially, the hernia is relatively small because it is contained within the femoral canal, but it can enlarge by passing through the saphenous opening into the subcutaneous tissue of the thigh. *Strangulation of a femoral hernia* may occur and interfere with the blood supply to the herniated intestine, and vascular impairment may result in death of the tissues.

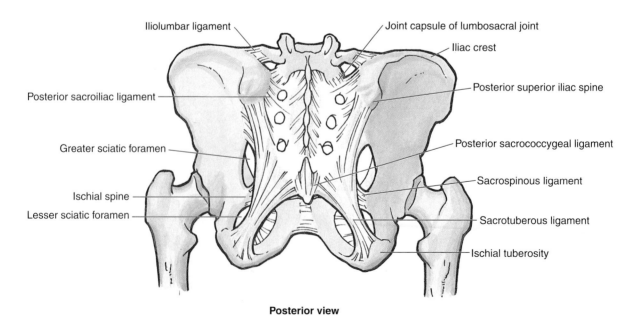

Iliolumbar ligament

Joint capsule of lumbosacral joint

Iliac crest

Posterior superior iliac spine

Posterior sacroiliac ligament

Posterior sacrococcygeal ligament

Greater sciatic foramen

Sacrospinous ligament

Ischial spine

Sacrotuberous ligament

Lesser sciatic foramen

Ischial tuberosity

Posterior view

Figure 5.14. Lumbar and pelvic ligaments.

sciatic notches in the hip bones into the greater and lesser sciatic foramina. The **greater sciatic foramen** is the passageway for structures entering or leaving the pelvis, whereas the **lesser sciatic foramen** is a passageway for structures entering or leaving the perineum (Fig. 5.14).

It is helpful to think of the greater sciatic foramen as the "door" through which arteries and nerves leave the pelvis and enter the gluteal region.

Gluteal Muscles

The gluteal muscles are organized into two layers: superficial and deep (Fig. 5.15; Table 5.4). The superficial layer consist of three large glutei (maximus, medius, and minimus) and the tensor of fascia lata. The main actions of the **gluteus maximus** are extension and lateral rotation of the thigh. It functions primarily between the flexed and the standing positions, as when rising from the sitting position, straightening from the bending position, walking uphill and up stairs, and running. The **gluteus medius** and **minimus,** are fan-shaped muscles that lie deep to the gluteus maximus. They are abductors and medial rotators of the thigh. The **tensor of fascia lata** (L. *tensor fasciae latae*) lies on the lateral side of the hip, enclosed between two layers of fascia lata. The tensor of fascia lata is primarily a flexor of the thigh; however, it generally does not act independently. To produce flexion, it acts in concert with the iliopsoas and rectus femoris. The tensor of fascia lata also tenses the fascia lata and iliotibial tract, thereby helping support the femur on the tibia when standing. The deep layer consists of smaller muscles, the **piriformis, obturator internus, superior** and **inferior gemelli,** and **quadratus femoris.** These muscles, covered by the inferior half of the gluteus maximus, are lateral rotators of the thigh, but they also stabilize the hip joint, working with the strong ligaments of the hip joint to steady the femoral head in the acetabulum.

Gluteal Bursae

Gluteal bursae, membranous sacs containing a capillary layer of synovial fluid, separate the gluteus maximus from adjacent structures. The bursae are located in areas subject to friction—for example, between a muscle and a bony prominence—to reduce friction and permit free movement. Usually, three bursae are associated with the gluteus maximus:

* The **trochanteric bursa** separates the superior fibers of the gluteus maximus from the greater trochanter of the femur.
* The **ischial bursa** separates the inferior part of the gluteus maximus from the ischial tuberosity.
* The **gluteofemoral bursa** separates the iliotibial tract from the superior part of the proximal attachment of the vastus lateralis.

Posterior Thigh Muscles

Three of the four muscles in the posterior aspect of the thigh are **hamstrings** (Fig. 5.16; Table 5.5): **semitendinosus, semimembranosus,** and **biceps femoris (long head).** The hamstrings span and act on two joints (extension at the hip joint and flexion at the knee joint), arise from the ischial tuberosity deep to the gluteus maximus, and are innervated by the tibial division of the sciatic nerve. Both actions cannot be performed maximally at the same time. A fully flexed knee shortens the hamstrings so they cannot further contract to extend the thigh. Similarly, a fully extended hip shortens the hamstrings so they cannot act on the knee. When the thighs and legs are fixed, the hamstrings can help extend the trunk at the hip joint. They are active in thigh extension under all situations except full flexion of the knee, including maintenance of the relaxed standing posture (standing at ease). The **short head of biceps femoris,** the fourth muscle in the posterior compartment, is not a hamstring as it crosses only the knee joint and is innervated by the fibular division of the sciatic nerve.

Trochanteric and Ischial Bursitis

Diffuse deep pain in the lateral thigh region, especially during stair climbing or rising from a seated position, may be caused by **trochanteric bursitis.** This type of **friction bursitis** is characterized by point tenderness over the greater trochanter; however, the pain radiates along the iliotibial tract, which extends from the iliac tubercle to the tibia. **Ischial bursitis** is a friction bursitis resulting from excessive friction between the ischial bursae and the ischial tuberosities (e.g., as from cycling or rowing). Because the tuberosities bear the body weight during sitting, these pressure points may lead to *pressure sores* in debilitated people, particularly paraplegic persons with poor nursing care.

Hamstring Injuries

Hamstrings strains (pulled and/or torn hamstrings) are common in people who run and/or kick hard (e.g., in running, jumping and quick-start sports such as baseball and soccer). The violent muscular exertion required to excel in these sports may tear part of the proximal attachments of the hamstrings to the ischial tuberosity. Hamstring injuries may result from inadequate warming up before practice or competition.

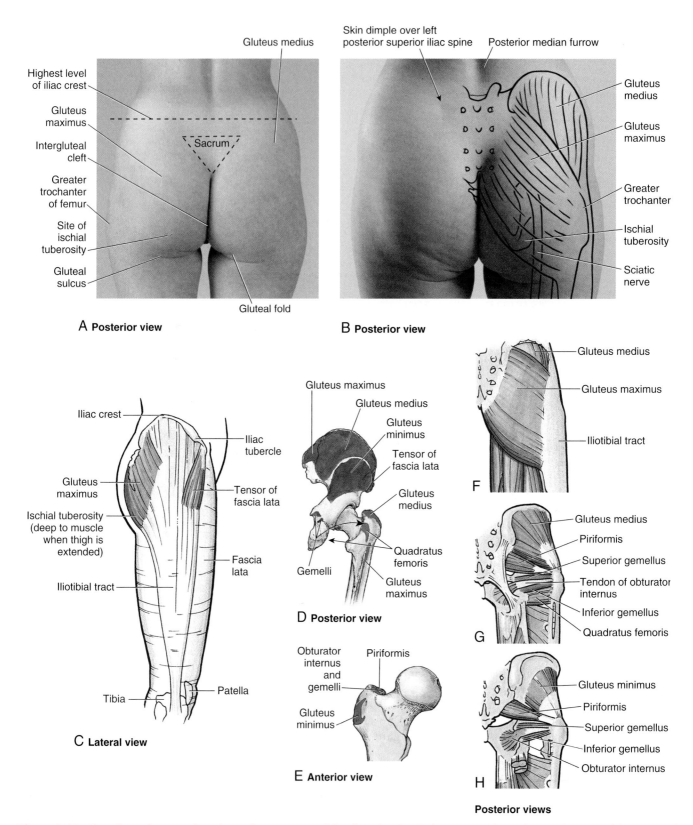

Figure 5.15. Gluteal muscles. A and B. The surface anatomy of the gluteal region is demonstrated. **C.** The attachments of the tensor of fascia lata and the gluteus maximus into the iliotibial tract are shown. **D and E.** The attachments of the muscles are identified. **F.** A superficial dissection of the gluteus maximus is shown. **G.** This deep dissection shows the gluteus medius and lateral rotators of the hip joint. **H.** A deeper dissection shows the gluteus minimus and obturator internus.

Table 5.4 Muscles of the Gluteal Region

Muscle	Proximal Attachment	Distal Attachment	Innervation[a]	Main Action(s)
Gluteus maximus	Ilium posterior to posterior gluteal line; dorsal surface of sacrum and coccyx; and sacrotuberous ligament	Most fibers end in iliotibial tract, which inserts into lateral condyle of tibia; some fibers insert on gluteal tuberosity of femur	Inferior gluteal nerve (L5, **S1, S2**)	Extends thigh and assists in its lateral rotation; steadies thigh and assists in rising from sitting position
Gluteus medius	External surface of ilium between anterior and posterior gluteal lines	Lateral surface of greater trochanter of femur	Superior gluteal nerve (L4, **L5**, S1)	Abduct and medially rotate thigh; keep pelvis level when opposite leg is raised
Gluteus minimus	External surface of ilium between anterior and inferior gluteal lines	Anterior surface of greater trochanter of femur		
Tensor of fascia lata	Anterior superior iliac spine; anterior part of iliac crest	Iliotibial tract, which attaches to lateral condyle of tibia		
Piriformis	Anterior surface of sacrum and sacrotuberous ligament	Superior border of greater trochanter of femur	Branches of anterior rami of **S1**, S2	Laterally rotate extended thigh; abduct flexed thigh; steady femoral head in acetabulum
Obturator internus	Pelvic surface of obturator membrane and surrounding bones	Medial surface of greater trochanter (trochanteric fossa) of femur[b]	Nerve to obturator internus (L5, **S1**)	
Gemelli, superior and inferior	*Superior:* ischial spine *Inferior:* ischial tuberosity		*Superior:* same as obturator internus *Inferior:* same as quadratus femoris	
Quadratus femoris	Lateral border of ischial tuberosity	Quadrate tubercle on intertrochanteric crest of femur and area inferior to it	Nerve to quadratus femoris (L5, S1)	Laterally rotates thigh;[c] steadies femoral head in acetabulum

[a]The spinal cord segmental innervation is indicated (e.g., "S1, S2" means that the nerves supplying the piriformis are derived from the first two sacral segments of the spinal cord). Numbers in boldface (**S1**) indicate the main segmental innervation. Damage to one or more of the listed spinal cord segments or to the motor nerve roots arising from them results in paralysis of the muscles concerned.

[b]Gemelli muscles blend with the tendon of the obturator internus muscle as it attaches to the greater trochanter of the femur.

[c]There are six lateral rotators of the thigh: piriformis, obturator internus, gemelli (superior and inferior), quadratus femoris, and obturator externus. These muscles also stabilize the hip joint.

Nerves of Gluteal Region and Posterior Thigh

Several nerves arise from the sacral plexus and either supply the gluteal region (e.g., superior and inferior gluteal nerves) or pass through it to supply the perineum (e.g., pudendal nerve) and thigh (e.g., sciatic nerve). The skin of the gluteal region is richly innervated by the superficial gluteal nerves, the **superior, middle,** and **inferior clunial nerves** (L. *clunes,* buttocks) (Fig. 5.9). The deep gluteal nerves are the **sciatic, posterior cutaneous nerve of the thigh, superior gluteal** and **inferior gluteal nerves, nerve to the quadratus femoris, pudendal nerve,** and **nerve to the obturator internus** (Fig. 5.17; Table 5.6). All of these nerves are branches of the sacral plexus and leave the pelvis through the greater sciatic foramen (Fig. 5.17C). Except for the superior gluteal nerve, they all emerge inferior to the piriformis muscle. The pudendal nerve supplies no structures in the gluteal region; it supplies structures in the perineum (see Chapter 3).

The **sciatic nerve** is the largest nerve in the body and is the continuation of the main part of the sacral plexus (Fig. 5.17D). The sciatic nerve runs inferolaterally under cover of the gluteus maximus, midway between the greater trochanter and the ischial tuberosity, and descends from the

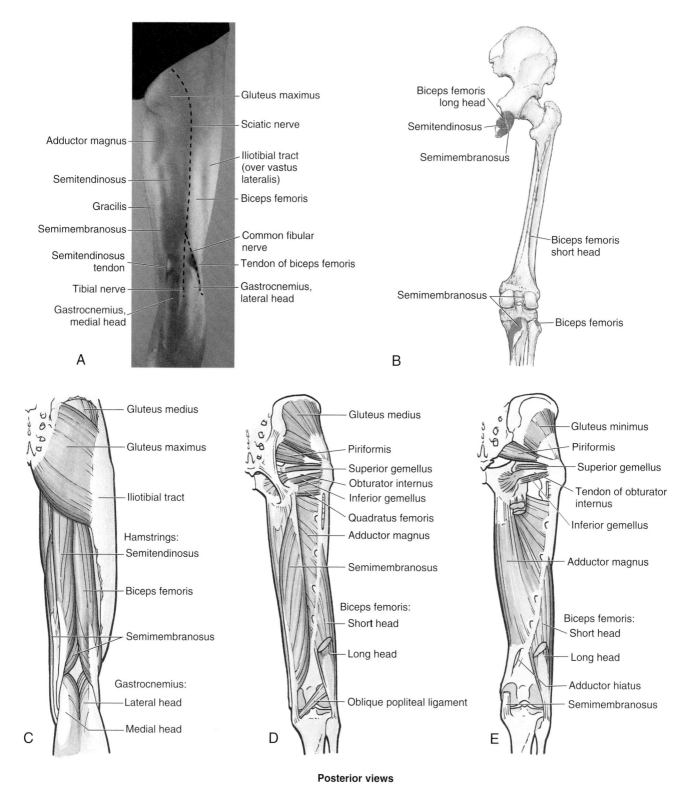

Posterior views

Figure 5.16. Muscles of posterior aspect of thigh. A. The surface anatomy is demonstrated. **B.** The attachments of the muscles are shown. **C.** A superficial dissection of the hamstrings is shown. **D.** A deep dissection shows the semimembranosus and the short head of the biceps femoris. **E.** A deeper dissection reveals the gluteus minimus and adductor magnus.

Table 5.5 Posterior Thigh Muscles

Muscle[a]	Proximal Attachment[b]	Distal Attachment[b]	Innervation[c]	Main Action(s)
Semitendinosus	Ischial tuberosity	Medial surface of superior part of tibia	Tibial division of sciatic nerve (**L5, S1**, S2)	Extend thigh; flex leg and rotate it medially when knee is flexed; when thigh and leg are flexed, can extend trunk
Semimembranosus		Posterior part of medial condyle of tibia; reflected attachment forms oblique popliteal ligament (to lateral femoral condyle)		
Biceps femoris, long and short heads	*Long head:* ischial tuberosity *Short head:* linea aspera and lateral supracondylar line of femur	Lateral side of head of fibula; tendon is split at this site by fibular collateral ligament of knee	*Long head:* tibial division of sciatic nerve (L5, **S1**, S2) *Short head:* common fibular division of sciatic nerve (L5, **S1**, S2)	Flexes leg and rotates it laterally when knee is flexed; extends thigh (e.g., when starting to walk)

[a]Collectively these three muscles are known as hamstrings.

[b]See Figure 5.16*B* for muscle attachments.

[c]The spinal cord segmental innervation is indicated (e.g., "L5, **S1**, S2" means that the nerves supplying the biceps femoris are derived from the fifth lumbar segment and first two sacral segments of the spinal cord). Numbers in boldface (**S1**) indicate the main segmental innervation. Damage to one or more of the listed spinal cord segments or to the motor nerve roots arising from them results in paralysis of the muscles concerned.

gluteal region into the posterior thigh, where it lies on the adductor magnus and is crossed posteriorly by the long head of the biceps femoris. The sciatic nerve is so large that it receives a named branch of the inferior gluteal artery, **the artery to the sciatic nerve.** The sciatic nerve is really two nerves loosely bound together in the same connective tissue sheath: the *tibial nerve,* derived from anterior (preaxial) divisions of anterior rami, and the *common fibular nerve,* derived from posterior (postaxial) divisions of the anterior rami (Figs. 5.17 *D,* 5.18 and 5.19). The two nerves separate in the inferior third of the thigh; however, in 12% of people, the nerves separate as they leave the pelvis. In these cases, the tibial nerve passes inferior to the piriformis, and the common fibular nerve pierces this muscle or passes superior to it. The sciatic nerve supplies no structures in the gluteal region; it innervates the posterior thigh muscles, all leg and foot muscles, and the skin of most of the leg and foot. It also supplies articular branches to all lower limb joints.

Vasculature of Gluteal Region and Posterior Thigh

The *arteries of the gluteal region* arise, directly or indirectly, from the *internal iliac arteries,* but the patterns of origin of the arteries are variable (Fig. 5.17; Table 5.7). The major gluteal branches of the internal iliac artery are the superior and inferior gluteal arteries and the internal pudendal artery. The **superior** and **inferior gluteal arteries** leave the pelvis through the greater sciatic foramen and pass superior and inferior to the piriformis, respectively. The

internal pudendal artery enters the gluteal region through the greater sciatic foramen inferior to the piriformis and enters the perineum through the lesser sciatic foramen. It does not supply the buttock. After birth, the posterior compartment of the thigh has no major artery exclusive to the compartment; it receives blood from the inferior gluteal, medial circumflex femoral, and perforating and popliteal arteries. The *deep artery of the thigh* is the chief artery of the thigh, giving off *perforating arteries* (Fig. 5.18; Table 5.7), which pierce the adductor magnus to enter the posterior compartment and supply the hamstrings. A continuous anastomotic chain thus extends from the gluteal to the popliteal region, which gives rise to branches to the muscles and to the sciatic nerve.

The *veins of the gluteal region* are tributaries of the **internal iliac veins** that drain blood from the gluteal region (Fig. 5.17 *B*). The **superior** and **inferior gluteal veins** accompany the corresponding arteries through the greater sciatic foramen, superior and inferior to the piriformis, respectively. They communicate with tributaries of the femoral vein, thereby providing an alternate route for the return of blood from the lower limb if the femoral vein is occluded or has to be ligated. The **internal pudendal veins** accompany the internal pudendal arteries and join to form a single vein that enters the internal iliac vein. The pudendal veins drain blood from the perineum (see Chapter 3). *Perforating veins* accompany the arteries of the same name to drain blood from the posterior compartment of the thigh into the *deep vein of the thigh.* They also communicate inferiorly with the popliteal vein and superiorly with the inferior gluteal vein.

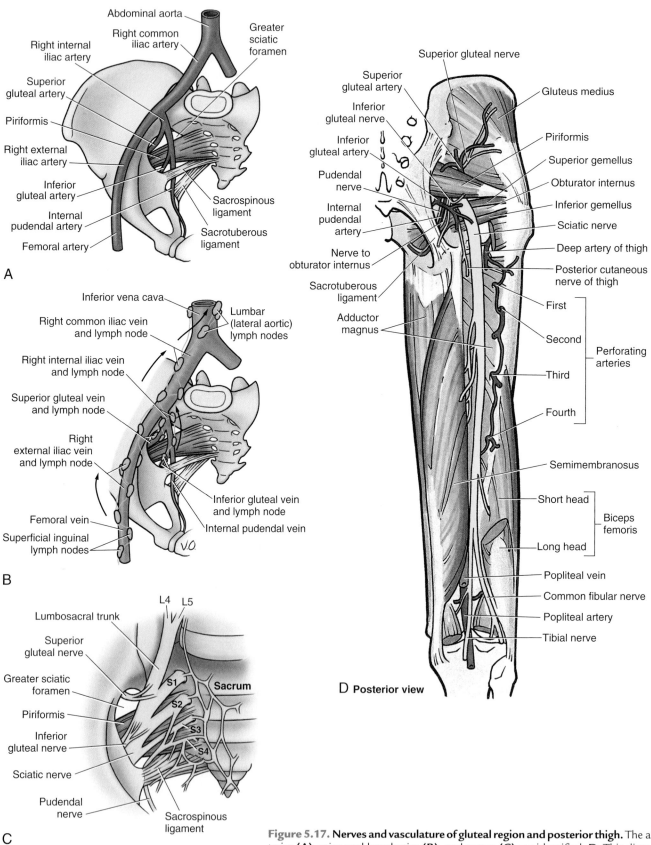

A

B

C

Anteromedial views

D Posterior view

Figure 5.17. Nerves and vasculature of gluteal region and posterior thigh. The arteries **(A)**, veins and lymphatics **(B)**, and nerves **(C)** are identified. **D.** This dissection shows the relation of the vessels and nerves to the muscles.

Table 5.6 Nerves of the Gluteal Region and Posterior Thigh

Nerve	Origin	Course	Distribution[a]
Clunial: superior, middle, and inferior	*Superior:* posterior rami of L1–L3 nerves *Middle:* posterior rami of S1–S3 nerves *Inferior:* posterior cutaneous nerve of thigh (anterior rami of S2–S3)	*Superior:* cross iliac crest *Middle:* exit through posterior sacral foramina and enter gluteal region *Inferior:* curve around inferior border of gluteus maximus	Supplies skin of gluteal region (buttocks) as far as greater trochanter
Sciatic	Sacral plexus (L4–S3)	Leaves pelvis through greater sciatic foramen inferior to piriformis; enters gluteal region; descends deep to biceps femoris; bifurcates into tibial and common fibular nerves at apex of popliteal fossa	Supplies no muscles in gluteal region; supplies all muscles in posterior compartment of thigh
Posterior cutaneous nerve of thigh	Sacral plexus (S1–S3)	Leaves pelvis through greater sciatic foramen inferior to piriformis, runs deep to gluteus maximus; emerges from its inferior border; descends in posterior thigh deep to fascia lata	Supplies skin of buttock through inferior clunial branches and skin over posterior aspect of thigh and calf; lateral perineum, upper medial thigh via perineal branch
Superior gluteal	Sacral plexus (L4–S1)	Leaves pelvis through greater sciatic foramen superior to piriformis; runs between gluteus medius and minimus	Innervates gluteus medius, gluteus minimus, and tensor of fascia lata
Inferior gluteal	Sacral plexus (L5–S2)	Leaves pelvis through greater sciatic foramen inferior to piriformis; divides into several branches	Innervates gluteus maximus
Nerve to quadratus femoris	Sacral plexus (L4, L5–S1)	Leaves pelvis through greater sciatic foramen deep to sciatic nerve	Innervates hip joint, inferior gemellus, and quadratus femoris
Pudendal	Sacral plexus (S2–S4)	Enters gluteal region through greater sciatic foramen inferior to piriformis; descends posterior to sacrospinous ligament; enters perineum through lesser sciatic foramen	Supplies most innervation to the perineum; supplies no structures in gluteal region
Nerve to obturator internus	Sacral plexus (L5–S2)	Enters gluteal region through greater sciatic foramen inferior to piriformis; descends posterior to ischial spine; enters lesser sciatic foramen; passes to obturator internus	Supplies superior gemellus and obturator internus

See Figure 5.9 for cutaneous innervation of the lower limb.

Table 5.7 Arteries of the Gluteal Region and Posterior Thigh

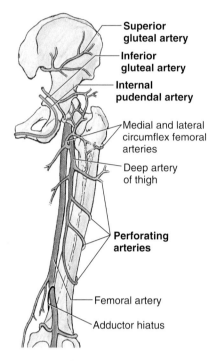

Posterior view

Artery	Course	Distribution
Superior gluteal[a]	*Superficial branch:* enters gluteal region through greater sciatic foramen, superior to piriformis; divides into superficial and deep branches; anastomoses with inferior gluteal and medial circumflex femoral arteries *Deep branch:* runs between gluteus medius and minimus	*Superficial branch:* gluteus maximus *Deep branch:* gluteus medius and minimus and tensor of fascia lata
Inferior gluteal[a]	Enters gluteal region through greater sciatic foramen, inferior to piriformis; descends on medial side of sciatic nerve; anastomoses with superior gluteal artery and participates in cruciate anastomosis of thigh, involving first perforating artery of deep femoral and medial and lateral circumflex femoral arteries	Gluteus maximus, obturator internus, quadratus femoris, and superior parts of hamstrings
Internal pudendal[a]	Enters gluteal region through greater sciatic foramen; descends posterior to ischial spine ; enters perineum through lesser sciatic foramen	External genitalia and muscles in the perineal region; does not supply gluteal region
Perforating[b]	Enters posterior compartment by perforating aponeurotic portion of adductor magnus attachment and medial intermuscular septum; after providing muscular branches to hamstrings, continues on to anterior compartment by piercing lateral intermuscular septum	Supplies majority (central portions) of hamstring muscles, then continues to supply vastus lateralis in anterior compartment

[a]Arise from the internal iliac artery.
[b]Arise from deep artery of thigh.

Injury to Superior Gluteal Nerve

Injury to the superior gluteal nerve results in a characteristic motor loss, resulting in a disabling *gluteus medius limp,* to compensate for weakened abduction of the thigh by the gluteus medius and minimus, and/or a *gluteal gait,* a compensatory list of the body to the weakened gluteal side. As a result of this compensation, the center of gravity is placed over the supporting lower limb. Medial rotation of the thigh is also severely impaired. When a person is asked to stand on one leg, the gluteus medius and minimus normally contract as soon as the contralateral foot leaves the floor, preventing tipping of the pelvis to the unsupported side (Fig. B5.5A). When a person with paralysis of the superior gluteal nerve is asked to stand on one leg, the pelvis descends on the unsupported side (Fig. B5.5B), indicating that the gluteus medius on the contralateral (supported) side is weak or non-functional. This observation is referred to clinically as a **positive Trendelenburg test.**

When the pelvis descends on the unsupported side, the lower limb becomes, in effect, too long and does not clear the ground when the foot is brought forward in the swing phase of walking. To compensate, the individual leans away from the unsupported side, raising the pelvis to allow adequate room for the foot to clear the ground as it swings forward. This results in a characteristic "waddling" or gluteal gait. Other ways to compensate is to lift the foot higher as it is brought forward, resulting in the so-called steppage gait, or to swing the foot outward (laterally), the so-called swing-out gait. These same gaits are adopted in the presence of *foot-drop,* which results from common fibular nerve paralysis.

Injury to Sciatic Nerve

A pain in the buttock may result from compression of the sciatic nerve by the piriformis muscle (**piriformis syndrome**). *Incomplete section of the sciatic nerve* (e.g., from a stab wound) may also involve the inferior gluteal and/or the posterior femoral cutaneous nerves. Recovery from a sciatic lesion is slow and usually incomplete. With respect to the sciatic nerve, the buttock has a side of safety (its lateral side) and a side of danger (its medial side). Wounds or surgery on the medial side may injure the sciatic nerve and its branches to the hamstrings. Paralysis of these muscles results in impairment of thigh extension and leg flexion.

Intragluteal Injections

The gluteal region is a common site for intramuscular injection of drugs because the gluteal muscles are thick and large, providing a large area for venous absorption of drugs. Injections into the buttock are safe only in the superolateral quadrant of the buttock (Fig. B5.5C, *green*). Complications of improper technique include nerve injury, hematoma, and abscess formation.

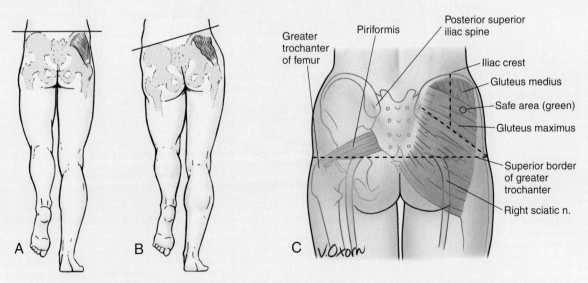

Figure B5.5 Clinical concerns of gluteal region. A. The pelvis is shown during normal gait. **B.** A positive Trendelenburg test indicates paralysis of the superior gluteal nerve. **C.** The safe area (*green*) for intragluteal injections is shown.

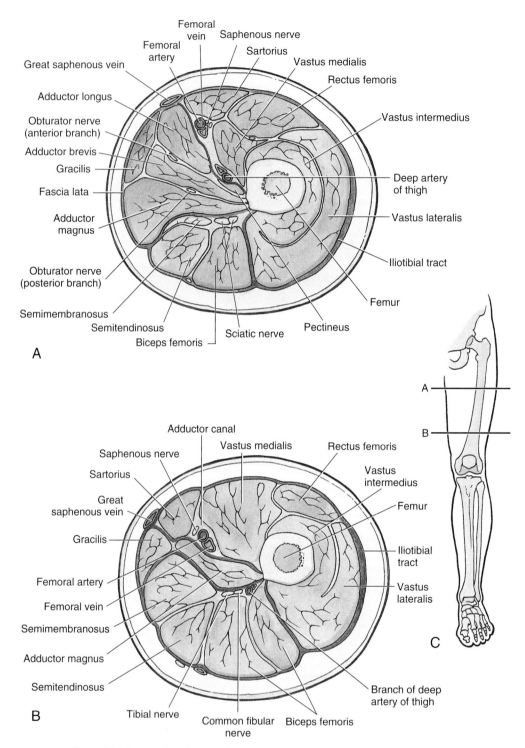

Figure 5.18. Transverse sections of thigh. A and B. The muscles, vessels, and nerves are shown. **C.** The orientation drawing shows the levels of the sections in parts A and B.

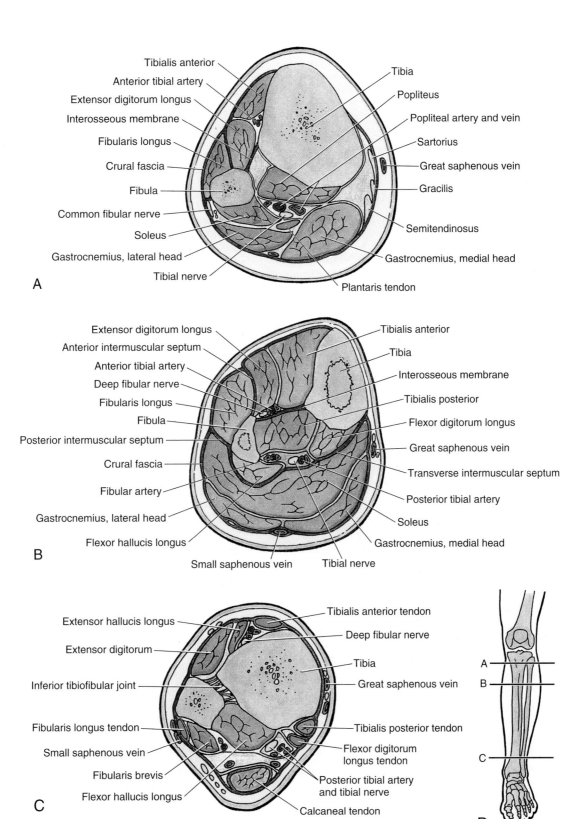

Transverse sections

Figure 5.19. Bones, muscles, vessels, and nerves of leg. The orientation drawing (**D**) shows the level of sections (**A–C**).

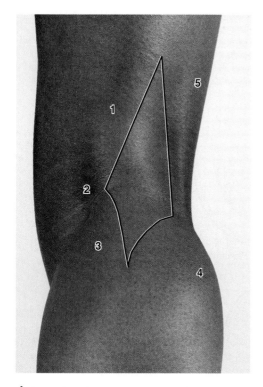

A **Posterior view**

Semimembranosus (1) ——————————————— Biceps femoris (5)

Semitendinosus (2) ——————

Gastrocnemius, ——————————— Head of fibula
medial head (3)
——————————— Gastrocnemius,
lateral head (4)

——————————— Fibularis longus

——————————— Soleus

——————————— Fibularis brevis

——————————— Calcaneal tendon

——————————— Fibularis longus
tendon

——————————— Lateral malleolus

B **Posterolateral view**

Semitendinosus ——————————— Sciatic nerve
(2)

Tibial nerve ——————— Common fibular
nerve

Popliteal vein
and artery ——————— Biceps
femoris (5)
Semi-
membranosus ——————— Superior lateral
(1) genicular vein
and artery
Superior
medial genicular
artery and vein ——————— Gastrocnemius,
lateral head (4)
Gastrocnemius,
medial head (3) ——————— Lateral sural
cutaneous nerve
Medial sural
cutaneous nerve ———————

Small saphenous vein ——————— Sural nerve

C **Posterior view**

Descending ——————— Femoral artery
branch of
lateral femoral ——————— Descending
circumflex genicular artery
artery
——————— Musculoarterial
Popliteal artery ——————— branch

Superior lateral ——————— Saphenous
genicular artery branch

——————— Superior medial
Inferior lateral genicular artery
genicular artery ———————
——————— Middle
Anterior tibial genicular artery
recurrent artery ———————
——————— Inferior medial
Anterior tibial genicular artery
artery ———————
——————— Posterior
tibial artery

D **Anterior view**

Figure 5.20. Popliteal fossa. A and B. The surface anatomy is demonstrated. *Line,* diamond-shaped gap in the muscles overlying the fossa; *numbers,* defined in part C. **C.** This dissection shows the boundaries and contents of the fossa. **D.** The genicular anastomosis is detailed.

Lymph from the deep tissues of the gluteal region follows the gluteal vessels to the **gluteal lymph nodes** and from them to the internal, external, and common **iliac lymph nodes** and then to the **lumbar (caval) lymph nodes** (Fig. 5.17 *B*). *Lymph from superficial tissues* of the gluteal region enters the *superficial inguinal nodes*. All the superficial inguinal nodes send efferent lymphatic vessels to the **external iliac nodes**.

Popliteal Fossa

The **popliteal fossa** is a mostly fat-filled diamond-shaped space posterior to the knee (Fig. 5.20). All important vessels and nerves from the thigh to the leg pass through this fossa.

The popliteal fossa is bound

- Superolaterally by the biceps femoris (superolateral border).
- Superomedially by the semimembranosus, lateral to which is the semitendinosus (superomedial border).
- Inferolaterally and inferomedially by the lateral and medial heads of the gastrocnemius, respectively (inferolateral and inferomedial borders).
- Posteriorly by skin and popliteal fascia (roof).
- Anteriorly by the popliteal surface of the femur, posterior capsule of the knee joint, and the popliteus fascia covering the popliteus muscle (floor).

The contents of the popliteal fossa include the (Fig. 5.20*C*):

- Termination of the small saphenous vein.
- Popliteal artery and vein and their branches and tributaries.
- Tibial and common fibular nerves.
- Posterior cutaneous nerve of the thigh.
- Popliteal lymph nodes and lymphatic vessels.

Fascia of Popliteal Fossa

The *subcutaneous tissue* overlying the fossa contains fat, the small saphenous vein (unless it has penetrated the deep fascia at a more inferior level), and three cutaneous nerves: the terminal branch(es) of the *posterior cutaneous nerve of the thigh* and the *medial and lateral sural cutaneous nerves*. The **popliteal fascia** is a strong sheet of deep fascia that forms a protective covering for neurovascular structures passing from the thigh through the popliteal fossa to the leg. The popliteal fascia is continuous with the *fascia lata* superiorly and the *deep fascia of the leg* inferiorly. When the leg is extended, the popliteal fascia stretches and the semimembranosus moves laterally, providing further protection to the contents of the fossa.

Vessels in Popliteal Fossa

The **popliteal artery**, the continuation of the femoral artery, begins where the femoral artery passes through the adductor hiatus (Fig. 5.20 *D;* Table 5.8). The popliteal artery passes through the popliteal fossa and ends at the inferior border of the popliteus by dividing into the **anterior** and **posterior tibial arteries**. The deepest structure in the popliteal fossa, the popliteal artery, runs close to the joint capsule of the knee joint. Five genicular branches of the popliteal artery supply the joint capsule and ligaments of the knee joint. The genicular arteries are the **superior lateral, superior medial, middle, inferior lateral,** and **inferior medial genicular arteries** (Fig. 5.20 *D*). They participate in the formation of the **genicular anastomosis** (L. *genu,* knee), a network of vessels around the knee that provide collateral circulation capable of maintaining blood supply to the leg during full knee flexion, which may kink the popliteal artery. Other contributions to the anastomosis are shown in Figure 5.20 *D*. The muscular branches of the popliteal artery supply the hamstring, gastrocnemius, soleus, and plantaris muscles. The superior muscular branches of the popliteal artery have clinically important anastomoses with the terminal part of the deep artery of thigh and gluteal arteries (Table 5.3).

The **popliteal vein** is formed at the distal border of the popliteus as a continuation of the *posterior tibial vein* (Fig. 5.8 *E*). Throughout its course, the vein is close to the popliteal artery and lies superficial to and in the same fibrous sheath as the artery (Fig. 5.20 *C*). Superiorly, the popliteal vein becomes the *femoral vein* as it traverses the adductor hiatus. The small saphenous vein passes from the posterior aspect of the lateral malleolus to the popliteal fossa, where it pierces the deep popliteal fascia and enters the popliteal vein.

The **superficial popliteal lymph nodes** are usually small and lie in the subcutaneous tissue. The **deep popliteal lymph nodes** surround the vessels and receive lymph from the joint capsule of the knee and the lymphatic vessels that accompany the deep veins of the leg (Fig. 5.8 *A* & *C*). Lymphatic vessels from the popliteal lymph nodes follow the femoral vessels to the *deep inguinal lymph nodes*.

Nerves in Popliteal Fossa

The *sciatic nerve* usually ends at the superior angle of the popliteal fossa by dividing into the tibial and common fibular nerves (Fig. 5.20 *C*; Table 5.6). The **tibial nerve**—the medial, larger terminal branch of the sciatic nerve—is the most superficial of the three main central components of the popliteal fossa (nerve, vein, and artery); however, it is still deep and in a protected position. The tibial nerve bisects the fossa as it passes from its superior to its inferior angle. While in the fossa, the tibial nerve gives branches to the soleus, gastrocnemius, plantaris, and popliteus muscles. A **medial sural cutaneous nerve** is also derived from the tibial nerve in the popliteal fossa and is joined by the **sural communicating branch** of the common fibular nerve at a highly variable level to form the **sural nerve**. This nerve supplies the lateral side of the leg and ankle.

Popliteal Pulse

Because the popliteal artery is deep in the popliteal fossa, it may be difficult to feel the *popliteal pulse.* Palpation of this pulse is commonly performed by placing the person in the prone position with the knee flexed to relax the popliteal fascia and hamstrings. The pulsations are best felt in the inferior part of the fossa. Weakening or loss of the popliteal pulse is a sign of femoral artery obstruction.

Popliteal Aneurysm

A *popliteal aneurysm* (abnormal dilation of all or part of the popliteal artery) usually causes edema (swelling) and pain in the popliteal fossa. If the femoral artery has to be ligated, blood can bypass the occlusion through the genicular anastomosis and reach the popliteal artery distal to the ligation.

Compartment Syndromes in Leg

Trauma to muscles and/or vessels in the compartments may produce hemorrhage, edema, and inflammation of the muscles. Because the septa and deep fascia of the leg forming the boundaries of the leg compartments are strong, the increased volume as a consequence of any of these processes increases intracompartmental pressure. This results in **compartment syndromes,** in which structures within or distal to the compressed area may become ischemic and permanently injured (e.g., loss of motor function in the muscles whose blood supply and/or innervation is affected). A **fasciotomy** (incision of the overlying fascia or a septum) may be performed to relieve the pressure in the compartment(s) concerned.

The **common fibular nerve** (Fig. 5.19*C*)—the lateral, smaller terminal branch of the sciatic nerve—begins at the superior angle of the popliteal fossa and follows closely the medial border of the biceps femoris and its tendon along the superolateral boundary of the popliteal fossa. The common fibular nerve leaves the fossa by passing superficial to the lateral head of the gastrocnemius and then passes over the posterior aspect of the head of the fibula. The common fibular nerve winds around the fibular neck, where it is vulnerable to injury. Here it divides into its terminal branches, the superficial and deep fibular nerves. The most inferior branches of the *posterior cutaneous nerve of the thigh* supply the skin that overlies the popliteal fossa.

Leg

The leg contains the *tibia* and *fibula,* bones that connect the knee and ankle. The tibia, the weight-bearing bone, is larger and stronger than the fibula. The leg bones are connected by the *interosseous membrane.* The leg is divided into three compartments, anterior, lateral, and posterior, which are formed by the anterior and posterior *intermuscular septa,* the *interosseous membrane,* and the two leg bones (Fig. 5.19).

Anterior Compartment of Leg

The anterior compartment, or dorsiflexor (*extensor) compartment*) is located anterior to the *interosseous membrane,* between the lateral surface of the tibial shaft and the medial surface of the fibular shaft. The anterior compartment is bounded anteriorly by the deep fascia of the leg and skin. Inferiorly, two band-like thickenings of the deep fascia form retinacula that bind the tendons of the anterior compartment muscles, preventing them from bow stringing anteriorly during dorsiflexion of the ankle joint. The **superior extensor retinaculum** is a strong, broad band of deep fascia (Fig. 5.21*A* & *C*) passing from the fibula to the tibia, proximal to the malleoli. The **inferior extensor retinaculum**, a Y-shaped band of deep fascia, attaches laterally to the anterosuperior surface of the calcaneus. It forms a strong loop around the tendons of the fibularis tertius and extensor digitorum longus muscles. The four muscles in the anterior compartment are (Figs. 5.19 and 5.21)

- Tibialis anterior.
- Extensor digitorum longus.
- Extensor hallucis longus.
- Fibularis tertius.

These muscles are mainly dorsiflexors of the ankle joint and extensors of the toes (Table 5.10).

The **deep fibular nerve**, one of the two terminal branches of the common fibular nerve, is the nerve of the anterior compartment (Fig. 5.21*C*; Table 5.8). The deep fibular nerve arises between the fibularis longus muscle and the neck of the fibula. After entering the compartment, the nerve accompanies the anterior tibial artery.

The **anterior tibial artery** supplies structures in the anterior compartment (Fig. 5.21*C*; Table 5.9). The smaller

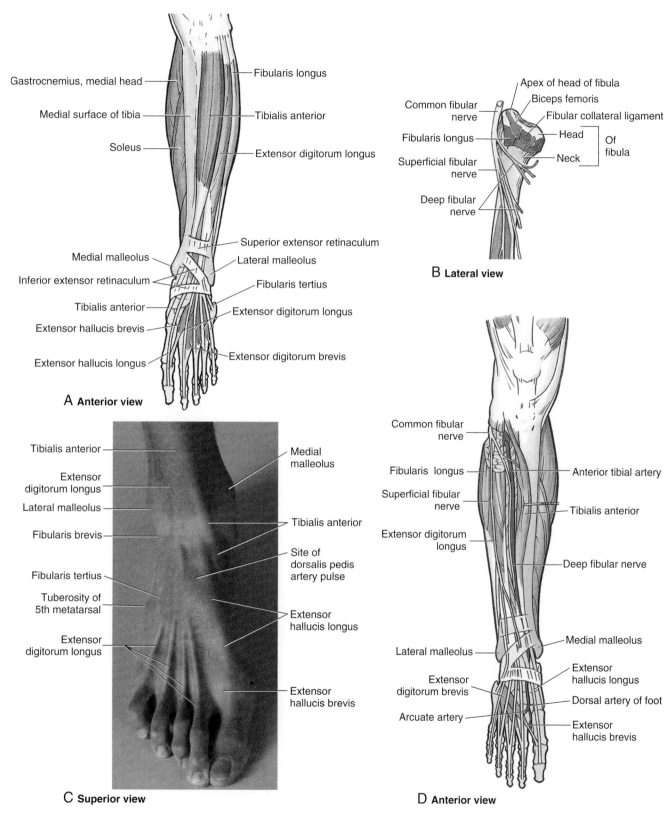

Figure 5.21. Anterior compartment of leg and dorsum of foot. The muscles (**A**), nerves (**B**), surface anatomy (**C**), and vessels (**D**) are shown. The muscles have been separated to display these structures.

A Anterior view

- Gastrocnemius, medial head
- Medial surface of tibia
- Soleus
- Medial malleolus
- Inferior extensor retinaculum
- Tibialis anterior
- Extensor hallucis brevis
- Extensor hallucis longus
- Fibularis longus
- Tibialis anterior
- Extensor digitorum longus
- Superior extensor retinaculum
- Lateral malleolus
- Fibularis tertius
- Extensor digitorum longus
- Extensor digitorum brevis

B Lateral view

- Common fibular nerve
- Fibularis longus
- Superficial fibular nerve
- Deep fibular nerve
- Apex of head of fibula
- Biceps femoris
- Fibular collateral ligament
- Head
- Neck
- Of fibula

C Superior view

- Tibialis anterior
- Extensor digitorum longus
- Lateral malleolus
- Fibularis brevis
- Fibularis tertius
- Tuberosity of 5th metatarsal
- Extensor digitorum longus
- Medial malleolus
- Tibialis anterior
- Site of dorsalis pedis artery pulse
- Extensor hallucis longus
- Extensor hallucis brevis

D Anterior view

- Common fibular nerve
- Fibularis longus
- Superficial fibular nerve
- Extensor digitorum longus
- Lateral malleolus
- Extensor digitorum brevis
- Arcuate artery
- Anterior tibial artery
- Tibialis anterior
- Deep fibular nerve
- Medial malleolus
- Extensor hallucis longus
- Dorsal artery of foot
- Extensor hallucis brevis

Table 5.8 Nerves of the Leg

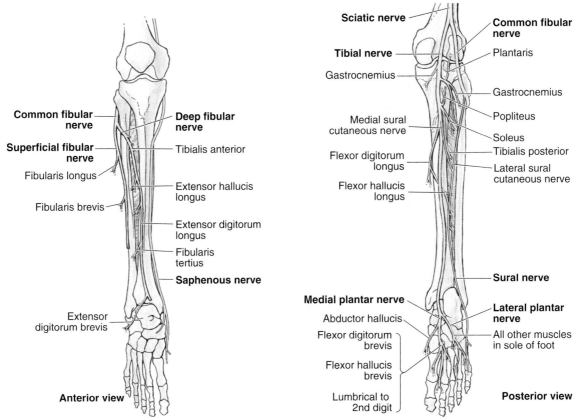

Anterior view

Posterior view

Nerve	Origin	Course	Distribution
Saphenous	Femoral nerve	Descends with femoral vessels through femoral triangle and adductor canal; then descends with great saphenous vein	Supplies skin on medial side of leg and foot
Sural	Usually arises from both tibial and common fibular nerves	Descends between heads of gastrocnemius; becomes superficial at middle of leg; descends with small saphenous vein; passes inferior to lateral malleolus to lateral side of foot	Supplies skin on posterior and lateral aspects of leg and lateral side of foot
Tibial	Sciatic nerve	Forms as sciatic bifurcates at apex of popliteal fossa; descends through popliteal fossa and lies on popliteus; runs inferiorly on tibialis posterior with posterior tibial vessels; terminates beneath flexor retinaculum by dividing into medial and lateral plantar nerves	Supplies posterior muscles of leg and knee joint
Common fibular		Forms as sciatic bifurcates at apex of popliteal fossa and follows medial border of biceps femoris and its tendon; passes over posterior aspect of head of fibula; then winds around neck of fibula deep to fibularis longus, where it divides into deep and superficial fibular nerves	Supplies skin on lateral part of posterior aspect of leg via its branch, the lateral sural cutaneous nerve; also supplies knee joint via its articular branch
Superficial fibular	Common fibular nerve	Arises between fibularis longus and neck of fibula; descends in lateral compartment of leg; pierces deep fascia at distal third of leg to become subcutaneous	Supplies fibularis longus and brevis and skin on distal third of anterior surface of leg and dorsum of foot
Deep fibular		Arises between fibularis longus and neck of fibula; passes through extensor digitorum longus and descends on interosseous membrane; crosses distal end of tibia and enters dorsum of foot	Supplies anterior muscles of leg, dorsum of foot, and skin of first interdigital cleft; sends articular branches to joints it crosses

Table 5.9 Arteries of the Leg

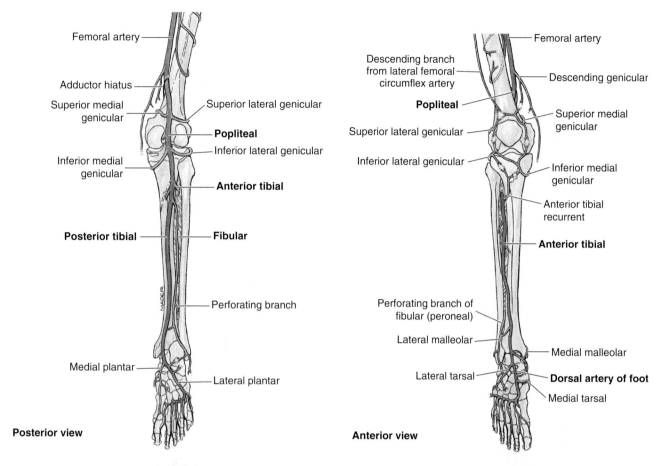

Posterior view

Anterior view

Artery	Origin	Course	Distribution
Popliteal	Continuation of femoral artery at adductor hiatus in adductor magnus	Passes through popliteal fossa to leg; ends at inferior border of popliteus muscle by dividing into anterior and posterior tibial arteries	Superior, middle, and inferior genicular arteries to knee
Anterior tibial	Popliteal artery	Passes into anterior compartment through gap in superior part of interosseous membrane; descends on this membrane between tibialis anterior and extensor digitorum longus	Anterior compartment of leg
Dorsal artery of foot (L. *dorsalis pedis*)	Continuation of anterior tibial artery distal to inferior extensor retinaculum	Descends anteromedially to first interosseous space; divides into plantar and arcuate arteries	Muscles on dorsum of foot; pierces first dorsal interosseous muscle as deep plantar artery to contribute to formation of plantar arch
Posterior tibial	Popliteal	Passes through posterior compartment of leg; terminates distal to flexor retinaculum by dividing into medial and lateral plantar arteries	Posterior and lateral compartments of leg; circumflex fibular branch joins anastomoses around knee; nutrient artery passes to tibia
Fibular	Posterior tibial	Descends in posterior compartment adjacent to posterior intermuscular septum	Posterior compartment of leg: perforating branches supply lateral compartment of leg

Injury to Common Fibular Nerve

The common fibular nerve is the most commonly injured nerve in the lower limb, mainly because it winds superficially around the neck of the fibula, leaving it vulnerable to direct trauma. This nerve may also be severed during fracture of the fibular neck or severely stretched when the knee joint is injured or dislocated. *Severance of the common fibular nerve* results in paralysis of all muscles in the anterior and lateral compartments of the leg. The loss of dorsiflexion of the ankle causes *footdrop,* which is further exacerbated by unopposed inversion of the foot. The toes do not clear the ground during the swing phase of walking. To compensate for this problem, the individual may adopt (1) a *waddling gait,* in which the individual leans to the side opposite the long limb, "hiking " the hip; (2) a *swing-out gait,* in which the long limb is swung out laterally (abducted) to allow the toes to clear the ground, or (3) a high–stepping *steppage gait,* in which extra flexion at the hip and knee raises the foot to keep the toe from hitting the ground. In addition, the braking action normally produced by eccentric contraction of the dorsiflexors is also lost, resulting in the foot slapping down when the heel is planted, producing a distinctive "clop." There also is a variable loss of sensation on the anterolateral aspect of the leg and the dorsum of the foot.

Anterior Tibialis Strain (Shin Splints)

Shin splints, edema and pain in the area of the distal third of the tibia, results from repetitive microtrauma of the tibialis anterior. These splints are a mild form of anterior compartment syndrome. The pain commonly occurs during traumatic injury or athletic overexertion of muscles in the anterior compartment, especially the tibialis anterior. Muscles in the anterior compartment swell from sudden overuse and the edema and muscle–tendon inflammation reduce blood flow to the muscles. The swollen muscles are painful and tender to pressure.

---

terminal branch of the popliteal artery, the anterior tibial artery, begins at the inferior border of the popliteus muscle. It passes anteriorly through a gap in the superior part of the interosseous membrane and descends on the anterior surface of this membrane between the tibialis anterior and the extensor digitorum longus. It ends at the ankle joint, midway between the malleoli (Fig. 5.21*C*), where it becomes the **dorsal artery of the foot** (L. *arteria dorsalis pedis*).

Lateral Compartment of Leg

The **lateral compartment,** or *evertor compartment,* is bounded by the lateral surface of the fibula, the anterior and posterior intermuscular septa, and the deep fascia of the leg (Fig. 5.22; Table 5.10). The lateral compartment contains two muscles: the **fibularis longus** and **brevis** that pass posterior to the lateral malleolus.

The **superficial fibular nerve,** the nerve in the lateral compartment, is a terminal branch of the common fibular nerve (Table 5.8). After supplying the two muscles, it continues as a cutaneous nerve, supplying the skin on the distal part of the anterior surface of the leg and nearly all the dorsum of the foot.

The lateral compartment of the leg does not have an artery coursing through it. The muscles are supplied proximally by perforating branches of the **anterior tibial artery** and distally by perforating branches of the **fibular artery** (Table 5.9). These perforating arteries have accompanying veins (L. *venae comitantes*).

Posterior Compartment of Leg

The **posterior compartment,** or plantarflexor compartment, is the largest of the three leg compartments. The posterior compartment and the *calf muscles* within it are divided into superficial and deep subcompartments/muscle groups by the **transverse intermuscular septum** (Fig. 5.19*B*). The tibial nerve and posterior tibial and fibular vessels supply both parts of the posterior compartment but run in the deep part, just deep (anterior) to the transverse intermuscular septum.

SUPERFICIAL MUSCLE GROUP IN THE POSTERIOR COMPARTMENT

The superficial muscle group, including the **gastrocnemius, soleus,** and **plantaris,** forms a powerful muscular mass in the calf (Fig. 5.23; Table 5.11). The two-headed **gastrocnemius** and the **soleus** share a common tendon, the **calcaneal tendon** (L. *tendo calcaneus,* Achilles tendon), which attaches to the calcaneus. Collectively, these two muscles form the three-headed **triceps surae** (L. *sura,* calf). The triceps surae elevates the heel and thus depresses the forefoot, generating as much as 93% of the plantarflexion force.

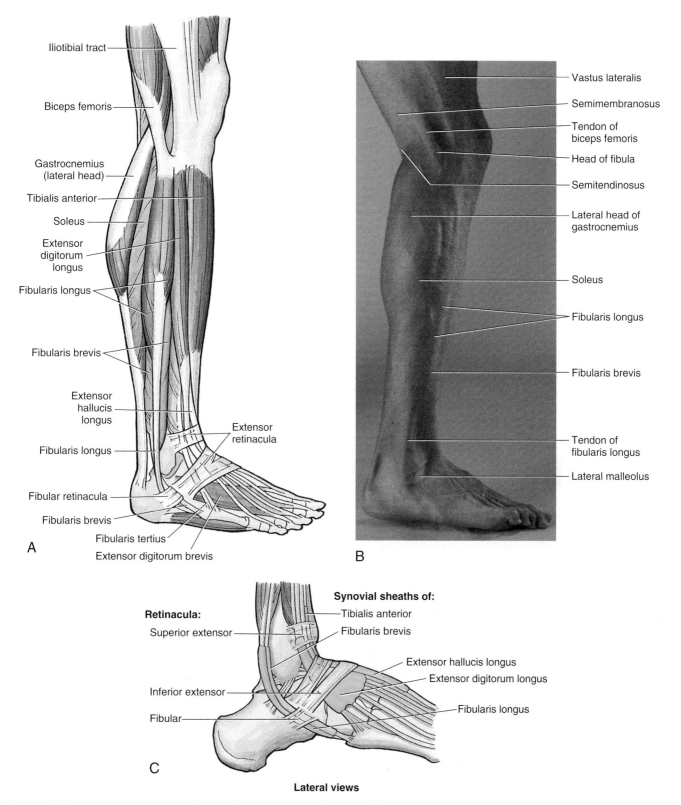

Figure 5.22. Lateral compartment of leg and lateral aspect of foot. A. The muscles of the leg and foot are identified. **B.** The surface anatomy is demonstrated. **C.** The retinacula and synovial sheaths of the tendons (*blue*) at the ankle are shown.

Table 5.10 Muscles of the Anterior and Lateral Compartments of the Leg

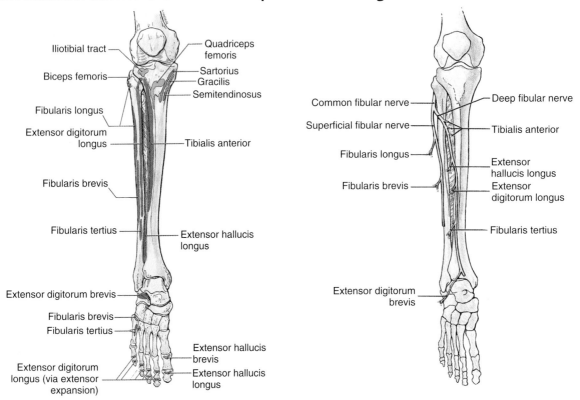

Anterior view of muscle attachments   Anterior view of nerves of leg

Muscle	Proximal Attachment	Distal Attachment	Innervation[a]	Main Action(s)
Anterior compartment				
Tibialis anterior	Lateral condyle and superior half of lateral surface of tibia and interosseous membrane	Medial and inferior surfaces of medial cuneiform and base of 1st metatarsal	Deep fibular nerve (**L4**, L5)	Dorsiflexes ankle; inverts foot
Extensor hallucis longus	Middle part of anterior surface of fibula and interosseous membrane	Dorsal aspect of base of distal phalanx of great toe (hallux)	Deep fibular nerve (**L5**, **S1**)	Extends great toe; dorsiflexes ankle
Extensor digitorum longus	Lateral condyle of tibia and superior three fourths of anterior surface of interosseous membrane	Middle and distal phalanges of lateral four digits		Extends lateral four digits; dorsiflexes ankle
Fibularis tertius	Inferior third of anterior surface of fibula and interosseous membrane	Dorsum of base of 5th metatarsal		Dorsiflexes ankle; aids in eversion of foot
Lateral compartment				
Fibularis longus	Head and superior two thirds of lateral surface of fibula	Base of 1st metatarsal and medial cuneiform	Superficial fibular nerve (**L5**, **S1**, S2)	Evert foot and weakly plantarflex ankle
Fibularis brevis	Inferior two thirds of lateral surface of fibula	Dorsal surface of tuberosity of base of 5th metatarsal		

[a]The spinal cord segmental innervation is indicated (e.g., "**L4**, L5" means that the nerves supplying the tibialis anterior are derived from the fourth and fifth lumbar segments of the spinal cord). Numbers in boldface (**L4**) indicate the main segmental innervation. Damage to one or more of the listed spinal cord segments or to the motor nerve roots arising from them results in paralysis of the muscles concerned.

Table 5.11 **Muscles of the Posterior Compartment of the Leg**

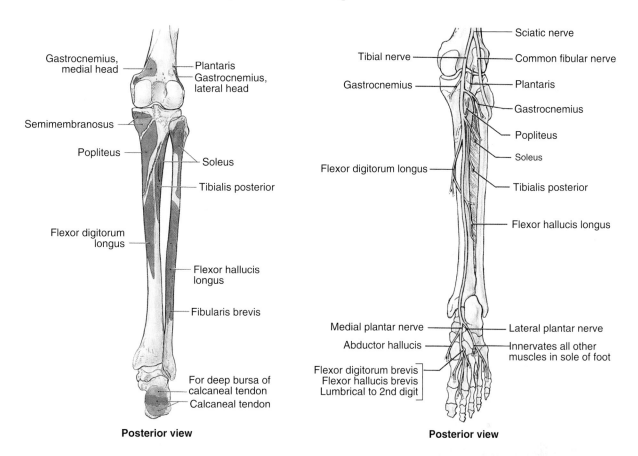

Posterior view

Posterior view

Muscle	Proximal Attachment	Distal Attachment	Innervation[a]	Main Action(s)
Superficial muscle group				
Gastrocnemius	*Lateral head:* lateral aspect of lateral condyle of femur *Medial head:* popliteal surface of femur, superior to medial condyle	Posterior surface of calcaneus via calcaneal tendon	Tibial nerve (S1, S2)	Plantarflexes ankle when knee is extended; raises heel during walking, and flexes leg at knee joint
Soleus	Posterior aspect of head of fibula, superior quarter of posterior surface of fibula, soleal line and medial border of tibia			Plantarflexes ankle; steadies leg on foot
Plantaris	Inferior end of lateral supracondylar line of femur and oblique popliteal ligament			Weakly assists gastrocnemius in plantarflexing ankle
Deep muscle group				
Popliteus	Lateral surface of lateral condyle of femur and lateral meniscus	Posterior surface of tibia, superior to soleal line	Tibial nerve (L4, L5, S1)	Weakly flexes knee and unlocks it

Table 5.11 Muscles of the Posterior Compartment of the Leg *(continued)*

Muscle	Proximal Attachment	Distal Attachment	Innervation[a]	Main Action(s)
Flexor hallucis longus	Inferior two thirds of posterior surface of fibula and inferior part of interosseous membrane	Base of distal phalanx of great toe (hallux)	Tibial nerve (**S2,** S3)	Flexes great toe at all joints; weakly plantarflexes ankle; supports medial longitudinal arch of foot
Flexor digitorum longus	Medial part of posterior surface of tibia inferior to soleal line and by a broad tendon to fibula	Bases of distal phalanges of lateral four digits		Flexes lateral four digits; plantarflexes ankle; supports longitudinal arches of foot
Tibialis posterior	Interosseous membrane, posterior surface of tibia inferior to soleal line, and posterior surface of fibula	Primarily to tuberosity of navicular; also to cuneiforms, cuboid and bases of 2nd–4th metatarsals	Tibial nerve (L4, L5)	Plantarflexes ankle; inverts foot

[a]The spinal cord segmental innervation is indicated (e.g., "**S2,** S3" means that the nerves supplying the flexor hallucis longus are derived from the second and third sacral segments of the spinal cord). Numbers in boldface (**S2**) indicate the main segmental innervation. Damage to one or more of the listed spinal cord segments or to the motor nerve roots arising from them results in paralysis of the muscles concerned.

The *soleus* is an antigravity muscle (the predominant plantarflexor for standing and strolling), which contracts antagonistically but cooperatively (alternately) with the dorsiflexor muscles of the leg to maintain balance. The soleus has a continuous proximal attachment in the shape of an inverted *U* to the posterior aspects of the tibia and fibula and the tendinous arch between them, the **tendinous arch of the soleus** (L. *arcus tendineus soleus*). The *plantaris* is a small muscle with a short belly and a long tendon; it is absent in 5–10% of people. Because of its minor role, the plantaris tendon can be removed for grafting (e.g., during reconstructive surgery of the tendons of the hand) without causing disability.

A *subcutaneous calcaneal bursa* lies between the skin and the calcaneal tendon, and a deep *bursa of the calcaneal tendon* (retrocalcaneal bursa) is located between the tendon and the calcaneus.

Inflammation and Rupture of Calcaneal Tendon

Inflammation of the calcaneal tendon constitutes 9–18% of running injuries. Microscopic tears of collagen fibers in the tendon, particularly just superior to its attachment to the calcaneus, result in *tendinitis,* which causes pain during walking. Calcaneal tendon rupture is probably the most severe acute muscular problem of the leg. After complete rupture of the tendon, passive dorsiflexion is excessive, and the person cannot plantarflex against resistance.

Calcaneal Tendon Reflex

The *ankle (jerk) reflex* is elicited by striking the calcaneal tendon briskly with a reflex hammer while the person's legs are dangling over the side of the examining table. This tendon reflex tests the S1 and S2 nerve roots. If the S1 nerve root is cut or compressed, the ankle reflex is virtually absent.

Gastrocnemius Strain

Gastrocnemius strain (tennis leg) is a painful calf injury resulting from partial tearing of the medial belly of the gastrocnemius at or near its musculotendinous junction. It is caused by overstretching the muscle by concomitant full extension of the knee and dorsiflexion of the ankle joint.

Calcaneal Bursitis

Calcaneal bursitis results from inflammation of the bursa of the calcaneal tendon located between the calcaneal tendon and the superior part of the posterior surface of the calcaneus. Calcaneal bursitis causes pain posterior to the heel and occurs commonly during long-distance running, basketball, and tennis. It is caused by excessive friction on the bursa as the calcaneal tendon continuously slides over it.

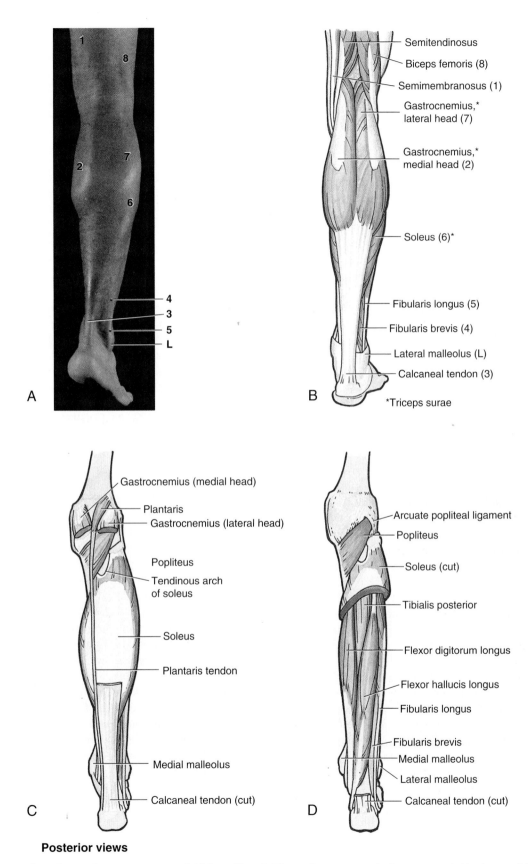

Posterior views

Figure 5.23. Muscles of posterior compartment of thigh and leg. A. The surface anatomy is demonstrated. *Numbers* are identified in part B. The gastrocnemius (**B**); soleus, popliteus, and plantaris (**C**); and deep muscles (**D**) are shown.

DEEP MUSCLE GROUP

Four muscles make up the deep group in the posterior compartment (Fig. 5.23; Table 5.11):

- Popliteus.
- Flexor digitorum longus.
- Flexor hallucis longus.
- Tibialis posterior.

The **popliteus** is a thin, triangular muscle in the floor of the popliteal fossa (Fig. 5.23*C* & *D*). The popliteus acts on the knee joint, whereas the other muscles act on the ankle and foot joints. The **flexor hallucis longus** is the powerful flexor of all the joints of the great toe. Immediately after the triceps surae has delivered the thrust of plantarflexion to the ball of the foot (the prominence of the sole underlying the heads of the 1st and 2nd metatarsals), the flexor hallucis longus delivers a final thrust via flexion of the great toe for the preswing (toe off) of the gait cycle. The **flexor digitorum longus** is smaller than the flexor hallucis longus, even though it moves four digits. It passes diagonally into the sole of the foot, superficial to the tendon of the flexor hallucis longus, and divides into four tendons, which pass to the distal phalanges of the lateral four toes. The **tibialis posterior**, the deepest muscle in the group, lies between the flexor digitorum longus and the flexor hallucis longus in the same plane as the tibia and fibula within the deep subcompartment. When the foot is off the ground, it can act synergistically with the tibialis anterior to invert the foot, their otherwise antagonistic functions canceling each other. However, the primary role of the tibialis posterior is to support or maintain (fix) the medial longitudinal arch during weight bearing; consequently the muscle contracts statically throughout the stance phase of gait.

The **tibial nerve** (L4, L5, and S1–S3) is the larger of the two terminal branches of the *sciatic nerve* (Fig. 5.24*A*). It runs through the popliteal fossa with the popliteal artery, and vein passing between the heads of the gastrocnemius. These structures pass deep to the tendinous arch of the soleus. The tibial nerve supplies all muscles in the posterior compartment of the leg (Table 5.8). At the ankle, the nerve lies between the flexor hallucis longus and the flexor digitorum longus. Posteroinferior to the medial malleolus, the tibial nerve divides into the medial and lateral plantar nerves. A branch of the tibial nerve, the *medial sural cutaneous nerve*, usually unites with the *sural communicating branch of the common fibular nerve* to form the **sural nerve** (Table 5.8). This nerve supplies the skin of the lateral and posterior part of the inferior third of the leg and the lateral side of the foot. Articular branches of the tibial nerve supply the knee joint and medial calcaneal branches supply the skin of the heel.

The **posterior tibial artery** (Fig. 5.24*A*; Table 5.9), the larger terminal branch of the popliteal artery, provides the

Posterior Tibial Pulse

The posterior tibial pulse can usually be palpated between the posterior surface of the medial malleolus and the medial border of the calcaneal tendon. Because the posterior tibial artery passes deep to the flexor retinaculum, it is important when palpating this pulse to have the person relax the retinaculum by inverting the foot. Failure to do this may lead to the erroneous conclusion that the pulse is absent.

blood supply to the posterior compartment of the leg and to the foot. It begins at the distal border of the popliteus and passes deep to the tendinous arch of the soleus. After giving off the **fibular artery**, its largest branch, the posterior tibial artery passes inferomedially on the posterior surface of the tibialis posterior. During its descent, it is accompanied by the tibial nerve and veins. The posterior tibial artery runs posterior to the medial malleolus. Deep to the flexor retinaculum and the origin of the abductor hallucis, the posterior tibial artery divides into *medial* and *lateral plantar arteries*, the arteries of the sole of the foot.

The fibular artery arises inferior to the distal border of the popliteus and the tendinous arch of soleus (Fig. 5.24*A*). It descends obliquely toward the fibula and then passes along its medial side, usually within the flexor hallucis longus. The fibular artery gives muscular branches to the muscles in the posterior and lateral compartments of the leg. It also gives rise to the *nutrient artery of the fibula*. Distally, the fibular artery gives rise to a perforating branch and terminal *lateral malleolar* and *lateral calcaneal branches*. The perforating branch pierces the *interosseous membrane* and passes to the dorsum of the foot. The **circumflex fibular artery** usually arises from the origin of the anterior or posterior tibial artery at the knee and passes laterally over the neck of the fibula to join the *genicular anastomosis* around the knee. The large **nutrient artery of the tibia** arises from the origin of the anterior or posterior tibial artery. It pierces the tibialis posterior and enters the nutrient foramen in the proximal third of the posterior surface of the tibia.

Foot

The **foot**, distal to the ankle, provides a platform for supporting the weight of the body when standing and has an

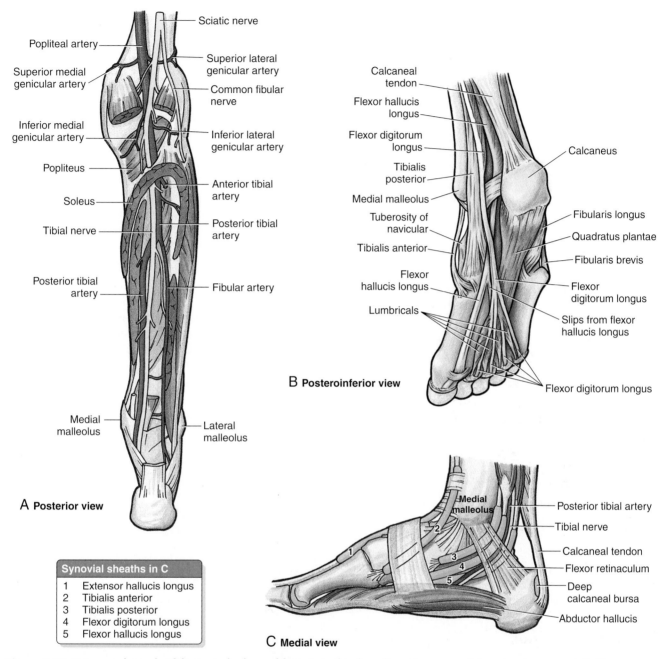

A Posterior view

Synovial sheaths in C
1   Extensor hallucis longus
2   Tibialis anterior
3   Tibialis posterior
4   Flexor digitorum longus
5   Flexor hallucis longus

B Posteroinferior view

C Medial view

Figure 5.24. Nerves and vessels of the posterior leg and foot. A. In this deep dissection, most of the soleus is cut away. **B.** The structures of the ankle and sole of the foot are shown. **C.** The retinacula and synovial sheaths of the tendons at the ankle are identified.

important role in locomotion. The skeleton of the foot consists of 7 tarsals, 5 metatarsals, and 14 phalanges (Fig. 5.25). The foot and its bones may be considered in terms of three anatomical and functional parts:

- The **hindfoot**: talus and calcaneus.
- The **midfoot**: navicular, cuboid, and cuneiforms.
- The **forefoot**: metatarsals and phalanges.

The regions of the foot include

- The **plantar region** (sole): the part contacting the ground.
- The **dorsal region of foot** (dorsum of the foot): the part directed superiorly.
- The **heel region** (heel): the sole underlying the calcaneus.
- The **ball of the foot**: the sole underlying the heads of the medial two metatarsals.

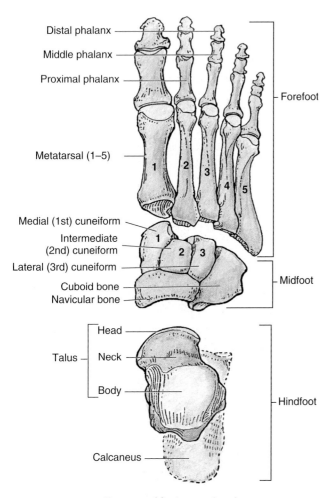

Dorsum of foot, superior view

Figure 5.25. Parts of foot.

superficial transverse metatarsal ligament. In the forefoot and midfoot, vertical intermuscular septa extend superiorly from the margins of the plantar aponeurosis toward the 1st and 5th metatarsals, forming three *compartments of the sole* (Figs. 5.26 and 5.27A):

- **Medial compartment of the sole**, covered superficially by *medial plantar fascia,* contains the abductor hallucis, flexor hallucis brevis, tendon of the flexor hallucis longus, and medial plantar nerve and vessels.
- **Central compartment of the sole**, covered by the *plantar aponeurosis,* contains the flexor digitorum brevis, flexor digitorum longus, quadratus plantae, lumbricals, adductor hallucis, distal part of tendon flexor hallucis longus, and lateral plantar nerve and vessels
- **Lateral compartment of the sole**, covered by the thinner *lateral plantar fascia,* contains the abductor and flexor digiti minimi brevis.

In the forefoot only, a fourth compartment, the **interosseous compartment of the foot**, contains the metatarsals, the dorsal and plantar interosseous muscles, and the deep plantar and metatarsal vessels.

Muscles of Foot

From the plantar aspect, the muscles of the sole are arranged in four layers within the compartments (Fig. 5.27; Table 5.12). The plantar muscles function primarily as a group during the support phase of stance, maintaining the arches of the foot. Concurrently, they are also able to refine further the ef-

The *great toe* (L. *hallux*) is also called the **1st toe** (L. *digitus primus*); the *little toe* (L. *digitus minimus*) is also called the **5th toe** (L. *digitus quintus*).

Deep Fascia of Foot

The **deep fascia** is thin on the dorsum of the foot, where it is continuous with the *inferior extensor retinaculum* (Fig. 5.21A). Over the lateral and posterior aspects, the deep fascia of the foot is continuous with the **plantar fascia**, the deep fascia of the sole, which has a thick central part (the **plantar aponeurosis**) and weaker medial and lateral parts (Fig. 5.27A). The plantar fascia holds parts of the foot together, helps protect the sole from injury, and helps support the longitudinal arches of the foot. The plantar aponeurosis arises posteriorly from the calcaneus and distally divides into five bands that become continuous with the fibrous digital sheaths that enclose the flexor tendons that pass to the toes. Inferior to the heads of the metatarsals, the aponeurosis is reinforced by transverse fibers forming the

Plantar Fasciitis

Straining and inflammation of the plantar aponeurosis, a condition called *plantar fasciitis,* may result from running and high-impact aerobics, especially when inappropriate footwear is worn. It causes pain on the plantar surface of the heel and on the medial aspect of the foot. Point tenderness is located at the proximal attachment of the plantar aponeurosis to the medial tubercle of the calcaneus and on the medial surface of this bone. The pain increases with passive extension of the great toe and may be further exacerbated by dorsiflexion of the ankle and/or weight bearing. If a *calcaneal spur* (abnormal bony process) protrudes from the medial tubercle, plantar fasciitis is likely to cause pain on the medial side of the foot when walking. Usually, a bursa develops at the end of the spur, which may become inflamed and tender.

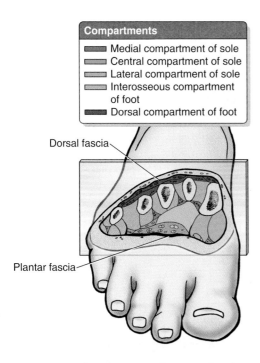

Compartments

■ Medial compartment of sole
■ Central compartment of sole
■ Lateral compartment of sole
■ Interosseous compartment of foot
■ Dorsal compartment of foot

Dorsal fascia

Plantar fascia

Transverse section, anterior view

Figure 5.26. Fascia and compartments of foot.

when the toes are extended. Both muscles on the dorsum of the foot help the long extensors to extend the toes.

Nerves of Foot

The *tibial nerve* divides posterior to the medial malleolus into the **medial** and **lateral plantar nerves** (Fig. 5.27C; Table 5.13). These nerves supply the intrinsic muscles of the foot, except for the extensor digitorum brevis and extensor hallucis brevis, which are supplied by the **deep fibular nerve**. The cutaneous innervation of the foot is supplied:

- Medially by the **saphenous nerve**, which extends distally to the head of the 1st metatarsal.
- Superiorly (dorsum of foot) by the **deep fibular nerve** (the web of skin between the contiguous sides of the 1st and 2nd toes) and the **superficial fibular nerve** (remainder of dorsum of foot).
- Inferiorly (sole of foot) by the **medial** and **lateral plantar nerves**; the common border of their distribution extends along the 4th metatarsal and digit.
- Laterally by the **sural nerve**, including part of the heel.
- Posteriorly (heel) by the **calcaneal branches of the tibial and sural nerves.**

forts of the long muscles, producing supination and pronation in enabling the foot to adjust to uneven ground. The muscles are of little importance individually because fine control of the individual toes is not important to most people.

The muscles on the dorsum of the foot are the **extensor digitorum brevis** and **extensor hallucis brevis** (Fig. 5.21A). These thin, broad muscles form a fleshy mass on the lateral part of the dorsum of the foot, anterior to the lateral malleolus. The extensor hallucis brevis is actually a part of the extensor digitorum brevis. Its small fleshy belly may be felt

Contusion of Extensor Digitorum Brevis

Clinically, knowing the location of the belly of the extensor digitorum brevis is important for distinguishing this muscle from abnormal edema. Contusion and tearing of the muscle fibers and associated blood vessels result in a *hematoma,* producing edema anteromedial to the lateral malleolus. Most people who have not seen this inflamed muscle assume they have a severely sprained ankle.

Sural Nerve Grafts

Pieces of the sural nerve are often used for nerve grafts in procedures such as repairing nerve defects resulting from wounds. The surgeon is usually able to locate this nerve in relation to the small saphenous vein. Because of variations in the level of formation of the sural nerve, the surgeon may have to make incisions in both legs and then select the better specimen.

Plantar Reflex

The **plantar reflex** (L4, L5, S1, and S2 nerve roots) is a myotatic (deep tendon) reflex. The lateral aspect of the sole is stroked with a blunt object, such as a tongue depressor, beginning at the heel and crossing to the base of the great toe. Flexion of the toes is a normal response. Slight fanning of the lateral four toes and dorsiflexion of the great toe is an abnormal response (*Babinski sign*), indicating brain injury or cerebral disease, except in infants. Because the corticospinal tracts (motor function), are not fully developed in newborns, a Babinski sign is usually elicited and may be present until children are 4 years of age.

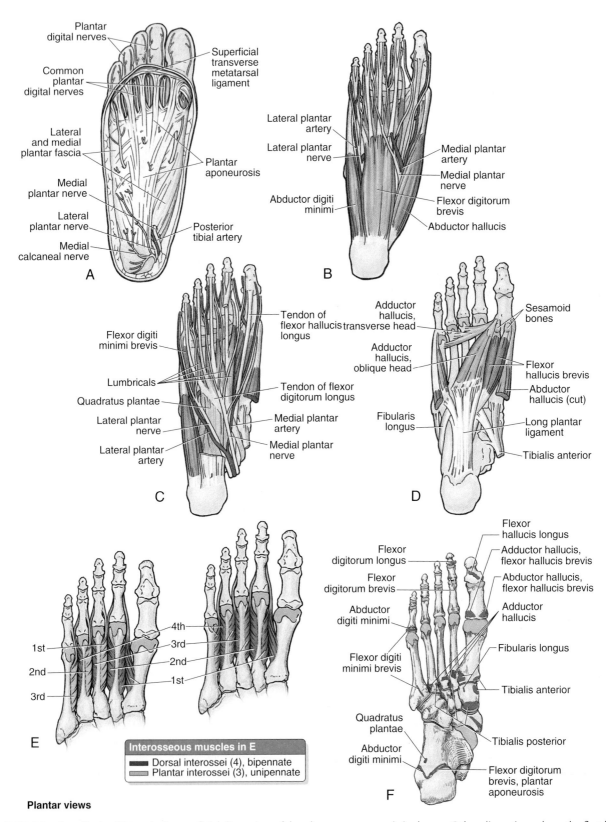

Plantar views

Figure 5.27. Muscles of sole of foot. A. A superficial dissection of the plantar aponeurosis is shown. Other dissections show the first layer (**B**), second layer (**C**), third layer (**D**), fourth layer (**E**), and muscle attachments (**F**).

Table 5.12 Muscles in the Sole of the Foot

Muscle	Proximal Attachment	Distal Attachment	Innervation[a]	Main Action(s)
First layer				
Abductor hallucis	Medial tubercle of tuberosity of calcaneus, flexor retinaculum, and plantar aponeurosis	Medial side of base of proximal phalanx of 1st digit	Medial plantar nerve (S2, **S3**)	Abducts and flexes 1st digit (great toe, hallux)
Flexor digitorum brevis	Medial tubercle of tuberosity of calcaneus, plantar aponeurosis, and intermuscular septa	Both sides of middle phalanges of lateral four digits		Flexes lateral four digits
Abductor digiti minimi	Medial and lateral tubercles of tuberosity of calcaneus, plantar aponeurosis, and intermuscular septa	Lateral side of base of proximal phalanx of 5th digit	Lateral plantar nerve (S2, **S3**)	Abducts and flexes 5th digit
Second layer				
Quadratus plantae	Medial surface and lateral margin of plantar surface of calcaneus	Posterolateral margin of tendon of flexor digitorum longus	Lateral plantar nerve (S2, **S3**)	Assists flexor digitorum longus in flexing lateral four digits
Lumbricals	Tendons of flexor digitorum longus	Medial aspect of expansion over lateral four digits	*Medial one:* medial plantar nerve (S2, **S3**) *Lateral three:* lateral plantar nerve (S2, **S3**)	Flex proximal phalanges; extend middle and distal phalanges of lateral four digits
Third layer				
Flexor hallucis brevis	Plantar surfaces of cuboid and lateral cuneiform	Both sides of base of proximal phalanx of 1st digit	Medial plantar nerve (S2, **S3**)	Flexes proximal phalanx of 1st digit
Adductor hallucis	*Oblique head:* bases of metatarsals 2–4 *Transverse head:* plantar ligaments of metatarsophalangeal joints	Tendons of both heads attach to lateral side of base of proximal phalanx of 1st digit	Deep branch of lateral plantar nerve (S2, **S3**)	Adducts 1st digit; assists in maintaining transverse arch of foot
Flexor digiti minimi brevis	Base of 5th metatarsal	Base of proximal phalanx of 5th digit	Superficial branch of lateral plantar nerve (S2, **S3**)	Flexes proximal phalanx of 5th digit, thereby assisting with its flexion
Fourth layer				
Plantar interossei (three muscles)	Bases and medial sides of metatarsals 3–5	Medial sides of bases of proximal phalanges of 3rd–5th digits	Lateral plantar nerve (S2, **S3**)	Adduct digits (2–4) and flex metatarsophalangeal joints
Dorsal interossei (four muscles)	Adjacent sides of metatarsals 1–5	*First:* medial side of proximal phalanx of 2nd digit *Second to fourth:* lateral sides of 2nd–4th digits		Abduct digits (2–4) and flex metatarsophalangeal joints

[a]The spinal cord segmental innervation is indicated (e.g., "S2, **S3**" means that the nerves supplying the abductor hallucis are derived from the second and third sacral segments of the spinal cord). Numbers in boldface (**S3**) indicate the main segmental innervation. Damage to one or more of the listed spinal cord segments or to the motor nerve roots arising from them results in paralysis of the muscles concerned.

Table 5.13 Nerves of the Foot

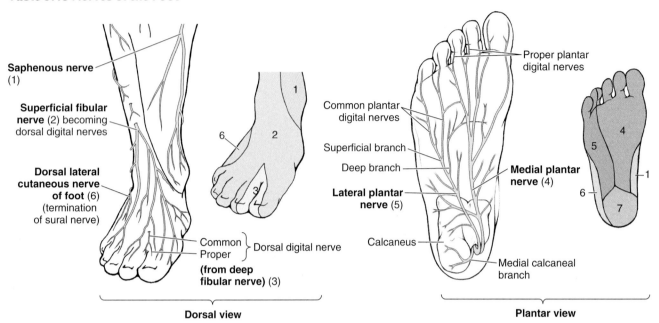

Dorsal view   **Plantar view**

Nerve[a]	Origin	Course	Distribution in Foot
Saphenous (1)	Femoral nerve	Arises in femoral triangle and descends through thigh and leg; accompanies great saphenous vein anterior to medial malleolus; ends on medial side of foot	Supplies skin on medial side of foot as far anteriorly as head of 1st metatarsal
Superficial fibular (2)	Common fibular nerve	Pierces deep fascia in distal third of leg to become cutaneous; then sends branches to foot and digits	Supplies skin on dorsum of foot and all digits, except lateral side of 5th and adjoining sides of 1st and 2nd digits
Deep fibular (3)	Common fibular nerve	Passes deep to extensor retinaculum to enter dorsum of foot	Supplies extensor digitorum brevis and skin on contiguous sides of 1st and 2nd digits
Medial plantar (4)	Larger terminal branch of tibial nerve	Passes distally in foot between abductor hallucis and flexor digitorum brevis; divides into muscular and cutaneous branches	Supplies skin of medial side of sole of foot and sides of first three digits; also supplies abductor hallucis, flexor digitorum brevis, flexor hallucis brevis, and first lumbrical
Lateral plantar (5)	Smaller terminal branch of tibial nerve	Passes laterally in foot between quadratus plantae and flexor digitorum brevis muscles; divides into superficial and deep branches	Supplies quadratus plantae, abductor digiti minimi, and flexor digiti minimi brevis; deep branch supplies plantar and dorsal interossei, lateral three lumbricals, and adductor hallucis; supplies skin on sole lateral to a line splitting 4th digit
Sural (6)	Usually arises from both tibial and common fibular nerves	Passes inferior to lateral malleolus to lateral side of foot	Lateral aspect of hindfoot and midfoot
Calcaneal branches (7)	Tibial and sural nerves	Pass from distal part of posterior aspect of leg to skin on heel	Skin of heel

[a]Numbers refer to the figure.

Arteries of Foot

The arteries of the foot are terminal branches of the anterior and posterior tibial arteries (Table 5.14), the dorsal and plantar arteries, respectively. The **dorsal artery of foot** (L. *arteria dorsalis pedis*), often a major source of blood supply to the forefoot, is the direct continuation of the anterior tibial artery. The dorsal artery begins midway between the malleoli (at the ankle joint) and runs anteromedially, deep to the inferior extensor retinaculum between the extensor hallucis longus and the extensor digitorum longus tendons on the dorsum of the foot. The dorsal artery gives off the **lateral tarsal artery** and then passes distally to the 1st interosseous space, where it gives off the **arcuate artery** and then divides into the **1st dorsal metatarsal artery** and a **deep plantar artery** (Table 5.14). The deep plantar artery passes deeply between the heads of the first dorsal interosseous muscle to enter the sole of the foot, where it joins the lateral plantar artery to form the **deep plantar arch.** The arcuate artery gives off the **2nd, 3rd,** and **4th dorsal metatarsal arteries**, which run to the clefts of the toes, where each of them divides into two **dorsal digital arteries.**

The sole of the foot has prolific blood supply from the **posterior tibial artery**, which divides deep to the flexor retinaculum. The terminal branches pass deep to the abductor hallucis as the *medial* and *lateral plantar arteries*, which accompany similarly named nerves. The **medial plantar**

artery supplies the muscles of the great toe and the skin on the medial side of the sole and has digital branches that accompany digital branches of the medial plantar nerve.

There are two neurovascular planes between the muscle layers in the sole of the foot: a superficial one between the 1st and 2nd muscular layers, and a deep one between the 3rd and 4th muscular layers.

Initially, the **lateral plantar artery** and nerve course laterally between the muscles of the 1st and 2nd layers of plantar muscles (Fig. 5.27 *B*). The **deep plantar arch** begins opposite the base of the 5th metatarsal as the continuation of the *lateral plantar artery*, coursing between the third and the fourth muscle layers. The arch is completed medially by union with the *deep plantar artery*, a branch of the dorsal artery of the foot. As it crosses the foot, the deep plantar arch gives rise to four **plantar metatarsal arteries;** three **perforating branches;** and many branches to the skin, fascia, and muscles in the sole (Table 5.14). The plantar digital arteries arise from the plantar metatarsal arteries near the base of the proximal phalanx, supplying adjacent digits. The more medial metatarsal arteries are joined by superficial digital branches of the medial plantar artery.

Venous Drainage of Foot

There are both superficial and deep veins in the foot. The deep veins consist of interanastomosing paired veins accompanying all the arteries internal to the deep fascia. The superficial veins are subcutaneous, are unaccompanied by arteries, and drain most of the blood from the foot. Dorsal digital veins continue proximally as **dorsal metatarsal veins**, which join to form the subcutaneous *dorsal venous arch*, proximal to which a **dorsal venous network** covers the remainder of the dorsum of the foot. Superficial veins from a **plantar venous network** drain around either the medial or the lateral border of the foot to converge with the dorsal venous arch and network to form medial and lateral marginal veins, which become the *great* and *small saphenous veins*, respectively.

Table 5.14 Arterial Supply to Foot

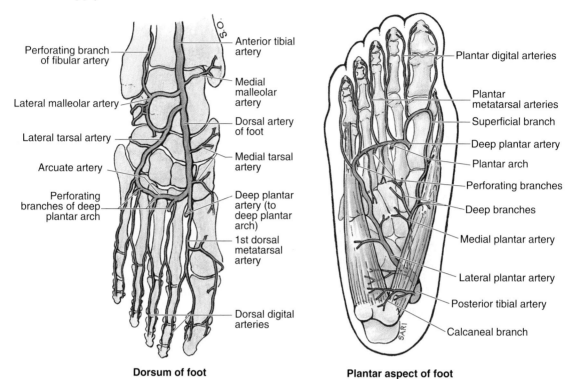

Dorsum of foot **Plantar aspect of foot**

Artery	Origin	Course and Distribution
Dorsum of foot		
Dorsal artery of foot (L. *dorsalis pedis*)	Continuation of anterior tibial artery distal to inferior extensor retinaculum	Descends anteromedially to 1st interosseous space; divides into plantar and arcuate arteries
Lateral tarsal artery	Dorsal artery of foot	Runs an arched course laterally beneath extensor digitorum brevis to anastomose with branches of arcuate artery
Arcuate artery		Runs laterally from 1st interosseous space across bases of lateral four metatarsals, deep to extensor tendons
Deep plantar artery		Passes to sole of foot; joins plantar arch
Metatarsal arteries		Run between metatarsals to clefts of toes where each vessel divides into two dorsal digital arteries; also connected to plantar arch and plantar metatarsal arteries by perforating arteries
1st	Deep plantar artery	
2nd–4th	Arcuate artery	
Dorsal digital arteries	Metatarsal arteries	Pass to sides of adjoining toes
Sole of foot		
Medial plantar artery	Posterior tibial artery	Runs deep to abductor hallucis; then between it and flexor digitorum brevis
Lateral plantar artery		Runs anterolaterally deep to abductor hallucis and flexor digitorum brevis; then arches medially to form deep plantar arch
Deep plantar arch	Continuation of lateral plantar artery	Begins opposite base of 5th metatarsal and is completed medially by deep plantar artery
Perforating arteries (three)	Deep plantar arch	Pass to dorsum of foot
Plantar metatarsal arteries (four)		Supply toes
Plantar digital arteries	Plantar metatarsal arteries	

Table 5.15 Muscle Action during the Gait Cycle

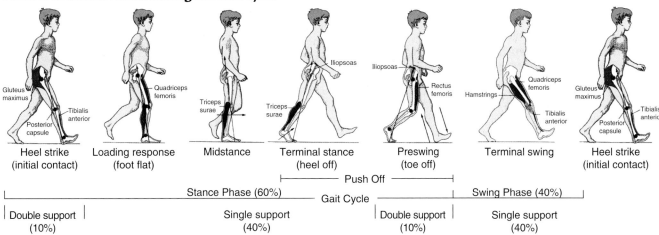

	Phase of Gait	Mechanical Goals	Active Muscle Groups
S T A N C E	Heel strike (initial contact)	Lower forefoot to ground	Ankle dorsiflexors (eccentric contraction)
		Continue deceleration (reverse forward swing)	Hip extensors
		Preserve longitudinal arch of foot	Intrinsic muscles of foot
			Long tendons of foot
	Loading response (flat foot)	Accept weight	Knee extensors
		Decelerate mass (slow dorsiflexion)	Ankle plantarflexors
		Stabilize pelvis	Hip abductors
		Preserve longitudinal arch of foot	Intrinsic muscles of foot
			Long tendons of foot
	Midstance	Stabilize knee	Knee extensors
		Control dorsiflexion (preserve momentum)	Ankle plantarflexors (eccentric contraction)
P H A S E		Stabilize pelvis	Hip abductors
		Preserve longitudinal arch of foot	Intrinsic muscles of foot
			Long tendons of foot
	Terminal stance (heel off)	Accelerate mass	Ankle plantarflexors (concentric contraction)
		Stabilize pelvis	Hip abductors
		Preserve arches of foot; fix forefoot	Intrinsic muscles of foot
			Long tendons of foot
	Preswing (toe off)	Accelerate mass	Long flexors of digits
		Preserve arches of foot; fix forefoot	Intrinsic muscles of foot
			Long tendons of foot
		Decelerate thigh; prepare for swing	Flexor of hip (eccentric contraction)
S W I N G	Initial swing	Accelerate thigh, vary cadence	Flexor of hip (concentric contraction)
		Clear foot	Ankle dorsiflexors
	Midswing	Clear foot	Ankle dorsiflexors
G	Terminal swing	Decelerate thigh	Hip extensors (eccentric contraction)
P H A S E		Decelerate leg	Knee flexors (eccentric contraction)
		Position foot	Ankle dorsiflexors
		Extend knee to place foot (control stride); prepare for contact	Knee extensors

Modified from Rose J, Gamble JG: *Human Walking,* 2nd ed. Baltimore, Lippincott Williams & Wilkins, 1994.

Lymphatic Drainage of Foot

The lymphatics of the foot begin in the subcutaneous plexuses. The collecting vessels consist of superficial and deep lymphatic vessels, which follow the superficial veins and major vascular bundles, respectively. Superficial lymphatic vessels are most numerous in the sole. The *medial superficial lymphatic vessels* leave the foot medially along the *great saphenous vein* and accompany it to the *superficial inguinal lymph nodes* (Fig. 5.8A), located along the vein's termination, and then to the *deep inguinal lymph nodes*. The *lateral superficial lymphatic vessels* drain the lateral side of the foot and accompany the *small saphenous vein* to the popliteal fossa, where they enter the *popliteal lymph nodes* (Fig. 5.8C). The *deep lymphatic vessels* from the foot also drain into the popliteal lymph nodes. Lymphatic vessels from them follow the femoral vessels to the deep inguinal lymph nodes. All lymph from the lower limb then passes to the iliac lymph nodes.

Walking: The Gait Cycle

Locomotion is a complex function. The movements of the lower limb during walking on a level surface may be divided into alternating swing and stance phases. The **gait cycle** consists of one cycle of swing and stance by one limb. The **stance phase** begins with **heel strike**, when the heel strikes the ground and begins to assume the body's full weight, and ends with **push off** from the forefoot. The **swing phase** begins after push off, when the toes leave the ground, and ends when the heel strikes the ground. The swing phase occupies approximately 40% of the walking cycle and the stance phase, 60%. In running, the time and percentage of the gait cycle represented by the stance phase are reduced. Walking is a remarkably efficient activity, taking advantage of gravity and momentum so that a minimum of physical exertion is required. The muscle actions during the gait cycle are summarized in Table 5.15.

Joints of Lower Limb

The joints of the lower limb include the articulations of the pelvic girdle (lumbosacral joints, sacroiliac joints, and pubic symphysis), which are discussed in Chapter 3. The remaining joints of the lower limb are the hip joint, knee joint, tibiofibular joints, ankle joint, and foot joints.

Hip Joint

The **hip joint** forms the connection between the lower limb and the pelvic girdle. It is a strong and stable multiaxial ball and socket type of synovial joint. The femoral head is the ball, and the acetabulum is the socket (Fig. 5.28). The hip joint is designed for stability over a wide range of movement. During standing, the entire weight of the upper body is transmitted through the hip bones to the heads and necks of the femurs.

ARTICULAR SURFACES

The round **head of the femur** articulates with the cup-like acetabulum of the hip bone. The head is covered with **articular cartilage**, except for the pit or *fovea for the ligament of the femoral head*. The rim of the acetabulum consists of a semilunar articular part covered with articular cartilage, the **lunate surface of the acetabulum.** Because the depth of the acetabulum is increased by the fibrocartilaginous **acetabular labrum** (L. *labrum,* lip) and the **transverse acetabular ligament** (bridging the *acetabular notch*), more than half of the head fits within the acetabulum (Fig. 5.28). Centrally, a deep non-articular part, the **acetabular fossa**, is thin and formed mainly by the ischium.

JOINT CAPSULE

The external **fibrous layer of the joint capsule** attaches proximally on the hip bone to the bony rim of the acetabulum and the transverse acetabular ligament. Distally, it attaches to the femoral neck only anteriorly at the intertrochanteric line and at the root of the greater trochanter (Fig. 5.28). Posteriorly, the fibrous layer has an arched border that crosses the neck proximal to the intertrochanteric crest but is not attached to it (Fig. 5.29B). The joint capsule covers approximately the proximal two thirds of the neck of the femur posteriorly. A protrusion of the **synovial membrane** beyond the free posterior margin of the joint capsule onto the femoral neck forms a bursa for the obturator externus tendon.

Most fibers of the fibrous layer take a spiral course from the hip bone to the intertrochanteric line; some deep fibers, most marked in the posterior part of capsule, wind circularly around the neck, forming an **orbicular zone** (Fig. 5.29B). Thick parts of the fibrous layer form the ligaments of the hip joint, which pass in a spiral fashion from the pelvis to the femur. Extension winds the spiraling ligaments and fibers more tightly, constricting the capsule and drawing the femoral head tightly into the acetabulum.

The hip joint is reinforced (Fig. 5.29):

- *Anteriorly and superiorly* by the strong Y-shaped **iliofemoral ligament** (Bigelow ligament), which attaches to the anterior inferior iliac spine and acetabular rim proximally and the intertrochanteric line distally. The iliofemoral ligament prevents hyperextension of the hip joint during

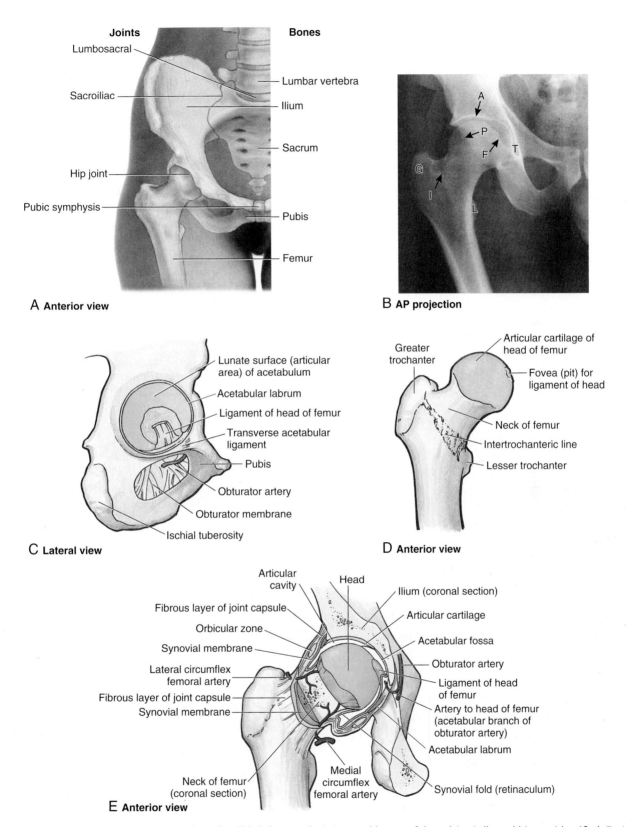

Figure 5.28. Articular surfaces and blood supply of hip joint. A. The joints and bones of the pelvic girdle and hip are identified. **B.** A radiograph of the hip joint is shown. *A*, roof; *F*, fovea (pit) for the ligament of the femoral head; *G*, greater trochanter; *I*, intertrochanteric crest; *L*, lesser trochanter; *P*, posterior rim of the acetabulum; *T*, "teardrop" appearance caused by superimposition of structures at the inferior margin of the acetabulum. **C.** The hip bone and associated structures are defined. **D.** The proximal femur is shown. **E.** The blood supply of the head and neck of the femur is detailed. A section of bone has been removed from the femoral neck.

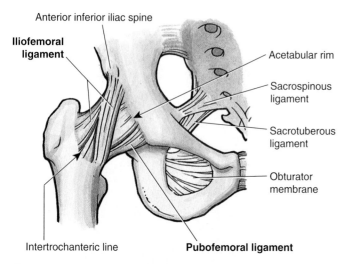

A **Anterior view**

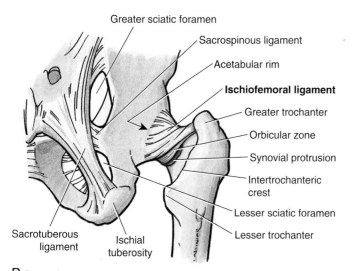

B **Posterior view**

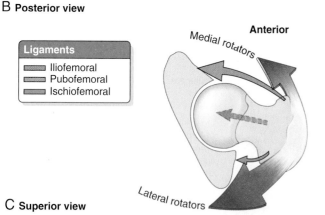

C **Superior view**

Figure 5.29. Ligaments of hip joint. The iliofemoral and pub-ofemoral (**A**) and ischiofemoral (**B**) ligaments are shown. **C.** This transverse section through the right hip joint demonstrates the re-ciprocal pull of the medial and lateral rotators (*reddish brown arrows*) and the intrinsic ligaments of the hip joint (see key). Relative strengths are indicated by arrow width.

standing by screwing the femoral head into the ace-tabulum.

- *Inferiorly and anteriorly* by the **pubofemoral ligament**, which arises from the obturator crest of the pubic bone and passes laterally and inferiorly to merge with the fi-brous layer of the joint capsule. This ligament blends with the medial part of the iliofemoral ligament and tightens during extension and abduction of the hip joint. The pubofemoral ligament prevents overabduction of the hip joint.

- *Posteriorly* by the weak **ischiofemoral ligament**, which arises from the ischial part of the acetabular rim and spi-rals superolaterally to the neck of the femur, medial to the base of the greater trochanter.

Both muscles (medial and lateral rotators of the thigh) and ligaments pull the femoral head medially into the ace-tabulum. They are reciprocally balanced when doing so (Fig. 5.29*C*).

The **synovial membrane of the hip joint** lines the fibrous layer as well as any intracapsular bony surfaces not lined with articular cartilage (Fig. 5.28*D*). Thus, where the fi-brous layer attaches to the femur, the synovial membrane reflects proximally along the femoral neck to the edge of the femoral head. The **synovial folds** (retinacula), which reflect superiorly along the femoral neck as longitudinal bands, contain subsynovial **retinacular arteries** (branches of the medial and a few from the lateral femoral circumflex artery), which supply the head and neck of the femur. The **ligament of the head of femur**, primarily a synovial fold conducting a blood vessel, is weak and of little importance in strengthening the hip joint (Fig. 5.28*D*). Its wide end at-taches to the margins of the acetabular notch and the *trans-verse acetabular ligament;* its narrow end attaches to the fe-mur at the *fovea for the ligament of the head.* Usually, the ligament contains a small artery to the head of the femur. A fat-pad in the acetabular fossa fills the part of the fossa that is not occupied by the ligament of the femoral head. Both the ligament and the fat-pad are covered with synovial membrane.

HIP MOVEMENTS

Hip movements are flexion–extension, abduction–adduc-tion, medial–lateral rotation, and circumduction (Fig. 5.30; Table 5.16). Movements of the trunk at the hip joints are also important, such as those occurring when a person lifts the trunk from the supine position during sit-ups or keeps the pelvis level when one foot is off the ground. The degree of flexion and extension possible at the hip joint depends on the position of the knee. If the knee is flexed relaxing the hamstrings, the thigh can be actively flexed until it almost reaches the anterior abdominal wall. Not all this movement

Functional groups of muscles
acting at hip joint

Flexors
Iliopsoas Sartorius Tensor of fascia lata Rectus femoris Pectineus Adductor longus Adductor brevis Adductor magnus, anterior part Gracilis
Adductors
Adductor longus Adductor brevis Adductor magnus Gracilis Pectineus Obturator externus
Lateral rotators
Obturator externus Obturator internus Gemelli Piriformis Quadratus femoris Gluteus maximus
Extensors

Hamstrings:
    Semitendinosus
    Semimembranosus
    Long head of biceps femoris
Adductor magnus, posterior part
Gluteus maximus

Abductors
Gluteus medius Gluteus minimus Tensor of fascia lata
Medial rotators
Gluteus medius } Gluteus minimus } Anterior parts Tensor of fascia lata

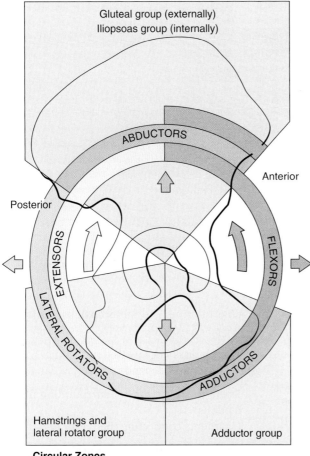

Circular Zones

The zones represent the position of origin of the functional groups relative to the center of the femoral head in the acetabulum (point of rotation). Pull is applied on the femur (femoral trochanters or shaft) from these positions.

Colored Arrows

The arrows show the direction of rotation of the femoral head caused by activity of the functional groups.

Figure 5.30. Lateral view of hip joint. The relative positions of the muscles producing the movements of the joint and the direction of the movement are demonstrated.

occurs at the hip joint; some results from flexion of the vertebral column. During extension of the hip joint, the fibrous layer of the joint capsule, especially the iliofemoral ligament, is taut; therefore, the hip can usually be extended only slightly beyond the vertical except by movement of the bony pelvis (flexion of the lumbar vertebrae). Abduction of the hip joint is usually somewhat freer than adduction. Lateral rotation is much more powerful than medial rotation.

BLOOD SUPPLY

The arteries supplying the hip joint are the (Fig. 5.28D):

- **Medial** and **lateral circumflex femoral arteries**, which are usually branches of the *deep artery of thigh* but occasionally branches of the femoral artery. The main blood supply is from the retinacular arteries arising as branches from the circumflex femoral arteries (especially the *medial circumflex femoral artery*).

Table 5.16 Structures Limiting the Movements of the Hip Joint

Movement	Limiting Structures
Flexion	Soft tissue apposition Tension of joint capsule posteriorly Tension of gluteus maximus
Extension	*Ligaments:* iliofemoral, ischiofemoral, and pubofemoral Tension of iliopsoas
Abduction	*Ligaments*: pubofemoral, ischiofemoral, and inferior band of iliofemoral Tension of hip adductors
Adduction	Soft tissue apposition (thighs) Tension of iliotibial band, superior joint capsule, superior band of iliofemoral ligament, and hip abductors (especially when contralateral hip joint is abducted or flexed)
Internal rotation	*Ligaments:* ischiofemoral and posterior joint capsule Tension of external rotators of hip joint
External rotation	*Ligaments:* iliofemoral, pubofemoral, and anterior joint capsule Tension of medial rotators of hip joint

Modified from Clarkson HM: *Musculoskeletal Assessment. Joint Range of Motion and Manual of Muscle Strength,* 2nd ed. Baltimore, Lippincott Williams & Wilkins, 2000.

- **Artery to the head of the femur,** a branch of the obturator artery that traverses the ligament of the head.

NERVE SUPPLY

Hilton's law states that the nerve supplying the muscles extending directly across and acting at a given joint also innervate the joint. Therefore, the nerve supply of the hip joint is from the:

- *Femoral nerve* or its muscular branches, anteriorly.
- *Obturator nerve,* inferiorly.
- *Superior gluteal nerve,* superiorly.
- *Nerve to quadratus femoris,* posteriorly.

Knee Joint

The knee is primarily a hinge type of synovial joint, allowing flexion and extension; however, the hinge movements are combined with gliding and rolling and with rotation about a vertical axis. Although the knee joint is well constructed, its function is commonly impaired when it is hyperextended (e.g., in body-contact sports such as hockey).

ARTICULAR SURFACES

The **articular surfaces of the knee joint** are characterized by their large size and their complicated and incongruent shapes (Fig. 5.31). The knee joint consists of three articulations:

- Two **femorotibial articulations (lateral** and **medial)** between the lateral and the medial femoral and tibial condyles.

- One intermediate **femoropatellar articulation** between the patella and the femur.

The fibula is not involved in the knee joint. The stability of the knee joint depends on the:

- Strength and actions of surrounding muscles and their tendons.
- Ligaments connecting the femur and tibia.

Of these supports, the muscles are most important; therefore, many sport injuries are preventable through appropriate conditioning and training. The most important muscle in stabilizing the knee joint is the large *quadriceps femoris,* particularly the inferior fibers of the vastus medialis and lateralis.

JOINT CAPSULE

The **joint capsule** is typical in consisting of an external *fibrous layer* (fibrous capsule) and an internal *synovial membrane* that lines all internal surfaces of the articular cavity not covered with articular cartilage. The fibrous layer has a few thickened parts that make up intrinsic ligaments but, for the main part, is thin. The fibrous layer attaches to the femur superiorly (Fig. 5.31*A*), just proximal to the articular margins of the condyles. Posteriorly, it encloses the condyles and the *intercondylar fossa.* The fibrous layer has an opening posterior to the lateral tibial condyle to allow the popliteus tendon to pass out of the joint capsule to attach to the tibia. Inferiorly, the fibrous layer attaches to the margin of the articular surface of the tibia (tibial plateau), except where the popliteus tendon crosses the bone. The quadriceps tendon, patella, and patellar ligament serve as a cap-

Fractures of the Femoral Neck ("Hip Fractures")

Fracture of the neck of the femur often disrupts the blood supply to the head of the femur. The medial circumflex femoral artery supplies most of the blood to the head and neck of the femur. Its retinacular arteries often are torn when the femoral neck is fractured or the hip joint is dislocated. In some cases, the blood supplied to the femoral head through the artery to the ligament of the femoral head may be the only remaining source of blood to the proximal fragment. This artery is frequently inadequate for maintaining the femoral head; consequently, the fragment may undergo *aseptic vascular necrosis*. These fractures are especially common in individuals > 60 years, especially in women because their femoral necks are often weak and brittle as a result of *osteoporosis*.

Surgical Hip Replacement

The hip joint is subject to severe traumatic injury and degenerative disease. *Osteoarthritis of the hip joint*, characterized by pain, edema, limitation of motion, and erosion of articular cartilage, is a common cause of disability. During hip replacement, a metal prosthesis anchored to the person's femur by bone cement replaces the femoral head and neck (Fig. B5.6). A plastic socket is cemented to the hip bone to replace the acetabulum.

Dislocation of Hip Joint

Congenital dislocation of the hip joint is common, occurring in approximately 1.5 per 1000 live births; it affects more girls and is bilateral in approximately half the cases. Dislocation occurs when the femoral head is not properly located in the acetabulum. The affected limb appears (and functions as if) shorter because the dislocated femoral head is more superior than on the normal side,

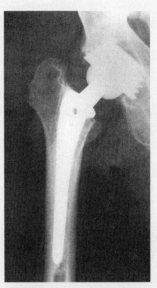

Figure B5.6 Hip prosthesis.

resulting in a positive *Trendelenburg sign* (hip appears to drop to one side during walking). Inability to abduct the thigh is characteristic of congenital dislocation.

Acquired dislocation of the hip joint is uncommon because this joint is so strong and stable. Nevertheless, dislocation may occur during an automobile accident when the hip is flexed, adducted, and medially rotated, the usual position of the lower limb when a person is riding in a car. Posterior dislocations are most common. The fibrous layer of the joint capsule ruptures inferiorly and posteriorly, allowing the femoral head to pass through the tear in the capsule and over the posterior margin of the acetabulum onto the lateral surface of the ilium, shortening and medially rotating the affected limb. Because of the close relationship of the *sciatic nerve* to the hip joint, it may be injured (stretched and/or compressed) during posterior dislocation or fracture–dislocation of the hip joint.

sule anteriorly—that is, the fibrous layer is continuous with the lateral and medial margins of these structures (Fig. 5.31*A*).

The extensive *synovial membrane* lines the internal aspect of the fibrous capsule and attaches to the periphery of the patella and the edges of the *menisci*. It lines the fibrous layer laterally and medially, but centrally it becomes separated from the fibrous layer. The synovial membrane reflects from the posterior aspect of the joint anteriorly into

the intercondylar region, covering the cruciate ligaments and the **infrapatellar fat-pad**, so they are excluded from the articular cavity (Fig. 5.32*A*). This creates a median infrapatellar synovial fold, a vertical fold of synovial membrane that approaches the posterior aspect of the patella. Thus it almost subdivides the articular cavity into right and left femorotibial articular cavities. Fat-filled lateral and medial alar folds cover the inner surface of the fat-pads that occupy the space on each side of the patellar ligament internal to

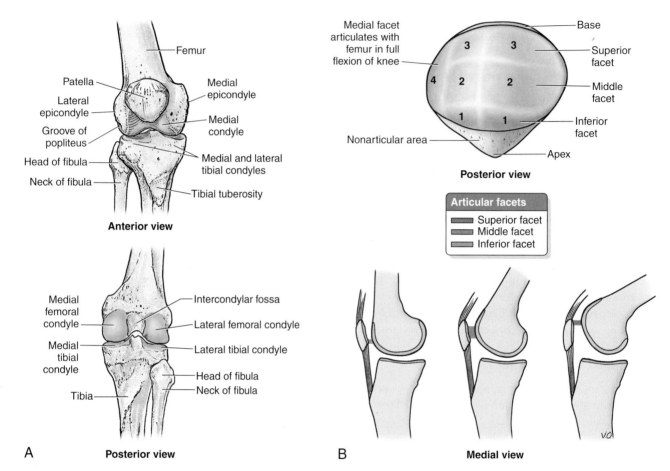

Figure 5.31. Bones of right knee joint. A. The bony landmarks are defined. **B.** The articular surfaces of the patella (*top*) and positions of the patella during knee movements (*bottom*) are shown.

the fibrous layer. Superior to the patella, the knee joint cavity extends deep to the vastus intermedius as the **suprapatellar bursa.** The synovial membrane of the joint capsule is continuous with the synovial lining of this bursa. Muscle slips deep to the vastus intermedius form the *articular muscle of the knee,* which attaches to the synovial membrane and retracts the bursa during extension of the knee.

LIGAMENTS

The joint capsule is strengthened by five extracapsular or capsular (intrinsic) ligaments (Fig. 5.32): patellar ligament, fibular collateral ligament, tibial collateral ligament, oblique popliteal ligament, and arcuate popliteal ligament.

The **patellar ligament,** the distal part of the quadriceps tendon, is a strong, thick fibrous band passing from the apex and adjoining margins of the patella to the tibial tuberosity. Laterally, it receives the *medial and lateral patellar retinacula,* aponeurotic expansions of the vastus medialis and lateralis and overlying deep fascia. The retinacula play an important role in maintaining alignment of the patella relative to the patellar articular surface of the femur.

The *collateral ligaments of the knee* are taut when the knee is fully extended; but as flexion proceeds, they become increasingly slack, permitting rotation at the knee.

The **fibular collateral ligament** (FCL), rounded and cord-like, is strong. It extends inferiorly from the lateral epicondyle of femur to the lateral surface of the head of the fibula (Fig. 5.32B & C). The tendon of the popliteus passes deep to the FCL, separating it from the lateral meniscus. The tendon of the biceps femoris is split into two parts by this ligament.

The **tibial collateral ligament** (TCL) is a strong flat band that extends from the medial epicondyle of the femur to the medial condyle and superior part of the medial surface of the tibia. At its midpoint, the deep fibers of the TCL are firmly attached to the medial meniscus.

The **oblique popliteal ligament** is a reflected expansion of the tendon of the semimembranosus that strengthens the joint capsule posteriorly. It arises posterior to the medial tibial condyle and passes superolaterally to attach to the central part of the posterior aspect of the joint capsule.

The **arcuate popliteal ligament** strengthens the fibrous capsule posterolaterally (Fig. 5.23D). It arises from the pos-

Genu Valgum and Genu Varum

The femur is placed diagonally within the thigh, whereas the tibia is almost vertical within the leg, creating an angle, the **Q-angle,** at the knee between the long axes of the bones. The Q-angle is assessed by drawing a line from the ASIS to the middle of the patella and extrapolating a second (vertical) line through the middle of the patella and tibial tuberosity (Fig. B5.7A). The Q-angle is typically greater in adult females, owing to their wider pelves. A medial angulation of the leg in relation to the thigh, in which the femur is abnormally vertical and the Q-angle is

small, is a deformity called *genu varum* (bowleg) that causes unequal weight distribution (Fig. B5.7B). Excess pressure is placed on the medial aspect of the knee joint, which results in *arthrosis* (destruction of knee cartilage). A lateral angulation of the leg (Fig. B5.7C) in relation to the thigh (exaggeration of knee angle) is *genu valgum* (knock-knee). Consequently, in genu valgum, excess stress is placed on the lateral structures of the knee The patella, normally pulled laterally by the tendon of the vastus lateralis, is pulled even farther laterally when the leg is extended in the presence of genu varum so that its articulation with the femur is abnormal.

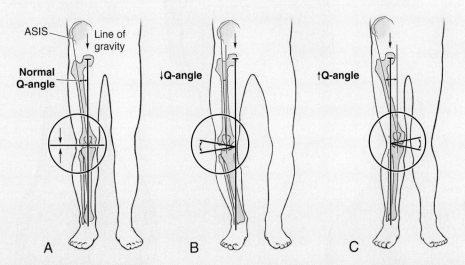

Figure B5.7. Alignment of lower limb bones. Normal alignment (**A**), genu varum (**B**), and genu valgum (**C**) are shown. *ASIS,* anterior superior iliac spine.

terior aspect of the fibular head, passes superomedially over the tendon of the popliteus, and spreads over the posterior surface of the knee joint.

The *intra-articular ligaments* within the knee joint consist of the cruciate ligaments and menisci. The popliteus tendon is also intra-articular during part of its course.

The **cruciate ligaments** (L. *crux,* a cross) join the femur and tibia, criss-crossing within the joint capsule but outside the articular cavity (Figs. 5.32 and 5.33). The cruciate ligaments cross each other obliquely like the letter X. During medial rotation of the tibia on the femur, the cruciate ligaments wind around each other; thus the amount of medial rotation possible is limited to about 10°. Because they become unwound during lateral rotation, nearly 60° of lateral rotation is possible when the knee is flexed

> 90°. The crossing-over point of the cruciate ligaments serves as the pivot for rotatory movements at the knee. Because of their oblique orientation, in every position one cruciate ligament, or parts of one or both ligaments, is tense.

The **anterior cruciate ligament** (ACL), the weaker of the two cruciate ligaments, arises from the anterior intercondylar area of the tibia, just posterior to the attachment of the medial meniscus (Fig. 5.33A). It extends superiorly, posteriorly, and laterally to attach to the posterior part of the medial side of the lateral condyle of the femur. The ACL has a relatively poor blood supply and limits posterior rolling of the femoral condyles on the tibial plateau during flexion, converting it to spin. It also prevents posterior displacement of the femur on the tibia and hyperextension of the

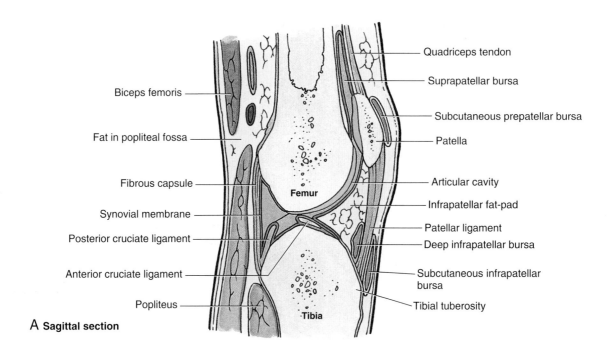

A Sagittal section

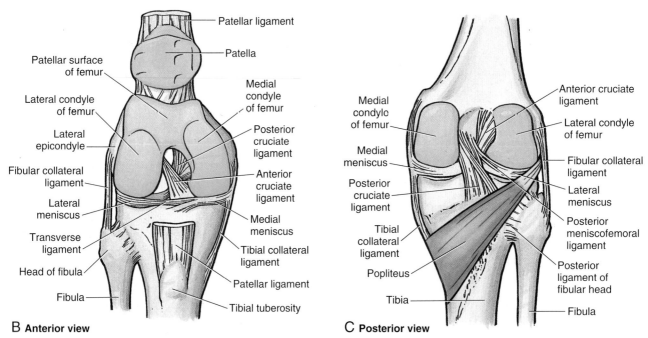

B Anterior view

C Posterior view

Figure 5.32. Relations and ligaments of knee joint.

knee joint. When the joint is flexed at a right angle, the tibia cannot be pulled anteriorly because it is held by the ACL.

The **posterior cruciate ligament** (PCL), the stronger of the two cruciate ligaments, arises from the posterior intercondylar area of the tibia (Fig. 5.33B). The PCL passes superiorly and anteriorly on the medial side of the ACL to attach to the anterior part of the lateral surface of the medial condyle of the femur. The PCL limits anterior rolling of the

femur on the tibial plateau during extension, converting it to spin. It also prevents anterior displacement of the femur on the tibia or posterior displacement of the tibia on the femur and helps prevent hyperflexion of the knee joint. In the weight-bearing flexed knee, the PCL is the main stabilizing factor for the femur (e.g., when walking downhill).

The **menisci of the knee joint** are crescentic plates of fibrocartilage on the articular surface of the tibia that deepen

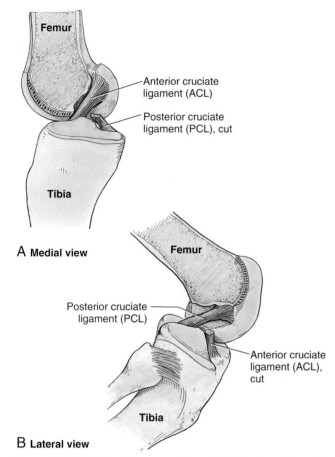

Figure 5.33. Cruciate ligaments of knee joint. In these views, the femur has been sectioned longitudinally and the near half has been removed with the proximal part of the corresponding cruciate ligament.

the surface and play a role in shock absorption (Fig. 5.34). The menisci are thicker at their external margins and taper to thin, unattached edges in the interior of the joint. Wedge-shaped in transverse section, the menisci are firmly attached at their ends to the *intercondylar area of the tibia*. Their external margins attach to the fibrous layer of the capsule of the knee joint. The **coronary ligaments** are capsular fibers that attach the margins of the menisci to the tibial condyles. A slender fibrous band, the **transverse ligament of knee**, joins the anterior edges of the menisci (Fig. 5.34A), allowing them to move together during knee movements. The **medial meniscus** is C-shaped and broader posteriorly than anteriorly. Its anterior end (horn) attaches to the anterior intercondylar area of the tibia, anterior to the attachment of the ACL. Its posterior end attaches to the posterior intercondylar area, anterior to the attachment of the PCL. The medial meniscus firmly adheres to the deep surface of the tibial collateral ligament. The **lateral meniscus** is nearly circular and is smaller and more freely movable than the medial meniscus. The tendon of the popliteus separates the lateral meniscus from the fibular collateral ligament. A

strong tendinous slip, the **posterior meniscofemoral ligament,** joins the lateral meniscus to the PCL and the medial femoral condyle (Fig. 5.32C).

MOVEMENTS OF THE KNEE JOINT

Flexion and extension are the main knee movements; some rotation occurs when the knee is flexed (Table 5.17). When the leg is fully extended with the foot on the ground, the knee passively "locks" because of medial rotation of the femur on the tibia. This position makes the lower limb a solid column and more adapted for weight bearing. When the knee is locked, the thigh and leg muscles can relax briefly without making the knee joint too unstable. To "unlock" the knee, the popliteus contracts, rotating the femur laterally about 5° on the tibial plateau so that flexion of the knee can occur. The menisci must be able to move on the tibial plateau as the points of contact between the femur and the tibia change.

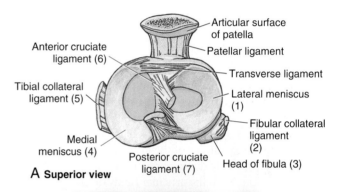

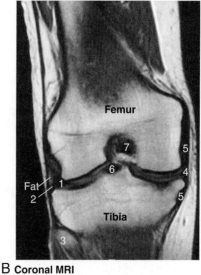

Figure 5.34. Cruciate ligaments and menisci of knee joint. A. The attachments to the tibial plateau are shown. The patella and quadriceps tendon are transected, and the patellar fragment and patellar ligament are reflected anteriorly. **B.** The numbers on this image of the right knee are defined in part A.

Table 5.17 Structures Limiting the Movements of the Knee Joint

Movement	Limiting Structures
Flexion (femoropatellar and femorotibial)	Soft tissue apposition posteriorly Tension of vastus lateralis, medialis, and intermedius Tension of rectus femoris (especially with hip joint extended)
Extension (femoropatellar and femorotibial)	*Ligaments:* anterior cruciate and posterior cruciate, fibular and tibial collateral, posterior joint capsule, and oblique popliteal ligament
Internal rotation (femorotibial with knee flexed)	*Ligaments:* anterior cruciate and posterior cruciate
External rotation (femorotibial with knee flexed)	*Ligaments:* fibular and tibial collateral

Modified from Clarkson HM: *Musculoskeletal Assessment. Joint Range of Motion and Manual of Muscle Strength,* 2nd ed. Baltimore, Lippincott Williams & Wilkins 2000.

BURSAE AROUND KNEE

There are at least 12 bursae around the knee joint because most tendons run parallel to the bones and pull lengthwise across the joint during knee movements (Table 5.18). The **subcutaneous prepatellar** and **infrapatellar bursae** are located at the convex surface of the joint, allowing the skin to be able to move freely during knee movements. Four bursae communicate with the articular cavity of the knee joint: *suprapatellar bursa* (deep to the distal quadriceps), *popliteus bursa, anserine bursa,* and *gastrocnemius bursa.*

ARTERIES AND NERVES

The arteries supplying the knee joint are the 10 vessels that form the periarticular *genicular anastomosis* around the knee: the genicular branches of the femoral, popliteal, and anterior and posterior recurrent branches of the anterior tibial recurrent and circumflex fibular arteries (Fig. 5.19D). The middle genicular branches of the popliteal artery penetrate the fibrous layer of the joint capsule and supply the cruciate ligaments, synovial membrane, and peripheral margins of the menisci. The nerves of the knee joint are articular branches from the femoral, tibial, and common fibular nerves and the obturator and saphenous nerves.

Tibiofibular Joints

The tibia and fibula are connected by two joints: the *superior tibiofibular joint* and the *tibiofibular syndesmosis* (inferior tibiofibular joint). In addition, an *interosseous membrane* joins the shafts of the two bones (Fig. 5.35A & B). Move-

ment at the proximal joint is impossible without movement at the distal one. The fibers of the interosseous membrane and all ligaments of tibiofibular articulations run inferiorly from the tibia to the fibula, resisting the downward pull placed on the fibula by most muscles attached to it. However, they allow slight upward movement of the fibula during dorsiflexion of the ankle.

The **superior tibiofibular joint** (proximal tibiofibular joint) is a plane type of synovial joint between the flat facet on the fibular head and a similar facet located posterolaterally on the lateral tibial condyle. The tense joint capsule surrounds the joint and attaches to the margins of the articular surfaces of the fibula and tibia. The joint capsule is strengthened by **anterior** and **posterior ligaments of fibular head**. The synovial membrane lines the fibrous capsule. Slight gliding movements occur during dorsiflexion of the foot. The arteries of the superior tibiofibular joint are from the inferior lateral genicular and anterior tibial recurrent arteries (Table 5.9). The nerves of the proximal tibiofibular joint are from the common fibular nerve and the nerve to the popliteus.

The **tibiofibular syndesmosis** is a compound fibrous joint (Fig. 5.35A & C). The integrity of this articulation is essential for stability of the ankle joint because it keeps the lateral malleolus firmly against the lateral surface of the talus. The strong **interosseous tibiofibular ligament** is continuous superiorly with the interosseous membrane and forms the principal connection between the distal ends of the tibia and fibula. The joint is also strengthened anteriorly and posteriorly by the **anterior** and **posterior tibiofibular ligaments**. The distal, deep continuation of the posterior inferior tibiofibular ligament, the **inferior transverse (tibiofibular) ligament**, forms a strong connection between the distal ends of the tibia (medial malleolus) and fibula (lateral malleolus) and the posterior "wall" of the malleolar mortise, for the trochlea of the talus. Slight movement of the joint occurs to accommodate the talus during dorsiflexion of the foot.

The arteries are from the perforating branch of the fibular artery and from the medial malleolar branches of the anterior and posterior tibial arteries (Table 5.9). The nerves are from the deep fibular, tibial, and saphenous nerves.

Ankle Joint

The **ankle joint (talocrural articulation)** is a hinge-type synovial joint. It is located between the distal ends of the tibia and fibula and the superior part of the talus (Fig. 5.36).

ARTICULAR SURFACES

The distal ends of the tibia and fibula (along with the inferior transverse part of the posterior tibiofibular ligament) form a *malleolar mortise* (deep socket) into which the pulley-shaped

Table 5.18 Bursae around the Knee

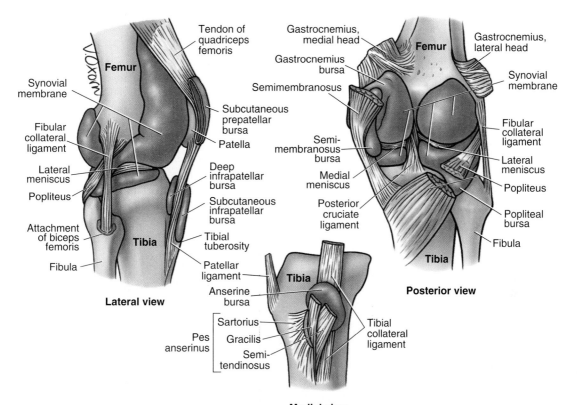

Lateral view

Posterior view

Medial view

Bursae	Locations	Comments
Suprapatellar	Between femur and tendon of quadriceps femoris	Held in position by articular muscle of knee; communicates freely with synovial cavity of knee joint
Popliteus	Between tendon of popliteus and lateral condyle of tibia	Opens into synovial cavity of knee joint inferior to lateral meniscus
Anserine	Separates tendons of sartorius, gracilis, and semitendinosus from tibia and tibial collateral ligament	Area where tendons of these muscles attach to tibia; resembles a goose's foot (L. *pes*, foot; L. *anserinus*, goose)
Gastrocnemius	Lies deep to proximal attachment of tendon of medial head of gastrocnemius	An extension of synovial cavity of knee joint
Semimembranosus	Between medial head of gastrocnemius and semimembranosus tendon	Related to distal attachment of semimembranosus
Subcutaneous prepatellar	Between skin and anterior surface of patella	Allows free movement of skin over patella during movements of leg
Subcutaneous infrapatellar	Between skin and tibial tuberosity	Helps knee withstand pressure when kneeling
Deep infrapatellar	Between patellar ligament and anterior surface of tibia	Separated from knee joint by infrapatellar fat-pad

Knee Joint Injuries

Knee joint injuries are common because the knee is a low-placed, mobile, weight-bearing joint and its stability depends almost entirely on its associated ligaments and muscles. To perform activities, the knee joint must be mobile; however, this mobility makes it susceptible to injuries. The most common knee injuries in contact sports are ligament sprains, which occur when the foot is fixed on the ground. If a force is applied against the knee when the foot cannot move, ligament injuries are likely to occur. The TCL and FCL are tightly stretched when the leg is extended, preventing disruption of the sides of the knee joint. The firm attachment of the TCL to the medial meniscus is of considerable clinical significance because tearing of this ligament frequently results in concomitant tearing of the medial meniscus. The injury is frequently caused by a blow to the lateral side of the extended knee or excessive lateral twisting of the flexed knee, which disrupts the TCL and concomitantly tears and/or detaches the medial meniscus from the joint capsule. This injury is common in athletes who twist their flexed knees while running (e.g., in football and soccer).

The ACL, which serves as a pivot for rotatory movements of the knee, is taut during flexion and may also tear subsequent to the rupture of the TCL, creating an

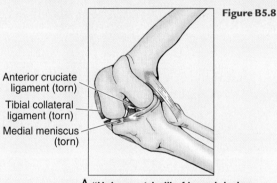

Figure B5.8

Anterior cruciate ligament (torn)
Tibial collateral ligament (torn)
Medial meniscus (torn)

A **"Unhappy triad" of knee injuries**

A **"Unhappy triad" of knee injuries**

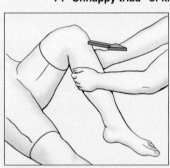

B **Anterior drawer sign (ACL)**

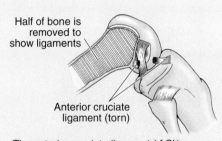

Half of bone is removed to show ligaments

Anterior cruciate ligament (torn)

The anterior cruciate ligament (*ACL*) prevents the femur from sliding posteriorly on the tibia and hyperextension of the knee and limits medial rotation of the femur when the foot is on the ground and the leg is flexed.

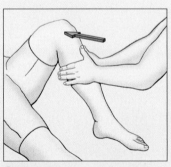

C **Posterior drawer sign (PCL)**

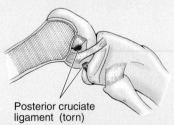

Posterior cruciate ligament (torn)

The posterior cruciate ligament (*PCL*) prevents the femur from sliding anteriorly on the tibia, particularly when the knee is flexed.

continued >

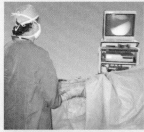

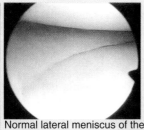

Normal lateral meniscus of the knee

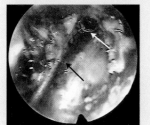

ACL graft (*black arrow*) with femoral anchoring screw visible (*white arrow*)

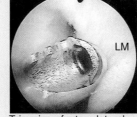

LM

Trimming of a torn lateral meniscus (*LM*)

D

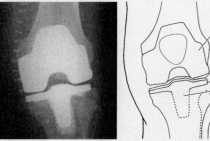

Metal femoral component

Plastic tibial component

Metal tibial component

E

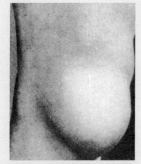

F Prepatellar bursitis

Figure B5.8 (continued)

rupture may occur when a person lands on the tibial tuberosity when the knee is flexed (e.g., when falling on the floor in basketball). PCL ruptures usually occur in conjunction with tibial or fibular ligament tears. The *posterior drawer sign,* in which the free tibia slides posteriorly under the fixed femur occurs as a result of PCL rupture.

Arthroscopy of the Knee Joint

Arthroscopy is an endoscopic examination that allows visualization of the interior of the knee joint cavity with minimal disruption of tissue (Fig. B5.8D). The arthroscope and one (or more) additional canula(e) are inserted through tiny incisions, known as portals. The second canula is for passage of specialized tools (e.g., manipulative probes or forceps) or equipment for trimming, shaping, or removing damaged tissue. This technique allows removal of torn menisci, loose bodies in the joint such as bone chips, and débridement (the excision of devitalized articular cartilaginous material in advanced cases of arthritis). Ligament repair or replacement may also be performed using an arthroscope.

Knee Replacement

If a person's knee is diseased, resulting from osteoarthritis, for example, an artificial knee joint may be inserted (*total knee replacement arthroplasty*) (Fig. B5.8E). The artificial knee joint consists of plastic and metal components that are cemented to the femoral and tibial bone ends after removal of the defective areas.

Bursitis in the Knee Region

Prepatellar bursitis (housemaid's knee) is usually a friction bursitis caused by friction between the skin and the patella. If the inflammation is chronic, the bursa becomes distended with fluid and forms a swelling anterior to the knee (Fig. B5.8F). *Subcutaneous infrapatellar bursitis* results from excessive friction between the skin and the tibial tuberosity; the edema occurs over the proximal end of the tibia. *Deep infrapatellar bursitis* results in edema between the patellar ligament and the tibia, superior to the tibial tuberosity.

The suprapatellar bursa communicates with the articular cavity of the knee joint; consequently, abrasions or penetrating wounds (e.g., a stab wound) superior to the patella may result in *suprapatellar bursitis* caused by bacteria entering the bursa from the torn skin. The infection may spread to the knee joint.

"unhappy triad" of knee injuries (Fig. B5.8A). *ACL rupture,* one of the most common knee injuries in skiing accidents, for example, causes the free tibia to slide anteriorly under the femur, a sign known as the *anterior drawer sign* (Fig. 5.8B). Although the PCL is strong, *PCL*

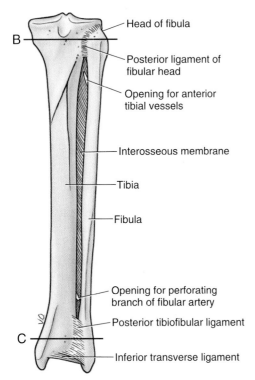

B — Head of fibula

Posterior ligament of fibular head

Opening for anterior tibial vessels

Interosseous membrane

Tibia

Fibula

Opening for perforating branch of fibular artery

Posterior tibiofibular ligament

C

Inferior transverse ligament

A Posterior view

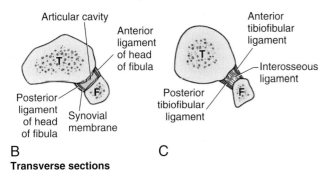

Articular cavity

Anterior ligament of head of fibula

Posterior ligament of head of fibula

Synovial membrane

B

Anterior tibiofibular ligament

Interosseous ligament

Posterior tibiofibular ligament

C

Transverse sections

Figure 5.35. Tibiofibular joints. A. The sections shown in parts B and C are identified. The superior tibiofibular joint (**B**) and tibiofibular syndesmosis (**C**) are shown. *F*, fibula; *T*, tibia.

trochlea of the talus fits. The trochlea (L. pulley) is the rounded superior articular surface of the talus. The medial surface of the lateral malleolus articulates with the lateral surface of the talus. The tibia articulates with the talus in two places:

- Its inferior surface forms the roof of the malleolar mortise, transferring the body's weight to the talus.
- Its medial malleolus articulates with the medial surface of the talus.

The malleoli grip the talus tightly as it rocks in the mortise during movements of the ankle joint. The grip of the malleoli on the trochlea is strongest during dorsiflexion of the foot because this movement forces the wider, anterior part of the trochlea posteriorly, spreading the tibia

and fibula slightly apart. This spreading is limited by the strong interosseous tibiofibular ligament and the anterior and posterior tibiofibular ligaments that unite the tibia and fibula. The ankle joint is relatively unstable during plantarflexion because the trochlea is narrower posteriorly and therefore lies loosely within the mortise.

JOINT CAPSULE

The joint capsule is thin anteriorly and posteriorly but is supported on each side by strong collateral ligaments. The fibrous layer of the capsule is attached superiorly to the borders of the articular surfaces of the tibia and malleoli and inferiorly to the talus. The synovial membrane lining the fibrous layer of the joint capsule extends superiorly between the tibia and the fibula as far as the interosseous tibiofibular ligament.

LIGAMENTS

The ankle joint is reinforced laterally by the **lateral ligament of the ankle**, which consists of three separate ligaments (Fig. 5.37):

- **Anterior talofibular ligament**, a flat, weak band that extends anteromedially from the lateral malleolus to the neck of the talus.
- **Posterior talofibular ligament**, a thick, fairly strong band that runs horizontally medially, and slightly posteriorly from the malleolar fossa of the fibula to the lateral tubercle of the talus.
- **Calcaneofibular ligament**, a round cord that passes posteroinferiorly from the tip of the lateral malleolus to the lateral surface of the calcaneus.

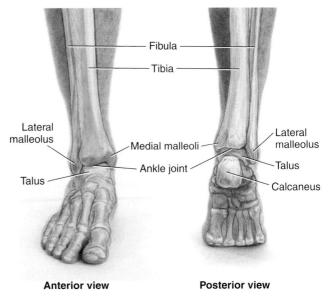

Fibula

Tibia

Lateral malleolus

Medial malleoli

Ankle joint

Talus

Lateral malleolus

Talus

Calcaneus

Anterior view   **Posterior view**

Figure 5.36. Bones of leg and ankle joint.

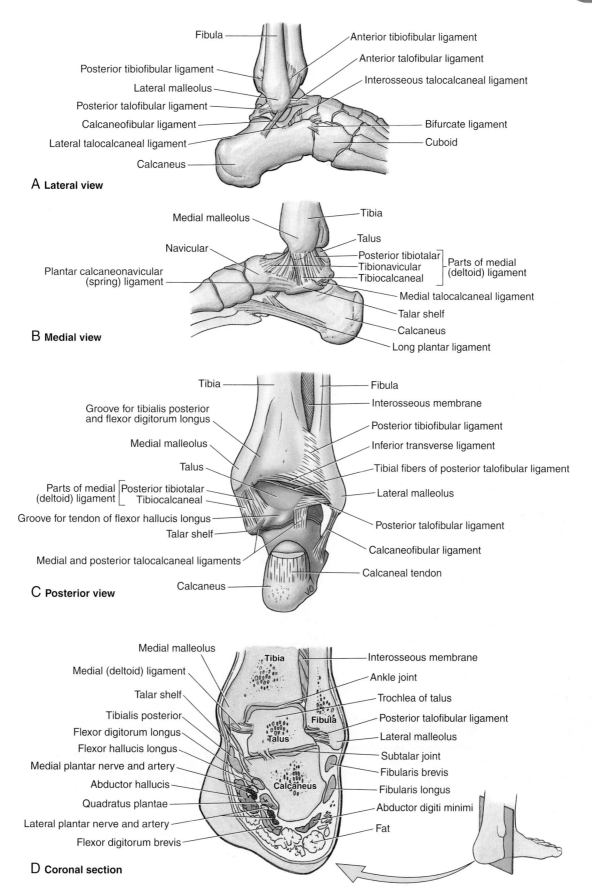

A **Lateral view**

Fibula
Anterior tibiofibular ligament
Posterior tibiofibular ligament
Anterior talofibular ligament
Lateral malleolus
Interosseous talocalcaneal ligament
Posterior talofibular ligament
Calcaneofibular ligament
Lateral talocalcaneal ligament
Bifurcate ligament
Cuboid
Calcaneus

B **Medial view**

Medial malleolus
Tibia
Navicular
Talus
Plantar calcaneonavicular (spring) ligament
Posterior tibiotalar
Tibionavicular
Tibiocalcaneal
Parts of medial (deltoid) ligament
Medial talocalcaneal ligament
Talar shelf
Calcaneus
Long plantar ligament

C **Posterior view**

Tibia
Fibula
Groove for tibialis posterior and flexor digitorum longus
Interosseous membrane
Posterior tibiofibular ligament
Medial malleolus
Inferior transverse ligament
Talus
Tibial fibers of posterior talofibular ligament
Parts of medial (deltoid) ligament Posterior tibiotalar Tibiocalcaneal
Lateral malleolus
Groove for tendon of flexor hallucis longus
Talar shelf
Posterior talofibular ligament
Medial and posterior talocalcaneal ligaments
Calcaneofibular ligament
Calcaneus
Calcaneal tendon

D **Coronal section**

Medial malleolus
Tibia
Interosseous membrane
Medial (deltoid) ligament
Ankle joint
Talar shelf
Trochlea of talus
Tibialis posterior
Fibula
Posterior talofibular ligament
Flexor digitorum longus
Talus
Lateral malleolus
Flexor hallucis longus
Subtalar joint
Medial plantar nerve and artery
Fibularis brevis
Abductor hallucis
Fibularis longus
Quadratus plantae
Calcaneus
Lateral plantar nerve and artery
Abductor digiti minimi
Flexor digitorum brevis
Fat

Figure 5.37. Ligaments of ankle and talocalcaneal joints.

The joint capsule of the ankle joint is reinforced medially by the large, strong **medial ligament of the ankle (deltoid ligament)** that attaches proximally to the medial malleolus and fans out from it to attach distally to the talus, calcaneus, and navicular via four adjacent and continuous parts (Fig. 5.37): the **tibionavicular part**, the **tibiocalcaneal part**, and the **anterior** and **posterior tibiotalar parts**. The medial ligament stabilizes the ankle joint during eversion of the foot and prevents subluxation (partial dislocation) of the ankle joint.

MOVEMENTS

The main movements of the ankle joint are dorsiflexion and plantarflexion of the foot. When the foot is plantarflexed, some "wobble" (small amounts of abduction, adduction, inversion, and eversion) is possible in this unstable position. Structures limiting movements of the ankle joint are outlined in Table 5.19.

- *Dorsiflexion of the ankle* is produced by muscles in the anterior compartment of the leg (Table 5.10). Dorsiflexion is usually limited by passive resistance of the triceps surae to stretching and by tension in the medial and lateral ligaments.
- *Plantarflexion of ankle* is produced by muscles in the posterior compartment of the leg (Table 5.11).

ARTERIES AND NERVES

The arteries are derived from malleolar branches of the fibular and anterior and posterior tibial arteries (Table 5.9). The nerves are derived from the tibial nerve and deep fibular nerve.

Joints of Foot

The joints of the foot involve the tarsals, metatarsals, and phalanges (Fig. 5.37D; Table 5.20). The important inter-

Table 5.19 Structures Limiting Movements of Ankle Joint

Movement	Limiting Structures
Plantarflexion	*Ligaments:* anterior talofibular, anterior part of medial, anterior joint capsule Contact of talus with tibia Tension of dorsiflexors of ankle
Dorsiflexion	*Ligaments:* medial, calcaneofibular, posterior talofibular, posterior joint capsule Contact of talus with tibia Tension of plantarflexors of ankle

Modified from Clarkson HM: *Musculoskeletal Assessment. Joint Range of Motion and Manual of Muscle Strength,* 2nd ed. Baltimore, Lippincott Williams & Wilkins 2000.

Ankle Injuries

The ankle is the most frequently injured major joint in the body. *Ankle sprains* (torn fibers of ligaments) are most common. A sprained ankle is nearly always an *inversion injury,* involving twisting of the weight-bearing plantarflexed foot. The *anterior talofibular ligament* (part of the lateral ligament) is most commonly torn during ankle sprains, either partially or completely, resulting in instability of the ankle joint. The *calcaneofibular ligament* may also be torn. A **Pott fracture–dislocation of the ankle** occurs when the foot is forcibly everted. This action pulls on the extremely strong medial ligament, often tearing off the medial malleolus (Fig. B5.9). The talus then moves laterally, shearing off the lateral malleolus or, more commonly, breaking the fibula superior to the tibiofibular syndesmosis. If the tibia is carried anteriorly, the posterior margin of the distal end of the tibia is also sheared off by the talus.

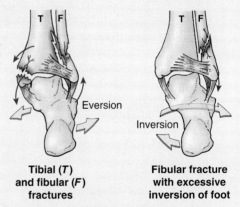

Tibial (*T*) and fibular (*F*) fractures

Fibular fracture with excessive inversion of foot

Posterior views

Figure B5.9

Tibial Nerve Entrapment

Entrapment and compression of the tibial nerve (*tarsal tunnel syndrome*) occurs when there is edema and tightness in the ankle involving the synovial sheaths of the tendons of muscles in the posterior compartment of the leg. The area involved is from the medial malleolus to the calcaneus. The heel pain results from compression of the tibial nerve by the flexor retinaculum.

Table 5.20 Joints of Foot

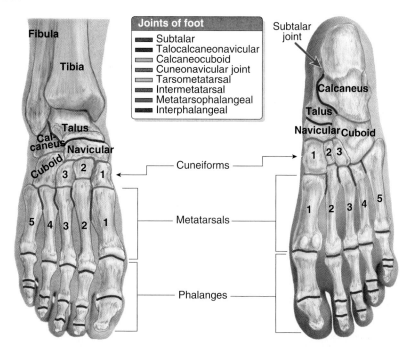

Dorsal surface   **Plantar surface**

Joint	Articulating Surfaces	Joint Capsule	Ligaments	Blood Supply	Nerve Supply
Subtalar (talocalcaneal, anatomical subtalar joint) Type: Plane synovial joint Movements: Inversion and eversion of foot	Inferior surface of body of talus (posterior calcaneal articular facet articulates with superior surface (posterior talar articular surface) of calcaneus	Attached to margins of articular surfaces	Medial, lateral, and posterior talocalcaneal ligaments support capsule; interosseous talocalcaneal ligament binds bones together	Posterior tibial and fibular arteries	
Talocalcaneonavicular Type: Synovial joint; talonavicular part is ball and socket type Movements: Gliding and rotatory	Head of talus articulates with calcaneus and navicular bones	Incompletely encloses joint	Plantar calcaneonavicular (spring) ligament supports head of talus		Plantar aspect: medial or lateral plantar nerve: Dorsal aspect: deep fibular nerve
Calcaneocuboid Type: Plane synovial joint Movements: Inversion and eversion of foot; circumduction	Anterior end of calcaneus articulates with posterior surface of cuboid	Encloses joint	Dorsal and plantar calcaneocuboid, and long plantar ligaments support joint capsule	Anterior tibial artery via lateral tarsal artery, a branch of dorsal artery of foot	
Cuneonavicular joint Type: Plane synovial joint Movements: Little	Anterior navicular articulates with bases of cuneiform bones	Common capsule encloses joint	Dorsal and plantar cuneonavicular ligaments		
Tarsometatarsal Type: Plane synovial joint(s) Movements: Gliding or sliding	Anterior tarsal bones articulate with bases of metatarsal bones	Separate joint capsules enclose each joint	Dorsal, plantar, and interosseous tarsometatarsal ligaments bind bones together		Deep fibular; medial and lateral plantar nerves; sural nerve

Table 5.20 Joints of Foot *(continued)*

Joint	Articulating Surfaces	Joint Capsule	Ligaments	Blood Supply	Nerve Supply
Intermetatarsal Type: Plane synovial joint Movements: Little	Bases of metatarsal bones articulate with each other	Separate joint capsules enclose each joint	Dorsal, plantar, and interosseous tarsometatarsal ligaments bind bones together	Lateral metatarsal artery, (a branch of dorsal artery of foot)	Digital nerves
Metatarsophalangeal Type: Condyloid synovial joint Movements: Flexion, extension, and some abduction, adduction, and circumduction	Heads of metatarsal bones articulate with bases of proximal phalanges		Collateral ligaments support capsule on each side; plantar ligaments support plantar part of capsule		
Interphalangeal Type: Hinge synovial joint Movements: Flexion and extension	Head of one phalanx articulates with base of one distal to it		Collateral and plantar ligaments support joints	Digital branches of plantar arch	

tarsal joints are the *subtalar (talocalcaneal) joint* and the *transverse tarsal joint (calcaneocuboid and talonavicular joints)*. Inversion and eversion of the foot are the main movements involving these joints. The other intertarsal joints and the *tarsometatarsal* and *intermetatarsal joints* are relatively small and are so tightly joined by ligaments that only slight movement occurs between them. In the foot, flexion and extension occurs in the forefoot at the metatarsophalangeal and interphalangeal joints. All of the foot bones proximal to the metatarsophalangeal joints are united by dorsal and plantar ligaments.

The **subtalar joint** occurs where the talus rests on and articulates with the calcaneus. The subtalar joint is a synovial joint that is surrounded by a weak joint capsule that is supported by medial, lateral, posterior, and interosseous *talocalcaneal ligaments*. The **interosseous talocalcaneal ligament** lies within the *tarsal sinus,* which separates the subtalar and calcaneonavicular joints and is especially strong. The **transverse tarsal joint** is a compound joint formed by the **talonavicular part of the talocalcaneonavicular** and the **calcaneocuboid joints**—two separate joints aligned transversely. Transection across the transverse tarsal joint is a standard method for *surgical amputation of the foot.*

The major ligaments of the plantar aspect of the foot are (Fig. 5.38; Table 5.21) the:

- **Plantar calcaneonavicular (spring) ligament,** which extends across and fills a wedge-shape gap between the talar shelf and the inferior margin of the posterior articular surface of the navicular. This ligament supports the head of the talus and plays important roles in the trans-

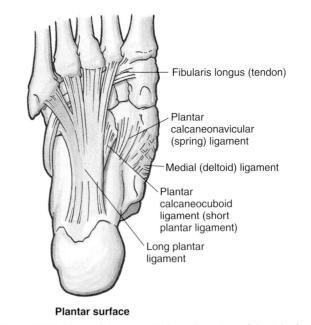

Plantar surface

Fibularis longus (tendon)

Plantar calcaneonavicular (spring) ligament

Medial (deltoid) ligament

Plantar calcaneocuboid ligament (short plantar ligament)

Long plantar ligament

Figure 5.38. Plantar ligaments. A deep dissection of the right foot is shown.

Table 5.21 Structures Limiting the Movements of Foot and Toes

Movement	Joint	Limiting Structures
Inversion	Subtalar, transverse tarsal	*Ligaments:* lateral ligament of ankle, talocalcaneal ligament, lateral joint capsule Tension of evertor muscles of ankle
Eversion	Subtalar, transverse tarsal	*Ligaments:* medial ligament of ankle, medial talocalcaneal ligament, medial joint capsule Tension of tibialis posterior, flexor hallucis longus, flexor digitorum longus Contact of talus with calcaneus
Flexion	MTP, PIP, DIP	*MTP:* tension of posterior joint capsule, extensor muscles, collateral ligaments *PIP:* soft tissue apposition, tension of collateral ligaments and posterior joint capsule *DIP:* tension in collateral and oblique retinacular ligaments, and posterior joint capsule
Extension	MTP. PIP, DIP	*MTP:* tension of plantar joint capsule, plantar ligaments, and flexor muscles *PIP:* tension in plantar joint capsule *DIP:* ligaments and plantar joint capsule
Abduction	MTP	*Ligaments:* collateral ligaments, medial joint capsule Tension of adductor muscles Skin between web spaces
Adduction	MTP	Apposition of toes

DIP, distal interphalangeal joints (toes 2–5); *MTP,* metatarsophalangeal joints; *PIP,* proximal interphalangeal joints.
Modified from Clarkson HM: *Musculoskeletal Assessment. Joint Range of Motion and Manual of Muscle Strength,* 2nd ed. Baltimore, Lippincott Williams & Wilkins 2000.

fer of weight from the talus and in maintaining the longitudinal arch of the foot.

- **Long plantar ligament**, which passes from the plantar surface of the calcaneus to the groove on the cuboid. Some of its fibers extend to the bases of the metatarsals, thereby forming a tunnel for the tendon of the fibularis longus. The long plantar ligament is important in maintaining the longitudinal arch of the foot.
- **Plantar calcaneocuboid (short plantar) ligament**, which is located deep to the long plantar ligament. It extends from the anterior aspect of the inferior surface of the calcaneus to the inferior surface of the cuboid. It is also involved in maintaining the longitudinal arch of the foot.

Arches of Foot

The foot is composed of numerous bones connected by ligaments that provide considerable flexibility that allow it to deform with each ground contact, thereby absorbing much of the shock. Furthermore, the tarsal and metatarsal bones are arranged in longitudinal and transverse arches passively supported and actively restrained by flexible tendons that add to the weight-bearing capabilities and resiliency of the foot. The arches distribute weight over the foot (*pedal platform*) acting not only as shock absorbers but also as springboards for propelling it during walking, running, and jumping. The resilient arches add to the foot's ability to adapt to changes in surface contour. The weight of the body is transmitted to the talus from the tibia. Then it is transmitted posteriorly to the calcaneus and anteriorly to the "ball of the foot" (the sesamoid bones of the 1st metatarsal and the head of the 2nd metatarsal), and that weight/pressure is shared laterally with the heads of the 3rd–5th metatarsals as necessary for balance and comfort (Fig. 5.39*A*). Between these weight-bearing points are the relatively elastic arches of the foot, which become slightly flattened by the body weight during standing, but they normally resume their curvature (recoil) when body weight is removed.

The **longitudinal arch of the foot** is composed of medial and lateral parts (Fig. 5.39*B*). Functionally, both parts act as a unit, with the transverse arch spreading the weight in all directions. The **medial longitudinal arch** is higher and more important than the lateral longitudinal arch. The medial longitudinal arch is composed of the calcaneus, talus, navicular, three cuneiforms, and three metatarsals. *The talar head is the keystone of the medial longitudinal arch.* The tibialis anterior, attaching to the 1st metatarsal and medial cuneiform (Fig. 5.39*C*), helps strengthen the medial longitudinal arch. The fibularis longus tendon, passing from lateral to medial, also helps support this arch. The **lateral longitudinal arch** is much flatter than the medial part of the arch and rests on the ground during standing. It is composed of the calcaneus, cuboid, and lateral two metatarsals.

The **transverse arch of the foot** runs from side to side. It is formed by the cuboid, cuneiforms, and bases of the metatarsals. The medial and lateral parts of the longitudinal arch serve as pillars for the transverse arch. The tendon of

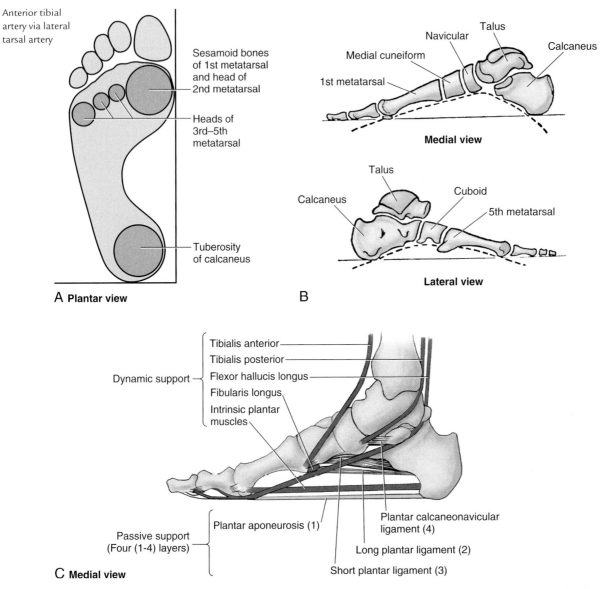

Figure 5.39. Arches of foot. A. The weight-bearing areas of the foot are defined. **B.** The medial and lateral longitudinal arches of the foot are shown. **C.** The passive (*purple*) and dynamic (*gray*) supports of the foot are identified.

the fibularis longus and tibialis posterior, crossing the sole of the foot obliquely, help maintain the curvature of the transverse arch.

The integrity of the bony arches of the foot is maintained by both passive factors and dynamic supports (Fig. 5.39C). The passive factors include the shape of the united bones and the four successive layers of fibrous tissue: plantar aponeurosis, long plantar ligament, plantar calcaneocuboid (short plantar) ligament, and calcaneonavicular (spring) lig-

ament. The dynamic supports include the active (reflexive) bracing action of the intrinsic muscles of the foot and the active and tonic contraction of the muscles with long tendons extending into the foot (flexor hallucis and flexor digitorum longus for the longitudinal arch and fibularis longus and tibialis anterior for the transverse arch). Of these factors, the plantar ligaments and plantar aponeurosis bear the greatest stress and are most important in maintaining the arches.

Hallux Valgus

Hallux valgus is a foot deformity caused by pressure from footwear and degenerative joint disease; it is characterized by lateral deviation of the great toe (L. *hallux*). In some people, the deviation is so great that the 1st toe overlaps the 2nd toe. These individuals are unable to move their 1st digit away from their 2nd digit because the sesamoid bones under the head of the 1st metatarsal are displaced and lie in the space between the heads of the 1st and 2nd metatarsals. In addition, a subcutaneous bursa may form owing to pressure and friction against the shoe. When tender and inflamed, the bursa is called a bunion (Fig. B5.10A).

Hammer Toe

Hammer toe is a deformity in which the proximal phalanx is permanently dorsiflexed (hyperextended) at the metatarsophalangeal joint and the middle phalanx is plantarflexed at the interphalangeal joint. The distal phalanx is also flexed or extended, giving the digit (usually the 2nd) a hammer-like appearance. This deformity may result from weakness of the lumbricals and interossei, which flex the metatarsophalangeal joints and extend the interphalangeal joints.

Pes Planus (Flatfeet)

Acquired flatfeet ("fallen arches") are likely to be secondary to dysfunction of the tibialis posterior owing to trauma, degeneration with age, or denervation (Fig. B5.10B & C). In the absence of normal passive or dynamic support, the plantar calcaneonavicular ligament fails to support the head of the talus. Consequently, the talar head displaces inferomedially and becomes prominent. As a result, some flattening of the medial part of the longitudinal arch occurs, along with lateral deviation of the forefoot. Flatfeet are common in older people, particularly if they undertake much unaccustomed standing or gain weight rapidly, adding stress on the muscles and increasing the strain on the ligaments supporting the arches.

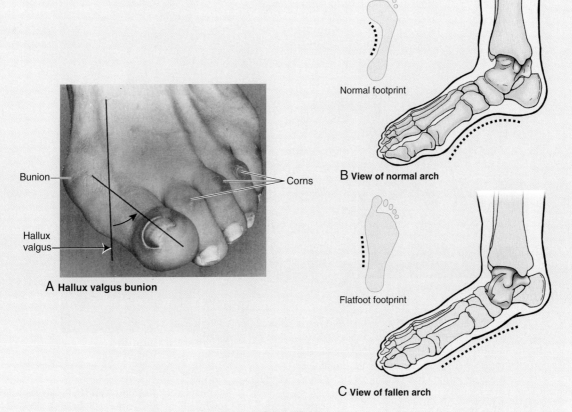

Bunion

Corns

Hallux valgus

A **Hallux valgus bunion**

Normal footprint

B **View of normal arch**

Flatfoot footprint

C **View of fallen arch**

Figure B5.10

Medical Imaging of Lower Limb

Radiographs of the pelvis and hip show bone and joint abnormalities or malalignment. In an antero-posterior (AP) projection of the hip joint (Fig. 5.40), the person is in the supine position on the radiographic table. The central X-ray beam is centered over the hip joint. Superimposed on the femoral head is the posterior rim of the acetabulum. At the junction of the femoral neck and shaft, the greater and lesser trochanters may be seen. Between the trochanters is an oblique line cast by the superimposed intertrochanteric line and crest. Extrapolated lines and curves superimposed on radiographic images in specific views are used to assess normal alignment of bony features.

Several radiographic projections (e.g., AP and lateral) are necessary to evaluate a joint properly. In an AP projection of the knee joint, the knee is extended and the central X-ray beam is directed through the joint cavity (Fig. 5.41A). Outlines of the femoral and tibial condyles and the shadows of patella are superimposed over the distal end of the femur. The joint cavity appears large because the menisci are not visible. In a lateral projection, the knee is slightly flexed (Fig. 5.41B). The menisci can be visualized if air or an opaque fluid is injected into the joint cavity. When a contrast medium is

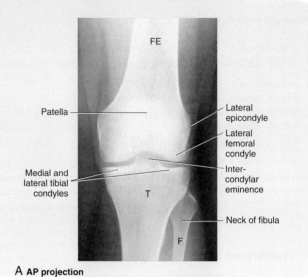

A AP projection

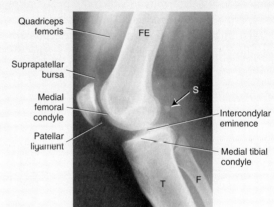

B Lateral projection

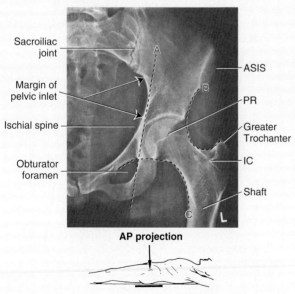

AP projection

Figure 5.40. Radiograph of normal hip joint. Several different lines and curvatures are used to detect hip abnormalities (dislocations, fractures, or slipped epiphyses). *A,* Köhler line; *B,* Shenton line; *C,* femoral line; *ASIS,* anterior superior iliac spine; *IC,* intertrochanteric crest; *PR,* posterior rim of the acetabulum.

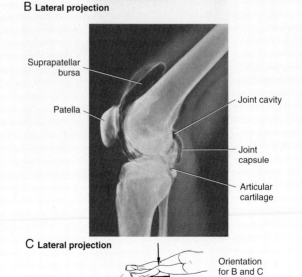

C Lateral projection

Orientation for B and C

Figure 5.41. Images of knee joint. A and B. Radiographs of the knee are shown. *F,* fibula; *FE,* femur; *S,* fabella; *T,* tibia. **C.** This arthrogram of the knee joint shows the joint slightly flexed.

continued >

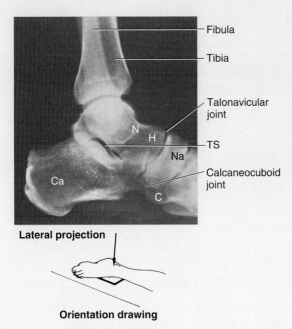

Lateral projection

Orientation drawing

Figure 5.42. **Radiograph of left ankle.** *C,* cuboid; *Ca,* calcaneus; *H,* head of talus; *N,* neck of talus; *Na,* navicular; *TS,* tarsal sinus.

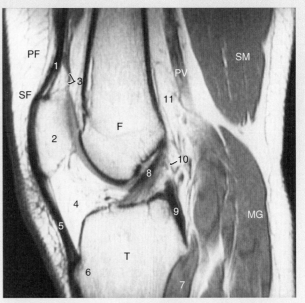

Sagittal MRI

Figure 5.43. **MRI study through lateral aspect of intercondylar notch of femur.** *1,* Quadriceps tendon; *2,* patella; *3,* suprapatellar bursa; *4,* infrapatellar fat-pad; *5,* patellar ligament; *6,* tibial tuberosity; *7,* popliteus; *8,* anterior cruciate ligament; *9,* posterior cruciate ligament; *10,* joint capsule; *11,* fat in popliteal fossa; *MG,* medial head of gastrocnemius; *PF,* prefemoral fat; *PV,* popliteal vessels; *SF,* suprapatellar fat; *SM,* semimembranosus.

injected into the knee joint cavity (arthrogram), the joint cavity and the extent of the synovial membrane are visible (Fig. 5.41*C*). Although MRI has largely replaced arthrography, it is sometimes useful for detecting loose bodies if the MRI study is inconclusive.

The common radiographs of the ankle and foot are lateral and AP projections. A lateral radiograph is taken with the lateral malleolus placed against the X-ray film cassette. In Figure 5.42, observe the convex surface of the trochlea of talus articulating with the malleoli of the tibia and fibula (the shadows of the malleoli are visible). Also observe the neck and head of the talus, the disc-shaped navicular, and the talonavicular joint. The calcaneus and cuboid articulate at the calcaneocuboid joint. The tarsal sinus—the space between the calca-

neus and the talus—contains the interosseous talocalcaneal ligament (Fig. 5.37*A*).

MRI produces images of exquisite resolution of the limbs without the use of radiation. MRI scanning requires the patient to keep the limbs motionless for 5–10 min. These studies show much more detail of the soft tissues than do radiographs or CT scans. MRI studies are helpful in evaluating the menisci, collateral ligaments, and cruciate ligaments of the knee joint. MRI is the procedure of choice for assessing internal derangements of the knee (Fig. 5.43). ●

6

Upper Limb

Chapter Outline

The upper limb is characterized by its mobility and ability to grasp, strike, and conduct fine motor skills (*manipulation*). These characteristics are especially marked in the hand. Efficiency of hand function results in a large part from the ability to place it in the proper position by movements at the scapulothoracic, glenohumeral, elbow, radioulnar, and wrist joints. The upper limb consists of four segments (Fig. 6.1):

- **Shoulder,** which includes the pectoral, scapular, and lateral supraclavicular regions and is built on half of the pectoral girdle. The **pectoral (shoulder) girdle** is a bony ring, incomplete posteriorly, formed by the scapulae and clavicles and completed anteriorly by the manubrium of the sternum.
- **Arm** (L. *brachium*), which is the part between the shoulder and the elbow and is centered around the humerus.
- **Forearm** (L. *antebrachium*), which is the part between the elbow and the wrist and contains the ulna and radius.

- **Hand** (L. *manus*), which is the part distal to the forearm and contains the carpus, metacarpus, and phalanges. It is composed of the wrist, palm, dorsum of hand, and fingers (including the opposable thumb) and is richly supplied with sensory endings for touch, pain, and temperature.

Bones of Upper Limb

The pectoral girdle and bones of the free part of the upper limb form the **superior appendicular skeleton,** which articulates with the axial skeleton only at the sternoclavicular joint, allowing great mobility (Fig. 6.2). The pectoral girdle is supported, stabilized, and propelled by **axioappendicular muscles,** which attach to the ribs, sternum, and vertebrae of the *axial skeleton.*

Clavicle

The **clavicle** (collar bone) connects the upper limb to the trunk. Its **sternal end** articulates with the **manubrium of the sternum** at the *sternoclavicular* (SC) *joint.* Its **acromial end** articulates with the *acromion of the scapula* at the *acromioclavicular* (AC) *joint.* The medial two thirds of the shaft of the clavicle are convex anteriorly (Figs. 6.2 and 6.3), whereas the lateral third is flattened and concave anteriorly. These curvatures increase the resilience of the clavicle and give it the appearance of an elongated capital S. The clavicle:

- Serves as a strut (rigid support) from which the scapula and free limb are suspended, keeping the limb away from the thorax so that the arm has maximum freedom of motion. Fixing the strut in position, especially after its elevation, enables elevation of the ribs for deep inspiration.
- Forms one of the boundaries of the *cervicoaxillary canal* (passageway between neck and arm), affording protection to the neurovascular bundle supplying the upper limb.
- Transmits shocks (traumatic impacts) from the upper limb to the axial skeleton.

Although designated as a long bone, the clavicle has no medullary (marrow) cavity. It consists of spongy (trabecular) bone with a shell of compact bone.

Scapula

The **scapula** (shoulder blade) is a triangular flat bone that lies on the posterolateral aspect of the thorax, overlying the 2nd–7th ribs (Figs. 6.2 and 6.4). The convex **posterior surface** of the scapula is unevenly divided by the **spine of the scapula** into a small **supraspinous fossa** and a much larger **infraspinous fossa.** The concave **costal surface** of the scapula has a large **subscapular fossa.** The triangular **body (blade) of the scapula** is thin and translucent superior and inferior to the scapular spine.

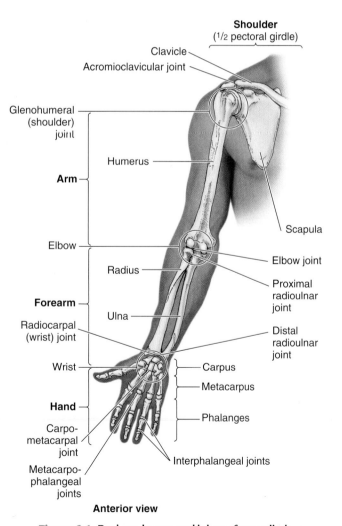

Figure 6.1. Regions, bones, and joints of upper limb.

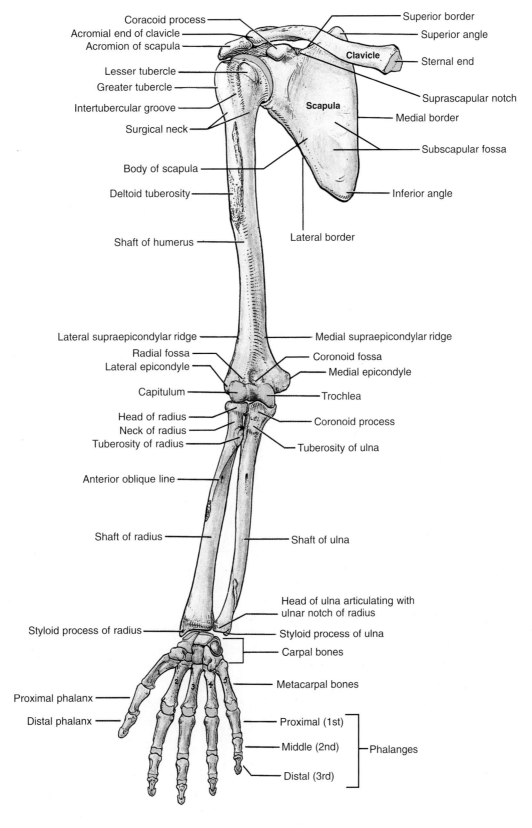

Coracoid process
Acromial end of clavicle
Acromion of scapula
Lesser tubercle
Greater tubercle
Intertubercular groove
Surgical neck
Body of scapula
Deltoid tuberosity
Shaft of humerus
Lateral supraepicondylar ridge
Radial fossa
Lateral epicondyle
Capitulum
Head of radius
Neck of radius
Tuberosity of radius
Anterior oblique line
Shaft of radius
Styloid process of radius
Proximal phalanx
Distal phalanx

Superior border
Superior angle
Clavicle
Sternal end
Suprascapular notch
Scapula
Medial border
Subscapular fossa
Inferior angle
Lateral border
Medial supraepicondylar ridge
Coronoid fossa
Medial epicondyle
Trochlea
Coronoid process
Tuberosity of ulna
Shaft of ulna
Head of ulna articulating with ulnar notch of radius
Styloid process of ulna
Carpal bones
Metacarpal bones
Proximal (1st)
Middle (2nd)
Phalanges
Distal (3rd)

A Anterior view

Figure 6.2. Bones of upper limb.

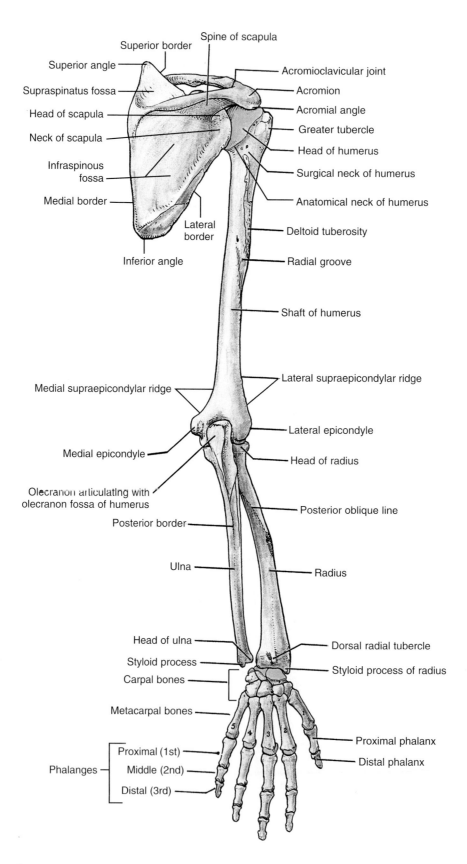

Spine of scapula
Superior border
Superior angle
Supraspinatus fossa
Head of scapula
Neck of scapula
Infraspinous fossa
Medial border
Lateral border
Inferior angle

Acromioclavicular joint
Acromion
Acromial angle
Greater tubercle
Head of humerus
Surgical neck of humerus
Anatomical neck of humerus
Deltoid tuberosity
Radial groove

Shaft of humerus

Medial supraepicondylar ridge
Lateral supraepicondylar ridge

Medial epicondyle
Lateral epicondyle
Head of radius

Olecranon articulating with olecranon fossa of humerus
Posterior oblique line

Posterior border

Ulna
Radius

Head of ulna
Dorsal radial tubercle
Styloid process
Styloid process of radius
Carpal bones

Metacarpal bones

Proximal phalanx
Distal phalanx

Phalanges
Proximal (1st)
Middle (2nd)
Distal (3rd)

B Posterior view

Figure 6.2. (continued)

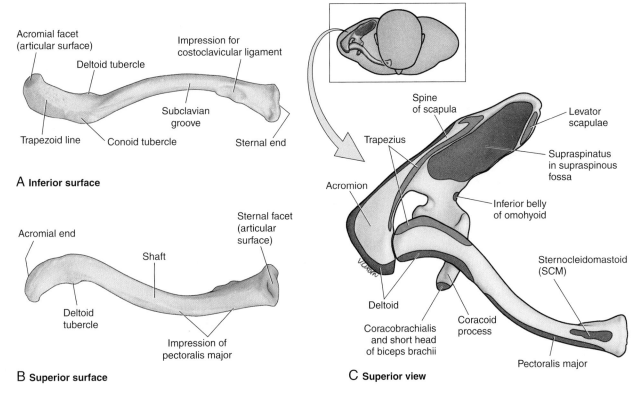

A **Inferior surface**

Acromial facet (articular surface)
Deltoid tubercle
Impression for costoclavicular ligament
Subclavian groove
Trapezoid line
Conoid tubercle
Sternal end

B **Superior surface**

Acromial end
Shaft
Sternal facet (articular surface)
Deltoid tubercle
Impression of pectoralis major

C **Superior view**

Spine of scapula
Levator scapulae
Trapezius
Supraspinatus in supraspinous fossa
Acromion
Inferior belly of omohyoid
Sternocleidomastoid (SCM)
Deltoid
Coracobrachialis and short head of biceps brachii
Coracoid process
Pectoralis major

Figure 6.3. Clavicle. The superior (**A**) and inferior (**B**) surfaces are shown. **C.** The muscle attachments to the clavicle and scapula are identified.

Fracture of Clavicle

The clavicle is commonly fractured, often caused by an indirect force transmitted from an outstretched hand through the bones of the forearm and arm to the shoulder during a fall. A fracture may also result from a fall directly on the shoulder. The weakest part of the clavicle is at the junction of its middle and lateral thirds. After fracture of the clavicle, the sternocleidomastoid (SCM) muscle elevates the medial fragment of bone (Fig. B6.1).

The trapezius muscle is unable to hold up the lateral fragment owing to the weight of the upper limb, and thus the shoulder drops. In addition to being depressed, the lateral fragment of the clavicle may be pulled medially by the adductor muscles of the arm, such as the pectoralis major. Overriding of the bone fragments shortens the clavicle.

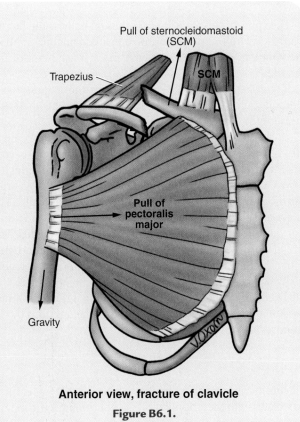

Pull of sternocleidomastoid (SCM)
Trapezius
SCM
Pull of pectoralis major
Gravity

Anterior view, fracture of clavicle

Figure B6.1.

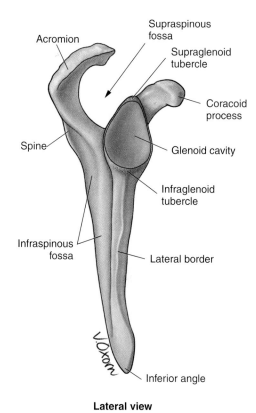

Lateral view
Figure 6.4. Right scapula.

The spine of the scapula continues laterally as the flat expanded acromion, which forms the subcutaneous point of the shoulder and articulates with the acromial end of the clavicle.

Superolaterally, the lateral surface of the scapula has a **glenoid cavity**, which articulates with the head of the humerus at the glenohumeral (shoulder) joint. The glenoid (G. socket) cavity is a shallow, concave, oval fossa, which is directed anterolaterally and slightly superiorly and is considerably smaller than the head of the humerus for which it serves as a socket. The beak-like **coracoid process** is superior to the glenoid cavity and projects anterolaterally. The scapula has **medial** (axillary), **lateral** (vertebral), and **superior borders** and **superior, lateral,** and **inferior angles.** The lateral border of scapula is the thickest part of the bone, which includes the **head of the scapula** where the glenoid cavity is located. The **neck of the scapula** is just inferior to the head. The superior border of the scapula is marked near the junction of its medial two thirds and lateral third by the **suprascapular notch** (Fig. 6.2A).

Humerus

The humerus (arm bone), the largest bone in the upper limb, articulates with the scapula at the glenohumeral joint and the radius and ulna at the elbow joint (Figs. 6.1 and 6.2).

Proximally, the ball-shaped **head of the humerus** articulates with the glenoid cavity of the scapula. The **intertubercular groove** (bicipital groove) of the proximal end of the humerus separates the **lesser tubercle** from the **greater tubercle.** Just distal to the humeral head, the **anatomical neck of the humerus** separates the head from the tubercles. Distal to the tubercles is the narrow **surgical neck of the humerus.**

The **shaft (body) of the humerus** has two prominent features: the **deltoid tuberosity** laterally and the **radial groove** (groove for radial nerve, spiral groove) posteriorly for the radial nerve and deep artery of the arm. The inferior end of the humeral shaft widens as the sharp medial and lateral **supraepicondylar** (supracondylar) **ridges** form and then end distally in the prominent **medial epicondyle** and **lateral epicondyle** (Fig. 6.2B).

The distal end of the humerus, including the trochlea, capitulum, olecranon, coronoid, and radial fossae, makes up the **condyle of the humerus.** It has two articular surfaces: a lateral **capitulum** (L. little head) for articulation with the head of the radius and a medial **trochlea** (L. pulley) for articulation with the trochlear notch of the ulna (Fig. 6.2A). Superior to the trochlea anteriorly is the **coronoid fossa,** which receives the coronoid process of the ulna during full flexion of the elbow. Posteriorly, the **olecranon fossa** accommodates the olecranon of the ulna during extension of the elbow. Superior to the capitulum anteriorly, the shallow **radial fossa** accommodates the edge of the head of the radius when the elbow is fully flexed.

Ulna and Radius

The **ulna**, the stabilizing bone of the forearm, is the medial and longer of the two forearm bones (Fig. 6.2). Its proximal end has two prominent projections—the **olecranon** posteriorly and the **coronoid process** anteriorly—which form the walls of the **trochlear notch.** The trochlear notch of the ulna articulates with the trochlea of the humerus. Inferior to the coronoid process is the **tuberosity of the ulna.** On the lateral side of the coronoid process is a smooth, rounded concavity, the **radial notch,** which articulates with the head of radius (Fig. 6.5A). Inferior to the radial notch is a prominent ridge, the **supinator crest,** and between it and the distal part of the coronoid process is a concavity, the **supinator fossa.** Proximally, the **shaft (body) of the ulna** is thick, but it tapers, diminishing in diameter distally. At its narrow distal end is the rounded **head of ulna** with the small, conical **ulnar styloid process** (Fig. 6.2). The ulna does not reach, and therefore does not participate in, the wrist (radiocarpal) joint.

The **radius** is the lateral and shorter of the two forearm bones. Its proximal end consists of a cylindrical head, a short neck, and a projection from the medial surface (the radial tuberosity) (Fig. 6.2A). Proximally, the smooth superior aspect of the **head of the radius** is concave for articulation with the capitulum of humerus. The head also

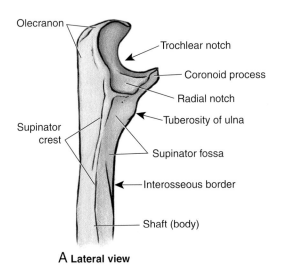

A Lateral view

- Olecranon
- Trochlear notch
- Coronoid process
- Radial notch
- Tuberosity of ulna
- Supinator crest
- Supinator fossa
- Interosseous border
- Shaft (body)

B Posterior view

- Dorsal tubercle of radius
- Groove for extensor pollicis longus
- Groove for extensor carpi radialis longus and brevis
- Groove for extensor digitorum and extensor indicis
- Groove for abductor pollicis longus and extensor pollicis brevis
- Ulnar notch
- Styloid process

Figure 6.5. Ulna and radius. A. The proximal part of the ulna is shown. **B.** The distal end of the radius is shown.

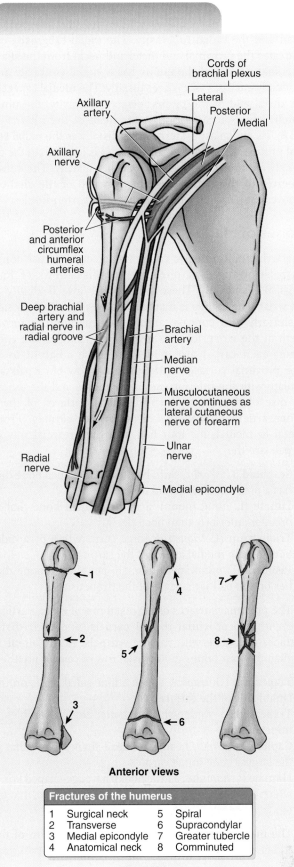

Anterior views

Fractures of the humerus			
1	Surgical neck	5	Spiral
2	Transverse	6	Supracondylar
3	Medial epicondyle	7	Greater tubercle
4	Anatomical neck	8	Comminuted

Figure B6.2.

Fractures of Humerus

Fractures of the surgical neck of the humerus are especially common in elderly people with *osteoporosis* (Fig. B6.2). The injuries usually result from a minor fall on the hand, with the force being transmitted up the forearm bones of the extended limb. *Transverse fractures of the shaft of humerus* frequently result from a direct blow to the arm. Fracture of the distal part of the humerus, near the supracondylar ridges, is a *supracondylar fracture*. Because nerves are in contact with the humerus, they may be injured when the associated part of the humerus is fractured: surgical neck, axillary nerve; radial groove, radial nerve; distal humerus, median nerve; and medial epicondyle, ulnar nerve.

articulates medially with the radial notch of ulna (Fig. 6.5*A*). The **neck of the radius** is the narrow part between the head and the radial tuberosity. The **radial tuberosity** demarcates the proximal end (head and neck) from the shaft. The **shaft (body) of the radius** has a lateral convexity and gradually enlarges as it passes distally. The medial aspect of the distal end of the radius forms a concavity, the **ulnar notch**, which accommodates the head of the ulna (Fig. 6.5*B*). Its lateral aspect terminates distally as the **radial styloid process**. The radial styloid process is larger than the ulnar styloid process and extends farther distally. The **dorsal tubercle of the radius** lies between two of the shallow grooves for passage of the tendons of forearm muscles.

Bones of Hand

The **wrist**, or **carpus**, is composed of eight **carpal bones** (carpals) arranged in proximal and distal rows of four (Figs. 6.1 and 6.6). These small bones give flexibility to the wrist. The carpus is markedly convex from side to side posteriorly and concave anteriorly. Augmenting movement at the wrist, the two rows of carpals glide on each other; each carpal also glides on those adjacent to it. The proximal surfaces of the proximal row of carpals articulate with the inferior end of the radius and the articular disc of the wrist joint. The distal surfaces of these bones articulate with the distal row of carpals. From lateral to medial, the four bones in the proximal row of carpals are the:

- **Scaphoid** (G. *skaphé,* skiff, boat): a boat-shaped bone that has a prominent **scaphoid tubercle.**
- **Lunate** (L. *luna,* moon): a moon-shaped bone that is broader anteriorly than posteriorly.
- **Triquetrum** (L. *triquetrus,* three cornered): a pyramidal bone on the medial aspect of the carpus.
- **Pisiform** (L. *pisum,* pea): a small, pea-shaped bone that lies on the palmar surface of the triquetrum.

The proximal surfaces of the distal row of carpals articulate with the proximal row of carpals, and their distal surfaces articulate with the metacarpals. From lateral to medial, the four bones in the distal row of carpals are the:

- **Trapezium** (G. *trapeze,* table): a four-sided bone, on the lateral side of the carpus.
- **Trapezoid:** a wedge-shaped bone, that resembles a trapezium.
- **Capitate** (L. *caput,* head): the head-shaped bone that is the largest bone in the carpus.
- **Hamate** (L. *hamulus,* a little hook): a wedge-shaped bone, which has a hooked process, the **hook of hamate,** that extends anteriorly.

The **metacarpus** forms the skeleton of the palm of the hand between the carpus and the phalanges (Fig. 6.6). It is

Fracture of Ulna and Radius

Fractures of both the ulna and the radius are the result of severe injury. A direct injury usually produces transverse fractures at the same level, often in the middle third of the bones. Because the shafts of these bones are firmly bound together by the interosseous membrane, a fracture of one bone is likely to be associated with dislocation of the nearest joint. *Fracture of the distal end of the radius is the most common fracture in people older than 50 years.* A complete fracture of the distal 2 cm of the radius, called a **Colles fracture,** is the most common fracture of the forearm (Fig. B6.3). The distal fragment of the radius is displaced dorsally and often **comminuted** (broken into pieces). The fracture results from forced dorsiflexion of the hand, usually as the result of trying to ease a fall by outstretching the upper limb. Often, the ulnar styloid process is **avulsed** (broken off). Normally, the radial styloid process projects farther distally than the ulnar styloid process; consequently, when a Colles fracture occurs, this relationship is reversed because of shortening of the radius. This clinical condition is often referred to as a *dinner fork* (silver fork) *deformity* because a posterior angulation occurs in the forearm just proximal to the wrist and the normal anterior curvature of the relaxed hand. The posterior bending is produced by the posterior displacement and tilt of the distal fragment of the radius.

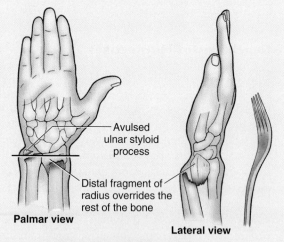

Avulsed ulnar styloid process

Distal fragment of radius overrides the rest of the bone

Palmar view

Lateral view

Colles fracture of distal radius ("dinner fork deformity")

Figure B6.3.

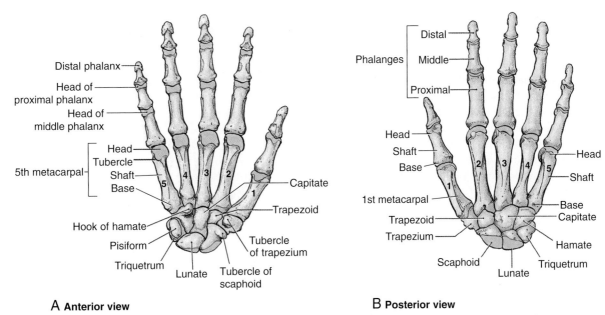

A Anterior view   **B Posterior view**

Figure 6.6. Bones of hand.

composed of five **metacarpal bones.** Each metacarpal consists of a base, shaft, and head. The proximal **bases of the metacarpals** articulate with the carpal bones, and the distal **heads of the metacarpals** articulate with the proximal phalanges and form the knuckles. The 1st metacarpal (of the thumb) is the thickest and shortest of these bones.

Each digit has three **phalanges (proximal, middle,** and **distal)** except for the first (thumb), which has only two **(proximal** and **distal).** Each phalanx has a **base** proximally, a **shaft (body),** and a **head** distally. The distal phalanges are flattened and expanded at their distal ends, which underlie the nail beds.

Fractures of Hand

Fracture of the scaphoid often results from a fall on the palm with the hand abducted (Fig. B6.4). The fracture occurs across the narrow part ("waist") of the scaphoid. Pain occurs primarily on the lateral side of the wrist, especially during dorsiflexion and abduction of the hand. Initial radiographs of the wrist may not reveal a fracture, but radiographs taken 10–14 days later reveal a fracture because bone resorption has occurred. Owing to the poor blood supply to the proximal part of the scaphoid, union of the fractured parts may take several months. *Avascular necrosis of the proximal fragment of the scaphoid* (pathological death of bone resulting from poor blood supply) may occur and produce *degenerative joint disease of the wrist.*

Severe crushing injuries of the hand may produce multiple metacarpal fractures, resulting in instability of the hand. Similar injuries of the distal phalanges are common

(e.g., when a finger is caught in a car door). A *fracture of a distal phalanx* is usually comminuted, and a painful hematoma (collection of blood) develops. Fractures of the proximal and middle phalanges are usually the result of crushing or hyperextension injuries.

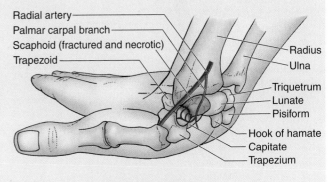

Fracture of scaphoid

Figure B6.4.

Surface Anatomy of Upper Limb Bones

Most bones of the upper limb offer a palpable segment or surface, enabling the skilled examiner to discern abnormalities owing to trauma or malformation (Fig. SA6.1A). The **clavicle** is subcutaneous and can be palpated throughout its length. Its sternal end projects superior to the manubrium. Between the elevated sternal ends of the clavicle is the **jugular notch** (suprasternal notch). The acromial end of the clavicle often rises higher than the acromion, forming a palpable elevation at the **acromioclavicular joint.** The acromial end can be palpated 2–3 cm medial to the lateral border of the acromion, particularly when the arm is alternately flexed and extended.

The **coracoid process of scapula** can be felt deeply at the lateral end of the clavicle in the clavipectoral (deltopectoral) triangle. The **acromion of the scapula** is felt easily and is often visible. The lateral and posterior borders of the acromion meet to form the **acromial angle** (Fig. SA6.1A). Inferior to the acromion, the *deltoid muscle* forms the rounded curve of the shoulder. The

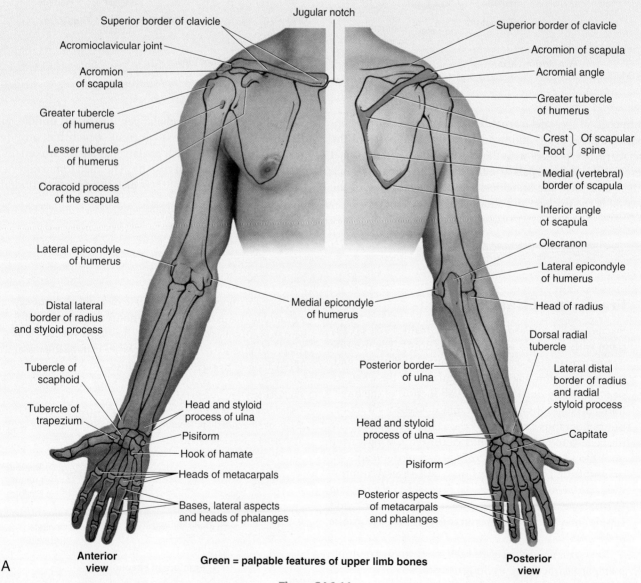

Figure SA6.1A.

Green = palpable features of upper limb bones

Anterior view

Posterior view

A

continued >

crest of the spine of scapula is subcutaneous throughout and can be easily palpated. When the upper limb is in the anatomical position, the:

* Superior angle of the scapula lies at the level of the T2 vertebra.
* Medial end of the root of the scapular spine is opposite the spinous process of the T3 vertebra.
* Inferior angle of the scapula lies at the level of the T7 vertebra, near the inferior border of the 7th rib and 7th intercostal space.

The **medial border of scapula** is palpable inferior to the root of the spine of the scapula as it crosses the 3rd–7th ribs. The **lateral border of scapula** is not easily palpated because it is covered by the teres major and minor muscles. The **inferior angle of scapula** is easily felt and is often visible.

The **greater tubercle of humerus** may be felt with the person's arm by the side on deep palpation through the deltoid muscle, inferior to the lateral border of the acromion. In this position, the tubercle is the most lateral bony point of the shoulder. When the arm is abducted, the greater tubercle is pulled beneath the acromion and is no longer palpable. The **lesser tubercle of the humerus** may be felt with difficulty by deep palpation through the anterior deltoid, approximately 1 cm laterally and slightly inferior to the tip of the coracoid process. Rotation of the arm fa-

cilitates palpation of this tubercle. The location of the **intertubercular groove**, between the greater and the lesser tubercles, is identifiable during flexion and extension of the elbow joint by palpating in an upward direction along the tendon of the long head of the biceps brachii as it moves through the intertubercular groove. The **shaft of humerus** may be felt with varying distinctness through the muscles surrounding it. The **medial** and **lateral epicondyles** of the humerus are palpated on the medial and lateral aspects of the elbow region.

The **olecranon** and posterior border of the ulna can be palpated easily. When the elbow joint is extended, observe that the tip of the olecranon and the humeral epicondyles lie in a straight line. When the elbow is flexed, the olecranon forms the apex of an approximately equilateral triangle, of which the epicondyles form the angles at its base. The **head of radius** can be palpated and felt to rotate in the depression on the posterolateral aspect of the extended elbow, just distal to the lateral epicondyle of the humerus. The **radial styloid process** can be palpated on the lateral side of the wrist in the **anatomical snuff box**; it is larger and approximately 1 cm more distal than the ulnar styloid process. The **dorsal radial tubercle** is easily felt around the middle of the dorsal aspect of the distal end of the radius (Fig. SA6.1B). The **head of ulna** forms a rounded subcutaneous prominence that can be easily

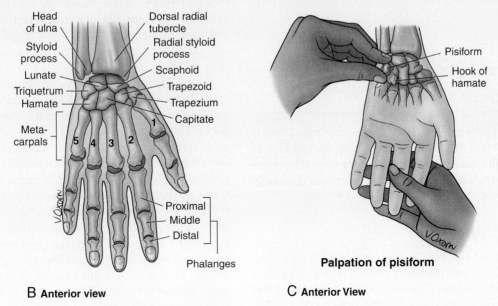

B Anterior view

C Anterior View

Figure SA6.1B.

continued >

seen and palpated on the medial side of the dorsal aspect of the wrist. The pointed subcutaneous ulnar styloid process may be felt slightly distal to the ulnar head when the hand is supinated.

The **pisiform** can be felt on the anterior aspect of the medial border of the wrist and can be moved from side to side when the hand is relaxed (Fig. SA6.1*C*). The **hook of hamate** can be palpated on deep pressure over the medial side of the palm, about 2 cm distal and lateral to the pisiform. The **tubercles of the scaphoid** and **trapezium** can be palpated at the base and medial aspect of the **thenar eminence** (ball of thumb) when the hand is extended.

The **metacarpals**, although overlain by the long extensor tendons of the digits, can be palpated on the dorsum of the hand (Fig. SA6.1*B*). The **heads of the metacarpals** form the knuckles; the 3rd metacarpal head is the most prominent. The dorsal aspects of the phalanges can be palpated easily. The knuckles of the fingers are formed by the **heads of the proximal and middle phalanges**.

When measuring upper limb length, or segments of it, the acromial angle, lateral epicondyle of the humerus, styloid process of the radius, and tip of the third finger are most commonly used as measuring points, with the limb relaxed (dangling) but with the palm directed anteriorly. ●

Superficial Structures of Upper Limb

Deep to the skin is subcutaneous tissue (superficial fascia) containing fat and deep fascia surrounding the muscles. If no structure (no muscle or tendon, for example) intervenes between the skin and the bone, the deep fascia usually attaches to bone.

Fascia of Upper Limb

The **pectoral fascia** invests the pectoralis major and is continuous inferiorly with the fascia of the anterior abdominal wall. The pectoral fascia leaves the lateral border of the pectoralis major and becomes the **axillary fascia** (Fig. 6.7*A*), which forms the floor of the axilla. Deep to the pectoral fascia and the pectoralis major, another fascial layer, the

clavipectoral fascia, descends from the clavicle, enclosing the subclavius and then the pectoralis minor, becoming continuous inferiorly with the axillary fascia. The part of the clavipectoral fascia between the pectoralis minor and the subclavius, the **costocoracoid membrane**, is pierced by the lateral pectoral nerve, which primarily supplies the pectoralis major. The part of the clavipectoral fascia inferior to the pectoralis minor, the **suspensory ligament of axilla** (Fig. 6.7*A*), supports the axillary fascia and pulls it and the skin inferior to it upward during abduction of the arm, forming the **axillary fossa**.

The scapulohumeral muscles that cover the scapula and form the bulk of the shoulder are also ensheathed by deep fascia. The **deltoid fascia** invests the deltoid and is continuous with the pectoral fascia anteriorly and the dense infraspinous fascia posteriorly. The muscles that cover the anterior and posterior surfaces of the scapula are covered superficially by deep fascia, which is attached to the margins of the scapula. This arrangement creates osseofibrous *subscapular, supraspinous,* and *infraspinous compartments.*

The **brachial fascia**, a sheath of deep fascia, encloses the arm like a snug sleeve (Fig. 6.7*B*); it is continuous superiorly with the deltoid, pectoral, axillary, and infraspinous fasciae. The brachial fascia is attached inferiorly to the epicondyles of the humerus and the olecranon of the ulna and is continuous with the antebrachial fascia, the deep fascia of the forearm. Two intermuscular septa, the **medial** and **lateral intermuscular septa**, extend from the deep surface of the brachial fascia and attach to the central shaft and medial and lateral supraepicondylar ridges of the humerus. These septa divide the arm into **anterior (flexor)** and **posterior (extensor) fascial compartments**, each of which contains muscles serving similar functions and sharing common innervation (Fig. 6.7*B*).

In the forearm, similar fascial compartments are surrounded by the **antebrachial fascia** and separated by the *interosseous membrane* connecting the radius and ulna (Fig. 6.7*C*). The antebrachial fascia thickens posteriorly over the distal ends of the radius and ulna to form a transverse band, the **extensor retinaculum**, which holds the extensor tendons in position. The antebrachial fascia also forms an anterior thickening, which is continuous with the extensor retinaculum but is officially unnamed; some authors identify it as the *palmar carpal ligament.* Immediately distal, but at a deeper level to the latter, the antebrachial fascia is also continued as the **flexor retinaculum** (transverse carpal ligament). This fibrous band extends between the anterior prominences of the outer carpal bones and converts the anterior concavity of the carpus into the *carpal tunnel* through which the flexor tendons and median nerve pass (Fig. 6.7*D*).

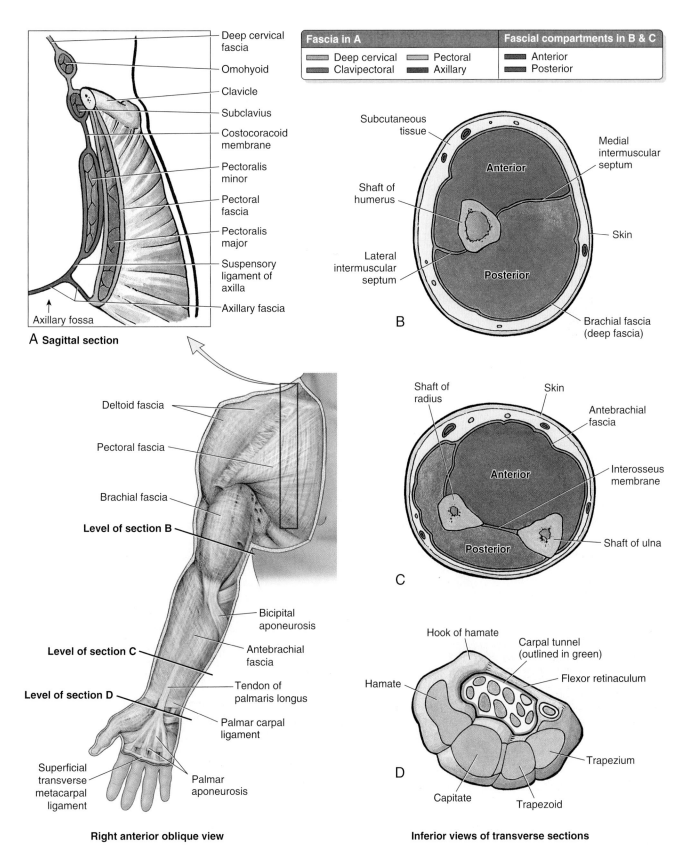

Fascia in A		**Fascial compartments in B & C**
Deep cervical	Pectoral	Anterior
Clavipectoral	Axillary	Posterior

A Sagittal section

B

C

Right anterior oblique view

D

Inferior views of transverse sections

Figure 6.7. Fascia of upper limb. A. *Inset,* The axillary fascia and fascia of the pectoral region are shown. **B.** This section of the arm shows its fascial compartments. **C.** This section of the forearm shows its fascial compartments. **D.** This section through the distal row of the carpal bones and flexor retinaculum shows the carpal tunnel.

The deep fascia of the upper limb continues beyond the extensor and flexor retinacula as the *palmar fascia*. The central part of the palmar fascia, the *palmar aponeurosis,* is thick, tendinous, and triangular. The aponeurosis forms four distinct thickenings that radiate to the bases of the fingers and become continuous with the fibrous tendon sheaths of the digits. The bands are traversed distally by the **superficial transverse metacarpal ligament**, which forms the base of the palmar aponeurosis. Strong *skin ligaments* extend from the palmar aponeurosis to the skin, holding the palmar skin close to the aponeurosis.

Cutaneous Nerves of the Upper Limb

Cutaneous nerves in the subcutaneous tissue supply the skin of the upper limb. The **dermatomes** of the limb follow a general pattern that is easy to understand if one notes that developmentally the limbs grow as lateral protrusions of the trunk, with the 1st digit (thumb or great toe) located on the cranial side. Thus the lateral surface of the upper limb is more cranial than the medial surface. There are two dermatome maps in common use. One corresponds to the concepts of limb development (Keegan and Garrett, 1948), and the other is based on clinical findings and is generally preferred by neurologists (Foerster, 1933). Both maps are approximations, delineating dermatomes as distinct zones when actually there is much overlap between adjacent dermatomes and much variation. In both maps, observe the progression of the segmental innervation (dermatomes) of the various cutaneous areas around the limb (Fig. 6.8A):

- C3 and C4 nerves supply the region at the base of the neck, extending laterally over the shoulder.
- C5 nerve supplies the arm laterally (i.e., superior aspect of the abducted limb).

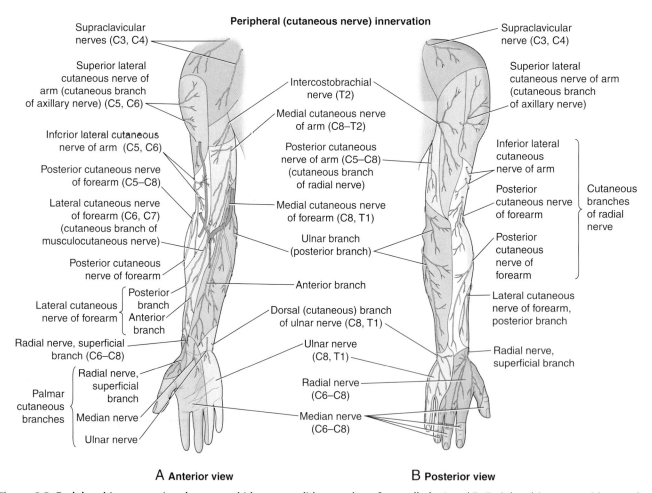

Peripheral (cutaneous nerve) innervation

Supraclavicular nerves (C3, C4)

Superior lateral cutaneous nerve of arm (cutaneous branch of axillary nerve) (C5, C6)

Inferior lateral cutaneous nerve of arm (C5, C6)

Posterior cutaneous nerve of forearm (C5–C8)

Lateral cutaneous nerve of forearm (C6, C7) (cutaneous branch of musculocutaneous nerve)

Posterior cutaneous nerve of forearm

Lateral cutaneous nerve of forearm { Posterior branch / Anterior branch

Radial nerve, superficial branch (C6–C8)

Palmar cutaneous branches { Radial nerve, superficial branch / Median nerve / Ulnar nerve

Intercostobrachial nerve (T2)

Medial cutaneous nerve of arm (C8–T2)

Posterior cutaneous nerve of arm (C5–C8) (cutaneous branch of radial nerve)

Medial cutaneous nerve of forearm (C8, T1)

Ulnar branch (posterior branch)

Anterior branch

Dorsal (cutaneous) branch of ulnar nerve (C8, T1)

Ulnar nerve (C8, T1)

Radial nerve (C6–C8)

Median nerve (C6–C8)

Supraclavicular nerve (C3, C4)

Superior lateral cutaneous nerve of arm (cutaneous branch of axillary nerve)

Inferior lateral cutaneous nerve of arm } Cutaneous branches of radial nerve

Posterior cutaneous nerve of forearm

Posterior cutaneous nerve of forearm

Lateral cutaneous nerve of forearm, posterior branch

Radial nerve, superficial branch

A **Anterior view**   B **Posterior view**

Figure 6.8. Peripheral (cutaneous) and segmental (dermatomal) innervation of upper limb. A and **B.** Peripheral (cutaneous) innervation.

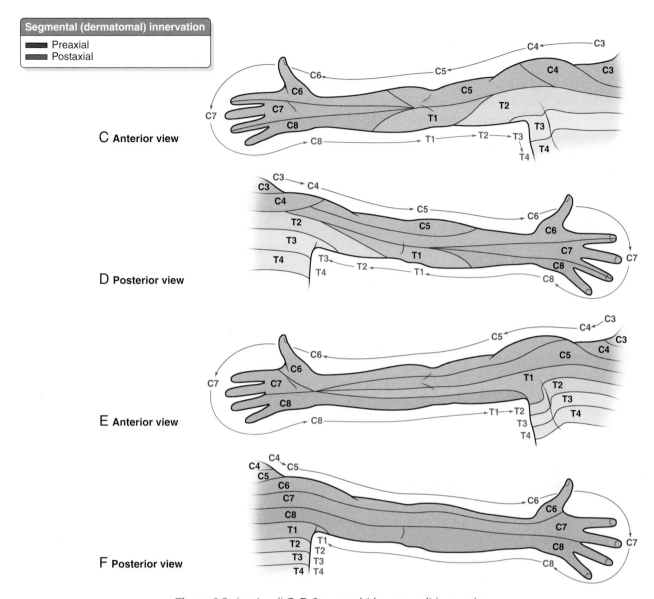

Segmental (dermatomal) innervation
- Preaxial
- Postaxial

C **Anterior view**

D **Posterior view**

E **Anterior view**

F **Posterior view**

Figure 6.8. *(continued)* **C–F.** Segmental (dermatomal) innervation.

- C6 nerve supplies the forearm laterally and the thumb.
- C7 nerve supplies the middle and ring fingers (or middle three fingers) and the middle of the posterior surface of the limb.
- C8 nerve supplies the little finger, the medial side of the hand, and the forearm (i.e., the inferior aspect of the abducted limb).
- T1 nerve supplies the middle of the forearm to the axilla.
- T2 nerve supplies a small part of the arm and the skin of the axilla.

Most cutaneous nerves of the upper limb are derived from the *brachial plexus,* a major nerve network formed by the anterior rami of the C5–T1 spinal nerves (Table 6.5). The cutaneous nerves to the shoulder are derived from the **cervical plexus,** a nerve network consisting of a series of nerve loops formed between adjacent anterior rami of the first four cervical nerves. The cervical plexus lies deep to the sternocleidomastoid (SCM) muscle on the lateral aspect of the neck. The cutaneous nerves of the arm and forearm are as follows (Fig. 6.8*B*):

- The **supraclavicular nerves** (C3, C4) pass anterior to the clavicle, immediately deep to the platysma, and supply the skin over the clavicle and the superolateral aspect of the pectoralis major.

- The **posterior cutaneous nerve of the arm** (C5–C8), a branch of the radial nerve, supplies the skin on the posterior surface of the arm.
- The **posterior cutaneous nerve of the forearm** (C5–C8), also a branch of the radial nerve, supplies the skin on the posterior surface of the forearm.
- The **superior lateral cutaneous nerve of the arm** (C5, C6), the terminal branch of the axillary nerve, emerges from beneath the posterior margin of the deltoid to supply the skin over the lower part of this muscle and on the lateral side of the midarm.
- The **inferior lateral cutaneous nerve of the arm** (C5, C6), a branch of the radial nerve, supplies the skin over the inferolateral aspect of the arm; it is frequently a branch of the posterior cutaneous nerve of the forearm.
- The **lateral cutaneous nerve of the forearm** (C6, C7), the terminal branch of the musculocutaneous nerve, supplies the skin on the lateral side of the forearm.
- The **medial cutaneous nerve of the arm** (C8–T2) arises from the medial cord of the brachial plexus, often uniting in the axilla with the lateral cutaneous branch of the 2nd intercostal nerve. It supplies the skin on the medial side of the arm.
- The **intercostobrachial nerve** (T2), a lateral cutaneous branch of the 2nd intercostal nerve, also contributes to the innervation of the skin on the medial surface of the arm.
- The **medial cutaneous nerve of the forearm** (C8, T1) arises from the medial cord of the brachial plexus and supplies the skin on the anterior and medial surfaces of the forearm.

Superficial Vessels of Upper Limb

The main superficial veins of the upper limb, the cephalic and basilic veins, originate in the subcutaneous tissue on the dorsum of the hand from the **dorsal venous network** (Fig. 6.9). **Perforating veins** form communications between the superficial and the deep veins.

The **cephalic vein** (G. *kephalé*, head) ascends in the subcutaneous tissue from the lateral aspect of the dorsal venous network, proceeding along the lateral border of the wrist and the anterolateral surface of the forearm and arm. Anterior to the elbow, the cephalic vein communicates with the **median cubital vein,** which passes obliquely across the anterior aspect of the elbow and joins the basilic vein. Superiorly, the cephalic vein passes between the deltoid and the pectoralis major muscles and enters the *clavipectoral (deltopectoral) triangle,* where it pierces the costocoracoid membrane, part of the clavipectoral fascia, and joins the terminal part of the axillary vein.

The **basilic vein** ascends in the subcutaneous tissue from the medial end of the dorsal venous network along the me-

dial side of the forearm and inferior part of the arm. It then passes deeply near the junction of the middle and inferior thirds of the arm, piercing the brachial fascia and running superiorly parallel to the brachial artery, where it merges with the accompanying veins (L. *venae comitantes*) of the axillary artery to form the axillary vein (Fig. 6.9). The highly variable **median antebrachial vein** (median vein of forearm) ascends in the middle of the anterior aspect of the forearm between the cephalic and the basilic veins; it sometimes divides into two branches that join the basilic and cephalic veins.

Superficial lymphatic vessels arise from **lymphatic plexuses** in the skin of the fingers, palm, and dorsum of the hand and ascend mostly with superficial veins, such as the cephalic and basilic veins (Fig. 6.9). Some lymphatic vessels accompanying the basilic vein enter the **cubital lymph nodes**, located proximal to the medial epicondyle. Efferent vessels from these nodes ascend in the arm and terminate in the **humeral (lateral) axillary lymph nodes.** Most lymphatic vessels accompanying the cephalic vein cross the proximal part of the arm and anterior aspect of the shoulder to enter the **apical axillary lymph nodes.** Some vessels enter the more superficial **deltopectoral lymph nodes.** Deep lymphatic vessels, less numerous than superficial vessels, accompany the major deep veins and terminate in the humeral axillary lymph nodes.

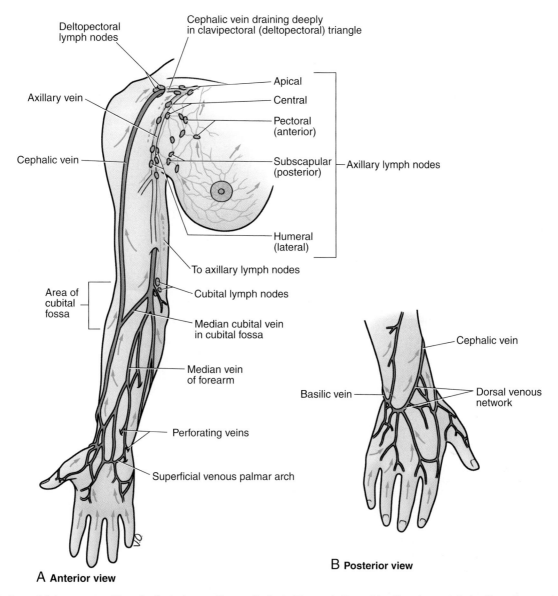

Figure 6.9. Superficial venous and lymphatic drainage of upper limb. A. The cephalic and basilic veins and their tributaries are shown. *Green arrows,* superficial lymphatic drainage to the lymph nodes. **B.** The dorsal venous network is identified.

Anterior Axioappendicular Muscles

Four **anterior axioappendicular (thoracoappendicular or pectoral) muscles** move the pectoral girdle: pectoralis major, pectoralis minor, subclavius, and serratus anterior (Fig. 6.10). The attachments, nerve supply, and main actions of these muscles are summarized in Table 6.1.

The fan-shaped **pectoralis major** covers the superior part of the thorax. It has **clavicular** and **sternocostal heads.** The latter head is much larger and its lateral border is responsible for the muscular mass that forms most of the ante-

rior wall of the axilla, with its inferior border forming the *anterior axillary fold* (see "Axilla," later in this chapter). The pectoralis major and adjacent deltoid form the narrow **deltopectoral groove,** in which the cephalic vein runs. However, the muscles diverge slightly from each other superiorly and, along with the clavicle, form the **clavipectoral (deltopectoral) triangle** (Fig. 6.10A).

The triangular **pectoralis minor** lies in the anterior wall of the axilla (Fig. 6.10B), where it is almost completely covered by the pectoralis major. The pectoralis minor stabilizes the scapula and is used when stretching the upper limb forward to touch an object that is just out of reach.

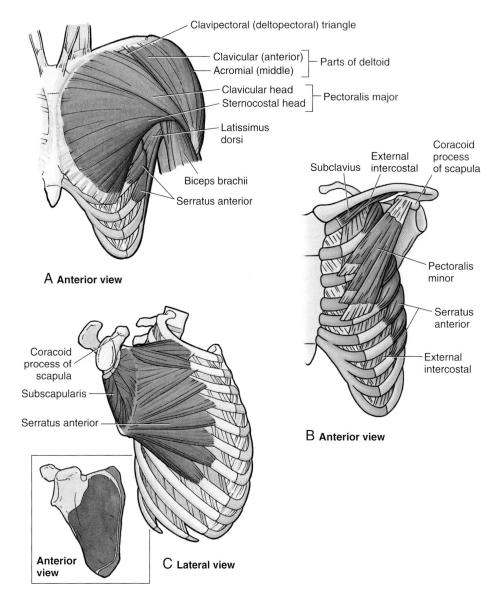

Figure 6.10. Pectoral region and axilla. A. The axioappendicular muscles are identified. **B.** The pectoralis minor and subclavius are shown. **C.** The serratus anterior and subscapularis are shown. *Inset,* the scapular attachments of the subscapularis (*red*) and serratus anterior (*blue*) are shown.

With the coracoid process, the pectoralis minor forms a "bridge" under which vessels and nerves pass to the arm (Fig. 6.15). Thus the pectoralis minor is a useful anatomical and surgical landmark for structures in the axilla (e.g., the axillary artery).

The **subclavius** lies almost horizontally when the arm is in the anatomical position. This small, round muscle is located inferior to the clavicle and affords some protection to the subclavian vessels and the superior trunk of the brachial plexus if the clavicle fractures.

The **serratus anterior** overlies the lateral part of the thorax and forms the medial wall of the axilla (Fig. 6.10C). This broad sheet of thick muscle was given its name because of

the sawtooth appearance of its fleshy slips or digitations (L. *serratus,* a saw). By keeping the scapula closely applied to the thoracic wall, the serratus anterior anchors this bone, enabling other muscles to use it as a fixed bone for movements of the humerus.

Posterior Axioappendicular and Scapulohumeral Muscles

The **posterior axioappendicular muscles** (superficial and intermediate groups of extrinsic back muscles) attach the su-

Table 6.1 Anterior Axioappendicular Muscles

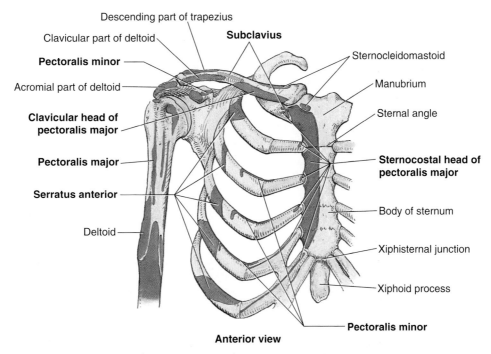

Anterior view

Muscle	Proximal Attachment	Distal Attachment	Innervation[a]	Main Action
Pectoralis major	*Clavicular head:* anterior surface of medial half of clavicle *Sternocostal head:* anterior surface of sternum, superior six costal cartilages, aponeurosis of external oblique muscle	Lateral lip of intertubercular groove of humerus	Lateral and medial pectoral nerves; clavicular head (C5, **C6**), sternocostal head (**C7, C8,** T1)	Adducts and medially rotates humerus; draws scapula anteriorly and inferiorly Acting alone, clavicular head flexes humerus and sternocostal head extends it from the flexed position
Pectoralis minor	3rd–5th ribs near their costal cartilages	Medial border and superior surface of coracoid process of scapula	Medial pectoral nerve (C8, T1)	Stabilizes scapula by drawing it inferiorly and anteriorly against thoracic wall
Subclavius	Junction of 1st rib and its costal cartilage	Inferior surface of middle third of clavicle	Nerve to subclavius (**C5**, C6)	Anchors and depresses clavicle
Serratus anterior	External surfaces of lateral parts of 1st–8th ribs	Anterior surface of medial border of scapula	Long thoracic nerve (C5, **C6, C7**)	Protracts scapula and holds it against thoracic wall; rotates scapula

[a] The spinal cord segmental innervation is indicated (e.g., "**C5,** C6" means that the nerves supplying the subclavius are derived from the fifth and sixth cervical segments of the spinal cord). Numbers in boldface (**C5**) indicate the main segmental innervation. Damage to one or more of the listed spinal cord segments or to the motor nerve roots arising from them results in paralysis of the muscles concerned.

perior appendicular skeleton (of the upper limb) to the axial skeleton (in the trunk). The *intrinsic back muscles,* which maintain posture and control movements of the vertebral column, are described in Chapter 4. The posterior shoulder muscles are divided into three groups (Tables 6.2 and 6.3):

- *Superficial posterior axioappendicular (extrinsic shoulder) muscles:* trapezius and latissimus dorsi.
- *Deep posterior axioappendicular (extrinsic shoulder) muscles:* levator scapulae and rhomboids.

- *Scapulohumeral (intrinsic shoulder) muscles:* deltoid, teres major, and the four rotator cuff muscles (supraspinatus, infraspinatus, teres minor, and subscapularis).

Superficial Posterior Axioappendicular Muscles

The **trapezius** provides a direct attachment of the pectoral girdle to the trunk. This large triangular muscle covers

Paralysis of Serratus Anterior

When the serratus anterior is paralyzed because of *injury to the long thoracic nerve* (Fig. 6.15*B*), the medial border of the scapula moves laterally and posteriorly away from the thoracic wall. This gives the scapula the appearance of a wing, especially when the person leans on the hand or presses the upper limb against a wall. When the arm is raised, the medial border and inferior angle of the scapula pull markedly away from the posterior thoracic wall, a deformation known as a *winged scapula* (Fig. B6.5). In addition, the arm cannot be abducted above the horizontal position because the serratus anterior is unable to rotate the glenoid cavity superiorly to allow complete abduction of the limb. Although protected when the limbs are at one's sides, the long thoracic nerve is exceptional in that it courses on the superficial aspect of the serratus anterior, which it supplies. Thus when the limbs are elevated, as in a knife fight, the nerve is especially vulnerable.

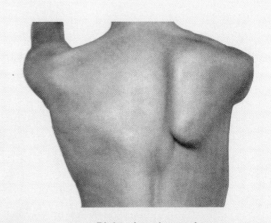

Right winged scapula

Figure B6.5.

the posterior aspect of the neck and the superior half of the trunk (Table 6.2). The trapezius attaches the pectoral girdle to the cranium and vertebral column and assists in suspending the upper limb. The fibers of the trapezius are divided into three parts that have different actions at the scapulothoracic joint between the scapula and the thoracic wall:

- Descending (superior) part elevates the scapula (e.g., when squaring shoulders).
- Middle part retracts the scapula (i.e., pulls it posteriorly).
- Ascending (inferior) fibers depress the scapula and lower the shoulder.

The descending (superior) and ascending (inferior) parts of trapezius act together in rotating the scapula on the thoracic wall. The trapezius also braces the shoulders by pulling the scapulae posteriorly and superiorly, fixing them in position with tonic contraction; consequently, weakness of this muscle causes drooping of the shoulders.

The **latissimus dorsi** is a large, fan-shaped muscle that covers a wide area of the back (Table 6.2). It passes from the trunk to the humerus and acts directly on the glenohumeral (shoulder) joint and indirectly on the pectoral girdle (scapulothoracic joint). In conjunction with the pectoralis major, the latissimus dorsi raises the trunk to the arm, which occurs when the limb is fixed and the body

moves, as when performing chin-ups (hoisting oneself so the chin touches an overhead bar) or climbing a tree. These movements are also used when the trunk is fixed and the limb moves, as when chopping wood, paddling a canoe, and swimming.

Deep Posterior Axioappendicular Muscles

The superior third of the **levator scapulae** lies deep to the SCM; the inferior third is deep to the trapezius (Table 6.2). True to its name, the levator scapulae acts with the superior part of trapezius to elevate the scapula. With the rhomboids and pectoralis minor, it rotates the scapula, depressing the glenoid cavity. Acting bilaterally, the levators extend the neck; acting unilaterally, the muscle may contribute to lateral flexion of the neck.

The two **rhomboids** (major and minor) lie deep to the trapezius and form parallel bands that pass inferolaterally from the vertebrae to the medial border of the scapula (Table 6.2). The thin flat **rhomboid major** is approximately two times wider than the thicker **rhomboid minor** lying superior to it. The rhomboids retract and rotate the scapula, depressing the glenoid cavity. They also assist the serratus anterior in holding the scapula against the thoracic wall and fixing the scapula during movements of the upper limb.

Table 6.2 Posterior Axioappendicular Muscles

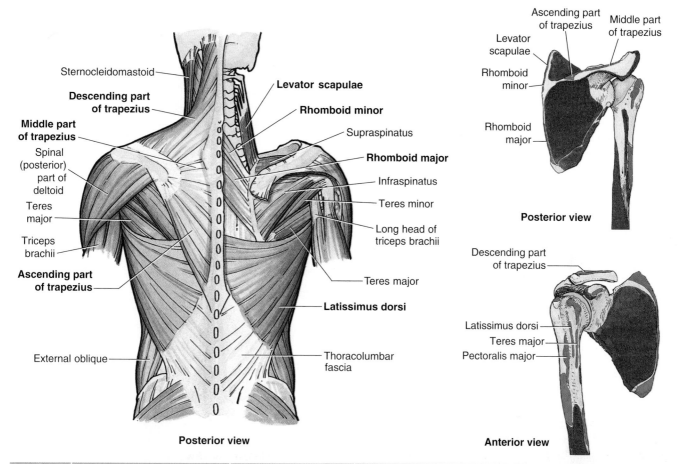

Posterior view

Posterior view

Anterior view

Muscle	Proximal Attachment	Distal Attachment	Innervation[a]	Main Action
Superficial posterior thoracoappendicular (extrinsic shoulder) muscles				
Trapezius	Medial third of superior nuchal line; external occipital protuberance; nuchal ligament; spinous processes of C7–C12 vertebrae	Lateral third of clavicle; acromion and spine of scapula	Spinal accessory nerve (CN XI) (motor fibers) and C3, C4 (pain and proprioceptive fibers)	Descending part elevates; ascending part depresses; and middle part (or all parts together) retracts scapula; descending and ascending parts act together to rotate glenoid cavity superiorly
Latissimus dorsi	Spinous processes of inferior 6 thoracic vertebrae, thoracolumbar fascia, iliac crest, and inferior 3 or 4 ribs	Floor of intertubercular groove of humerus	Thoracodorsal nerve (**C6, C7,** C8)	Extends, adducts, and medially rotates humerus; raises body toward arms during climbing
Deep posterior thoracoappendicular (extrinsic shoulder) muscles				
Levator scapulae	Posterior tubercles of transverse processes of C1–C4 vertebrae	Medial border of scapula superior to root of spine	Dorsal scapular (C5) and cervical (C3, C4) nerves	Elevates scapula and tilts its glenoid cavity inferiorly by rotating scapula
Rhomboid minor and major	*Minor:* nuchal ligament; spinous processes of C7 and T1 vertebrae *Major:* spinous processes of T2–T5 vertebrae	*Minor:* smooth triangular area at medial end of scapular spine *Major:* medial border of scapula from level of spine to inferior angle	Dorsal scapular nerve (C4, **C5**)	Retract scapula and rotate it to depress glenoid cavity; fix scapula to thoracic wall

[a]The spinal cord segmental innervation is indicated (e.g., "**C6, C7,** C8" means that the nerves supplying the latissimus dorsi are derived from the sixth through eighth cervical segments of the spinal cord). Numbers in boldface (**C6, C7**) indicate the main segmental innervation. Damage to one or more of the listed spinal cord segments or to the motor nerve roots arising from them results in paralysis of the muscles concerned.

Table 6.3 Scapulohumeral (Intrinsic Shoulder) Muscles

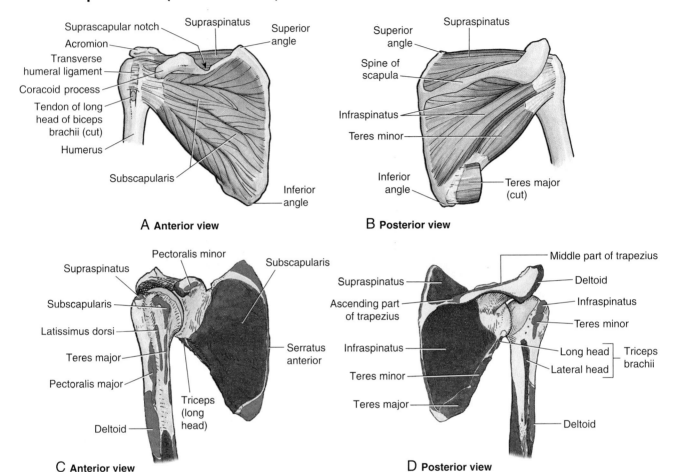

A **Anterior view**

B **Posterior view**

C **Anterior view**

D **Posterior view**

Muscle	Proximal Attachment	Distal Attachment	Innervation[a]	Main Action
Deltoid	Lateral third of clavicle; acromion and spine of scapula	Deltoid tuberosity of humerus	Axillary nerve (**C5**, C6)	Clavicular (anterior) part flexes and medially rotates arm; acromial (middle) part abducts arm; spinal (posterior) part extends and laterally rotates arm
Supraspinatus[b]	Supraspinous fossa of scapula	Superior facet	Suprascapular nerve (C4, **C5**, C6)	Initiates and assists deltoid in abduction of arm and acts with rotator cuff muscles[b]
Infraspinatus[b]	Infraspinous fossa of scapula	Middle facet — Of greater tubercle of humerus	Suprascapular nerve (**C5**, C6)	Laterally rotate arm; help hold humeral head in glenoid cavity of scapula
Teres minor[b]	Middle part of lateral border of scapula	Inferior facet	Axillary nerve (**C5**, C6)	
Teres major	Posterior surface of inferior angle of scapula	Medial lip of intertubercular groove of humerus	Lower subscapular nerve (C5, **C6**)	Adducts and medially rotates arm
Subscapularis[b]	Subscapular fossa (most of anterior surface of scapula)	Lesser tubercle of humerus	Upper and lower subscapular nerves (C5, **C6**, C7)	Medially rotates and adducts arm; helps hold humeral head in glenoid cavity

[a]The spinal cord segmental innervation is indicated (e.g., "**C5**, C6" means that the nerves supplying the deltoid are derived from the fifth and sixth cervical segments of the spinal cord). Numbers in boldface (**C5**) indicate the main segmental innervation. Damage to one or more of the listed spinal cord segments or to the motor nerve roots arising from them results in paralysis of the muscles concerned.

[b]Collectively, the supraspinatus, infraspinatus, teres minor, and subscapularis muscles are referred to as the rotator cuff, or SITS, muscles. Their primary function during all movements of the glenohumeral (shoulder) joint is to hold the humeral head in the glenoid cavity of the scapula.

Scapulohumeral Muscles

The six **scapulohumeral muscles** (the deltoid, teres major, supraspinatus, infraspinatus, subscapularis, and teres minor) are relatively short muscles that pass from the scapula to the humerus and act on the glenohumeral joint (Table 6.3).

The **deltoid** is a thick powerful muscle forming the rounded contour of the shoulder. The muscle is divided into clavicular (anterior), acromial (middle), and spinal (posterior) parts that can act separately or as a whole (Table 6.3). When all three parts contract simultaneously, the arm is abducted. The clavicular and spinal parts act like guy ropes to steady the arm as it is abducted. When the arm is fully adducted, the line of pull of the deltoid coincides with the axis of the humerus; thus it pulls directly upward on the bone and cannot initiate or produce abduction. The deltoid is, however, able to act as a shunt muscle, resisting inferior displacement of the head of the humerus from the glenoid cavity. From the fully adducted position, abduction must be initiated by the supraspinatus or by leaning to the side, allowing gravity to initiate the movement. The deltoid becomes fully effective as an abductor after the initial 15° of abduction.

The **teres major** is a thick rounded muscle that lies on the inferolateral third of the scapula (Table 6.3). It adducts and medially rotates the arm, but along with the deltoid and rotator cuff muscles it is an important stabilizer of the humeral head in the glenoid cavity during movement.

Four of the scapulohumeral muscles (intrinsic shoulder muscles)—**supraspinatus, infraspinatus, teres minor,** and **subscapularis** (referred to as SITS muscles)—are called **rotator cuff muscles** because they form a musculotendinous rotator cuff around the glenohumeral joint (Table 6.3). All except the supraspinatus are rotators of the humerus. The supraspinatus, besides being part of the rotator cuff, initiates and assists the deltoid in the first 15° of abduction of the arm. The tendons of the SITS or rotator cuff muscles blend with the joint capsule of the glenohumeral joint, reinforcing it as the musculotendinous rotator cuff, which protects the joint and gives it stability. Tonic contraction of these muscles holds the relatively large head of the humerus firmly against the small and shallow glenoid cavity during arm movements. Bursae around the glenohumeral joint, between the tendons of the rotator cuff muscles and the fibrous layer of the joint capsule, reduce friction on the tendons passing over the bones or other areas of resistance.

Axilla

The axilla is the pyramidal space inferior to the glenohumeral joint and superior to the skin and axillary fascia at the junction of the arm and thorax (Fig. 6.11). The shape

Injury to the Axillary Nerve

Atrophy of the deltoid occurs when the axillary nerve (C5 and C6) is severely damaged (e.g., as might occur when the surgical neck of the humerus is fractured). As the deltoid atrophies, the rounded contour of the shoulder disappears. This gives the shoulder a flattened appearance and produces a slight hollow inferior to the acromion. A loss of sensation may occur over the lateral side of the proximal part of the arm, the area supplied by the superior lateral cutaneous nerve of the arm. To test the deltoid (or the function of the axillary nerve) the arm is abducted, against resistance, starting from approximately 15°.

Rotator Cuff Injuries and the Supraspinatus

Injury or disease may damage the rotator cuff, producing instability of the glenohumeral joint. Rupture or tear of the supraspinatus tendon is the most common injury of the rotator cuff. *Degenerative tendonitis of the rotator cuff* is common, especially in older people. These syndromes are discussed in detail later in this chapter, in relationship to the glenohumeral joint.

and size of the axilla varies, depending on the position of the arm; it almost disappears when the arm is fully abducted. The axilla provides a passageway for vessels and nerves going to and from the upper limb. The axilla has an apex, base, and four walls, three of which are muscular:

- The *apex of the axilla* is the **cervicoaxillary canal,** the passageway between the neck and the axilla. It is bounded by the 1st rib, clavicle, and superior edge of the scapula. The arteries, veins, lymphatics, and nerves traverse this superior opening to pass to or from the arm.
- The *base of the axilla* is formed by the concave skin, subcutaneous tissue, and axillary (deep) fascia extending from the arm to the thoracic wall forming the **axillary fossa** (armpit).
- The *anterior wall of the axilla* is formed by the pectoralis major and minor and the pectoral and clavipectoral fascia associated with them. The **anterior axillary fold** is the inferiormost part of the anterior wall.

Surface Anatomy of Pectoral and Scapular Regions (Anterior and Posterior Axioappendicular and Scapulohumeral Muscles)

The large vessels and nerves to the upper limb pass posterior to the convexity in the clavicle. The **clavipectoral (deltopectoral) triangle** is the slightly depressed area just inferior to the lateral part of the clavicle (Fig. SA6.2*A*). The clavipectoral triangle is bounded by the clavicle superiorly, the deltoid laterally, and the **clavicular head of pectoralis major** medially. When the arm is abducted and then adducted against resistance, the two heads of the **pectoralis major** are visible and palpable. As this muscle extends from the thoracic wall to the arm, it forms the **anterior axillary fold**. Digitations of the **serratus anterior** appear inferolateral to the pectoralis major. The **coracoid process** of the scapula is covered by the **anterior part of deltoid**; however, the tip

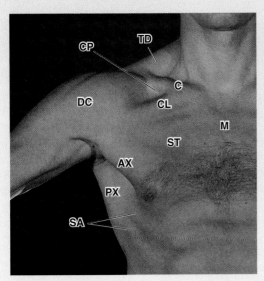

A Anterior view

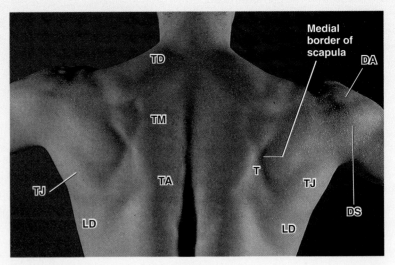

B Posterior view

Key	
AX	Anterior axillary fold
C	Clavicle
CL	Clavicular head of pectoralis major
CP	Clavipectoral triangle
DA	Acromial (middle) part of deltoid
DC	Clavicular (anterior) part of deltoid
DS	Spinal (posterior) part of deltoid
LD	Latissimus dorsi
M	Manubrium
PX	Posterior axillary fold
SA	Serratus anterior
ST	Sternocostal head of pectoralis major
T	Triangle of auscultation
TA	Ascending part of trapezius
TD	Descending part of trapezius
TJ	Teres major
TM	Middle part of trapezius

C Posterior view

Figure SA6.2.

continued >

of the process can be felt on deep palpation in the clavipectoral triangle. The **deltoid** forms the contour of the shoulder (Fig. SA6.2*B*); and as its name indicates, it is shaped like an inverted Greek letter delta.

The superior border of the **latissimus dorsi** and a part of the **rhomboid major** are overlapped by the **trapezius** (Fig. SA6.2*C*). The area formed by the superior border of latissimus dorsi, the medial border of the scapula, and the inferolateral border of the trapezius is called the *triangle of auscultation*. This gap in the thick back musculature is a good place to examine posterior segments of the lungs with a stethoscope. When the scapulae are drawn anteriorly by folding the arms across the thorax and the trunk is flexed, the auscultatory triangle enlarges. The **teres major** forms a raised oval area on the inferolateral third of the posterior aspect of the scapula when the arm is adducted against resistance. The **posterior axillary fold** is formed by the teres major and the tendon of the latissimus dorsi. ●

- The *posterior wall of the axilla* is formed chiefly by the scapula and subscapularis on its anterior surface and inferiorly by the teres major and latissimus dorsi. The **posterior axillary fold** is the inferiormost part of the posterior wall that may be grasped.
- The *medial wall of the axilla* is formed by the thoracic wall (1st–4th ribs and intercostal muscles) and the overlying serratus anterior.
- The *lateral wall of the axilla* is the narrow bony wall formed by the *intertubercular groove* in the humerus.

The axilla contains the axillary artery and its branches, axillary vein and its tributaries, nerves of the cords and branches of the brachial plexus, lymphatic vessels, and several groups of *axillary lymph nodes*, all embedded in *axillary fat*. Proximally, the neurovascular structures are ensheathed in a sleeve-like extension of the cervical fascia, the **axillary sheath** (Fig 6.15*D*).

Axillary Artery and Vein

The **axillary artery** begins at the lateral border of the 1st rib as the continuation of the subclavian artery and ends at the inferior border of the teres major (Table 6.4). It passes posterior to the pectoralis minor into the arm and becomes the brachial artery when it passes distal to the inferior border of the teres major. For descriptive purposes, the axillary artery is divided into three parts relative to the pectoralis minor (the part number also indicates the number of its branches):

- The **first part of the axillary artery** is located between the lateral border of the 1st rib and the medial border of the pectoralis minor; it is enclosed in the *axillary sheath* and has one branch: the *superior thoracic artery*.
- The **second part of the axillary artery** lies posterior to the pectoralis minor and has two branches: the *thoracoacromial artery* and *lateral thoracic artery*, which pass medial and lateral to the muscle, respectively.
- The **third part of the axillary artery** extends from the lateral border of the pectoralis minor to the inferior border of the teres major and has three branches. The *subscapular artery* is the largest branch of the axillary artery. Opposite the origin of this artery, the *anterior circumflex humeral artery* and *posterior circumflex humeral artery* arise.

The **axillary vein** lies initially (distally) on the anteromedial side of the axillary artery, with its terminal part anteroinferior to the artery (Fig. 6.12). This large vein is formed by the union of the *accompanying brachial veins* and the basilic vein at the inferior border of the teres major. The axillary vein ends at the lateral border of the 1st rib, where it becomes the **subclavian vein**. The veins of the axilla are more abundant than the arteries, are highly variable, and frequently anastomose.

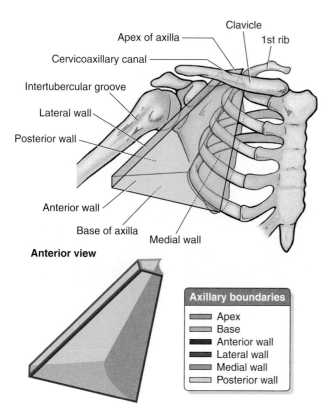

Anterior view

Clavicle
1st rib
Apex of axilla
Cervicoaxillary canal
Intertubercular groove
Lateral wall
Posterior wall
Anterior wall
Base of axilla
Medial wall

Axillary boundaries

- Apex
- Base
- Anterior wall
- Lateral wall
- Medial wall
- Posterior wall

Figure 6.11. Location and walls of axilla.

Axillary Lymph Nodes

Many lymph nodes are found in the axillary fat. There are five principal groups of axillary lymph nodes: pectoral, subscapular, humeral, central, and apical (Figs. 6.12 and 6.13).

The **pectoral (anterior) nodes** consist of three to five nodes that lie along the medial wall of the axilla, around the lateral thoracic vein and inferior border of the pectoralis minor. The pectoral nodes receives lymph mainly from the anterior thoracic wall, including most of the breast (see Chapter 1).

The **subscapular (posterior) nodes** consist of six to seven nodes that lie along the posterior axillary fold and subscapular blood vessels. These nodes receive lymph

Table 6.4 Arteries of the Proximal Upper Limb (Shoulder Region and Arm)

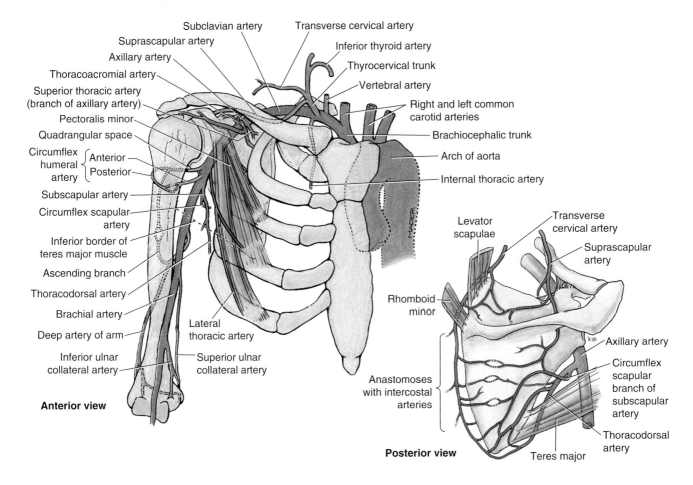

Anterior view

Posterior view

Artery	Origin		Course
Internal thoracic	Inferior surface of first part	Subclavian artery	Descends, inclining anteromedially, posterior to sternal end of clavicle and 1st costal cartilage; enters thorax to descend in parasternal plane; gives rise to perforating branches, anterior intercostal, musculophrenic, and superior epigastric arteries
Thyrocervical trunk	Anterior surface of first part		Ascends as a short, wide trunk, giving rise to four branches: suprascapular, transverse cervical, ascending cervical, and inferior thyroid arteries.
Suprascapular	Thyrocervical (or as direct branch of subclavian artery)		Passes inferolaterally crossing anterior scalene muscle, phrenic nerve, subclavian artery, and brachial plexus, running laterally posterior and parallel to clavicle; next passes over transverse scapular ligament to supraspinous fossa; then lateral to scapular spine (deep to acromion) to infraspinous fossa on posterior surface of scapula

Artery	Origin		Course
Superior thoracic	First part (as only branch)		Runs anteromedially along superior border of pectoralis minor; then passes between it and pectoralis major to thoracic wall; helps supply 1st and 2nd intercostal spaces and superior part of serratus anterior
Thoracoacromial	Second part (first branch)		Curls around superomedial border of pectoralis minor; pierces costocoracoid membrane (clavipectoral fascia); divides into four branches: pectoral, deltoid, acromial, and clavicular
Lateral thoracic	Second part (second branch)	Axillary artery	Descends along axillary border of pectoralis minor; follows it onto thoracic wall, supplying lateral aspect of breast
Circumflex humeral (anterior and posterior)	Third part (sometimes via a common trunk)		Encircle surgical neck of humerus, anastomosing with each other laterally; larger posterior branch traverses quadrangular space
Subscapular	Third part (as largest branch of any part)		Descends from level of inferior border of subscapularis along lateral border of scapula, dividing within 2–3 cm into terminal branches, the circumflex scapular and thoracodorsal arteries
Circumflex scapular	Subscapular artery		Curves around lateral border of scapula to enter infraspinous fossa, anastomosing with suprascapular artery
Thoracodorsal	Subscapular artery		Continues course of subscapular artery, descending with thoracodorsal nerve to enter apex of latissimus dorsi
Deep brachial artery of arm	Near its origin		Accompanies radial nerve along radial groove of humerus, supplying posterior compartment of arm and participating in periarticular arterial anastomoses around elbow joint
Superior ulnar collateral	Near middle of arm	Brachial artery	Accompanies ulnar nerve to posterior aspect of elbow; anastomoses with posterior ulnar recurrent artery
Inferior ulnar collateral	Superior to medial epicondyle of humerus		Passes anterior to medial epicondyle of humerus to anastomose with anterior ulnar collateral artery

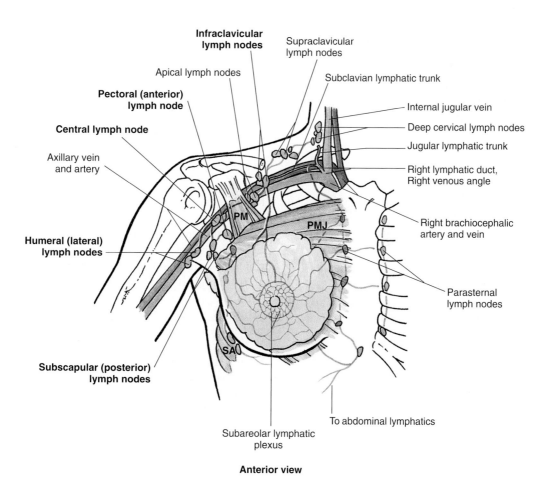

Anterior view

Figure 6.12. Axillary lymph nodes. *PM,* pectoralis minor; *PMJ,* pectoralis major; *SA,* serratus anterior.

Compression of the Axillary Artery

Compression of the third part of the axillary artery against the humerus may be necessary when profuse bleeding occurs (e.g., resulting from a stab or bullet wound in the axilla). If compression is required at a more proximal site, the axillary artery can be compressed at its origin at the lateral border of the 1st rib by exerting downward pressure in the angle between the clavicle and the attachment of the SCM.

Arterial Anastomoses Around the Scapula

Many arterial anastomoses (communications between arteries) occur around the scapula (Table 6.4). Several arteries join to form networks on the anterior and posterior surfaces of the scapula: the dorsal scapular, suprascapular, and subscapular (via the circumflex scapular branch). The importance of the *collateral circulation* made possible by these anastomoses becomes apparent when ligation of a lacerated subclavian or axillary artery is necessary. For example, the axillary artery may have to be ligated between the 1st rib and subscapular artery; in other cases, vascular stenosis (narrowing) of the axillary artery may result from an atherosclerotic lesion that causes reduced blood flow. In either case, the direction of blood flow in the subscapular artery is reversed, enabling blood to reach the third part of the axillary artery. Note that the subscapular artery receives blood through several anastomoses with the suprascapular artery, transverse cervical artery, and intercostal arteries. *Slow occlusion of an artery* (e.g., resulting from disease) often enables sufficient collateral circulation to develop, preventing *ischemia* (deficiency of blood). Sudden occlusion usually does not allow sufficient time for adequate collateral circulation to develop; as a result, ischemia of the upper limb occurs. *Surgical ligation of the axillary artery* between the origins of the subscapular artery and the deep artery of the arm will cut off the blood supply to the arm because the collateral circulation is inadequate.

Injury to the Axillary Vein

Wounds in the axilla often involve the axillary vein because of its large size and exposed position. When the arm is fully abducted, the axillary vein overlaps the axillary artery anteriorly. A wound in the proximal part of the vein is particularly dangerous, not only because of profuse bleeding but also because to the risk of air entering the vein and producing *air emboli* (air bubbles) in the blood.

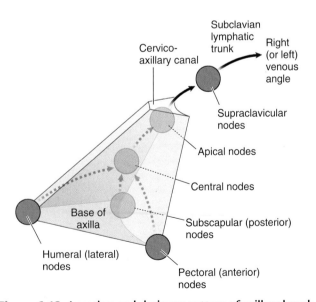

Figure 6.13. Location and drainage pattern of axillary lymph nodes.

from the posterior aspect of the thoracic wall and scapular region.

The **humeral (lateral) nodes** consist of four to six nodes that lie along the lateral wall of the axilla, medial and posterior to the axillary vein. These humeral nodes receive nearly all the lymph from the upper limb, except that carried by lymphatic vessels accompanying the cephalic vein, which primarily drain to the apical axillary and infraclavicular nodes.

Efferent lymphatic vessels from the pectoral, subscapular and humeral nodes pass to the **central nodes**. The central nodes consist of three to four large nodes situated deep to the pectoralis minor near the base of the axilla, in association with the second part of the axillary artery. Efferent vessels from the central nodes pass to the apical nodes.

The **apical nodes** are located at the apex of the axilla along the medial side of the axillary vein and the first part of the axillary artery. The apical nodes receive lymph from lymphatic trunk may be joined by the jugular and broncho-mediastinal trunks on the right side to form the **right lymphatic duct**, or it may enter the **right venous angle** independently. On the left side, the subclavian trunk most commonly joins the **thoracic duct**.

Brachial Plexus

The **brachial plexus** is a major network of nerves supplying the upper limb. It begins in the lateral cervical region (posterior triangle) and extends into the axilla. The brachial plexus is formed by the union of the anterior rami of the C5–T1 nerves, which constitute the **roots of brachial plexus** (Figs. 6.14; Table 6.5). The roots usually pass through the gap between the anterior and the middle scalene muscles with the subclavian artery. The sympathetic fibers carried by each root of the plexus are received from gray rami of the middle and inferior cervical ganglia as the roots pass between the scalene muscles.

In the inferior part of the neck, the roots of the brachial plexus unite to form three trunks (Fig. 6.15):

- A **superior trunk**, from the union of the C5 and C6 roots.
- A **middle trunk**, which is a continuation of the C7 root.
- An **inferior trunk**, from the union of the C8 and T1 roots.

Enlargement of Axillary Lymph Nodes

An infection in the upper limb can cause the axillary nodes to enlarge and become tender and inflamed, a condition called *lymphangitis* (inflammation of lymphatic vessels). The humeral group of nodes is usually the first ones to be involved. Lymphangitis is characterized by warm, red streaks in the skin of the limb. Infections in the pectoral region and breast, including the superior part of the abdomen, can also produce enlargement of the axillary nodes. These nodes are also the most common site of metastases (spread) of cancer of the breast.

all other groups of axillary nodes as well as from lymphatics accompanying the proximal cephalic vein. Efferent vessels from the apical nodes traverse the *cervicoaxillary canal* and unite to form the **subclavian lymphatic trunk**, although some vessels may drain en route through the **clavicular (infraclavicular and supraclavicular) nodes**. The subclavian

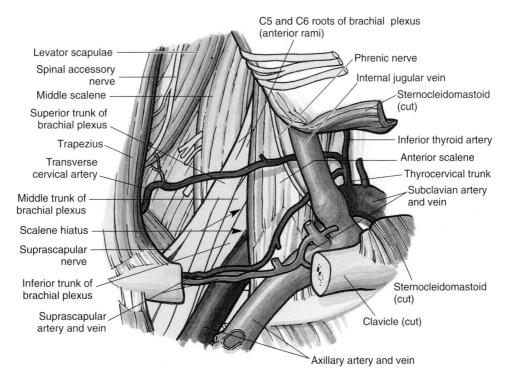

Anterolateral view

Figure 6.14. Brachial plexus and subclavian vessels.

Table 6.5 Brachial Plexus and Nerves of Upper Limb

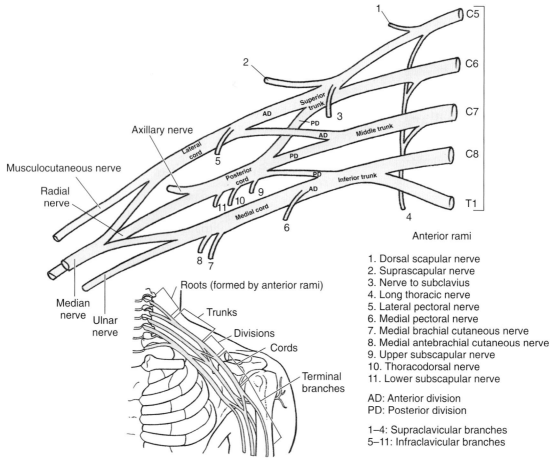

1. Dorsal scapular nerve
2. Suprascapular nerve
3. Nerve to subclavius
4. Long thoracic nerve
5. Lateral pectoral nerve
6. Medial pectoral nerve
7. Medial brachial cutaneous nerve
8. Medial antebrachial cutaneous nerve
9. Upper subscapular nerve
10. Thoracodorsal nerve
11. Lower subscapular nerve

AD: Anterior division
PD: Posterior division

1–4: Supraclavicular branches
5–11: Infraclavicular branches

Nerve	Origin[a]	Course	Structures Innervated
Supraclavicular branches			
Dorsal scapular	Posterior aspect of anterior ramus of **C5** with a frequent contribution from C4	Pierces middle scalene; descends deep to levator scapulae and rhomboids	Rhomboids; occasionally supplies levator scapulae
Long thoracic	Posterior aspect of anterior rami of **C5, C6,** C7	Passes through cervicoaxillary canal, descending posterior to C8 and T1 roots of plexus (anterior rami); runs inferiorly on superficial surface of serratus anterior	Serratus anterior
Suprascapular	Superior trunk, receiving fibers from **C5,** C6 and often C4	Passes laterally across lateral cervical region (posterior triangle of neck), superior to brachial plexus; then through scapular notch inferior to superior transverse cervical ligament	Supraspinatus and infraspinatus muscles; glenohumeral (shoulder) joint
Subclavian nerve (nerve to subclavius)	Superior trunk, receiving fibers from C5, **C6** and often C4	Descends posterior to clavicle and anterior to brachial plexus and subclavian artery; often giving an *accessory root to phrenic nerve*	Subclavius and sternoclavicular joint (accessory phrenic root innervates diaphragm)
Infraclavicular branches			
Lateral pectoral	Side branch of lateral cord, receiving fibers from C5, **C6,** C7	Pierces costocoracoid membrane to reach deep surface of pectoral muscles; a *communicating branch to the medial pectoral nerve* passes anterior to axillary artery and vein	Primarily pectoralis major; but some lateral pectoral nerve fibers pass to pectoralis minor via branch to medial pectoral nerve

Table 6.5 Brachial Plexus and Nerves of Upper Limb (continued)

Nerve	Origin[a]	Course	Structures Innervated
Musculocutaneous	Terminal branch of lateral cord, receiving fibers from C5–C7	Exits axilla by piercing coracobrachialis; descends between biceps brachii and brachialis, supplying both; continues as *lateral cutaneous nerve of forearm*	Muscles of anterior compartment of arm (coracobrachialis, biceps brachii and brachialis); skin of lateral aspect of forearm
Median	**Lateral root of median nerve** is a terminal branch of lateral cord (C6, C7 fibers); **medial root of median nerve** is a terminal branch of medial cord (C8, T1 fibers)	Lateral and medial roots merge to form median nerve lateral to axillary artery; descends through arm adjacent to brachial artery, with nerve gradually crossing anterior to artery to lie medial to artery in cubital fossa	Muscles of anterior forearm compartment (except for flexor carpi ulnaris and ulnar half of flexor digitorum profundus), five intrinsic muscles in thenar half of palm and palmar skin
Medial pectoral	Side branches of medial cord, receiving fibers from C8, T1	Passes between axillary artery and vein; then pierces pectoralis minor and enters deep surface of pectoralis major; although it is called *medial* for its origin from medial cord, it lies lateral to lateral pectoral nerve	Pectoralis minor and sternocostal part of pectoralis major
Medial cutaneous nerve of arm		Smallest nerve of plexus; runs along medial side of axillary and brachial veins; communicates with *intercostobrachial nerve*	Skin of medial side of arm, as far distal as medial epicondyle of humerus and olecranon of ulna
Median cutaneous nerve of forearm		Initially runs with ulnar nerve (with which it may be confused) but pierces deep fascia with basilic vein and enters subcutaneous tissue, dividing into anterior and posterior branches	Skin of medial side of forearm, as far distal as wrist
Ulnar	Larger terminal branch of medial cord, receiving fibers from C8, T1 and often C7	Descends medial arm; passes posterior to medial epicondyle of humerus; then descends ulnar aspect of forearm to hand	Flexor carpi ulnaris and ulnar half of flexor digitorum profundus (forearm); most intrinsic muscles of hand; skin of hand medial to axial line of digit 4
Upper subscapular	Side branch of posterior cord, receiving fibers from **C5**	Passes posteriorly, entering subscapularis directly	Superior portion of subscapularis
Lower subscapular	Side branch of posterior cord, receiving fibers from **C6**	Passes inferolaterally, deep to subscapular artery and vein	Inferior portion of subscapularis and teres major
Thoracodorsal	Side branch of posterior cord, receiving fibers from C6, **C7**, C8	Arises between upper and lower subscapular nerves and runs inferolaterally along posterior axillary wall to apical part of latissimus dorsi	Latissimus dorsi
Axillary	Terminal branch of posterior cord, receiving fibers from **C5**, C6	Exits axillary fossa posteriorly, passing through quadrangular space[b] with posterior circumflex humeral artery; gives rise to *superior lateral brachial cutaneous nerve;* then winds around surgical neck of humerus deep to deltoid	Glenohumeral (shoulder) joint; teres minor and deltoid muscles; skin of superolateral arm (over inferior part of deltoid)
Radial	Larger terminal branch of posterior cord (largest branch of plexus), receiving fibers from C5–T1	Exits axillary fossa posterior to axillary artery; passes posterior to humerus in radial groove with deep artery of arm, between lateral and medial heads of triceps; perforates lateral intermuscular septum; enters cubital fossa, dividing into *superficial* (cutaneous) and *deep* (motor) *radial nerves*	All muscles of posterior compartments of arm and forearm; skin of posterior and inferolateral arm, posterior forearm, and dorsum of hand lateral to axial line of digit 4

[a]Boldface (**C5**) indicates primary component of the nerve.
[b]Bounded superiorly by the subscapularis, head of humerus, and teres minor; inferiorly by the teres major; medially by the long head of the triceps; and laterally by the coracobrachialis and surgical neck of the humerus.

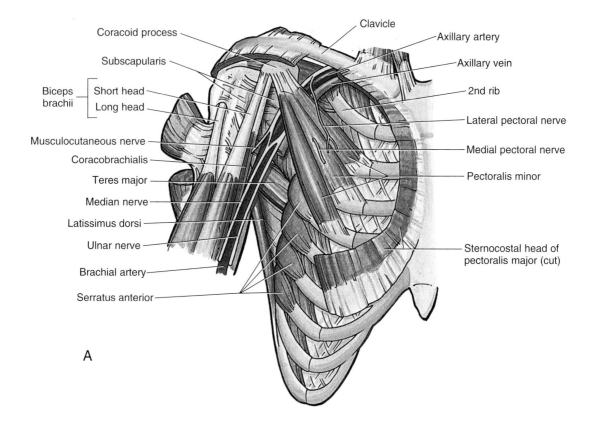

Coracoid process

Subscapularis

Biceps brachii — Short head / Long head

Musculocutaneous nerve

Coracobrachialis

Teres major

Median nerve

Latissimus dorsi

Ulnar nerve

Brachial artery

Serratus anterior

Clavicle

Axillary artery

Axillary vein

2nd rib

Lateral pectoral nerve

Medial pectoral nerve

Pectoralis minor

Sternocostal head of pectoralis major (cut)

A

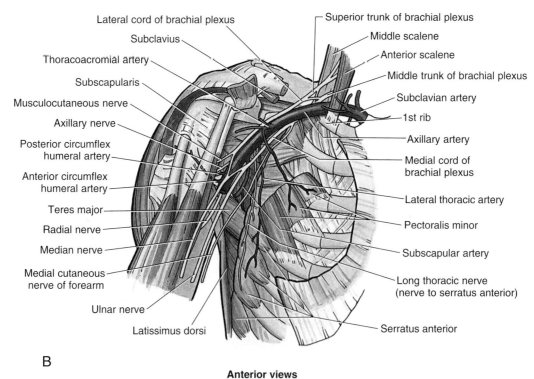

Lateral cord of brachial plexus

Subclavius

Thoracoacromial artery

Subscapularis

Musculocutaneous nerve

Axillary nerve

Posterior circumflex humeral artery

Anterior circumflex humeral artery

Teres major

Radial nerve

Median nerve

Medial cutaneous nerve of forearm

Ulnar nerve

Latissimus dorsi

Superior trunk of brachial plexus

Middle scalene

Anterior scalene

Middle trunk of brachial plexus

Subclavian artery

1st rib

Axillary artery

Medial cord of brachial plexus

Lateral thoracic artery

Pectoralis minor

Subscapular artery

Long thoracic nerve (nerve to serratus anterior)

Serratus anterior

B

Anterior views

Figure 6.15. Boundaries and contents of axilla. A. Note the relationship of nerves and vessels to the pectoralis minor. **B.** This view of the posterior and medial walls of the axilla shows the axillary artery and brachial plexus.

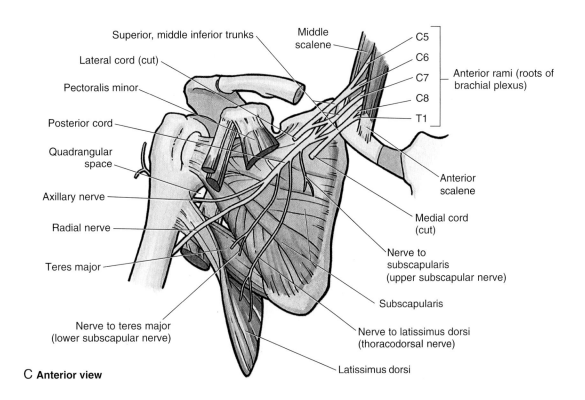

Superior, middle inferior trunks

Lateral cord (cut)

Pectoralis minor

Posterior cord

Quadrangular space

Axillary nerve

Radial nerve

Teres major

Nerve to teres major (lower subscapular nerve)

Middle scalene

C5

C6

C7

C8

T1

Anterior rami (roots of brachial plexus)

Anterior scalene

Medial cord (cut)

Nerve to subscapularis (upper subscapular nerve)

Subscapularis

Nerve to latissimus dorsi (thoracodorsal nerve)

Latissimus dorsi

C **Anterior view**

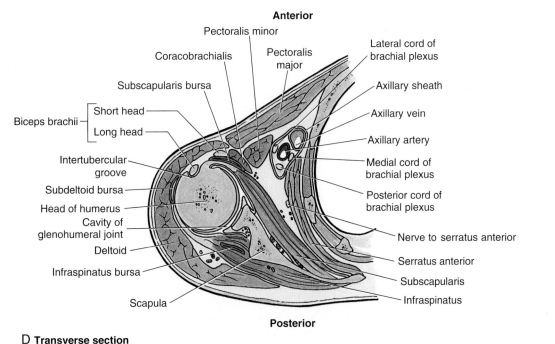

Anterior

Pectoralis minor

Coracobrachialis

Pectoralis major

Subscapularis bursa

Lateral cord of brachial plexus

Axillary sheath

Biceps brachii

Short head

Long head

Axillary vein

Axillary artery

Intertubercular groove

Medial cord of brachial plexus

Subdeltoid bursa

Posterior cord of brachial plexus

Head of humerus

Cavity of glenohumeral joint

Nerve to serratus anterior

Deltoid

Serratus anterior

Infraspinatus bursa

Subscapularis

Scapula

Infraspinatus

Posterior

D **Transverse section**

Figure 6.15. *(continued)* **C.** This view of the posterior wall of the axilla demonstrates the posterior cord of the brachial plexus and its branches. **D.** A transverse section of the shoulder and axilla is shown.

Each trunk of the brachial plexus divides into anterior and posterior divisions as the plexus passes through the *cervicoaxillary canal* posterior to the clavicle. **Anterior divisions of the trunks** supply the *anterior (flexor) compartments* of the upper limb, and **posterior divisions of the trunks** supply the *posterior (extensor) compartments* of the upper limb.

The divisions of the trunks form three cords of the brachial plexus, within the axilla (Fig. 6.15):

- Anterior divisions of the superior and middle trunks unite to form the **lateral cord.**
- Anterior division of the inferior trunk continues as the **medial cord.**
- Posterior divisions of all three trunks unite to form the **posterior cord.**

The cords of the brachial plexus are named for their position in relation to the second part of the axillary artery (e.g., the lateral cord is lateral to the axillary artery, most easily seen when the limb is abducted).

The brachial plexus is divided into **supraclavicular** and **infraclavicular parts** by the clavicle (Table 6.5).

- Four *branches of the supraclavicular part of the plexus* arise from the roots (anterior rami) and trunks of the plexus (dorsal scapular nerve, long thoracic nerve, nerve to the subclavius, and suprascapular nerve) and are approachable through the neck. *Muscular branches* arise from the anterior rami of C5–T1 to supply the scalene and longus colli muscles.
- *Branches of the infraclavicular part of the plexus* arise from the cords of the brachial plexus and are approachable through the axilla.

Variations of the Brachial Plexus

Variations in the brachial plexus formation are common. In addition to the five anterior rami (C5–T1) that form the roots of the plexus, small contributions may be made by the anterior rami of C4 or T2. When the superiormost root (anterior ramus) of the plexus is C4 and the inferiormost root is C8, it is called a *prefixed brachial plexus.* Alternatively, when the superior root is C6 and the inferior root is T2, it is a *postfixed brachial plexus.* In the latter type, the inferior trunk of the plexus may be compressed by the 1st rib, producing neurovascular symptoms in the upper limb. Variations also may occur in the formation of trunks, divisions, and cords; in the origin and/or combination of branches; and in the relationship to the axillary artery and scalene muscles.

Brachial Plexus Injuries

Injuries to the brachial plexus affect movements and cutaneous sensations in the upper limb. Disease, stretching, and wounds in the lateral cervical region (posterior triangle of the neck) or in the axilla may produce brachial plexus injuries (see Chapter 8). Signs and symptoms depend on which part of the plexus is involved. Injuries to the brachial plexus result in loss of muscular movement (*paralysis*) and loss of cutaneous sensation (*anesthesia*). In *complete paralysis,* no movement is detectable. In *incomplete*

paralysis, not all muscles are paralyzed; therefore, the person can move, but the movements are weak compared to those on the uninjured side.

Injuries to superior parts of the brachial plexus (C5 and C6) usually result from an excessive increase in the angle between the neck and the shoulder. These injuries can occur in a person who is thrown from a motorcycle or a horse and lands on the shoulder in a way that widely separates the neck and shoulder (Fig. B6.6A). When thrown, the person's shoulder often hits something (e.g., a tree or the ground) and stops, but the head and trunk continue to move. This stretches or ruptures superior parts of the brachial plexus or **avulses** (tears) the roots of the plexus from the spinal cord. Injury to the superior trunk is apparent by the characteristic position of the limb ("waiter's tip position") in which the limb hangs by the side in medial rotation (Fig. B6.6B). *Upper brachial plexus injuries* can also occur in a newborn when excessive stretching of the neck occurs during delivery (Fig. B6.6C). As a result of *injuries to the superior parts of the brachial plexus (Erb-Duchenne palsy),* paralysis of the muscles of the shoulder and arm supplied by C5–C6 occurs. The usual clinical appearance is an upper limb with an adducted shoulder, medially rotated arm, and extended elbow. The lateral aspect of the upper limb also experiences loss of sensation. Chronic microtrauma to the superior trunk of the brachial plexus from carrying a heavy backpack can produce motor and sensory deficits

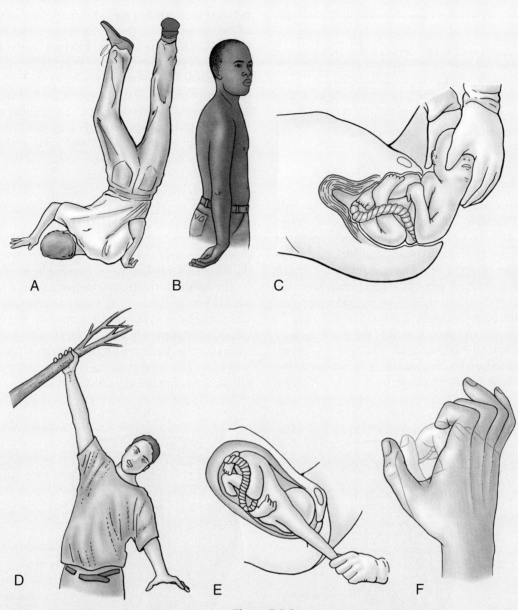

Figure B6.6.

in the distribution of the musculocutaneous and radial nerves.

Injuries to inferior parts of the brachial plexus (Klumpke paralysis) are much less common. These injuries may occur when the upper limb is suddenly pulled superiorly—for example, when a person grasps something to break a fall or when a baby's limb is pulled excessively during delivery (Fig. B6.6D & E). These events injure the inferior trunk of the plexus (C8 and T1) and may avulse the roots of the spinal nerves from the spinal cord. The short muscles of the hand are affected and a *claw hand* results (Fig. B6.6F).

Brachial Plexus Block

Injection of an anesthetic solution into or immediately surrounding the axillary sheath interrupts nerve impulses and produces anesthesia of the structures supplied by the branches of the cords of the plexus. Combined with an occlusive tourniquet technique to retain the anesthetic agent, this procedure enables surgeons to operate on the upper limb without using a general anesthetic. The brachial plexus can be anesthetized using a number of approaches, such as interscalene, supraclavicular, and axillary.

Arm

The arm extends from the shoulder to the elbow. Two types of movement occur between the arm and the forearm at the elbow joint: flexion–extension and pronation–supination. The muscles performing these movements are clearly divided into anterior (*flexor*) and posterior (*extensor*) groups. The chief action of both groups is at the elbow joint, but some muscles also act at the glenohumeral joint.

Muscles of Arm

Of the four arm muscles, three flexors (biceps brachii, brachialis, and coracobrachialis) are in the anterior (flexor) compartment and are supplied by the musculocutaneous nerve (Figs. 6.7*B*, 6.15*A*, and 6.16), and one extensor (triceps brachii) is in the posterior compartment, supplied by the radial nerve (Fig. 6.17). A small triangular muscle on the posterior aspect of the elbow, the anconeus, covers the posterior aspect of the ulna proximally. Table 6.6 lists the attachments, nerve supply, and main actions of the arm muscles.

The **biceps brachii** has two heads (*bi*, two + L. *caput*, head): a **long head** and a **short head.** A broad band, the transverse humeral ligament, passes from the lesser to the

greater tubercle of the humerus and converts the intertubercular groove into a canal for the tendon of the long head of the biceps. When the elbow is extended, the biceps is a simple flexor of the forearm; however, as the elbow flexion approaches 90° and more power is needed, the biceps with the forearm in supination produces flexion, but with the forearm in pronation the biceps is the primary (most powerful) supinator of the forearm. A triangular membranous band, the **bicipital aponeurosis** (Fig. 6.16), runs from the biceps tendon across the cubital fossa and merges with the antebrachial (deep) fascia covering the flexor muscles in the medial side of the forearm.

The **brachialis,** a flattened fusiform muscle, lies posterior (deep) to the biceps (Fig. 6.16*B*). It is the only pure flexor, producing the greatest amount of flexion force. It flexes the forearm in all positions and during slow and quick movements. When the forearm is extended slowly, the brachialis steadies the movement by slowly relaxing.

The **coracobrachialis,** an elongated muscle in the superomedial part of the arm, is a useful landmark for locating other structures in the arm (Fig. 6.16*B*). The musculocutaneous nerve pierces it, and the distal part of its attachment indicates the location of the nutrient foramen of the humerus. The coracobrachialis helps flex and adduct the arm and stabilize the glenohumeral joint.

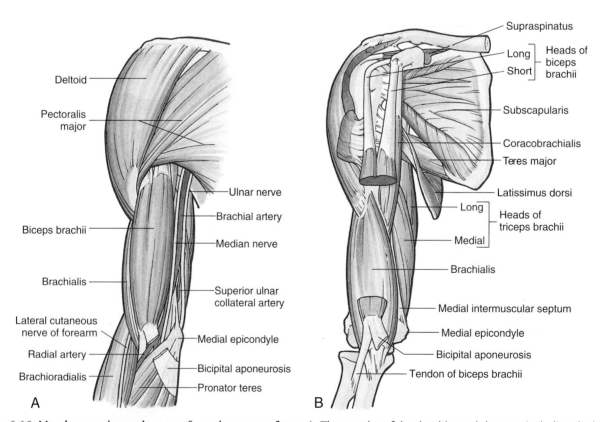

Figure 6.16. Muscles, arteries, and nerves of anterior aspect of arm. A. The muscles of the shoulder and the arm, including the brachial artery and associated nerves, are shown. **B.** A deep dissection of the muscles is shown.

The **triceps brachii** is a large fusiform muscle in the posterior compartment of the arm that arises by **long, lateral, and medial heads** (Figs. 6.17 and 6.18; Table 6.6). The triceps is the main extensor of the elbow. Because its long head crosses the glenohumeral joint, the triceps helps stabilize the adducted glenohumeral joint by serving as a shunt muscle, resisting inferior displacement of the head of the humerus along with the deltoid and coracobrachialis. Just proximal to the distal attachment of the triceps is a friction-reducing *subtendinous olecranon bursa*, between the

Table 6.6 **Muscles of Arm**

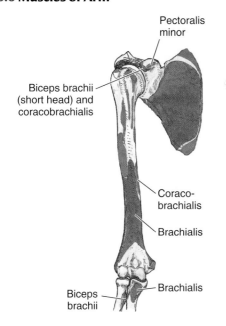

Anterior view

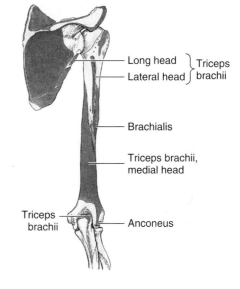

Posterior view

Muscle	Proximal Attachment	Distal Attachment	Innervation[a]	Main Action
Biceps brachii	*Short head:* tip of coracoid process of scapula *Long head:* supraglenoid tubercle of scapula	Tuberosity of radius and fascia of forearm via bicipital aponeurosis	Musculocutaneous nerve[b] (C5, **C6**)	Supinates forearm and, when it is supine, flexes forearm; short head resists dislocation of shoulder
Brachialis	Distal half of anterior surface of humerus	Coronoid process and tuberosity of ulna		Flexes forearm in all positions
Coracobrachialis	Tip of coracoid process of scapula	Middle third of medial surface of humerus	Musculocutaneous nerve (C5, **C6**, C7)	Helps flex and adduct arm; resists dislocation of shoulder
Triceps brachii	*Long head:* infraglenoid tubercle of scapula *Lateral head:* posterior surface of humerus, superior to radial groove *Medial head:* posterior surface of humerus, inferior to radial groove	Proximal end of olecranon of ulna and fascia of forearm	Radial nerve (C6, **C7, C8**)	Chief extensor of forearm; long head resists dislocation of humerus; especially important during abduction
Anconeus	Lateral epicondyle of humerus	Lateral surface of olecranon and superior part of posterior surface of ulna	Radial nerve (C7, C8, T1)	Assists triceps in extending forearm; stabilizes elbow joint; may abduct ulna during pronation

[a]The spinal cord segmental innervation is indicated (e.g., "C5, **C6**" means that the nerves supplying the biceps brachii are derived from the fifth and sixth cervical segments of the spinal cord). Numbers in boldface (**C6**) indicate the main segmental innervation. Damage to one or more of the listed spinal cord segments or to the motor nerve roots arising from them results in paralysis of the muscles concerned.
[b]Some of the lateral part of the brachialis is innervated by a branch of the radial nerve.

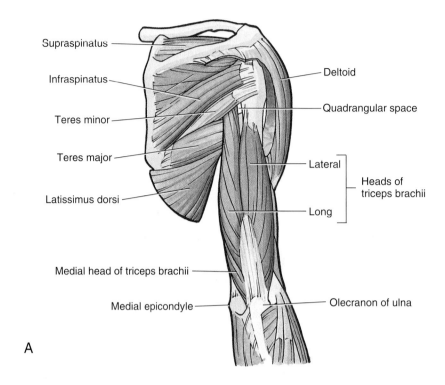

Supraspinatus

Infraspinatus

Teres minor

Teres major

Latissimus dorsi

Deltoid

Quadrangular space

Lateral — ⎫
            ⎬ Heads of
            ⎮ triceps brachii
Long — ⎭

Medial head of triceps brachii

Medial epicondyle

Olecranon of ulna

A

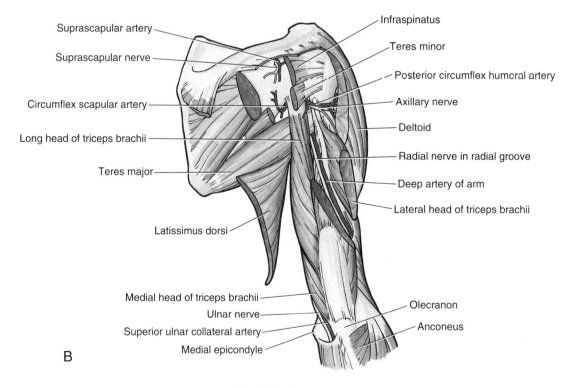

Suprascapular artery

Suprascapular nerve

Circumflex scapular artery

Long head of triceps brachii

Teres major

Latissimus dorsi

Infraspinatus

Teres minor

Posterior circumflex humeral artery

Axillary nerve

Deltoid

Radial nerve in radial groove

Deep artery of arm

Lateral head of triceps brachii

Medial head of triceps brachii

Ulnar nerve

Superior ulnar collateral artery

Medial epicondyle

Olecranon

Anconeus

B

Posterior views

Figure 6.17. Muscles, arteries, and nerves of posterior aspect of arm. A. The muscles of the shoulder and arm are shown. **B.** A deeper dissection shows the arteries and nerves.

triceps tendon and the olecranon. The **anconeus** muscle helps the triceps extend the forearm and is also said to abduct the humerus during pronation of the forearm.

Arteries and Veins of Arm

The **brachial artery** provides the main arterial supply to the arm and is the continuation of the axillary artery (Figs. 6.16*A* and 6.18*A;* Table 6.4). It begins at the inferior border of the teres major and ends in the cubital fossa opposite the neck of the radius under cover of the bicipital aponeurosis, where it divides into the radial and ulnar arteries. The brachial artery, relatively superficial and palpable throughout its course, lies anterior to the triceps and brachialis. At first, it lies medial to the humerus, where its pulsations are palpable in the **medial**

bicipital groove. It then passes anterior to the medial supraepicondylar ridge and trochlea of the humerus. As it passes inferolaterally, the brachial artery accompanies the median nerve, which crosses anterior to the artery. During its course through the arm, the brachial artery gives rise to unnamed *muscular branches* and the *humeral nutrient artery,* which arise from its lateral aspect. The main named branches of the brachial artery that arise from its medial aspect are the **deep artery of arm** (L. *arteria profunda brachii*) (Fig. 6.17*B*) and the **superior** and **inferior ulnar collateral arteries.** The latter vessels help form the periarticular **arterial anastomoses of the elbow region** (Table 6.4).

Two sets of *veins of the arm,* superficial and deep, anastomose freely with each other. The two main **superficial veins of the arm,** the *cephalic* and *basilic veins,* are described earlier

Measuring Blood Pressure

A *sphygmomanometer* is used to measure arterial blood pressure. A cuff is placed around the arm and inflated with air until it compresses the *brachial artery* against the humerus and occludes it. A stethoscope is placed over the artery in the *cubital fossa,* the pressure in the cuff is gradually released, and the examiner detects the sound of blood beginning to spurt through the artery. The first audible spurt indicates *systolic blood pressure.* As the

pressure is completely released, the point at which the pulse can no longer can heard indicates *diastolic blood pressure.*

Compression of Brachial Artery

The best place to compress the brachial artery to control hemorrhage is near the middle of the arm. The biceps must be pushed laterally to detect pulsations of the artery (Fig. B6.7). Because the arterial anastomoses around the elbow provide a functionally and surgically important collateral circulation, the brachial artery may be clamped distal to the inferior ulnar collateral artery without producing tissue damage (Table 6.3). The anatomical basis for this is that the ulnar and radial arteries still receive sufficient blood through the anastomoses. Ischemia of the elbow and forearm results from clamping the brachial artery proximal to the deep artery of the arm for an extended period.

Occlusion of Laceration of Brachial Artery

Although collateral pathways confer some protection against gradual temporary and partial occlusion, sudden complete occlusion or laceration of the brachial artery creates a surgical emergency because paralysis of muscles results from ischemia within a few hours. After this, fibrous scar tissue develops and causes the involved muscles to shorten permanently, producing a flexion deformity—*ischemic compartment syndrome* (Volkmann ischemic contracture). Contraction of the fingers and sometimes the wrist results in loss of hand power.

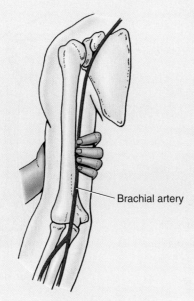

Brachial artery

Compression of brachial artery

Figure B6.7.

Biceps Tendinitis

The tendon of the long head of the biceps, enclosed by a synovial sheath, moves back and forth in the intertubercular groove of the humerus. Wear and tear of this mechanism can cause shoulder pain. Inflammation of the tendon (**biceps tendinitis**), usually is the result of repetitive microtrauma, in sports involving throwing (e.g., baseball).

Rupture of Tendon of Long Head of Biceps

Rupture of the tendon of the long head of the biceps usually results from wear and tear of an inflamed tendon (*biceps tendinitis*). Normally, the tendon is torn from its attachment to the supraglenoid tubercle of the scapula. The rupture is commonly dramatic and is associated with a snap or pop. The detached muscle belly forms a ball near the center of the distal part of the anterior aspect of the arm (Popeye deformity) (Fig. B6.8).

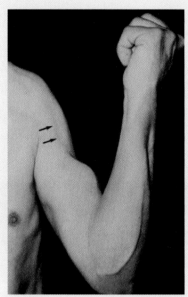

Rupture of biceps tendon (*arrows*)

Figure B6.8.

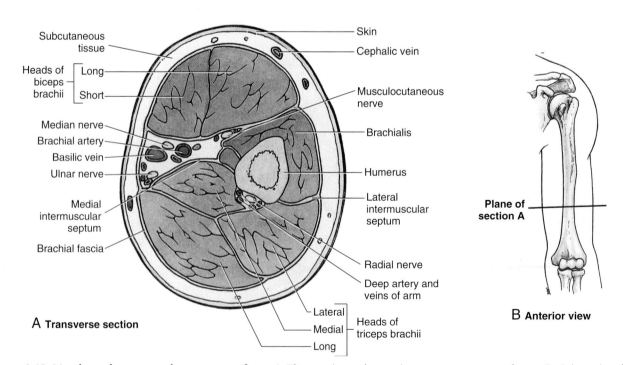

A Transverse section

B Anterior view

Figure 6.18. Muscles and neurovascular structures of arm. A. The anterior and posterior compartments are shown. **B.** Orientation drawing showing the level of the section shown in part A.

in this chapter (Figs. 6.9 and 6.18A). Paired deep veins, collectively constituting the **brachial vein**, accompany the brachial artery. The brachial vein begins at the elbow by union of the *accompanying veins of the ulnar and radial arteries* and ends by merging with the basilic vein to form the axillary vein. Both superficial and deep veins have valves, but the deep veins have more.

Nerves of Arm

Four main nerves pass through the arm: median, ulnar, musculocutaneous, and radial (Figs. 6.15–6.18; Table 6.5). The **median nerve** in the arm is formed in the axilla by the union of medial and lateral roots from the medial and lateral cords of the brachial plexus, respectively (Fig. 6.15A & B). The nerve runs distally in the arm, initially on the lateral side of the brachial artery until it reaches the middle of the arm, where it crosses to the medial side and contacts the brachialis. The median nerve then descends into the cubital fossa, where it lies deep to the bicipital aponeurosis and median cubital vein. The median and ulnar nerves supply no branches to the arm; however, they supply articular branches to the elbow joint.

The **ulnar nerve** in the arm arises from the medial cord of the brachial plexus, conveying fibers mainly from the C8 and T1 nerves (Fig. 6.15). It passes distally, anterior to the insertion of teres major and to the long head of triceps, on the medial side of the brachial artery. Around the middle of the arm, it pierces the medial intermuscular septum with the superior ulnar collateral artery and descends between the septum and the medial head of triceps. The ulnar nerve passes posterior to the medial humeral epicondyle of the humerus to enter the forearm (Figs. 6.16A and 6.17B).

The **musculocutaneous nerve** arises from the lateral cord of the brachial plexus, pierces the coracobrachialis, and then continues distally between the brachialis and the biceps (Fig. 6.15A & B). After supplying all three muscles of the anterior compartment of the arm, the nerve emerges lateral to the biceps as the *lateral cutaneous nerve of the forearm* (Fig. 6.16A).

The **radial nerve** enters the arm posterior to the brachial artery, medial to the humerus, and anterior to the long head of triceps (Figs. 6.15B & C and 6.17B). The radial nerve descends inferolaterally with the deep artery of arm and curves around the humeral shaft in the radial groove. The radial nerve pierces the lateral intermuscular septum and continues inferiorly in the anterior compartment between the brachialis and the brachioradialis. In the cubital fossa, it divides into *deep* and *superficial branches* (Fig. 6.23). The radial nerve supplies the muscles in the posterior compartments of the arm and forearm and the overlying skin.

Injury to Musculocutaneous Nerve

Injury to the musculocutaneous nerve in the axilla is usually inflicted by a weapon such as a knife. A musculocutaneous nerve injury results in *paralysis of the coracobrachialis, biceps, and brachialis;* consequently, flexion of the elbow and supination of the forearm are greatly weakened. Loss of sensation may occur on the lateral surface of the forearm supplied by the lateral cutaneous nerve of the forearm.

Injury to Radial Nerve

Injury to the radial nerve superior to the origin of its branches to the triceps brachii results in *paralysis of the triceps, brachioradialis, supinator, and extensor muscles of the wrist and fingers.* Loss of sensation occurs in areas of skin supplied by this nerve. When the radial nerve is injured in the radial groove, the triceps is usually not completely paralyzed but only weakened because only the medial head is affected; however, the muscles in the posterior compartment of the forearm that are supplied by more distal branches of the radial nerve are paralyzed. The characteristic clinical sign of radial nerve injury is **wrist-drop** (inability to extend the wrist and fingers at the metacarpophalangeal joints) (Fig. B6.9). Instead, the wrist is flexed because of unopposed tonus of the flexor muscles and gravity.

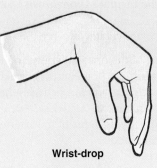

Wrist-drop

Figure B6.9.

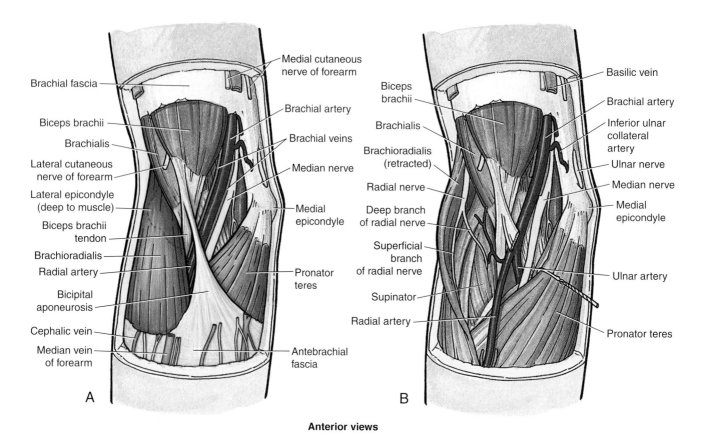

Anterior views

Figure 6.19. **Cubital fossa.** Superficial (**A**) and deep (**B**) dissections are shown.

Cubital Fossa

The **cubital fossa** is the shallow triangular depression on the anterior surface of the elbow (Fig. 6.19*A*). The boundaries of the cubital fossa are

- Superiorly, an imaginary line connecting the medial and lateral epicondyles.
- Medially, the pronator teres.
- Laterally, the brachioradialis.

The *floor of the cubital fossa* is formed by the brachialis and supinator muscles. The *roof of the cubital fossa* is formed by the continuity of brachial and antebrachial (deep) fascia, reinforced by the bicipital aponeurosis, subcutaneous tissue, and skin.

The *contents of the cubital fossa* are the (Fig. 6.19*B*):

- Terminal part of the brachial artery and the commencement of its terminal branches, the radial and ulnar arteries; the brachial artery lies between the biceps tendon and the median nerve.
- (Deep) accompanying veins of the arteries.
- Biceps brachii tendon.
- Median nerve.
- Radial nerve, dividing into its superficial and deep branches.

In the subcutaneous tissue overlying the cubital fossa are the *median cubital vein,* lying anterior to the brachial artery, and the *medial and lateral cutaneous nerves of the forearm,* related to the basilic and cephalic veins (Figs. 6.8 and 6.9*A*).

Forearm

The **forearm** lies between the elbow and the wrist and contains two bones, the *radius* and *ulna,* which are joined by an interosseous membrane. The role of forearm movement, occurring at the elbow and radioulnar joints, is to assist the shoulder in the application of force and in controlling the placement of the hand in space.

Muscles of Forearm

The tendons of the forearm muscles pass through the distal part of the forearm and continue into the wrist, hand, and fingers. The flexors and pronators of the forearm are in the anterior compartment and are served mainly by the *median nerve;* the one and a half exceptions are innervated by the *ulnar nerve.* The extensors and supinators of the forearm are in the posterior compartment and are all innervated by the *radial nerve* (Fig. 6.20).

Surface Anatomy of Arm and Cubital Fossa

The borders of the *deltoid* are visible when the arm is abducted against resistance. The **distal attachment of the deltoid** can be palpated on the lateral surface of the humerus. The **three heads of the triceps** form a bulge on the posterior aspect of the arm and are identifiable when the forearm is extended from the flexed position against resistance (Fig. SA6.3*A*). The **triceps tendon** may be felt as it descends along the posterior aspect of the arm to the **olecranon**. The **biceps brachii** forms a bulge on the anterior aspect of the arm; its belly becomes more prominent when the elbow is flexed and

supinated against resistance (Fig. SA6.3*B*). Medial and lateral **bicipital grooves** separate the bulges formed by the biceps and triceps. The cephalic vein runs superiorly in the lateral bicipital groove and the basilic vein ascends in the medial bicipital groove. The **biceps tendon** can be palpated in the cubital fossa, immediately lateral to the midline. The proximal part of the **bicipital aponeurosis** can be palpated where it passes obliquely over the brachial artery and median nerve. The **brachial artery** may be felt pulsating deep to the medial border of the biceps. ●

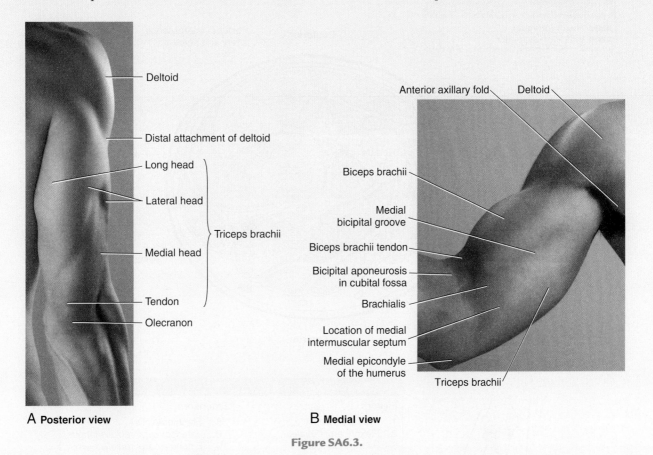

A **Posterior view**   B **Medial view**

Figure SA6.3.

FLEXOR–PRONATOR MUSCLES OF THE FOREARM

The **flexor–pronator muscles** are in the anterior compartment of the forearm (Figs. 6.20 and 6.21). The tendons of most flexor muscles pass across the anterior surface of the wrist and are held in place by the **palmar carpal ligament** and the *flexor retinaculum (transverse carpal ligament)*, thickenings of the antebrachial fascia. The

flexor muscles are arranged in three layers or groups (Table 6.7):

- A **superficial layer or group** of four muscles (**pronator teres, flexor carpi radialis, palmaris longus,** and **flexor carpi ulnaris**) These muscles are all attached proximally by a *common flexor tendon* to the medial epicondyle of the humerus, the *common flexor origin*.

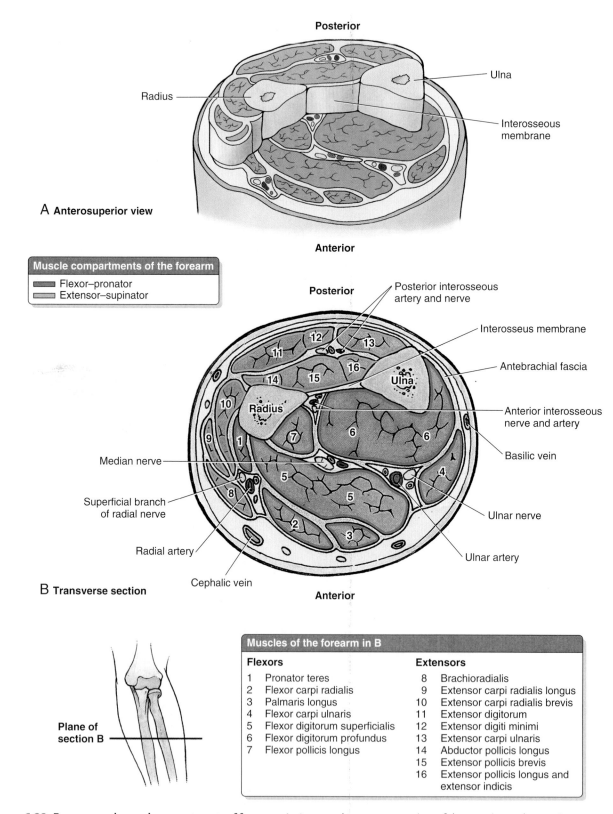

A Anterosuperior view

Posterior

Radius

Ulna

Interosseous membrane

Anterior

Muscle compartments of the forearm
- Flexor–pronator
- Extensor–supinator

Posterior

Posterior interosseous artery and nerve

Interosseus membrane

Antebrachial fascia

Anterior interosseous nerve and artery

Basilic vein

Median nerve

Superficial branch of radial nerve

Radial artery

Cephalic vein

B Transverse section

Anterior

Ulnar nerve

Ulnar artery

Plane of section B

Muscles of the forearm in B

Flexors		Extensors	
1	Pronator teres	8	Brachioradialis
2	Flexor carpi radialis	9	Extensor carpi radialis longus
3	Palmaris longus	10	Extensor carpi radialis brevis
4	Flexor carpi ulnaris	11	Extensor digitorum
5	Flexor digitorum superficialis	12	Extensor digiti minimi
6	Flexor digitorum profundus	13	Extensor carpi ulnaris
7	Flexor pollicis longus	14	Abductor pollicis longus
		15	Extensor pollicis brevis
		16	Extensor pollicis longus and extensor indicis

Figure 6.20. Bones, muscles, and compartments of forearm. A. A stepped transverse section of the anterior and posterior compartments is shown. **B.** The contents of the anterior and posterior compartments are identified.

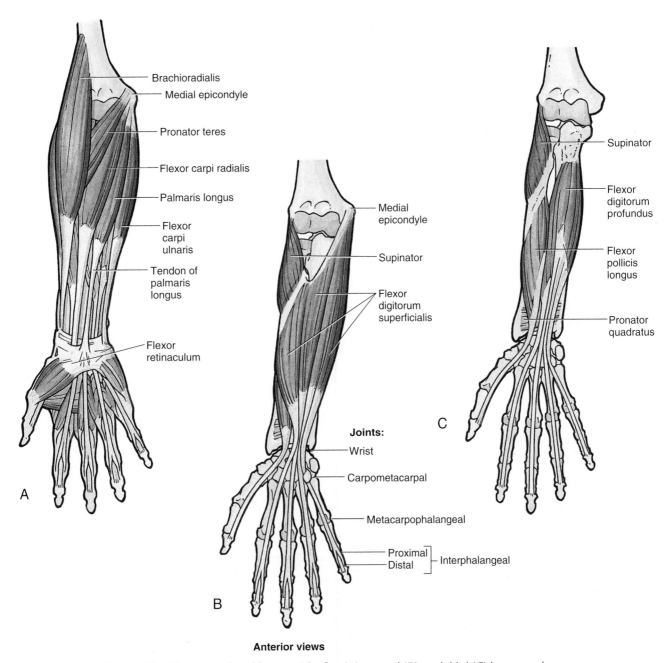

Brachioradialis

Medial epicondyle

Pronator teres

Flexor carpi radialis

Palmaris longus

Flexor carpi ulnaris

Tendon of palmaris longus

Flexor retinaculum

A

Medial epicondyle

Supinator

Flexor digitorum superficialis

Joints:

Wrist

Carpometacarpal

Metacarpophalangeal

Proximal
Distal   Interphalangeal

B

Supinator

Flexor digitorum profundus

Flexor pollicis longus

Pronator quadratus

C

Anterior views

Figure 6.21. Flexor muscles of forearm. The first (**A**), second (**B**), and third (**C**) layers are shown.

- An **intermediate layer or group**, consisting of one muscle (**flexor digitorum superficialis [FDS]**).
- A **deep layer or group** of three muscles (**flexor digitorum profundus [FDP] flexor pollicis longus**, and **pronator quadratus**).

The five superficial and intermediate muscles cross the elbow joint; the three deep muscles do not.

Functionally, the *brachioradialis* is a flexor of the forearm, but it is located in the posterior (posterolateral) or extensor compartment and is thus supplied by the radial nerve (Table 6.7). Therefore, the brachioradialis is a major exception to the generalization that the radial nerve supplies only extensor muscles and that all flexors lie in the anterior compartment.

The **long flexors of the digits** (FDS and FDP) also flex the metacarpophalangeal and wrist joints. The FDP flexes the fingers in slow action; this action is reinforced by the FDS when speed and flexion against resistance are required. When the wrist is flexed at the same time that

Table 6.7 Muscles of the Anterior Compartment of the Forearm

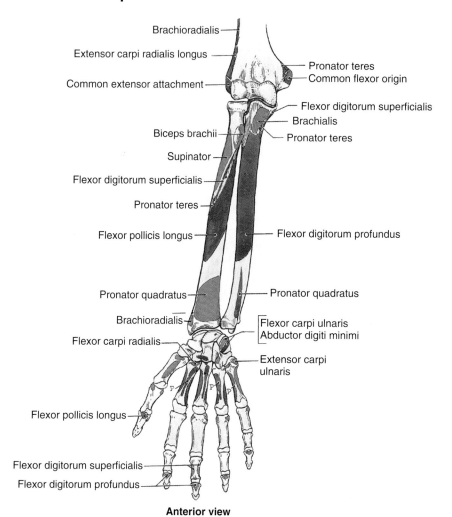

Anterior view

Muscle	Proximal Attachment	Distal Attachment	Innervation[a]	Main Action
Superficial (first) layer				
Pronator teres (PT): Ulnar head Humeral head	Coronoid process	Middle of convexity of lateral surface of radius	Median nerve (C6, **C7**)	Pronates and flexes forearm (at elbow)
Flexor carpi radialis (FCR)		Base of 2nd metacarpal		Flexes and abducts hand (at wrist)
Palmaris longus	Medial epicondyle of humerus (common flexor origin)	Distal half of flexor retinaculum and apex of palmar aponeurosis	Median nerve (C7, C8)	Flexes hand (at wrist) and tenses palmar aponeurosis
Flexor carpi ulnaris (FCU): Humeral head Ulnar head	Olecranon and posterior border (via aponeurosis)	Pisiform, hook of hamate, 5th metacarpal	Ulnar nerve (C7, **C8**)	Flexes and adducts hand (at wrist)

Table 6.7 Muscles of the Anterior Compartment of the Forearm (continued)

Muscle	Proximal Attachment	Distal Attachment	Innervation[a]	Main Action
Intermediate (second) layer				
Flexor digitorum superficialis (FDS): Humeroulnar head Radial head	Medial epicondyle (common flexor origin and coronoid process) Superior half of anterior border	Shafts (bodies) of middle phalanges of medial four fingers	Median nerve (C7, C8, T1)	Flexes middle phalanges at proximal interphalangeal joints of middle four fingers; acting more strongly, it also flexes proximal phalanges at metacarpophalangeal joints
Deep (third) layer				
Flexor digitorum profundus (FDP): Medial part Lateral part	Proximal three quarters of medial and anterior surfaces of ulna and interosseous membrane	Bases of distal phalanges of 4th and 5th fingers	Ulnar nerve (C8, **T1**)	Flexes distal phalanges 4 and 5 at distal interphalangeal joints
		Bases of distal phalanges of 2nd and 3rd fingers	Anterior interosseous nerve, from median nerve (**C8**, T1)	Flexes distal phalanges 2 and 3 at distal interphalangeal joints
Flexor pollicis longus (FPL)	Anterior surface of radius and adjacent interosseous membrane	Base of distal phalanx of thumb		Flexes phalanges of 1st digit (thumb)
Pronator quadratus	Distal quarter of anterior surface of ulna	Distal quarter of anterior surface of radius		Pronates forearm; deep fibers bind radius and ulna together

[a] The spinal cord segmental innervation is indicated (e.g., "C6, **C7**" means that the nerves supplying the pronator teres are derived from the sixth and seventh cervical segments of the spinal cord). Numbers in boldface (**C7**) indicate the main segmental innervation. Damage to one or more of the listed spinal cord segments or to the motor nerve roots arising from them results in paralysis of the muscles concerned.

the metacarpophalangeal and interphalangeal joints are flexed, the long flexor muscles of the fingers are operating over a shortened distance between attachments, and the action resulting from their contraction is consequently weaker. Extending the wrist increases their operating distance, and thus their contraction is more efficient in producing a strong grip. Tendons of the long flexors of the digits pass through the distal part of the forearm, wrist, and palm and continue to the medial four fingers. The FDS flexes the middle phalanges; the FDP flexes the distal phalanges.

The *pronator quadratus* is the prime mover for pronation. The pronator quadratus initiates pronation and is assisted by the *pronator teres* when more speed and power are needed. The pronator quadratus also helps the interosseous membrane hold the radius and ulna together, particularly when upward thrusts are transmitted through the wrist (e.g., during a fall on the hand).

EXTENSOR MUSCLES OF THE FOREARM

The extensor muscles are in the posterior (extensor–supinator) compartment of the forearm, and all are innervated by branches of the radial nerve (Figs. 6.20 and 6.22; Table 6.8). These muscles may be organized into three functional groups:

- Muscles that extend and abduct or adduct the hand at the wrist joint (extensor carpi radialis longus, extensor carpi radialis brevis, and extensor carpi ulnaris).
- Muscles that extend the medial four digits (extensor digitorum, extensor indicis, and extensor digiti minimi).
- Muscles that extend or abduct the thumb (abductor pollicis longus [APL], extensor pollicis brevis [EPB], and extensor pollicis longus [EPL]).

The extensor tendons are held in place in the wrist region by the **extensor retinaculum**, which prevents bowstringing

Muscle Testing of FDS and FDP

To *test the FDP*, the proximal interphalangeal joint is held in the extended position while the person attempts to flex the distal interphalangeal joint. To *test the FDP*, the proximal interphalangeal joint is held in the extended position while the person attempts to flex the distal interphalangeal joint (Fig. B6.10).

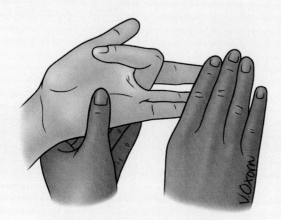

Flexor digitorum superficialis (FDS) muscle test

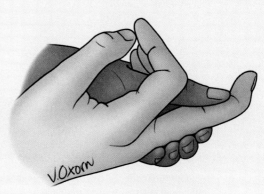

Flexor digitorum profundus (FDP) muscle test

Figure B6.10.

of the tendons when the hand is extended at the wrist joint. As the tendons pass over the dorsum of the wrist, they are covered with **synovial tendon sheaths**, which reduce friction for the extensor tendons as they traverse the osseofibrous tunnels formed by the attachment of the extensor retinaculum to the distal radius and ulna (Fig. 6.23).

The extensor muscles are organized anatomically into superficial and deep layers. Four *superficial extensors* (extensor carpi radialis brevis, extensor digitorum, extensor digiti minimi, and extensor carpi ulnaris) are attached proximally by a *common extensor tendon* to the lateral epicondyle (Fig. 6.22A; Table 6.8). The proximal attachment of the other two superficial extensors (brachioradialis and extensor carpi radialis longus) is to the lateral supraepicondylar ridge of the humerus and the adjacent lateral intermuscular septum. The four flat tendons of the extensor digitorum pass deep to the extensor retinaculum to the medial four fingers (Fig. 6.23A). The common tendons of the index and little fingers are joined on their medial sides near the knuckles by the respective tendons of the extensor indicis and extensor digiti minimi (extensors of index and little fingers, respectively). The extensor indicis tendon joins the tendons of extensor digitorum to pass deep to the extensor retinaculum through the **tendinous sheath**

of extensor digitorum and extensor indicis (common extensor synovial sheath). On the dorsum of the hand, the tendons of extensor digitorum spread out as they run toward the fingers. Adjacent tendons are linked proximal to the metacarpophalangeal joints by three oblique *intertendinous connections* that restrict independent extension of the fingers (Fig. 6.23A). Consequently, normally no finger can remain fully flexed as the other ones are fully extended.

On the distal ends of the metacarpals and along the phalanges, the four tendons of extensor digitorum flatten to form **extensor expansions** (Fig. 6.23). Each extensor expansion (dorsal expansion or hood) is a triangular tendinous aponeurosis that wraps around the dorsum and sides of a head of the metacarpal and base of the proximal phalanx. The visor-like "hood" of the extensor expansion over the head of the metacarpal is anchored on each side to the **palmar ligament** (a thickened portion of the fibrous layer of the joint capsule of the metacarpophalangeal joints). In forming the extensor expansion, each extensor digitorum tendon divides into a **median band**, which passes to the base of the middle phalanx and two **lateral bands**, which pass to the base of the distal phalanx. The tendons of the interosseous and lumbrical muscles of

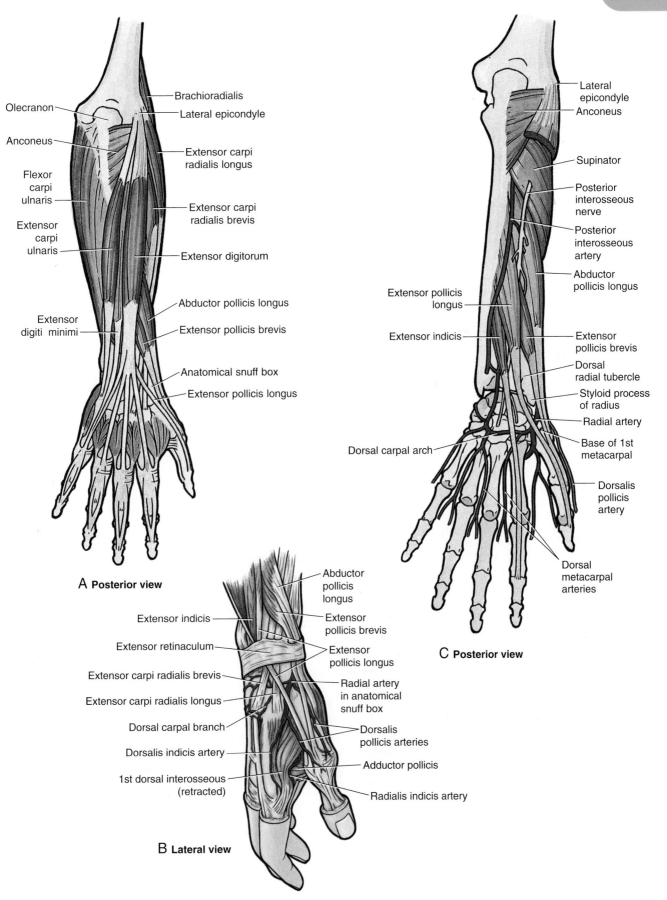

A Posterior view

Olecranon

Brachioradialis

Lateral epicondyle

Anconeus

Extensor carpi radialis longus

Flexor carpi ulnaris

Extensor carpi radialis brevis

Extensor carpi ulnaris

Extensor digitorum

Extensor digiti minimi

Abductor pollicis longus

Extensor pollicis brevis

Anatomical snuff box

Extensor pollicis longus

B Lateral view

Extensor indicis

Abductor pollicis longus

Extensor retinaculum

Extensor pollicis brevis

Extensor carpi radialis brevis

Extensor pollicis longus

Extensor carpi radialis longus

Radial artery in anatomical snuff box

Dorsal carpal branch

Dorsalis pollicis arteries

Dorsalis indicis artery

Adductor pollicis

1st dorsal interosseous (retracted)

Radialis indicis artery

C Posterior view

Lateral epicondyle

Anconeus

Supinator

Posterior interosseous nerve

Posterior interosseous artery

Abductor pollicis longus

Extensor pollicis longus

Extensor indicis

Extensor pollicis brevis

Dorsal radial tubercle

Styloid process of radius

Radial artery

Dorsal carpal arch

Base of 1st metacarpal

Dorsalis pollicis artery

Dorsal metacarpal arteries

Figure 6.22. Extensor muscles of forearm. A. A superficial dissection is shown. **B.** The anatomical snuff box is detailed. **C.** This deeper dissection of the supinator and outcropping muscles shows the arteries and the posterior interosseous nerve, the terminal part of the deep branch of the radial nerve.

Table 6.8 Muscles of the Posterior Compartment of the Forearm

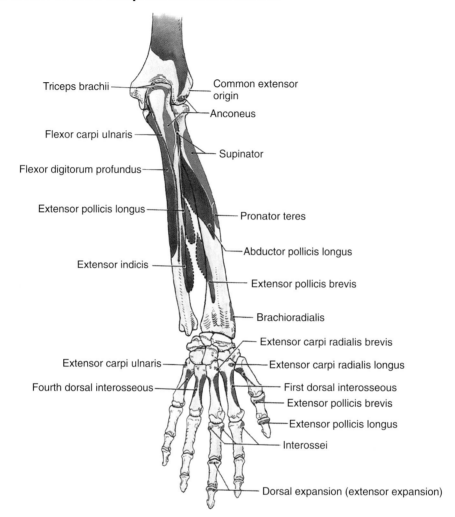

Muscle	Proximal Attachment	Distal Attachment	Innervation[a]	Main Action
Superficial layer				
Brachioradialis	Proximal two thirds of supraepicondylar ridge of humerus	Lateral surface of distal end of radius proximal to styloid process	Radial nerve (C5, **C6,** C7)	Relatively weak flexion of forearm, maximal when forearm is in midpronated position
Extensor carpi radialis longus	Lateral supraepicondylar ridge of humerus	Dorsal aspect of base of 2nd metacarpal	Radial nerve (C6, C7)	Extend and abduct hand at the wrist joint; extensor carpi radialis brevis active during fist clenching
Extensor carpi radialis brevis	Lateral epicondyle of humerus (common extensor origin)	Dorsal aspect of base of 3rd metacarpal	Deep branch of radial nerve (**C7,** C8)	
Extensor digitorum		Extensor expansions of medial four fingers	Posterior interosseous nerve (**C7,** C8), continuation of deep branch of radial nerve	Extends medial four fingers primarily at metacarpophalangeal joints, secondarily at interphalangeal joints
Extensor digiti minimi		Extensor expansion of 5th finger		Extends 5th finger primarily at metacarpophalangeal joint, secondarily at interphalangeal joint
Extensor carpi ulnaris	Lateral epicondyle of humerus; posterior border of ulna via a shared aponeurosis	Dorsal aspect of base of 5th metacarpal		Extends and adducts hand at wrist joint (also active during fist clenching)

Table 6.8 Muscles of the Posterior Compartment of the Forearm *(continued)*

Muscle	Proximal Attachment	Distal Attachment	Innervation[a]	Main Action
Deep layer				
Supinator	Lateral epicondyle of humerus; radial collateral and anular ligaments; supinator fossa; crest of ulna	Lateral, posterior, and anterior surfaces of proximal third of radius	Deep branch of radial nerve (C7, **C8**)	Supinates forearm; rotates radius to turn palm anteriorly or superiorly (if elbow is flexed)
"Outcropping" muscles of deep layer				
Abductor pollicis longus	Posterior surface of proximal halves of ulna, radius, and interosseous membrane	Base of 1st metacarpal	Posterior interosseous nerve (C7, **C8**), continuation of deep branch of radial nerve	Abducts thumb and extends it at carpometacarpal joint
Extensor pollicis longus	Posterior surface of middle third of ulna and interosseous membrane	Dorsal aspect of base of distal phalanx of thumb		Extends distal phalanx of thumb at interphalangeal joint; extends metacarpophalangeal and carpometacarpal joints
Extensor pollicis brevis	Posterior surface of distal third of radius and interosseous membrane	Dorsal aspect of base of proximal phalanx of thumb		Extends proximal phalanx of thumb at metacarpophalangeal joint; extends carpometacarpal joint
Extensor indicis	Posterior surface of distal third of ulna and interosseous membrane	Extensor expansion of 2nd finger		Extends 2nd finger (enabling its independent extension); helps extend hand at wrist

[a] The spinal cord segmental innervation is indicated (e.g., "C7, C8" means that the nerves supplying the extensor carpi radialis brevis are derived from the seventh and eighth cervical segments of the spinal cord). Numbers in boldface (**C7**) indicate the main segmental innervation. Damage to one or more of the listed spinal cord segments or to the motor nerve roots arising from them results in paralysis of the muscles concerned.

the hand join the lateral bands of the extensor expansion (Fig. 6.23).

The **retinacular ligament** is a delicate fibrous band that runs from the proximal phalanx and fibrous digital sheath obliquely across the middle phalanx and two interphalangeal joints (Fig. 6.23 *D*). During flexion of the distal interphalangeal joint, the retinacular ligament becomes taut and pulls the proximal interphalangeal joint into flexion. Similarly, on extending the proximal joint, the distal joint is pulled by the retinacular ligament into nearly complete extension.

The deep extensor muscles of forearm (APL, EPB, and **extensor pollicis longus**) act on the thumb. The extensor indicis confers independence to the index finger in that it may act alone or together with the extensor digitorum to extend the index finger (Figs. 6.20 *B* and 6.22; Table 6.8). The three muscles acting on the thumb (APL, EPB, and EPL) are deep to the superficial extensors and emerge ("crop out") from a furrow in the lateral part of the forearm that divides the extensors. Because of this characteristic, they are referred to as *outcropping muscles*. The tendons of the APL and EPB bound the triangular **anatomical snuff box** laterally, and the tendon of the EPL bounds it medially (Fig. 6.22 *A* & *B*). The snuff box is visible as a hollow on the lateral aspect of the wrist when the thumb is extended fully;

this draws the APL, EPB, and EPL tendons up and produces a concavity between them. Observe that the:

- *Radial artery* lies on the floor of the snuff box.
- *Radial styloid process* can be palpated proximally and the base of the 1st metacarpal can be palpated distally in the snuff box.
- *Scaphoid and trapezium* can be felt in the floor of the snuff box between the radial styloid process and the 1st metacarpal.

Nerves of Forearm

The major **nerves of the forearm** are the median, ulnar, and radial. Although the radial nerve appears in the cubital region, it soon enters the posterior compartment of the forearm. Besides the cutaneous branches, there are only two nerves of the anterior aspect of the forearm: the median and ulnar nerves. Their origins are described in Table 6.5 and their courses and distributions are described in Table 6.9.

The **median nerve** is the principal nerve of the anterior compartment of the forearm. It enters the forearm with the brachial artery and lies medial to it. The median nerve leaves the cubital fossa by passing between the heads of the pronator teres, giving branches to them and then passes

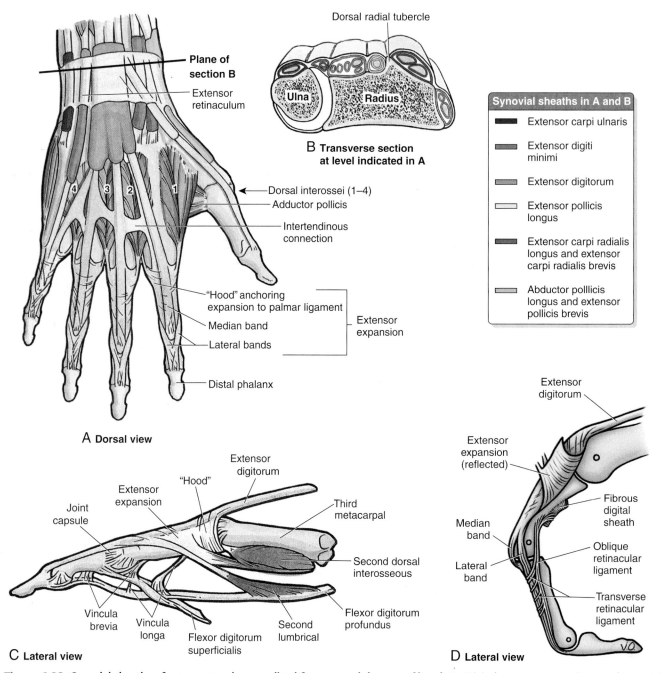

Figure 6.23. Synovial sheaths of extensor tendons on distal forearm and dorsum of hand. A. Digital extensor expansions and synovial sheaths of the extensor tendons are shown. **B.** This section of the distal end of the forearm shows the tendons in their synovial sheaths. **C.** The vincula are fibrous bands that convey small vessels to the tendons. **D.** The retinacular ligaments are identified.

deep to the FDS continuing distally through the middle of the forearm, between the FDS and the FDP (Fig. 6.24). Near the wrist, the median nerve becomes superficial by passing between the tendons of the FDS and flexor carpi radialis (FCR) deep to the palmaris longus tendon (Fig. 6.28A). The anterior interosseous nerve is its major branch (Fig. 6.24). Articular and muscular branches and a palmar cutaneous branch are also derived from the median nerve.

The **ulnar nerve** passes posterior to the medial epicondyle of the humerus and enters the forearm by passing between the heads of the flexor carpi ulnaris (Fig. 6.24), giving branches to them. It then passes inferiorly between the flexor carpi ulnaris and the FDP, supplying the ulnar (medial) part of the muscle that sends tendons to digits 4 and 5. The ulnar nerve becomes superficial at the wrist, running on the medial side of the ulnar artery and the

Table 6.9 Nerves of Forearm

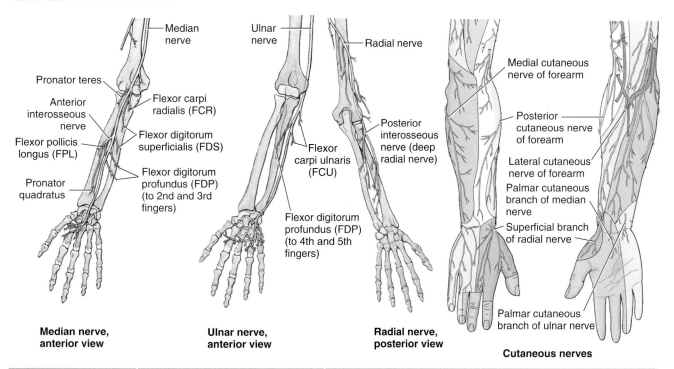

Median nerve, anterior view

Median nerve
Pronator teres
Anterior interosseous nerve
Flexor pollicis longus (FPL)
Pronator quadratus
Flexor carpi radialis (FCR)
Flexor digitorum superficialis (FDS)
Flexor digitorum profundus (FDP) (to 2nd and 3rd fingers)

Ulnar nerve, anterior view

Ulnar nerve
Flexor carpi ulnaris (FCU)
Flexor digitorum profundus (FDP) (to 4th and 5th fingers)

Radial nerve, posterior view

Radial nerve
Posterior interosseous nerve (deep radial nerve)

Cutaneous nerves

Medial cutaneous nerve of forearm
Posterior cutaneous nerve of forearm
Lateral cutaneous nerve of forearm
Palmar cutaneous branch of median nerve
Superficial branch of radial nerve
Palmar cutaneous branch of ulnar nerve

Nerve	Origin	Course in Forearm
Median	By union of lateral root of median nerve (C6, C7, from lateral cord of brachial plexus) with medial root (C8, T1) from medial cord	Enters cubital fossa medial to brachial artery; exits by passing between heads of pronator teres; descends in fascial plane between flexors digitorum superficialis and profundus; runs deep to palmaris longus tendon as it approaches flexor retinaculum to traverse carpal tunnel
Anterior interosseous	Median nerve in distal part of cubital fossa	Descends on anterior aspect of interosseous membrane with artery of same name, between FDP and FPL, to pass deep to pronator quadratus
Palmar cutaneous branch of median nerve	Median nerve of middle to distal forearm, proximal to flexor retinaculum	Passes superficial to flexor retinaculum to reach skin of central palm
Ulnar	Larger terminal branch of medial cord of brachial plexus (C8, T1, often receives fibers from C7)	Enters forearm by passing between heads of flexor carpi ulnaris, after passing posterior to medial epicondyle of humerus; descends forearm between FCU and FDP; becomes superficial in distal forearm
Palmar cutaneous branch of ulnar nerve	Ulnar nerve near middle of forearm	Descends anterior to ulnar artery; perforates deep fascia in distal forearm; runs in subcutaneous tissue to palmar skin medial to axis of 4th digit
Dorsal cutaneous branch of ulnar nerve	Ulnar nerve in distal half of forearm	Passes posteroinferiorly between ulna and flexor carpi ulnaris; enters subcutaneous tissue to supply skin of dorsum medial to axis of 4th digit
Radial	Larger terminal branch of posterior cord of brachial plexus (C5–T1)	Enters cubital fossa between brachioradialis and brachialis; anterior to lateral epicondyle divides into terminal superficial and deep branches
Posterior cutaneous nerve of forearm	Radial nerve, as it traverses radial groove of posterior humerus	Perforates lateral head of triceps; descends along lateral side of arm and posterior aspect of forearm to wrist
Superficial branch of radial nerve	Sensory terminal branch of radial nerve, in cubital fossa	Descends between pronator teres and brachioradialis, emerging from latter to arborize over anatomical snuff box and supply skin of dorsum lateral to axis of 4th finger
Deep branch of radial/ posterior interosseous nerve	Motor terminal branch of radial nerve, in cubital fossa	Deep branch exits cubital fossa winding around neck of radius, penetrating and supplying supinator; emerges in posterior compartment of forearm as posterior interosseous nerve; descends on membrane with artery of same name
Lateral cutaneous nerve of forearm	Continuation of musculocutaneous nerve distal to muscular branches	Emerges lateral to biceps brachii on brachialis, running initially with cephalic vein; descends along lateral border of forearm to wrist
Medial cutaneous nerve of forearm	Medial cord of brachial plexus, receiving C8 and T1 fibers	Perforates deep fascia of arm with basilic vein proximal to cubital fossa; descends medial aspect of forearm in subcutaneous tissue to wrist

FCU, flexor carpi ulnaris; *FDP,* flexor digitorum profundus; *FPL,* flexor pollicis longus.

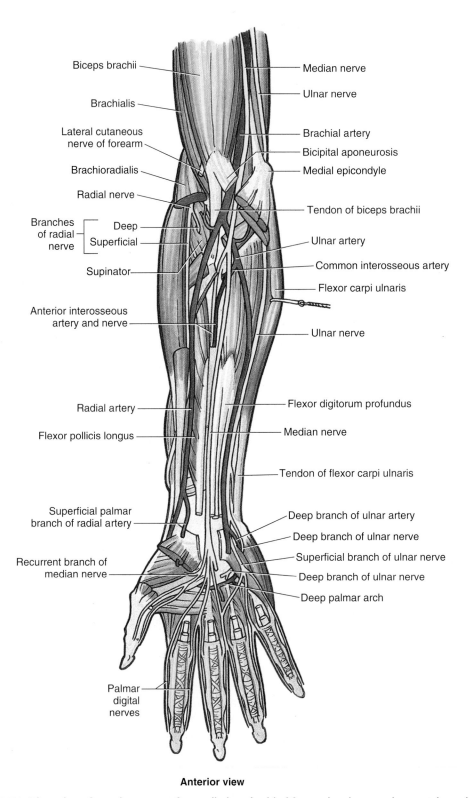

Biceps brachii

Brachialis

Lateral cutaneous
nerve of forearm

Brachioradialis

Radial nerve

Branches
of radial
nerve { Deep
Superficial

Supinator

Anterior interosseous
artery and nerve

Radial artery

Flexor pollicis longus

Superficial palmar
branch of radial artery

Recurrent branch of
median nerve

Palmar
digital
nerves

Median nerve

Ulnar nerve

Brachial artery

Bicipital aponeurosis

Medial epicondyle

Tendon of biceps brachii

Ulnar artery

Common interosseous artery

Flexor carpi ulnaris

Ulnar nerve

Flexor digitorum profundus

Median nerve

Tendon of flexor carpi ulnaris

Deep branch of ulnar artery

Deep branch of ulnar nerve

Superficial branch of ulnar nerve

Deep branch of ulnar nerve

Deep palmar arch

Anterior view

Figure 6.24. Dissection of anterior aspect of upper limb and cubital fossa, showing muscles, vessels, and nerves.

Table 6.10 Arteries of Forearm and Wrist

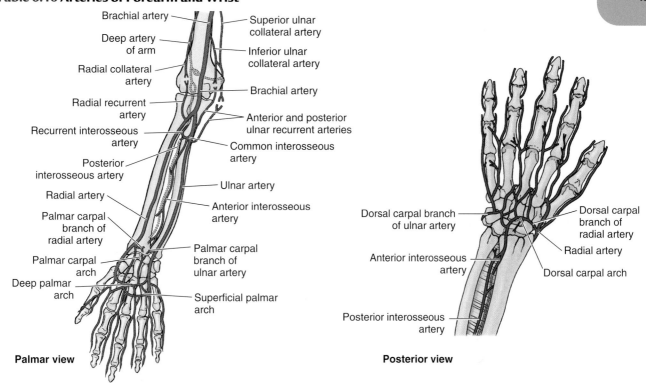

Palmar view

Posterior view

Artery	Origin	Course in Forearm
Ulnar	As larger terminal branch of brachial artery in cubital fossa	Descends inferomedially and then directly inferiorly deep to superficial pronator teres, palmaris longus and flexor digitorum superficialis to reach medial side of forearm; passes superficial to flexor retinaculum at wrist in ulnar (Guyon) canal to enter hand
Anterior ulnar recurrent artery	Ulnar artery just distal to elbow joint	Passes superiorly between brachialis and pronator teres, supplying both; then anastomoses with inferior ulnar collateral artery anterior to medial epicondyle
Posterior ulnar recurrent artery	Ulnar artery distal to anterior ulnar recurrent artery	Passes superiorly, posterior to medial epicondyle and deep to tendon of flexor carpi ulnaris; then anastomoses with superior ulnar collateral artery
Common interosseous	Ulnar artery in cubital fossa, distal to bifurcation of brachial artery	Passes laterally and deeply, terminating by dividing into anterior and posterior interosseous arteries
Anterior interosseous	As terminal branches of common interosseous artery, between radius and ulna	Passes distally on anterior aspect of interosseous membrane to proximal border of pronator quadratus; pierces membrane and continues distally to join dorsal carpal arch on posterior aspect of interosseous membrane
Posterior interosseous	As terminal branches of common interosseous artery, between radius and ulna	Passes to posterior aspect of interosseous membrane, giving rise to recurrent interosseous artery; runs distally between superficial and deep extensor muscles, supplying both
Recurrent interosseous	Posterior interosseous artery, between radius and ulna	Passes superiorly, posterior to proximal radioulnar joint, to anastomose with middle collateral artery (from deep artery of arm)
Palmar carpal branch	Ulnar artery in distal forearm	Runs across anterior aspect of wrist, deep to tendons of flexor digitorum profundus, to anastomose with the palmar carpal branch of the radial artery, forming **palmar carpal arch**
Dorsal carpal branch	Ulnar artery, proximal to pisiform	Passes across dorsal surface of wrist, deep to extensor tendons, to anastomose with dorsal carpal branch of radial artery, forming **dorsal carpal arch**
Radial	As smaller terminal branch of brachial artery in cubital fossa	Runs inferolaterally under cover of brachioradialis; lies lateral to flexor carpi radialis tendon in distal forearm; winds around lateral aspect of radius and crosses floor of anatomical snuff box to pierce 1st dorsal interosseous muscle
Radial recurrent	Lateral side of radial artery, just distal to brachial artery bifurcation	Ascends between brachioradialis and brachialis, supplying both (and elbow joint); then anastomoses with radial collateral artery (from deep brachial artery)
Palmar carpal branch	Distal radial artery near distal border of pronator quadratus	Runs across anterior wrist deep to flexor tendons to anastomose with the palmar carpal branch of ulnar artery to form palmar carpal arch
Dorsal carpal branch	Distal radial artery in proximal part of snuff box	Runs medially across wrist deep to pollicis and extensor radialis tendons, anastomoses with ulnar dorsal carpal branch forming dorsal carpal arch

lateral side of the flexor carpi ulnaris tendon. The ulnar nerve emerges from beneath the flexor carpi ulnaris tendon just proximal to the wrist and passes superficial to the flexor retinaculum to enter the hand, where it supplies the skin on the medial side of the hand. The branches of the ulnar nerve in the forearm (articular, muscular, and palmar and dorsal cutaneous branches) are described in Table 6.9.

The **radial nerve** leaves the posterior compartment of the arm to cross the anterior aspect of the lateral epicondyle of the humerus. In the cubital region, the radial nerve divides into deep and superficial branches (Fig. 6.24). The *deep branch of radial nerve* arises anterior to the lateral epicondyle and pierces the supinator. The deep branch winds around the lateral aspect of the neck of the radius and enters the posterior (extensor–pronator) compartment of the forearm where it continues as the *posterior interosseous nerve* (Fig. 6.22C; Table 6.9). The superficial branch of the radial nerve is a cutaneous and articular nerve that descends in the forearm under cover of the brachioradialis (Fig. 6.24). The *superficial branch of the radial nerve* (sensory or cutaneous) emerges in the distal part of the forearm and crosses the roof of the anatomical snuff box. It is distributed to skin on the dorsum of the hand and to a number of joints in the hand.

Arteries and Veins of Forearm

The brachial artery ends in the distal part of the cubital fossa opposite the neck of the radius by dividing into the ulnar and radial arteries, the main arteries of the forearm (Fig. 6.24). The branches of the ulnar and radial arteries are described in Table 6.10. The **ulnar artery** descends through the anterior (flexor–pronator) compartment of the forearm, deep to the pronator teres. Pulsations of the ulnar artery be palpated on the lateral side of the flexor carpi ulnaris tendon (FCU), where it lies anterior to the ulnar head. The ulnar nerve is on the medial side of the ulnar artery. The pulsations of the **radial artery** can be felt throughout the forearm. When the brachioradialis is pulled laterally, the entire length of the artery is visible until the distal part of the forearm. The radial artery leaves the forearm by winding around the lateral aspect of the wrist and crossing the floor of the anatomical snuff box to reach the hand. There are superficial and deep veins in the forearm: *superficial veins* ascend in the subcutaneous tissue; *deep veins* accompany the deep arteries (e.g., radial and ulnar).

Hand

The wrist, the proximal part of the hand, is at the junction of the forearm and hand. The *skeleton of the hand* consists of carpals in the wrist, metacarpals in the hand proper, and phalanges in the fingers, which are numbered from 1 to 5, beginning with the thumb and ending with the little finger. The palmar aspect of the hand features a central concavity that separates two eminences: a lateral more prominent **thenar eminence** at the base of the thumb, and a medial, smaller **hypothenar eminence** proximal to the base of the 5th finger (Fig. 6.25).

Fascia of Palm

The **fascia of the palm** is continuous with the antebrachial fascia and the fascia of the dorsum of the hand. The **palmar fascia** is thin over the thenar and hypothenar eminences, but it is thick centrally where it forms the fibrous palmar aponeurosis and in the fingers where it forms the digital sheaths (Fig. 6.25C). The **palmar aponeurosis**, a strong, well-defined part of the deep fascia of the palm, covers the soft tissues and overlies the long flexor tendons. The proximal end or apex of the triangular palmar aponeurosis is continuous with the flexor retinaculum and the palmaris longus tendon. Distal to the apex, the palmar aponeurosis forms four longitudinal digital bands that radiate from the apex and attach distally to the bases of the proximal phalanges, where they become continuous with the fibrous digital sheaths (Fig. 6.25C). The **fibrous digital sheaths** are ligamentous tubes that enclose the flexor tendon(s) and the synovial sheaths that surround them as they pass along the palmar aspect of their respective digit.

A **medial fibrous septum** extends deeply from the medial border of the palmar aponeurosis to the 5th metacarpal. Medial to this septum is the medial or **hypothenar compartment** containing the hypothenar muscles (Fig. 6.25B). Similarly, a **lateral fibrous septum** extends deeply from the lateral border of the palmar aponeurosis to the 3rd metacarpal. Lateral to the septum is the lateral or **thenar compartment** containing the thenar muscles. Between the hypothenar and the thenar compartments is the **central compartment** containing the flexor tendons and their sheaths, the lumbrical muscles, the superficial palmar arterial arch, and the digital vessels and nerves (Fig. 6.28A). The deepest muscular plane of the palm is the **adductor compartment** containing the adductor pollicis. Between the flexor tendons and the fascia covering the deep palmar muscles are two potential spaces: the **thenar space** and the **midpalmar space** (Fig. 6.25A). These spaces are bounded by fibrous septa passing from the edges of the palmar aponeurosis to the metacarpals. Between the two spaces is the especially strong lateral fibrous septum, which is attached to the 3rd metacarpal (Fig. 6.25B). The midpalmar space is continuous with the anterior compartment of the forearm via the carpal tunnel.

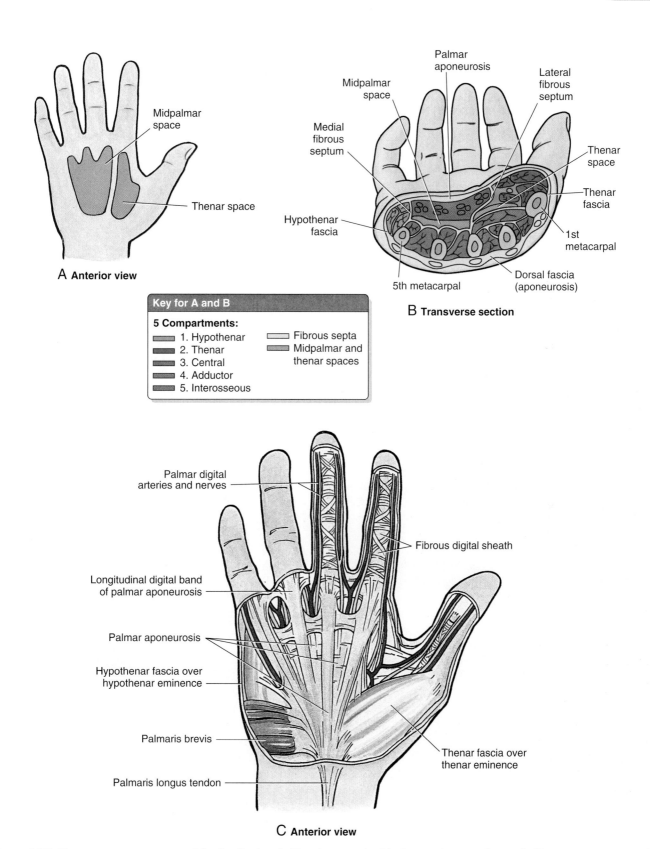

Key for A and B

5 Compartments:
- 1. Hypothenar
- 2. Thenar
- 3. Central
- 4. Adductor
- 5. Interosseous
- Fibrous septa
- Midpalmar and thenar spaces

A **Anterior view**

Midpalmar space

Thenar space

Palmar aponeurosis

Midpalmar space

Lateral fibrous septum

Medial fibrous septum

Thenar space

Thenar fascia

Hypothenar fascia

1st metacarpal

5th metacarpal

Dorsal fascia (aponeurosis)

B **Transverse section**

Palmar digital arteries and nerves

Fibrous digital sheath

Longitudinal digital band of palmar aponeurosis

Palmar aponeurosis

Hypothenar fascia over hypothenar eminence

Thenar fascia over thenar eminence

Palmaris brevis

Palmaris longus tendon

C **Anterior view**

Figure 6.25. Compartments, spaces, and fascia of palm. A. The thenar and midpalmar spaces are shown. **B.** The compartments and spaces of the palm are identified. **C.** The palmar aponeurosis, fibrous digital sheaths, and digital nerves and vessels are shown.

Elbow Tendinitis or Lateral Epicondylitis

Elbow tendinitis (tennis elbow) is a painful musculoskeletal condition that may follow repetitive use of the superficial extensor muscles of the forearm. Pain is felt over the lateral epicondyle and radiates down the posterior surface of the forearm. People with elbow tendinitis often feel pain when they open a door or lift a glass. Repeated forceful flexion and extension of the wrist strain the attachment of the common extensor tendon, producing inflammation of the periosteum of the lateral epicondyle (*lateral epicondylitis*) (Fig. 6.22A).

Mallet or Baseball Finger

Sudden severe tension on a long extensor tendon may avulse part of its attachment to the phalanx. The most common result of the injury is *mallet* or *baseball finger*. This deformity results from the distal interphalangeal joint suddenly being forced into extreme flexion (hyperflexion) when the tendon is attempting to extend the distal phalanx—for example, when a baseball is miscaught (hyperflexing it) or the finger is jammed into a base pad. These actions avulse the attachment of the tendon from the base of the distal phalanx. As a result, the person is unable to extend the distal interphalangeal joint (Fig. B6.11A).

Synovial Cyst of the Wrist

Sometimes a non-tender cystic swelling appears on the hand, most commonly on the dorsum of the wrist (Fig. B6.11B). The thin-walled cyst contains clear mucinous fluid. Clinically, this type of swelling is called a "ganglion" (G. swelling or knot). These synovial cysts are close to and often communicate with the synovial sheaths. The distal attachment of the extensor carpi radialis brevis (ECRB) tendon is a common site for such a cyst. A cystic swelling of the common flexor synovial sheath on the anterior aspect of the wrist can enlarge enough to produce compression of the median nerve by narrowing the carpal tunnel (*carpal tunnel syndrome*).

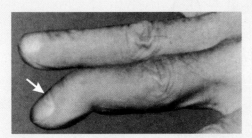

A **Mallet finger**

Figure B6.11.

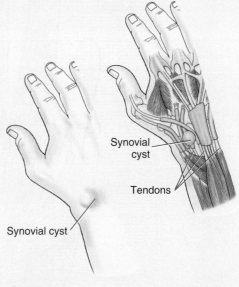

Synovial cyst

Tendons

Synovial cyst

B **Synovial cyst**

Dupuytren Contracture of Palmar Fascia

Dupuytren contracture is a disease of the palmar fascia resulting in progressive shortening, thickening, and fibrosis of the palmar fascia and palmar aponeurosis. The fibrous degeneration of the longitudinal digital bands of the aponeurosis on the medial side of the hand pulls the 4th and 5th fingers into partial flexion at the metacarpophalangeal and proximal interphalangeal joints (Fig. B6.12).

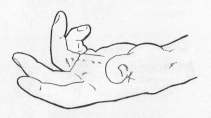

Dupuytren contracture

Figure B6.12.

The contracture is frequently bilateral. Treatment of Dupuytren contracture usually involves surgical excision of all fibrotic parts of the palmar fascia to free the fingers.

Hand Infections

Because the palmar fascia is thick and strong, swellings resulting from hand infections usually appear on the dorsum of the hand where the fascia is thinner. The potential fascial spaces of the palm are important because they may become infected. The fascial spaces determine the extent and direction of the spread of pus formed in the infected areas. Depending on the site of infection, pus will accumulate in the thenar, hypothenar, or adductor compartments. Antibiotic therapy has made infections that spread beyond one of these fascial compartments rare, but an untreated infection can spread proximally through the carpal tunnel into the forearm anterior to the pronator quadratus and its fascia.

Muscles of Hand

The intrinsic muscles of the hand are located in five compartments (Fig. 6.25; Table 6.11):

- Thenar muscles in the *thenar compartment:* abductor pollicis brevis, flexor pollicis brevis, and opponens pollicis.
- Hypothenar muscles in the *hypothenar compartment:* abductor digiti minimi, flexor digiti minimi brevis, and opponens digiti minimi.
- Adductor pollicis in the *adductor compartment.*
- The short muscles of the hand, the lumbricals, in the *central compartment* with the long flexor tendons.
- The interossei in separate *interosseous compartments* between the metacarpals.

THENAR MUSCLES

The **thenar muscles** form the *thenar eminence* on the lateral surface of the palm and are chiefly responsible for opposition of the thumb (Fig. 6.26). Normal movement of the thumb is important for the precise activities of the hand. The high degree of freedom of movements of the thumb results from the 1st metacarpal being independent,

with mobile joints at both ends. Several muscles are required to control its freedom of movement (Fig. 6.26):

- *Abduction:* **APL** and **abductor pollicis brevis** (APB).
- *Adduction:* **adductor pollicis** (AD) and 1st dorsal interosseous.
- *Extension:* EPL, EPB, and APL.
- *Flexion:* **flexor pollicis longus** (FPL) and **flexor pollicis brevis** (FPB).
- *Opposition:* **opponens pollicis.**

Opposition occurs at the carpometacarpal joint of the thumb. The complex movement of opposition begins with the thumb in the extended position and initially involves abduction and medial rotation of the 1st metacarpal ("cupping" of the palm) produced by the action of the opponens pollicis and then flexion at the metacarpophalangeal joint. The reinforcing action of the adductor pollicis and flexor pollicis longus increases the pressure that the opposed thumb can exert on the fingertips.

HYPOTHENAR MUSCLES

The **hypothenar muscles** (abductor digiti minimi, flexor digiti minimi brevis, and opponens digiti minimi) are in

Table 6.11 Intrinsic Muscles of Hand

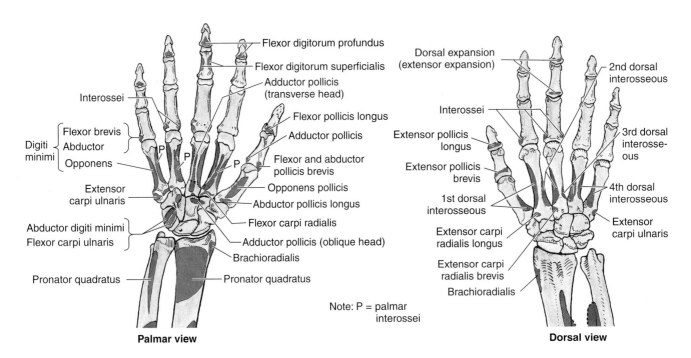

Palmar view

Dorsal view

Note: P = palmar interossei

Muscle	Proximal Attachment	Distal Attachment	Innervation[a]	Main Action
Thenar muscles				
Opponens pollicis		Lateral side of 1st metacarpal	Recurrent branch of medial nerve (**C8**, T1)	To oppose thumb, it draws 1st metacarpal medially to center of palm and rotates it medially
Abductor pollicis brevis	Flexor retinaculum and tubercles of scaphoid and trapezium			Abducts thumb; helps oppose it
Flexor pollicis brevis: Superficial head Deep head		Lateral side of base of proximal phalanx of thumb		Flexes thumb
Adductor pollicis: Oblique head Transverse head	Bases of 2nd and 3rd metacarpals, capitate, adjacent carpals Anterior surface of shaft of 3rd metacarpal	Medial side of base of proximal phalanx of thumb	Deep branch of ulnar nerve (C8, **T1**)	Adducts thumb toward lateral border of palm
Hypothenar muscles				
Abductor digiti minimi	Pisiform	Medial side of base of proximal phalanx of 5th finger	Deep branch of ulnar nerve (C8, **T1**)	Abducts 5th finger; assists in flexion of its proximal phalanx
Flexor digiti minimi brevis	Hook of hamate and flexor retinaculum			Flexes proximal phalanx of 5th finger
Opponens digiti minimi		Medial border of 5th metacarpal		Draws 5th metacarpal anterior and rotates it, bringing 5th finger into opposition with thumb

Table 6.11 **Intrinsic Muscles of Hand** (continued)

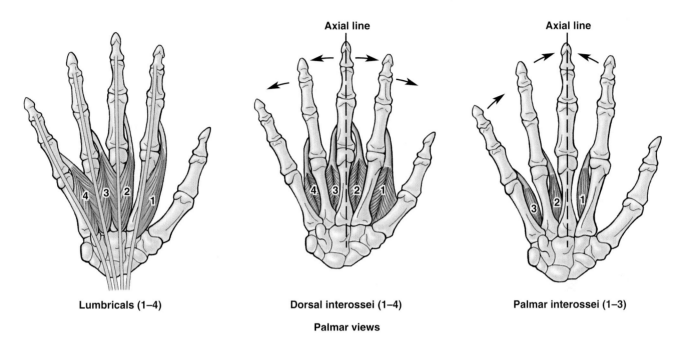

Lumbricals (1–4)   Dorsal interossei (1–4)   Palmar interossei (1–3)

Palmar views

Muscle	Proximal Attachment	Distal Attachment	Innervation[a]	Main Action
Short muscles				
Lumbricals			Median nerve (C8, **T1**)	
1 and 2	Lateral two tendons of flexor digitorum profundus (as unipennate muscles)	Lateral sides of extensor expansions of 2nd–5th fingers		Flex metacarpophalangeal joints; extend interphalangeal joints of 2nd–5th fingers
3 and 4	Medial three tendons of flexor digitorum profundus (as bipennate muscles)			
Dorsal interossei, 1–4	Adjacent sides of two metacarpals (as bipennate muscles)	Bases of proximal phalanges; extensor expansions of 2nd–4th fingers	Deep branch of ulnar nerve (C8, **T1**)	Abduct 2nd–4th fingers from axial line; act with lumbricals in flexing metacarpophalangeal joints and extending interphalangeal joints
Palmar interossei, 1–3	Palmar surfaces of 2nd, 4th, and 5th metacarpals (as unipennate muscles)	Bases of proximal phalanges; extensor expansions of 2nd, 4th, and 5th fingers		Adduct 2nd, 4th, and 5th fingers toward axial line; assist lumbricals in flexing metacarpophalangeal joints and extending interphalangeal joints

[a]The spinal cord segmental innervation is indicated (e.g., "**C8,** T1" means that the nerves supplying the opponens pollicis are derived from the eighth cervical segment and first thoracic segment of the spinal cord). Numbers in boldface (**C8**) indicate the main segmental innervation. Damage to one or more of the listed spinal cord segments or to the motor nerve roots arising from them results in paralysis of the muscles concerned.

the hypothenar compartment and produce the *hypothenar eminence* on the medial side of the palm (Fig. 6.27*A & B*). The **palmaris brevis** is a small muscle in the subcutaneous tissue of the hypothenar eminence (Fig. 6.25*C*); it is not in the hypothenar compartment. It wrinkles the skin of the hypothenar eminence, deepening the hollow of the palm, thereby aiding the palmar grip. The palmaris brevis covers and protects the ulnar nerve and artery. It is attached prox-

imally to the medial border of the palmar aponeurosis and to the skin on the medial border of the hand.

SHORT MUSCLES OF THE HAND

The **short hand muscles** are the lumbricals and interossei (Figs. 6.27 and 6.28; Table 6.11). The four slender **lumbrical muscles** were named because of their worm-like

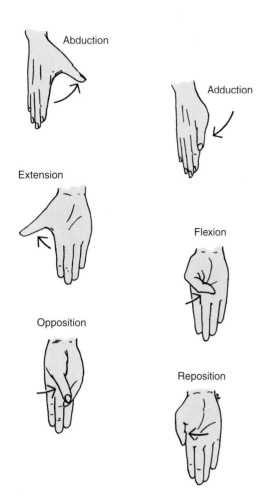

Figure 6.26. Thumb movements. The most complex movement, opposition, brings the tip of the thumb in contact with the pulps (pads) of the fingers (little finger pictured here).

appearance (L. *lumbricus,* earthworm). The lumbricals flex the fingers at the metacarpophalangeal joints and extend the interphalangeal joints. The four **dorsal interosseous muscles** (dorsal interossei) are located between the metacarpals; the three **palmar interosseous muscles** (palmar interossei) are on the palmar surfaces of the 2nd, 4th, and 5th metacarpals. The 1st dorsal interosseous muscle is easy to palpate; oppose the thumb firmly against the index finger and it can be felt easily in the web between them. The four dorsal interossei abduct the fingers and the three palmar interossei adduct them. As a mnemonic device use the following acronyms: *dorsal abduct* (**DAB**) and *palmar adduct* (**PAD**). Acting together, the dorsal and palmar interossei and lumbricals produce flexion at the metacarpophalangeal joints and extension of the interphalangeal joints (Z-movement). This occurs because of their attachment to the lateral bands of the extensor expansions.

Flexor Tendons of Extrinsic Muscles

The tendons of the flexor digitorum superficialis (FDS) and flexor digitorum profundus (FDP) enter the **common flexor sheath** deep to the flexor retinaculum (Fig. 6.27). The tendons enter the central compartment of the hand and fan out to enter the respective **digital synovial sheaths.** The common flexor and digital sheaths enable the tendons to slide freely past each other during movements of the fingers. Near the base of the proximal phalanx, the tendon of the FDS splits and surrounds the tendon of the FDP (Fig. 6.28*A*). The halves of the FDS tendon are attached to the margins of the anterior aspect of the base of the middle phalanx. The tendon of the FDP, after passing through the split in the FDS tendon, the *tendinous chiasm,* passes distally to attach to the anterior aspect of the base of the distal phalanx.

The **fibrous of sheaths of the digits of the hand** are strong ligamentous tunnels containing the flexor tendons and their synovial sheaths (Figs. 6.27 and 6.28). The sheaths extend from the heads of the metacarpals to the bases of the distal phalanges. These sheaths prevent the tendons from pulling away from the digits (bowstringing). The fibrous sheaths attach to the bones to form **osseofibrous tunnels** through which the tendons pass to reach the digits. The **anular** and **cruciform parts (ligaments) of the fibrous sheath** (often referred to clinically as "pulleys") are thickened reinforcements of these sheaths. The long flexor tendons are supplied by small blood vessels that pass to them within synovial folds (*vincula*) from the periosteum of the phalanges (Fig. 6.23*C*).

The tendon of FPL passes deep to the flexor retinaculum to the thumb within its own synovial sheath. At the head of the metacarpal, the tendon runs between two *sesamoid bones,* one in the combined tendon of the FPB and APB and the other in the tendon of the AD.

Arteries and Veins of Hand

The ulnar and radial arteries and their branches provide all the blood to the hand (Fig. 6.28; Table 6.12). The *ulnar artery* enters the hand anterior to the flexor retinaculum between the pisiform and the hook of hamate via the *ulnar canal* (Guyon canal). The **ulnar artery** lies lateral to the ulnar nerve. It divides into two terminal branches, the superficial palmar arch and the deep palmar branch. The **superficial palmar arch,** the main termination of the ulnar artery, gives rise to three **common palmar digital arteries** that anastomose with **palmar metacarpal arteries** from the deep palmar arch. Each common palmar digital artery divides into a pair of **proper palmar digital arteries** that run along the adjacent sides of the 2nd–4th fingers. The **radial artery** curves dorsally around the scaphoid and trapezium in the floor of the *anatomical snuff box* and enters the palm by passing between the heads of the 1st dorsal interosseous

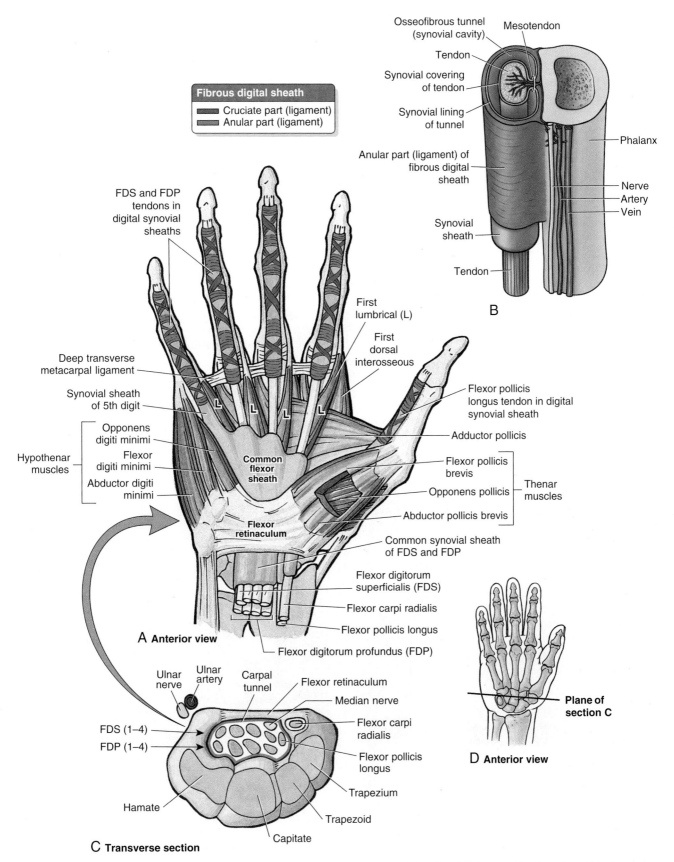

Fibrous digital sheath
- ▬ Cruciate part (ligament)
- ▬ Anular part (ligament)

Osseofibrous tunnel (synovial cavity)
Mesotendon
Tendon
Synovial covering of tendon
Synovial lining of tunnel
Anular part (ligament) of fibrous digital sheath
Synovial sheath
Tendon
Phalanx
Nerve
Artery
Vein

B

FDS and FDP tendons in digital synovial sheaths

First lumbrical (L)
First dorsal interosseous

Deep transverse metacarpal ligament

Synovial sheath of 5th digit

Hypothenar muscles
- Opponens digiti minimi
- Flexor digiti minimi
- Abductor digiti minimi

Common flexor sheath

Flexor pollicis longus tendon in digital synovial sheath
Adductor pollicis
Flexor pollicis brevis
Opponens pollicis
Abductor pollicis brevis

Thenar muscles

Flexor retinaculum

Common synovial sheath of FDS and FDP

Flexor digitorum superficialis (FDS)
Flexor carpi radialis
Flexor pollicis longus
Flexor digitorum profundus (FDP)

A Anterior view

Ulnar nerve
Ulnar artery
Carpal tunnel
Flexor retinaculum
Median nerve
Flexor carpi radialis
Flexor pollicis longus
Trapezium
Trapezoid
Capitate
Hamate

FDS (1–4)
FDP (1–4)

C Transverse section

Plane of section C

D Anterior view

Figure 6.27. Flexor tendons, common flexor sheath, fibrous sheaths, and synovial sheaths of digits. A. This dissection of the hand shows the muscles, common flexor sheath, and synovial sheaths of digits 1–5 (*blue*) of the long flexor tendons. **B.** A close-up of the anular part of a fibrous digital sheath is shown. **C.** This section of the wrist shows the carpal tunnel and its contents. **D.** Orientation drawing for part C.

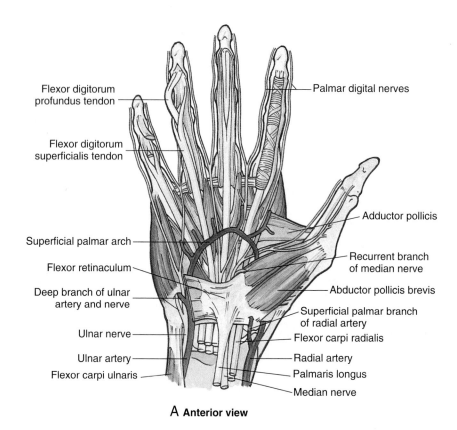

Flexor digitorum profundus tendon

Flexor digitorum superficialis tendon

Palmar digital nerves

Adductor pollicis

Superficial palmar arch

Flexor retinaculum

Deep branch of ulnar artery and nerve

Ulnar nerve

Ulnar artery

Flexor carpi ulnaris

Recurrent branch of median nerve

Abductor pollicis brevis

Superficial palmar branch of radial artery

Flexor carpi radialis

Radial artery

Palmaris longus

Median nerve

A Anterior view

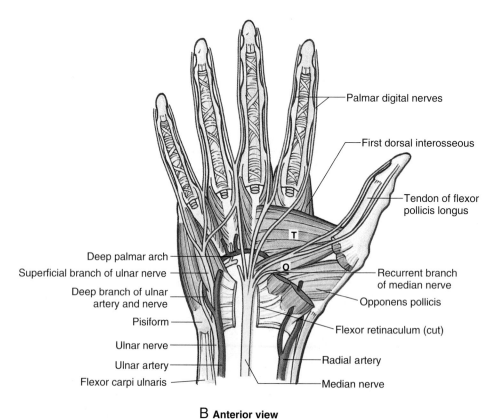

Palmar digital nerves

First dorsal interosseous

Tendon of flexor pollicis longus

Deep palmar arch

Superficial branch of ulnar nerve

Deep branch of ulnar artery and nerve

Pisiform

Ulnar nerve

Ulnar artery

Flexor carpi ulnaris

Recurrent branch of median nerve

Opponens pollicis

Flexor retinaculum (cut)

Radial artery

Median nerve

B Anterior view

Figure 6.28. Palmar arches and nerves. A. This superficial dissection of the palm of the hand shows the superficial palmar arch and the distribution of the median and ulnar nerves. **B.** Deeper dissection showing the deep palmar arch and the deep branch of the ulnar nerve. *T,* transverse head of adductor pollicis; *O,* oblique head of adductor pollicis.

Tenosynovitis

Injuries such as puncture of a finger by a rusty nail can cause infection of the digital synovial sheaths. When inflammation of the tendon and synovial sheath (**tenosynovitis**) occurs, the digit swells and movement becomes painful. Because the tendons of the 2nd–4th digits nearly always have separate synovial sheaths, the infection usually is confined to the infected digit. If the infection is untreated, however, the proximal ends of these sheaths may rupture, allowing the infection to spread to the midpalmar space (Fig. 6.25A). Because the synovial sheath of the little finger is usually continuous with the common flexor sheath, tenosynovitis in this finger may spread to the common sheath and thus through the palm and carpal tunnel to the anterior forearm. Likewise, tenosynovitis in the thumb may spread through the continuous

synovial sheath of FPL (radial bursa). How far an infection spreads from the digits depends on variations in their connections with the common flexor sheath.

The tendons of the APL and EPB are in the same tendinous sheath on the dorsum of the wrist. Excessive friction of these tendons results in fibrous thickening of the sheath and stenosis of the osseofibrous tunnel, **Quervain tenovaginitis stenosans.** This condition causes pain in the wrist that radiates proximally to the forearm and distally to the thumb.

If the tendons of the FDS and FDP enlarge (forming a nodule) proximal to the tunnel, the person is unable to extend the finger. When the finger is extended passively, a snap is audible. Flexion produces another snap as the thickened tendon moves. This condition is called **digital tenovaginitis stenosans** (trigger finger or snapping finger) (Fig. B6.13).

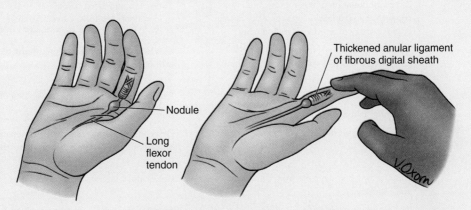

Digital tenovaginitis stenosans (trigger finger)
Figure B6.13.

muscle. It then turns medially and passes between the heads of the adductor pollicis (Fig. 6.28B). The radial artery ends by anastomosing with the deep branch of the ulnar artery to form the **deep palmar arch.** This arch, formed mainly by the radial artery, lies across the metacarpals just distal to their bases. The deep palmar arch gives rise to three *palmar metacarpal arteries* and the *princeps pollicis artery.* The *radialis indicis artery* passes along the lateral side of the index finger.

The *superficial* and *deep palmar venous arches,* associated with the superficial and deep palmar (arterial) arches, drain into the deep veins of the forearm. The dorsal digital veins drain into three dorsal metacarpal veins, which unite to

form the *dorsal venous network.* Superficial to the metacarpus, this network is prolonged proximally on the lateral side as the *cephalic vein.* The *basilic vein* arises from the medial side of the dorsal venous network (Fig. 6.9).

Nerves of Hand

The median, ulnar, and radial nerves supply the hand (Figs. 6.22C and 6.24). The **median nerve** enters the hand through the carpal tunnel, deep to the flexor retinaculum (Figs. 6.27 and 6.28), along with the tendons of the FDS, FDP, and FPL. The **carpal tunnel** is the passageway deep to the flexor retinaculum between the tubercles of the

Table 6.12 Arteries of Hand

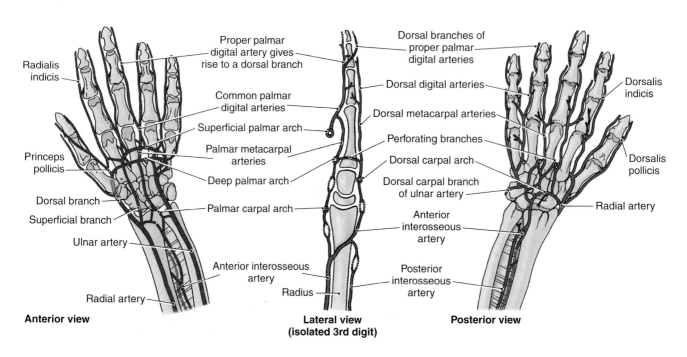

Anterior view

Radialis indicis

Proper palmar digital artery gives rise to a dorsal branch

Common palmar digital arteries

Superficial palmar arch

Palmar metacarpal arteries

Princeps pollicis

Deep palmar arch

Dorsal branch

Superficial branch

Palmar carpal arch

Ulnar artery

Anterior interosseous artery

Radial artery

Lateral view (isolated 3rd digit)

Dorsal branches of proper palmar digital arteries

Dorsal digital arteries

Dorsal metacarpal arteries

Perforating branches

Dorsal carpal arch

Dorsal carpal branch of ulnar artery

Anterior interosseous artery

Posterior interosseous artery

Radius

Posterior view

Dorsalis indicis

Dorsalis pollicis

Radial artery

Artery	Origin	Course
Superficial palmar arch	Direct continuation of ulnar artery; arch is completed on lateral side by superficial branch of radial artery or another of its branches	Curves laterally deep to palmar aponeurosis and superficial to long flexor tendons; curve of arch lies across palm at level of distal border of extended thumb
Deep palmar arch	Direct continuation of radial artery; arch is completed on medial side by deep branch of ulnar artery	Curves medially, deep to long flexor tendons; is in contact with bases of metacarpals
Common palmar digitals	Superficial palmar arch	Pass distally on lumbricals to webbing of fingers
Proper palmar digitals	Common palmar digital arteries	Run along sides of 2nd–5th fingers
Princeps pollicis	Radial artery as it turns into palm	Descends on palmar aspect of 1st metacarpal; divides at base of proximal phalanx into two branches that run along sides of thumb
Radialis indicis	Radial artery; but may arise from princeps pollicis artery	Passes along lateral side of index finger to its distal end
Dorsal carpal arch	Radial and ulnar arteries	Arches within fascia on dorsum of hand
Palmar carpal arch	Radial and ulnar arteries	Arches on anterior aspect of wrist

Laceration of Palmar Arches

Bleeding is usually profuse when the palmar (arterial) arches are lacerated. It may not be sufficient to ligate (tie off) only one forearm artery when the arches are lacerated because these vessels usually have numerous communications in the forearm and hand and thus bleed from both ends. To obtain a bloodless surgical operating field for treating complicated hand injuries, it may be necessary to compress the brachial artery and its branches proximal to the elbow (e.g., using a pneumatic tourniquet). This procedure prevents blood from reaching the ulnar and radial arteries through the anastomoses around the elbow.

The superficial and deep palmar (arterial) arches are not palpable, but their surface markings are visible. The superficial palmar arch occurs at the level of the distal border of the fully extended thumb. The deep palmar arch lies approximately 1 cm proximal to the superficial palmar arch. The location of these arches should be borne in mind in wounds of the palm and when palmar incisions are made.

scaphoid and the trapezoid bones on the lateral side and the pisiform and the hook of hamate on the medial side. Distal to the carpal tunnel, the median nerve supplies two and a half thenar muscles and the 1st and 2nd lumbricals (Table 6.11). It also sends sensory fibers to the skin on the entire palmar surface, the sides of the first three digits, the lateral half of the 4th digit, and the dorsum of the distal halves of these digits. Note, however, that the *palmar cutaneous branch of the median nerve,* which supplies the central palm, arises proximal to the flexor retinaculum and passes superficial to it (i.e., it does not pass through the carpal tunnel).

The **ulnar nerve** leaves the forearm by emerging from deep to the tendon of the FCU (Figs. 6.27 and 6.28). It continues distally to the wrist via the *ulnar (Guyon) canal.* Here the ulnar nerve is bound by fascia to the anterior surface of the flexor retinaculum. It then passes alongside the lateral border of the pisiform; the ulnar artery is on its lateral side. Just proximal to the wrist, the ulnar nerve gives off a *palmar cutaneous branch* that passes superficial to the flexor retinaculum and palmar aponeurosis; it supplies skin on the medial side of the palm. The ulnar nerve also gives off a *dorsal cutaneous branch,* which supplies the medial half of the dorsum of the hand, the 5th finger, and the medial half of the 4th finger. The ulnar nerve ends at the distal border of the flexor retinaculum by dividing into superficial and deep branches (Fig. 6.28*B*). The *superficial branch of the ulnar nerve* supplies cutaneous branches to the anterior surfaces of the medial one and a half fingers. The *deep branch of the ulnar nerve* supplies the hypothenar muscles, the medial two lumbricals, the adductor pollicis, the deep head of FPB and all the interossei (Table 6.11). The deep branch also supplies several joints (wrist, intercarpal, carpometacarpal, and intermetacarpal). The ulnar nerve is referred to as the *nerve of fine movements* because it innervates muscles that are concerned with intricate hand movements.

The **radial nerve** supplies no hand muscles. Its terminal branches, superficial and deep, arise in the cubital fossa (Fig. 6.24; Table 6.9). The *superficial branch of the radial nerve* is entirely sensory. It pierces the deep fascia near the dorsum of the wrist to supply the skin and fascia over the lateral two thirds of the dorsum of the hand, the dorsum of the thumb, and the proximal parts of the lateral one and a half digits.

Carpal Tunnel Syndrome

Carpal tunnel syndrome results from any lesion that significantly reduces the size of the carpal tunnel or, more commonly, increases the size of some of the structures (or their coverings) that pass through it (e.g., inflammation of the synovial sheaths). The median nerve is the most sensitive structure in the carpal tunnel and, therefore, is the most affected (Fig. 6.27C). The median nerve has two terminal sensory branches that supply the skin of the hand; hence **paresthesia** (tingling), **hypothesia** (diminished sensation), or **anesthesia** (absence of tactile sensation) may occur in the lateral three and a half digits. Recall however, that the palmar cutaneous branch of the median nerve arises proximal to and does not pass through the carpal tunnel; thus sensation in the central palm remains unaffected. This nerve also has one terminal motor branch, the recurrent branch, which innervates the three thenar muscles.

Wasting of the thenar eminence and progressive loss of coordination and strength in the thumb (owing to weakness of the APB and opponens pollicis) may occur if the cause of the compression is not alleviated. Individuals with carpal tunnel syndrome are unable to oppose the thumb (Fig. B6.14A). To relieve the compression and resulting symptoms, partial or complete surgical division of the flexor retinaculum, a procedure called **carpal tunnel release,** may be necessary. The incision for carpal tunnel release is made toward the medial side of the wrist and flexor retinaculum to avoid possible injury to the recurrent branch of the median nerve.

Trauma to Median Nerve

Lesions of the median nerve usually occur in two places: the forearm and wrist. The most common site is where the nerve passes through the carpal tunnel. Laceration of the wrist often causes median nerve injury because this nerve is relatively close to the surface. This results in paralysis of the thenar muscles and the first two lumbricals. Hence opposition of the thumb is not possible and fine control movements of the 2nd and 3rd digits are impaired. Sensation is also lost over the thumb and adjacent two and a half fingers.

Median nerve injury resulting from a perforating wound in the elbow region results in loss of flexion of the proximal and distal interphalangeal joints of the 2nd and 3rd digits. The ability to flex the metacarpophalangeal joints of these digits is also affected because digital branches of the median nerve supply the 1st and 2nd lumbricals. *Ape hand* refers to a deformity in which thumb movements are limited to flexion and extension of the thumb in the plane of the palm. This condition is caused by the inability to oppose and by limited abduction of the thumb (Fig. B6.14*B*).

Ulnar Nerve Injury

Ulnar nerve injury usually occurs in one of four places: (1) posterior to the medial epicondyle of the humerus (most common), (2) in the cubital fossa formed by the tendinous arch connecting the humeral and ulnar heads of the FCU, (3) at the wrist, and (4) in the hand. Ulnar nerve injury occurring at the elbow, wrist, or in the hand may result in extensive motor and sensory loss to the hand. An injury to the nerve in the distal part of the forearm denervates most intrinsic hand muscles. The power of wrist adduction is impaired, and when an attempt is made to flex the wrist joint, the hand is drawn to the lateral side by the FCR in the absence of the "balance" provided by the FCU. After ulnar nerve injury, the person has difficulty making a fist because, in the absence of opposition, the metacarpophalangeal joints become hyperextended, and he or she cannot flex the 4th and 5th fingers at the distal interphalangeal joints when trying to make a fist. Furthermore, the person cannot extend the interphalangeal joints when trying to straighten the fingers. This characteristic appearance of the hand, resulting from a distal lesion of the ulnar nerve, is known as a *claw hand*

(Fig. B6.14*C*). This deformity results from atrophy of the interosseous muscles of the hand. The claw is produced by the unopposed action of the extensors and FDP.

Compression of the ulnar nerve also may occur at the wrist where it passes between the pisiform and the hook of hamate. The depression between these bones is converted by the pisohamate ligament into an osseofibrous ulnar tunnel (Guyon tunnel). **Ulnar canal syndrome** is manifest by hypoesthesia in the medial one and one half fingers and weakness of the intrinsic hand muscles. Clawing of the 4th and 5th fingers may occur; but in contrast to proximal ulnar nerve injury, their ability to flex is unaffected and there is no radial deviation of the hand.

Radial Nerve Injury

Although the radial nerve supplies no muscles in the hand, radial nerve injury in the arm by a fracture of the humeral shaft can produce serious disability of the hand. This injury is proximal to the branches to the extensors of the wrist, so wrist drop is the primary clinical manifestation. The hand is flexed at the wrist and lies flaccid, and the digits also remain in the flexed position at the metacarpophalangeal joints. The extent of anesthesia is minimal, even in serious radial nerve injuries, and usually is confined to a small area on the lateral part of the dorsum of the hand. Severance of the deep branch of the radial nerve results in an inability to extend the thumb and the metacarpophalangeal joints of the other digits. Loss of sensation does not occur because the deep branch is entirely muscular and articular in distribution.

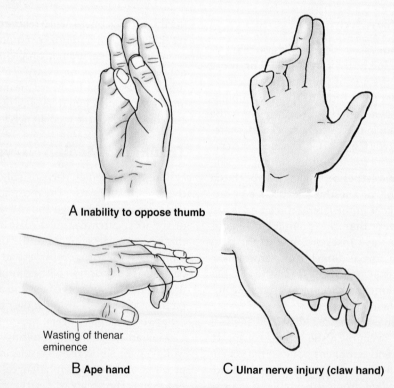

A **Inability to oppose thumb**

Wasting of thenar eminence

B **Ape hand**

C **Ulnar nerve injury (claw hand)**

Figure B6.14.

Surface Anatomy of Forearm and Hand

The cubital fossa, the triangular hollow area on the anterior surface of the elbow, is bounded medially by the prominence formed by the flexor–pronator group of muscles that are attached to the medial epicondyle. To estimate the position of these muscles, put your thumb posterior to your medial epicondyle and place your fingers on your forearm as shown in Figure SA6.4A.

A common place for measuring the radial pulse rate is where the radial artery lies on the anterior surface of the distal end of the radius, lateral to the FCR tendon

(Fig. SA6.4B). Here the artery can be felt pulsating between the tendons of the FCR and the APL and where it can be compressed against the radius. The **tendons of the FCR and palmaris longus** can be palpated anterior to the wrist, a little lateral to its middle, and are usually observed by flexing the closed fist against resistance. The tendon of the palmaris longus serves as a guide to the median nerve, which lies deep to it. The **FCU tendon** can be palpated as it crosses the anterior aspect of the wrist near the medial side and inserts into the pisiform. The

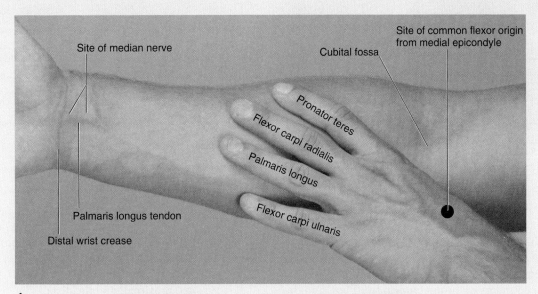

A **Anterior view of supinated forearm**

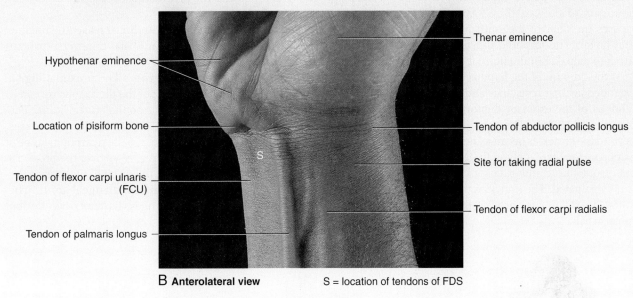

B **Anterolateral view**   S = location of tendons of FDS

Figure SA6.4.

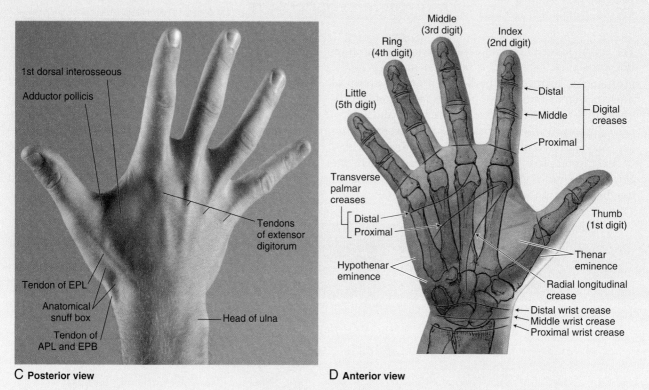

C Posterior view

D Anterior view

Figure SA6.4. (Continued)

FCU tendon serves as a guide to the ulnar nerve and artery. The **tendons of the FDS** can be palpated as the digits are alternately flexed and extended.

The **tendons of the APL and EPB** indicate the lateral (anterior) boundary of the **anatomical snuff box**, and the **tendon of the EPL** indicates the medial (posterior) boundary of the box (Fig. SA6.4*C*). The radial artery crosses the floor of the snuff box, where its pulsations may be felt. The scaphoid and, less distinctly, the trapezium are palpable in the floor of the snuff box.

If the dorsum of the hand is examined with the wrist extended against resistance and the digits abducted, the **tendons of the extensor digitorum** to the fingers stand out (Fig. SA6.4*C*). These tendons are not visible far beyond the knuckles because they flatten here to form the extensor expansions of the fingers. Under the loose subcutaneous tissue and extensor tendons, the metacarpals can be palpated. The knuckles that become visible when a fist is made are produced by the **heads of the metacarpals**.

The palmar skin presents several more or less constant *flexion creases* where the skin is firmly bound to the deep fascia (Fig. SA6.4*D*):

- *Wrist creases:* **proximal, middle, distal.** The *distal wrist crease* indicates the proximal border of the flexor retinaculum.
- *Palmar creases:* **radial longitudinal crease** (the life line of palmistry), proximal and distal transverse palmar creases:
- *Transverse digital flexion creases:* The **proximal digital crease** is located at the root of the digit, approximately 2 cm distal to the metacarpophalangeal joint. The proximal digital crease of the thumb crosses obliquely, proximal to the 1st metacarpophalangeal joint. The **middle digital crease** lies over the proximal interphalangeal joint, and the **distal digital crease** lies proximal to the distal interphalangeal joint. The thumb, having two phalanges, has only two flexion creases. ●

Joints of Upper Limb

Movement of the *pectoral girdle* involves the sternoclavicular, acromioclavicular, and glenohumeral joints, usually all moving simultaneously (Fig. 6.29). Functional defects in any of these joints impair movements of the pectoral girdle. Mobility of the scapula is essential for the freedom of movement of the upper limb. When testing *the range of motion of the pectoral girdle,* both scapulothoracic (movement of the scapula on the thoracic wall) and glenohumeral movements must be considered. Although the initial 30° may occur without scapular motion, in the overall movement of fully elevating the arm, the movement occurs in a 2:1 ratio. For every 3° of elevation, approximately 2° occurs at the glenohumeral joint and 1° at the scapulothoracic joint. This is known as *scapulohumeral rhythm.* The important movements of the pectoral girdle are scapular movements: elevation and depression, protraction (lateral or forward movement of the scapula), and retraction (medial or backward movement of the scapula) and rotation of the scapula.

Sternoclavicular Joint

This **sternoclavicular (SC) joint** is a synovial articulation between the sternal end of the clavicle and the manubrium of the sternum and the 1st costal cartilage. The SC joint is a saddle type of joint but functions as a ball and socket joint (Fig. 6.29). The SC joint is divided into two compartments by an **articular disc.** The disc is firmly attached to the *anterior and posterior SC ligaments,* thickenings of the fibrous layer of the joint capsule, as well as to the *interclavicular ligament.* The great strength of the SC joint is a consequence of these attachments. Thus, although the articular disc serves as a shock absorber of forces transmitted along the clavicle from the upper limb, dislocation of the clavicle is unusual whereas fracture of the clavicle is common. The SC joint, the only articulation between the upper limb and the axial skeleton, can be readily palpated because the sternal end of the clavicle lies superior to the manubrium of the sternum.

The **joint capsule** surrounds the SC joint, including the epiphysis at the sternal end of the clavicle. The *fibrous layer of the capsule* is attached to the margins of the articular surfaces, including the periphery of the articular disc. A *synovial membrane* lines the internal surfaces of the fibrous layer of the capsule. **Anterior** and **posterior SC ligaments** reinforce the joint capsule anteriorly and posteriorly. The **interclavicular ligament** strengthens the capsule superiorly. It extends from the sternal end of one clavicle to the sternal end of the other clavicle; it is also attached to the superior border of the manubrium. The **costoclavicular ligament** anchors the

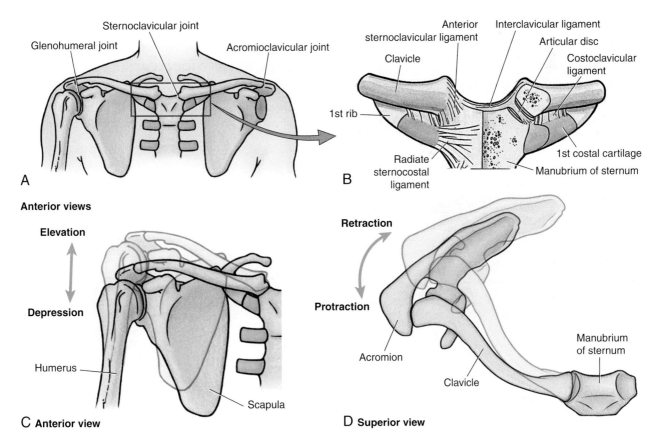

Figure 6.29. A. Pectoral girdle. Orientation drawing for B. **B.** Sternoclavicular joints. **C.** and **D.** Range of motion of clavicle permitted by movements at sternoclavicular joint. Elevation and depression (C), protraction and retraction (D).

inferior surface of the sternal end of the clavicle to the 1st rib and its costal cartilage, limiting elevation of the pectoral girdle.

Although the SC joint is extremely strong, it is significantly mobile to allow movements of the pectoral girdle and upper limb. During full elevation of the limb, the clavicle is raised to approximately a 60° angle. The SC joint can also be moved anteriorly or posteriorly over a range up to 25–30°.

The SC joint is supplied by internal thoracic and suprascapular arteries (Table 6.4). Branches of the medial supraclavicular nerve and the nerve to the subclavius supply the SC joint (Table 6.5).

Acromioclavicular Joint

The **acromioclavicular (AC) joint** is a plane synovial articulation (Fig. 6.30). It is located 2–3 cm from the "point" of the shoulder formed by the lateral part of the acromion of the scapula. The acromial end of the clavicle articulates with the acromion. The articular surfaces, covered with fibrocartilage, are separated by an incomplete wedge-shaped *articular disc.*

The sleeve-like, relatively loose *fibrous layer of the joint capsule* is attached to the margins of the articular surfaces. A *synovial membrane* lines the internal surface of the fibrous layer of the capsule. Although relatively weak, the joint capsule is strengthened superiorly by fibers of the trapezius.

The **AC ligament**, a fibrous band extending from the acromion to the clavicle, strengthens the AC joint superiorly (Fig. 6.32*C* & *D*). Most of its strength comes from coracoclavicular ligament. It maintains its integrity and prevents the acromion from being driven under the clavicle even when the AC joint is separated. The strong, extra-articular **coracoclavicular ligament** (subdivided into conoid

and trapezoid ligaments) is located several centimeters from the AC joint, which anchors the clavicle to the coracoid process of the scapula. The apex of the vertical **conoid ligament** is attached to the root of the *coracoid process*. Its wide attachment (base) is to the *conoid tubercle* on the inferior surface of the clavicle. The nearly horizontal **trapezoid ligament** is attached to the superior surface of the coracoid process and extends laterally and posteriorly to the trapezoid line on the inferior surface of the clavicle. In addition to augmenting the AC joint, the coracoclavicular ligament provides the means by which the scapula and free limb are (passively) suspended from the clavicle.

The acromion of the scapula rotates on the acromial end of the clavicle. These movements are associated with motion at the physiological scapulothoracic joint. The axioappendicular muscles that attach to and move the scapula cause the acromion to move on the clavicle (Fig. 6.31). Factors limiting scapular movements are listed in Table 6.13. The AC joint is supplied by the suprascapular and thoracoacromial arteries (Table 6.4). Supraclavicular, lateral pectoral, and axillary nerves supply the joint (Table 6.5).

Glenohumeral Joint

The **glenohumeral (shoulder) joint** is a ball and socket, synovial joint that permits a wide range of movement; however, its mobility makes the joint relatively unstable (Fig. 6.32).

ARTICULATION AND JOINT CAPSULE OF THE GLENOHUMERAL JOINT

The large *humeral head* articulates with the relatively shallow *glenoid cavity* of the scapula, which is deepened slightly

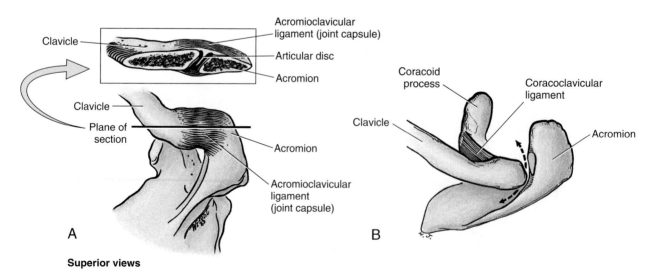

Figure 6.30. Acromioclavicular joints. The joint capsule and articular disc (**A**) and coracoclavicular ligament (**B**) are shown.

Table 6.13 Structures Limiting Movements of Pectoral Girdle

Movement	Joint(s)	Limiting Structures (Tension)
Flexion (0–180°)	Sternoclavicular Acromioclavicular Glenohumeral Scapulothoracic	*Ligaments:* posterior part of coracohumeral, trapezoid, and posterior part of joint capsule of glenohumeral joint *Muscles:* rhomboids, levator scapulae, extensor and external rotator muscles, rotator muscles of glenohumeral joint
Abduction (0–180°)	Sternoclavicular Acromioclavicular Glenohumeral Scapulothoracic	*Ligaments:* middle and inferior glenohumeral, trapezoid, and inferior part of joint capsule of glenohumeral joint *Muscles:* rhomboids, levator scapulae, adductor muscles of glenohumeral joint *Bony apposition* between greater tubercle of humerus and superior part of glenoid cavity/labrum or lateral aspect of acromion
Extension	Glenohumeral	*Ligaments:* anterior part of coracohumeral and anterior part of joint capsule of glenohumeral joint *Muscles:* clavicular head of pectoralis major
Medial (internal) rotation	Glenohumeral	*Ligaments:* posterior glenohumeral joint capsule *Muscles:* infraspinatus and teres minor
Lateral (external) rotation	Glenohumeral	*Ligaments:* glenohumeral, coracohumeral, anterior glenohumeral joint capsule *Muscles:* latissimus dorsi, teres major, pectoralis major, subscapularis

Modified from Clarkson HM: *Musculoskeletal Assessment. Joint Range of Motion and Manual of Muscle Strength,* 2nd ed. Baltimore, Lippincott Williams & Wilkins 2000.

Dislocation of AC Joint

Although its extrinsic (coracoclavicular) ligament is strong, the AC joint itself is weak and easily injured by a direct blow. In contact sports such as football, soccer, and hockey, it is not uncommon for *dislocation of the AC joint* to result from a hard fall on the shoulder or on the outstretched upper limb (Fig. B6.15). Dislocation of the AC joint also can occur when a hockey player is, for example, driven violently into the boards. An AC dislocation, often called a "shoulder separation," is severe when both the AC and the coracoclavicular ligaments are torn. When the coracoclavicular ligament tears, the shoulder separates from the clavicle and falls because of the weight of the upper limb. Dislocation of the AC joint makes the acromion more prominent, and the clavicle may move superior to this process.

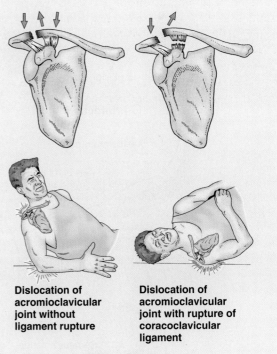

Dislocation of acromioclavicular joint without ligament rupture

Dislocation of acromioclavicular joint with rupture of coracoclavicular ligament

Figure B6.15.

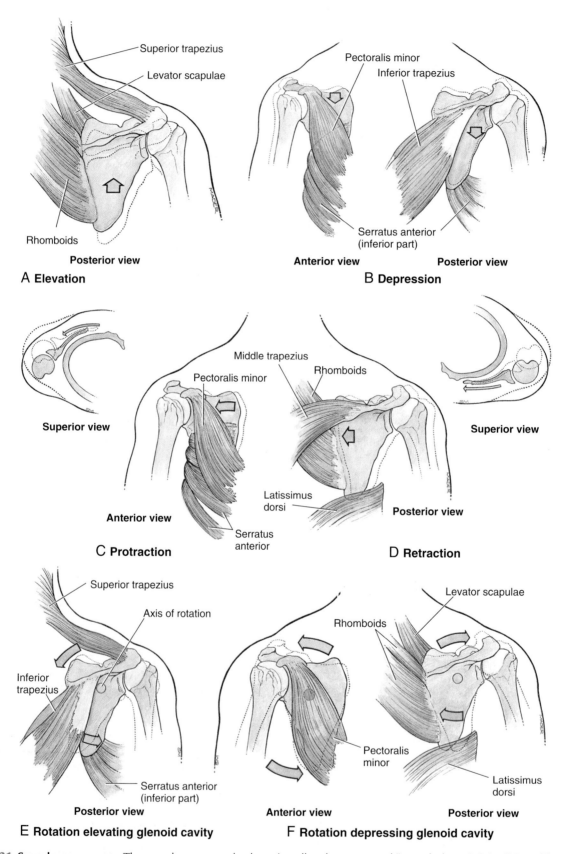

Figure 6.31. Scapular movements. The scapula moves on the thoracic wall at the conceptual "scapulothoracic joint." *Dotted lines*, the starting position of each movement.

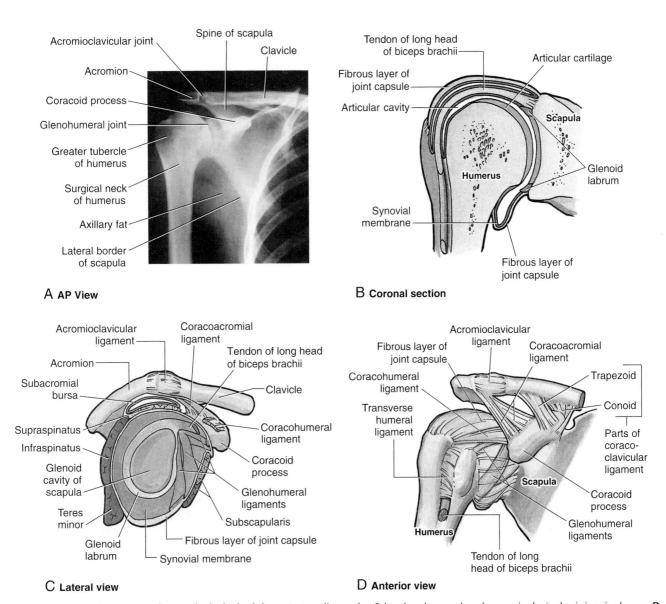

Figure 6.32. Glenohumeral and acromioclavicular joints. A. A radiograph of the glenohumeral and acromioclavicular joints is shown. **B.** Note the articulating bones and joint capsule of the glenohumeral joint. **C.** The glenoid cavity and the glenohumeral ligaments are demonstrated. **D.** The ligaments of the glenohumeral and sternoclavicular joints are identified.

by the ring-like, fibrocartilaginous **glenoid labrum** (L. lip). Both articular surfaces are covered with hyaline cartilage. The glenoid cavity accepts little more than a third of the humeral head, which is held in the cavity by the tonus of the musculotendinous rotator cuff (supraspinatus, infraspinatus, teres minor, and subscapularis).

The loose *fibrous layer of the joint capsule* surrounds the glenohumeral joint and is attached medially to the margin of the glenoid cavity and laterally to the anatomical neck of the humerus. Superiorly, the fibrous layer encloses the proximal attachment of the long head of biceps brachii to the supraglenoid tubercle of the scapula within the joint. The inferior part of the joint capsule, the only part not reinforced by the rotator cuff, muscles, is its weakest area. Here the capsule is

particularly lax and lies in folds when the arm is adducted; however, it becomes taut when the arm is abducted.

The *synovial membrane* lines the internal surface of the fibrous capsule and reflects from it onto the glenoid labrum and the humerus as far as the articular margin of the head. The synovial membrane also forms a tubular sheath for the tendon of the long head of the biceps brachii. Anteriorly, there is a communication between the *subscapular bursa* and the synovial cavity of the joint.

LIGAMENTS OF GLENOHUMERAL JOINT

The *glenohumeral ligaments*, evident only on the internal aspect of the capsule, strengthen the anterior aspect of the capsule. The **coracohumeral ligament**, a strong band that passes from the base of the coracoid process to the anterior aspect of the greater tubercle, strengthens the capsule superiorly (Fig. 6.32C & D). The glenohumeral ligaments are intrinsic ligaments that are part of the fibrous layer of the capsule. The **transverse humeral ligament** is a broad fibrous band that runs from the greater to the lesser tubercle, bridging over the intertubercular groove and converting the groove into a canal for the tendon of the long head of biceps brachii and its synovial sheath.

The **coracoacromial arch** is an extrinsic, protective structure formed by the smooth inferior aspect of the *acromion* and *coracoid process* of the scapula, with the **coracoacromial ligament** spanning between them (Fig. 6.32C). The coracoacromial arch overlies the head of the humerus, preventing its superior displacement from the glenoid cavity. The arch is so strong that a forceful superior thrust of the humerus will not fracture it; the shaft of the humerus or clavicle fractures first.

MOVEMENTS OF THE GLENOHUMERAL JOINT

The glenohumeral joint has more freedom of movement than any other joint in the body. This freedom results from the laxity of its joint capsule and the large size of the humeral head compared with the small size of the glenoid cavity. The glenohumeral joint allows movements around the three axes and permits flexion–extension, abduction-adduction, rotation (medial and lateral) of the humerus, and circumduction. Table 6.13 lists structures that limit movements of the glenohumeral joint. Lateral rotation of the humerus increases the range of abduction. When the arm is abducted without rotation, the greater tubercle contacts the *coracoacromial arch*, preventing further abduction. If the arm is then laterally rotated 180°, the tubercles are rotated posteriorly and more articular surface becomes available to continue elevation. Stiffening or fixation of the joints of the pectoral girdle (*ankylosis*) results in a much more restricted range of movement, even if the glenohumeral joint is normal.

The muscles moving the joint are the *axioappendicular muscles*, which may act indirectly on the joint (i.e., act on the pectoral girdle), and the *scapulohumeral muscles*, which act directly on the joint (Tables 6.1–6.3). Other muscles serve the glenohumeral joint as *shunt muscles*, acting to resist dislocation without producing movement at the joint, or maintain the head of the humerus in the glenoid cavity.

BLOOD SUPPLY AND INNERVATION OF THE GLENOHUMERAL JOINT

The glenohumeral joint is supplied by the *anterior* and *posterior circumflex humeral arteries* and branches of the *suprascapular artery* (Table 6.4). The *suprascapular, axillary,* and *lateral pectoral nerves* supply the glenohumeral joint.

BURSAE AROUND THE GLENOHUMERAL JOINT

Several **bursae** containing capillary films of *synovial fluid* are located near the joint where tendons rub against bone, ligaments, or other tendons and where skin moves over a bony prominence. Some bursae communicate with the joint cavity; hence, opening a bursa may mean entering the cavity of the joint.

The **subacromial bursa**, sometimes referred to as the *subdeltoid bursa* (Fig. 6.32C), is located between the acromion, coracoacromial ligament and deltoid superiorly and the supraspinatus tendon and joint capsule of the glenohumeral joint inferiorly. Thus it facilitates movement of the supraspinatus tendon under the coracoacromial arch and of the deltoid over the joint capsule and the greater tubercle of the humerus.

The **subscapular bursa** is located between the tendon of the subscapularis and the neck of the scapula. This bursa protects the tendon where it passes inferior to the root of the coracoid process and over the neck of the scapula. It usually communicates with the cavity of the glenohumeral joint through an opening in the fibrous layer of the joint capsule.

Dislocation of the Glenohumeral Joint

Because of its freedom of movement and instability, the glenohumeral joint is commonly dislocated by direct or indirect injury. Most dislocations of the humeral head occur in the downward (inferior) direction but are described clinically as anterior or (more rarely) posterior dislocations, indicating whether the humeral head has descended anterior or posterior to the infraglenoid tubercle and the long head of triceps. *Anterior dislocation of the glenohumeral joint* occurs most often in young adults (Fig. B6.16A), particularly athletes. It is usually caused by excessive extension and lateral rotation of the humerus. The head of the humerus is driven inferoanteriorly, and the fibrous layer of the joint capsule and glenoid labrum may be stripped from the anterior aspect of the glenoid cavity. A hard blow to the humerus when the glenohumeral joint is fully abducted tilts the head of the humerus inferiorly onto the inferior weak part of the joint capsule. This may tear the capsule and dislocate the joint so that the humeral head comes to lie inferior to the glenoid cavity and anterior to the infraglenoid tubercle. Subsequently, the strong flexor and adductor muscles of the glenohumeral joint usually pull the humeral head anterosuperiorly into a subcoracoid position. Unable to use the arm, the person commonly supports it with the other hand. The axillary nerve may be injured when the glenohumeral joint dislocates because of its close relation to the inferior part of the capsule of this joint (Fig. B6.16*B*).

Calcific Supraspinatus Tendinitis

Inflammation and calcification of the subacromial bursa result in pain, tenderness, and limitation of movement of the glenohumeral joint. This condition is also known as *calcific scapulohumeral bursitis*. Deposition of calcium in the supraspinatus tendon may irritate the overlying subacromial bursa, producing an inflammatory reaction, *subacromial bursitis*. As long as the glenohumeral joint is adducted, no pain usually results because in this position the painful lesion is away from the inferior surface of the acromion. In most people, the pain occurs during 50–130° of abduction (*painful arc syndrome*) because during this arc the supraspinatus tendon is in intimate contact with the inferior surface of the acromion. The pain usually develops in males 50 years of age and older after unusual or excessive use of the glenohumeral joint.

Rotator Cuff Injuries

The musculotendinous rotator cuff is commonly injured during repetitive use of the upper limb above the hori-zontal (e.g., during throwing and racquet sports, swimming, and weight lifting). Recurrent inflammation of the rotator cuff, especially the relatively avascular area of the supraspinatus tendon, is a common cause of shoulder pain and results in tears of the rotator cuff. Repetitive use of the rotator cuff muscles (e.g., by baseball pitchers) may allow the humeral head and rotator cuff to impinge on the coracoacromial arch, producing irritation of the arch and inflammation of the rotator cuff. As a result, *degenerative tendonitis of the rotator* cuff develops. Attrition of the supraspinatus tendon also occurs. Because the supraspinatus muscle is no longer functional with a complete tear of the rotator cuff, the person cannot initiate abduction of the upper limb. If the arm is passively abducted 15° or more, the person can usually maintain or continue the abduction using the deltoid.

Adhesive Capsulitis of the Glenohumeral Joint

Adhesive fibrosis and scarring between the inflamed capsule of the glenohumeral joint, rotator cuff, subacromial bursa, and deltoid usually cause **adhesive capsulitis** ("frozen shoulder"). A person with this condition has difficulty abducting the arm but can obtain an apparent abduction of up to 45° by elevating and rotating the scapula. Injuries that may initiate this condition include glenohumeral dislocations, calcific supraspinatus tendonitis, partial tearing of the rotator cuff, and bicipital tendonitis.

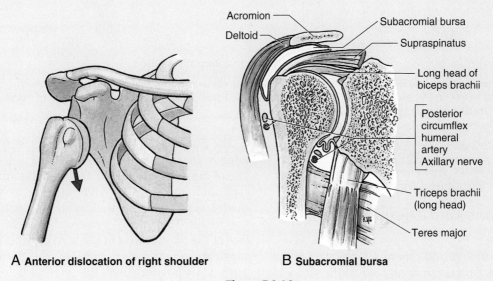

A Anterior dislocation of right shoulder   **B Subacromial bursa**

Figure B6.16.

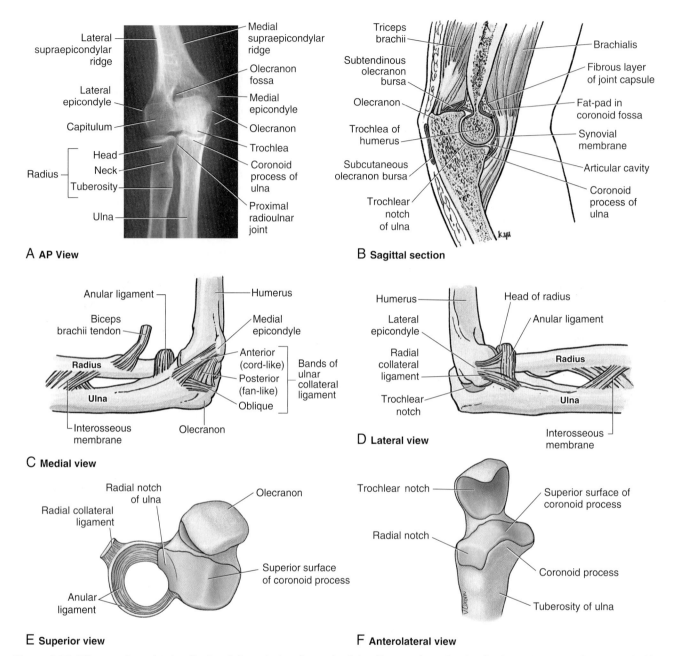

Figure 6.33. Elbow and proximal radioulnar joints. A. A radiograph of the elbow and proximal radioulnar joints. Bursae (**B**), medial ligaments (**C**), and lateral ligaments (**D**) are shown. **E.** Observe that the anular ligament attaches to the radial notch of the ulna. **F.** The articular surfaces of ulna are demonstrated.

Elbow Joint

The **elbow joint**, a hinge type of synovial joint, is located 2–3 cm inferior to the humeral epicondyles.

ARTICULATION AND JOINT CAPSULE OF THE ELBOW JOINT

The spool-shaped *trochlea* and spheroidal *capitulum* of the humerus articulate with the *trochlear notch* of the ulna and the slightly concave superior aspect of the *head of radius,* respectively; therefore, there are *humeroulnar* and *humeroradial articulations* (Fig. 6.33A & C).

The *fibrous layer of the joint capsule* surrounding the joint is attached to the humerus at the margins of the lateral and medial ends of the articular surfaces of the capitulum and trochlea. Anteriorly and posteriorly, it is carried superiorly, proximal to the coronoid and olecranon fossae. The *synovial membrane* lines the internal surface of the fibrous layer of the joint capsule and the intracapsular non-articular parts of the humerus. It is continuous inferiorly with the synovial membrane of the proximal radioulnar joint. The joint capsule is weak anteriorly and posteriorly but is strengthened on each side by ligaments.

LIGAMENTS OF ELBOW JOINT

The collateral ligaments of the elbow joint are strong triangular bands that are medial and lateral thickenings of the fibrous layer of the joint capsule (Fig. 6.33 B, D, & E). The lateral, fan-like **radial collateral ligament** extends from the lateral epicondyle of the humerus and blends distally with the **anular ligament of the radius**. This ligament encircles and holds the head of the radius in the radial notch of the ulna, forming the proximal radioulnar joint and permitting pronation and supination of the forearm. The medial, triangular **ulnar collateral ligament** extends from the medial epicondyle of the humerus to the coronoid process and olecranon of the ulna. It consists of three bands: (1) the *anterior cord-like band* is the strongest, (2) the *posterior fan-like band* is the weakest, and (3) the slender *oblique band* deepens the socket for the trochlea of the humerus (Fig. 6.33 C).

MOVEMENTS OF THE ELBOW JOINT

Flexion and extension occur at the elbow joint. The long axis of the fully extended ulna makes an angle of approximately 170° with the long axis of the humerus. This angle is called the **carrying angle** and is named for the way the forearm angles away from the body when something is carried, such as a pail of water (Fig. 6.34). The obliquity of the angle is more pronounced in women than in men. Table 6.14 lists structures limiting movements of the elbow joint

BLOOD SUPPLY AND INNERVATION OF THE ELBOW JOINT

The arteries supplying the elbow are derived from the anastomosis of arteries around the elbow joint (Table 6.10). The elbow joint is supplied by the musculocutaneous, radial, and ulnar nerves.

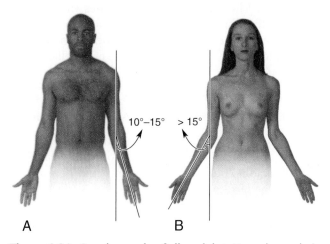

Figure 6.34. Carrying angle of elbow joint. Note the angle is greater in the woman.

Table 6.14 Structures Limiting Movements of the Elbow and Radioulnar Joints

Joint(s)	Movement	Limiting Structures (Tension)
Humeroulnar Humeroradial	Extension	*Muscles:* flexor muscles of elbow *Joint capsule:* anteriorly *Bony apposition* between olecranon of ulna and olecranon fossa of humerus
Humeroulnar Humeroradial	Flexion	*Muscle:* triceps brachii *Joint capsule:* posteriorly *Soft tissue apposition* between anterior forearm and arm *Bony apposition* between head of radius and radial fossa of humerus
Humeroradial Proximal radioulnar Distal radioulnar Interosseous membrane	Pronation	*Muscles:* supinator, biceps brachii *Ligaments:* quadrate, dorsal inferior radioulnar, interosseous membrane *Bony apposition* of the radius on ulna
Humeroradial Proximal radioulnar Distal radioulnar	Supination	*Muscles:* pronator teres, pronator quadratus *Ligaments:* quadrate, anterior inferior radioulnar, interosseous membrane

Modified from Clarkson HM: *Musculoskeletal Assessment. Joint Range of Motion and Manual of Muscle Strength,* 2nd ed. Baltimore, Lippincott Williams & Wilkins 2000.

BURSAE AROUND THE ELBOW JOINT

The three olecranon bursae are the (Figs. 6.33 C and 6.35):

- **Intratendinous olecranon bursa**, which is sometimes present in the tendon of triceps brachii.
- **Subtendinous olecranon bursa**, which is located between the olecranon and the triceps tendon, just proximal to its attachment to the olecranon.
- **Subcutaneous olecranon bursa**, which is located in the subcutaneous connective tissue over the olecranon.

The *bicipitoradial bursa* (biceps bursa) separates the biceps tendon from the anterior part of the radial tuberosity.

Proximal Radioulnar Joint

The **proximal (superior) radioulnar joint** is a pivot type of synovial joint that allows movement of the head of the radius on the ulna (Figs. 6.33 B & E and 6.36).

Bursitis of the Elbow

The subcutaneous olecranon bursa is exposed to injury during falls on the elbow and to infection from abrasions of the skin covering the olecranon. Repeated excessive pressure and friction produces a friction *subcutaneous olecranon bursitis* (e.g., "student's elbow") (Fig. B6.17). *Subtendinous olecranon bursitis* results from excessive friction between the triceps tendon and the olecranon, for example, resulting from repeated flexion–extension of the forearm as occurs during certain assembly-line jobs. The pain is severe during flexion of the forearm because of pressure exerted on the inflamed subtendinous olecranon bursa by the triceps tendon.

Avulsion of Medial Epicondyle

Avulsion of the medial epicondyle in children can result from a fall that causes severe abduction of the extended elbow. The resulting traction on the ulnar collateral ligament pulls the medial epicondyle distally. The anatomical basis of avulsion of the medial epicondyle is that the epiphysis for the medial epicondyle may not fuse with the distal end of the humerus until up to age 20. *Traction injury of the ulnar nerve* is a complication of the abduction type of avulsion of the medial epicondyle.

Dislocation of Elbow Joint

Posterior dislocation of the elbow joint may occur when children fall on their hands with their elbows flexed. Dislocations of the elbow may result from hyperextension or a blow that drives the ulna posteriorly or posterolaterally. The distal end of the humerus is driven through the weak anterior part of the fibrous layer of the joint capsule as the radius and ulna dislocate posteriorly. Injury to the ulnar nerve may also occur.

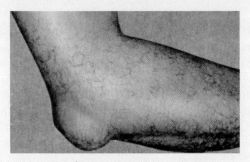

Subcutaneous olecranon bursitis

Figure B6.17.

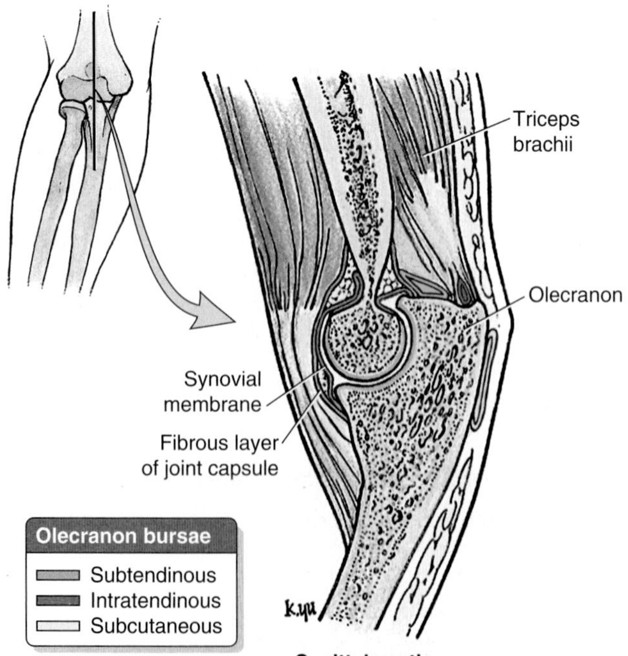

Figure 6.35. Bursae around elbow joint.

ARTICULATION AND JOINT CAPSULE OF THE PROXIMAL RADIOULNAR JOINT

The head of the radius articulates with the radial notch of the ulna. The radial head is held in place by the *anular ligament of the radius*. The *fibrous layer of the joint capsule* encloses the joint and is continuous with that of the elbow joint. The *synovial membrane* lines the internal surface of the fibrous layer and non-articulating aspects of the bones. The synovial membrane is an inferior prolongation of the synovial membrane of the elbow joint (Fig. 6.33C).

LIGAMENTS OF THE PROXIMAL RADIOULNAR JOINT

The *anular ligament* attaches to the ulna, anterior and posterior to the radial notch, which forms a collar that, with the radial notch, forms a ring that completely encircles the head of the radius. The deep surface of the anular ligament is lined with synovial membrane, which continues distally as a **sacciform recess of the proximal radioulnar joint** on the neck of the radius. This arrangement allows the radius to rotate within the anular

Triceps
brachii

Olecranon

Synovial
membrane

Fibrous layer
of joint capsule

Olecranon bursae

- Subtendinous
- Intratendinous
- Subcutaneous

Sagittal section

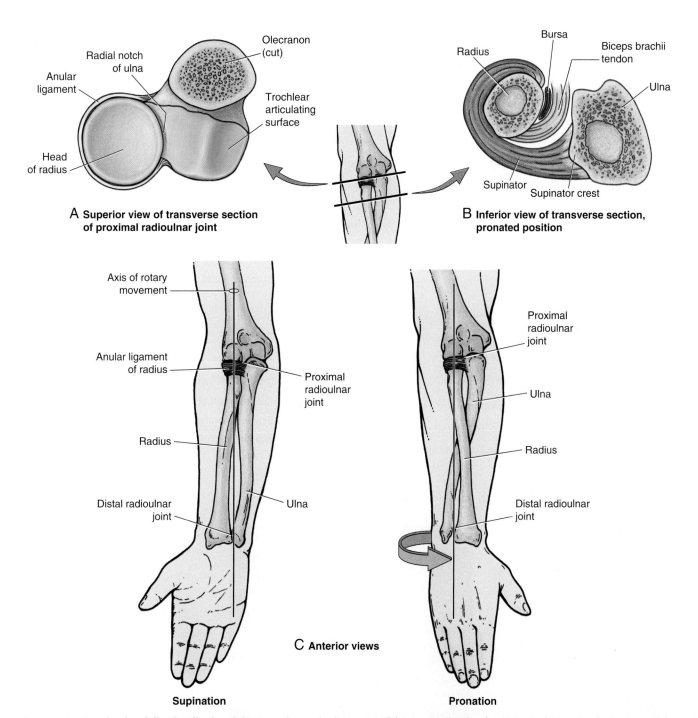

Figure 6.36. Proximal and distal radioulnar joints. A. The anular ligament of the proximal radioulnar joint is shown. **B.** The actions of the supinator and biceps brachii are shown. **C.** Supination and pronation of the forearm are demonstrated.

ligament without binding, stretching, or tearing of the synovial membrane.

MOVEMENTS OF THE PROXIMAL RADIOULNAR JOINT

During pronation and supination of the forearm, the head of the radius rotates within the cup-shaped anular ligament (Fig. 6.36). *Supination* turns the palm anteriorly, or superi-

orly when the forearm is flexed. **Pronation** turns the palm posteriorly, or inferiorly when the forearm is flexed. During pronation and supination, it is the radius that rotates. Table 6.15 lists the structures that limit movements of the proximal radioulnar joint.

Supination is produced by the supinator (when resistance is absent) and by the biceps brachii (when resistance is present), with some assistance from the EPL and exten-

Table 6.15 Wrist and Carpal Joints

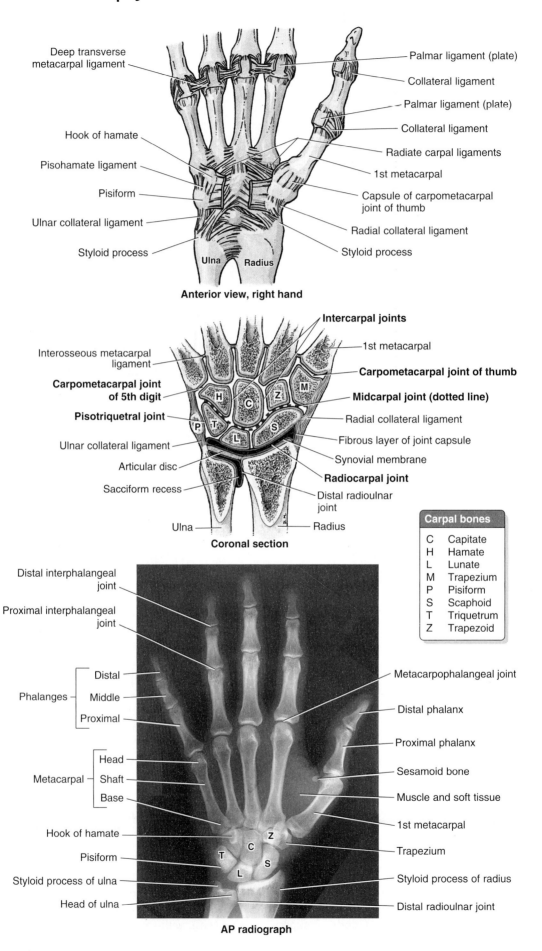

Deep transverse metacarpal ligament

Hook of hamate

Pisohamate ligament

Pisiform

Ulnar collateral ligament

Styloid process

Ulna   Radius

Anterior view, right hand

Palmar ligament (plate)

Collateral ligament

Palmar ligament (plate)

Collateral ligament

Radiate carpal ligaments

1st metacarpal

Capsule of carpometacarpal joint of thumb

Radial collateral ligament

Styloid process

Intercarpal joints

Interosseous metacarpal ligament

Carpometacarpal joint of 5th digit

Pisotriquetral joint

Ulnar collateral ligament

Articular disc

Sacciform recess

Ulna

1st metacarpal

Carpometacarpal joint of thumb

Midcarpal joint (dotted line)

Radial collateral ligament

Fibrous layer of joint capsule

Synovial membrane

Radiocarpal joint

Distal radioulnar joint

Radius

Coronal section

Carpal bones	
C	Capitate
H	Hamate
L	Lunate
M	Trapezium
P	Pisiform
S	Scaphoid
T	Triquetrum
Z	Trapezoid

Distal interphalangeal joint

Proximal interphalangeal joint

Phalanges — Distal / Middle / Proximal

Metacarpal — Head / Shaft / Base

Hook of hamate

Pisiform

Styloid process of ulna

Head of ulna

Metacarpophalangeal joint

Distal phalanx

Proximal phalanx

Sesamoid bone

Muscle and soft tissue

1st metacarpal

Trapezium

Styloid process of radius

Distal radioulnar joint

AP radiograph

Table 6.15 **Wrist and Carpal Joints** (*continued*)

Joint	Type	Articulation	Joint Capsule	Ligaments	Movements	Blood Supply	Nerve Supply
Wrist (radiocarpal)	Condyloid synovial joint	Distal end of radius and its articular disc with proximal row of carpal bones (except pisiform)	Fibrous layer of joint capsule surrounds joint and attaches to distal ends of radius and ulna and proximal row of carpal bones; lined by synovial membrane	Anterior and posterior ligaments strengthen fibrous capsule; ulnar collateral ligament attaches to styloid process of ulna and triquetrum; radial collateral ligament attaches to styloid process of radius and scaphoid	Flexion-extension, abduction-adduction, circumduction	Dorsal and palmar carpal arches	Anterior interosseous branch of median nerve, posterior interosseous branch of radial nerve, and dorsal and deep branches of ulnar nerve
Carpal (intercarpal)	Plane synovial joint	Between carpal bones of proximal row; joints between carpal bones of distal row *Midcarpal joint:* synovial joint between proximal and distal rows of carpal bones *Pisiform joint:* synovial joint between pisiform and triquetrum	Fibrous layer of joint capsule surrounds joints; lined by synovial membrane; pisiform joint is separate from other carpal joints	Carpal bones united by anterior, posterior, and interosseous ligaments	Small amount of gliding movement possible; flexion and abduction of hand occur at midcarpal joint	Dorsal and palmar carpal arches	
Carpometacarpal (CMC) and intermetacarpal (IM)	Plane synovial joints, except for CMC joint of thumb (saddle-shaped synovial joint)	Carpals and metacarpals with each other; CMC joint of thumb between trapezium and base of 1st metacarpal	Fibrous layer of joint capsule surrounds joints; lined on internal surface by synovial membrane	Bones united by anterior, posterior, and interosseous ligaments	Flexion-extension and abduction-adduction of CMC joint of 1st digit; almost no movement at 2nd and 3rd digits; 4th digit slightly mobile; 5th digit very mobile	Dorsal and palmar metacarpal arteries and deep carpal and deep palmar arches	

sor carpi radialis longus (ECRL). *Pronation* is produced by the pronator quadratus (primarily) and pronator teres (secondarily), with some assistance from the FCR, palmaris longus, and brachioradialis (when the forearm is in the midpronated position).

ARTERIES AND NERVES OF THE PROXIMAL RADIOULNAR JOINT

The proximal radioulnar joint is supplied by the radial portion of the periarticular arterial anastomosis of the elbow joint (Table 6.10). It is innervated by the musculocutaneous, median, and radial nerves (Table 6.9). Pronation is essentially a function of the median nerve, whereas supination is a function of the musculocutaneous and radial nerves.

Distal Radioulnar Joint

The **distal (inferior) radioulnar joint** is a pivot type of synovial joint. The radius moves around the relatively fixed distal end of the ulna (Fig. 6.36; Table 6.15).

ARTICULATION AND JOINT CAPSULE OF THE DISTAL RADIOULNAR JOINT

The rounded head of the ulna articulates with the ulnar notch on the medial side of the distal end of the radius. A fibrocartilaginous **articular disc of the distal radioulnar joint** binds the ends of the ulna and radius together and is the main uniting structure of the joint. The base of the disc attaches to the medial edge of the ulnar notch of the radius, and its apex is attached to the lateral side of the base of the

Subluxation and Dislocation of the Radial Head

Preschool children, particularly girls, are vulnerable to transient subluxation (incomplete temporary dislocation) of the head of the radius ("pulled elbow"). The history of these cases is typical. The child is suddenly lifted (jerked) by the upper limb when the forearm is pronated (e.g., when lifting a child into a bus) (Fig. B6.18). The child may cry out and refuse to use the limb, which is protected by holding it with the elbow flexed and the forearm pronated. The sudden pulling of the upper limb tears the distal attachment of the anular ligament, where it is loosely attached to the neck of the radius. The radial head then moves distally, partially out of the anular ligament. The proximal part of the torn ligament may become trapped between the head of the radius and the capitulum of the humerus. The source of pain is the pinched anular ligament. The treatment of subluxation consists of supination of the child's forearm while the elbow is flexed. The tear in the anular ligament soon heals when the limb is placed in a sling for about 2 weeks.

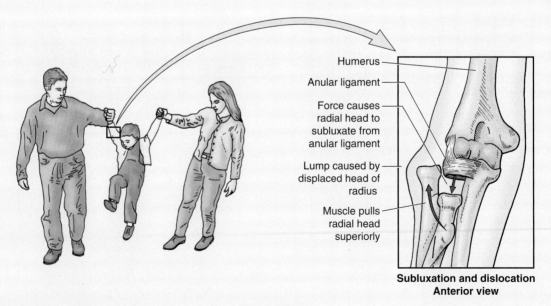

Humerus
Anular ligament
Force causes radial head to subluxate from anular ligament
Lump caused by displaced head of radius
Muscle pulls radial head superiorly

**Subluxation and dislocation
Anterior view**

Figure B6.18.

styloid process of ulna. The proximal surface of this triangular disc articulates with the distal aspect of the head of the ulna. Hence the joint cavity is L-shaped in a coronal section, with the vertical bar of the *L* between the radius and the ulna and the horizontal bar between the ulna and the articular disc. The articular disc separates the cavity of the distal radioulnar joint from the cavity of the wrist joint.

The *fibrous layer of the joint capsule* encloses the joint but is deficient superiorly. The *synovial membrane* extends superiorly between the radius and the ulna to form the **sacciform recess of the distal radioulnar joint** (Table 6.15). This redundancy of the synovial membrane accommodates the twisting of the capsule that occurs when the distal end of the radius travels around the relatively fixed distal end of the ulna during pronation and supination of the forearm.

LIGAMENTS OF THE DISTAL RADIOULNAR JOINT

Anterior and posterior ligaments strengthen the fibrous layer of the joint capsule. These relatively weak transverse bands extend from the radius to the ulna across the anterior and posterior surfaces of the joint.

MOVEMENTS OF THE DISTAL RADIOULNAR JOINT

The distal end of the radius rotates around the head of the ulna during pronation of the forearm and hand. The muscles producing movements of the distal radioulnar joint are discussed with the proximal radioulnar joint, and Table 6.14 lists the structures limiting movements of the distal radioulnar joint.

ARTERIES AND NERVES OF THE DISTAL RADIOULNAR JOINT

The anterior and posterior *interosseous arteries* and *nerves* supply the distal radioulnar joint.

Table 6.16 Structures Limiting Movements of the Wrist and Carpal Joints

Movement	Limiting Structures (Tension)
Flexion	*Ligaments:* posterior radiocarpal and posterior part of joint capsule
Extension	*Ligaments:* anterior radiocarpal and anterior part of joint capsule *Bony apposition* between radius and carpal bones
Abduction	*Ligaments:* ulnar collateral ligament and medial part of joint capsule *Bony apposition* between styloid process of radius and scaphoid
Adduction	*Ligaments:* radial collateral and lateral part of joint capsule

Modified from Clarkson HM: *Musculoskeletal Assessment. Joint Range of Motion and Manual of Muscle Strength,* 2nd ed. Baltimore, Lippincott Williams & Wilkins 2000.

Wrist fractures

Fractures of the distal end of the radius (*Colles fracture*) and *fracture of the scaphoid* are discussed earlier in this chapter. Anterior dislocation of the lunate is a serious injury that usually results from a fall on the dorsiflexed wrist. The lunate is pushed to the palmar surface of the wrist and may compress the median nerve and lead to carpal tunnel syndrome. Because of poor blood supply, avascular necrosis of the lunate may occur.

Joints of Hand

The wrist (carpus), the proximal segment of the hand, is a complex of eight carpal bones. The carpus articulates proximally with the forearm at the wrist joint and distally with the five metacarpals. The joints formed by the carpus include the *wrist (radiocarpal joint), intercarpal, carpometacarpal,* and *intermetacarpal joints.* Augmenting movement at the wrist joint, the two rows of carpals glide on each other; in addition, each bone glides on those adjacent to it. The joints are described in Table 6.15, and structures limiting movement are summarized in Table 6.16.

Each digit has three phalanges except the thumb, which has two. The proximal phalanges articulate with the metacarpal bones at the metacarpophalangeal joints. The joint between the proximal and the middle phalanx is the proximal interphalangeal joint and that between the middle and the distal phalanx is the distal interphalangeal joint. The thumb has one interphalangeal joint (Table 6.15). These joints are described in Table 6.17, and structures limiting movement are summarized in Table 6.18.

Skier's Thumb

Skier's thumb refers to the rupture or chronic laxity of the collateral ligament of the 1st metacarpophalangeal (MP) joint. The injury results from hyperextension of the joint, which occurs when the thumb is held by the ski pole while the rest of the hand hits the ground or enters the snow.

Table 6.17 Metacarpophalangeal and Interphalangeal Joints

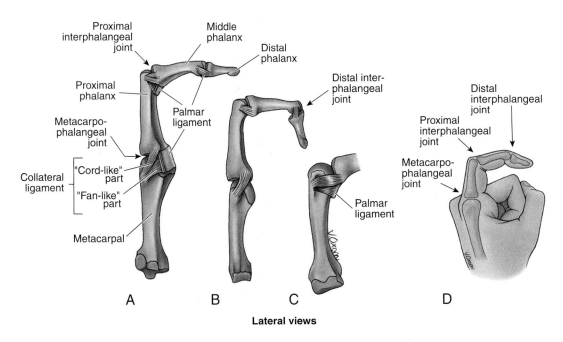

Lateral views

Joint	Type	Articulation	Joint Capsule	Ligaments	Movements	Blood Supply	Nerve Supply
Metacarpo-phalangeal	Condyloid synovial joints	Heads of metacarpals with base of proximal phalanges	Fibrous layer of joint capsule encloses each joint; lined on internal surface by synovial membrane	Strong palmar ligaments attached to phalanges and metacarpals; deep transverse metacarpal ligaments unite 2nd–5th joints holding heads of metacarpals together; collateral ligaments pass from heads of metacarpals to bases of phalanges	Flexion–extension, abduction–adduction, and circumduction of 2nd–5th digits; flexion–extension of thumb occurs but abduction–adduction is limited	Deep digital arteries arising from superficial palmar arches	Digital nerves arising from ulnar and median nerves
Interphalangeal	Hinge synovial joints	Heads of phalanges with bases of more distally located phalanges	Fibrous capsule encloses each joint; lined on internal surface by synovial membrane	Similar to metacarpopha-langeal joints, except they unite phalanges	Flexion–extension	Digital arteries	Digital nerves arising from ulnar and median nerves

Table 6.18 Structures Limiting Movements of the Hand Joints

Movement	Joint(s)	Limiting Structures (Tension)
Flexion	CMC (thumb)	*Ligaments:* posterior part of joint capsule *Muscles:* extensor and abductor pollicis brevis *Apposition* between thenar eminence and palm
	MCP (digits 1–5)	*Ligaments:* collateral, posterior part of joint capsule *Apposition* between proximal phalanx and metacarpal
	PIP (digits 2–5)	*Ligaments:* collateral, posterior part of joint capsule *Apposition* between middle and proximal phalanges
	DIP (digits 2–5)	*Ligaments:* collateral, oblique retinacular, and posterior part of joint capsule
	IP (thumb)	*Ligaments:* collateral and posterior part of joint capsule *Apposition* between distal and proximal phalanges
Extension	CMC (thumb)	*Ligaments:* anterior part of joint capsule *Muscles:* 1st dorsal interosseous, flexor pollicis brevis
	MCP (digits 1–5) PIP and DIP (digits 2–5) IP (thumb)	*Ligaments:* anterior part of joint capsule of joint, palmar ligament
Abduction	CMC and MCP	*Muscles:* 1st dorsal interosseous, adductor pollicis *Fascia and skin* of 1st web space
	MCP (digits 2–5)	*Ligaments:* collateral *Fascia and skin* of web spaces
Adduction	CMC and MCP (thumb)	*Apposition* between thumb and index finger
	MCP (digits 2–5)	*Apposition* between adjacent digits

Modified from Clarkson HM: *Musculoskeletal Assessment. Joint Range of Motion and Manual of Muscle Strength,* 2nd ed. Baltimore, Lippincott Williams & Wilkins 2000.

CMC, carpometacarpal joint; *DIP,* distal interphalangeal joint; *IP,* interphalangeal joint; *MCP,* metacarpophalangeal joint; *PIP,* proximal interphalangeal joint.

Medical Imaging of Upper Limb

Radiographs are often taken when an injury produces bone tenderness, angulation, rotation, or instability. Anteroposterior (AP), lateral, axial, and oblique views are usually sufficient to detect bony and other injuries. Radiological examinations of the upper limb focus mainly on bony structures because muscles, tendons, and nerves are not well visualized (Figs. 6.37*A* and 6.38). (Radiographs of the upper limb are also shown in Figures 6.32*A* and 6.33*A*). When examining radiographs of the upper limb, it is essential to know the median times of appearance of postnatal ossification centers and when fusion of epiphyses is radiographically complete in males and females. Without such knowledge, an epiphysial line could be mistaken for a fracture.

Angiography (visualization of the arteries) is used to detect vascular injuries, ischemia, and variations of arteries. *Angiograms* are produced by injecting a dye into an artery as a radiograph is taken (Fig. 6.37*B*). When interest is in a specific artery, the dye is injected directly into it, usually through a catheter. Angiography may be used to determine the patency of arteries before and after surgical procedures in the upper limb to repair injuries resulting from trauma.

CT scans are produced by X-rays, but the anatomical images are created by computer reconstructions of the electronic data (Fig. 6.38). The reconstructed images look like cross sections of the limb and can be reconstructed in the coronal and sagittal planes. Because the

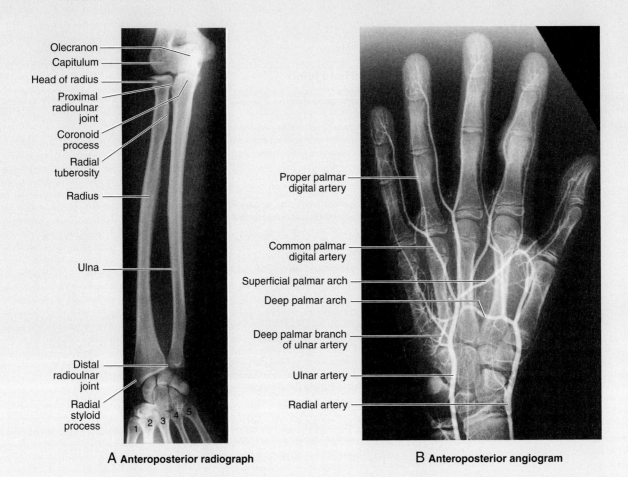

A Anteroposterior radiograph

B Anteroposterior angiogram

Figure 6.37. Imaging of upper limb. A. Note that the forearm is supinated. **B.** Observe the superficial and deep palmar arterial arches. (Courtesy of Dr. D. Armstrong, Associate Professor of Medical Imaging, University of Toronto, Toronto, Ontario, Canada.)

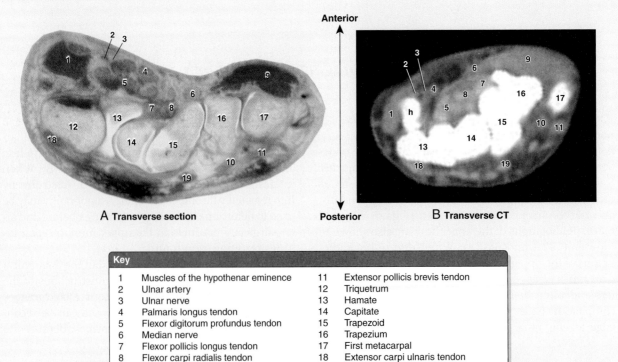

A Transverse section

B Transverse CT

Key			
1	Muscles of the hypothenar eminence	11	Extensor pollicis brevis tendon
2	Ulnar artery	12	Triquetrum
3	Ulnar nerve	13	Hamate
4	Palmaris longus tendon	14	Capitate
5	Flexor digitorum profundus tendon	15	Trapezoid
6	Median nerve	16	Trapezium
7	Flexor pollicis longus tendon	17	First metacarpal
8	Flexor carpi radialis tendon	18	Extensor carpi ulnaris tendon
9	Muscles of the thenar eminence	19	Extensor carpi radialis tendon
10	Abductor pollicis longus tendon	h	Hook of hamate

Figure 6.38. Carpal tunnel. A cadaveric specimen (**A**) and CT study (**B**) are shown.

person must be in the CT scanner for only brief periods, fast scans can be produced; consequently, involuntary movement produces minimal distortion of the images.

MRI produces images with good resolution of various soft tissues of the limbs (Fig. 6.39). The limb must be kept motionless for the 5–10 minutes required for scanning. This technique produces cross-sectional, coronal, and sagittal images. An advantage of MRI is that it does not involve the use of X-rays. ●

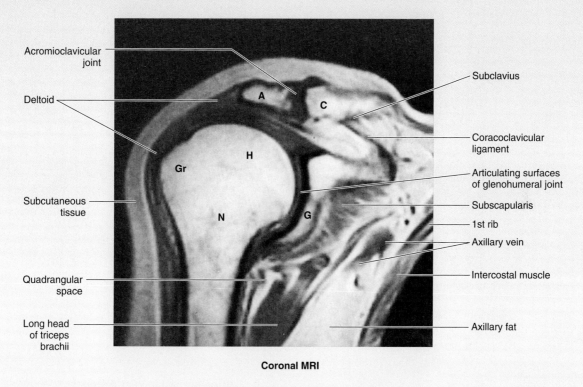

Coronal MRI

Figure 6.39. Imaging of glenohumeral and AC joints. The white (signal-intense) parts of the identified bones are the fatty matrix of cancellous bone; the thin black outlines (absence of signal) of the bones are the compact bone that forms their outer surface. *A,* acromion; *C,* clavicle; *G,* glenoid cavity; *GR,* greater tubercle of humerus; *H,* head of humerus; *N,* surgical neck of humerus

7 Head

Chapter Outline

The **head** consists of the *brain,* its protective coverings, and the *ears* and *face.* The **cranium** (skull) is the skeleton of the head. Learning the features of the cranium serves as an important framework to facilitate the understanding of the head region.

In the *anatomical position,* the cranium is oriented so that the inferior margin of the orbit (eye sockets or orbital cavity) and the superior margin of the external acoustic opening of the external acoustic meatus of both sides lie in the same horizontal plane (Fig. 7.1). This standard craniometric reference is the **orbitomeatal plane** (Frankfort horizontal plane).

Cranium

The *cranium* consists of two parts: the neurocranium and viscerocranium (Fig. 7.1*B*). The **neurocranium** (cranial vault) is the bony covering (case) of the brain and its membranous coverings, the cranial meninges. It also contains the proximal parts of the cranial nerves and the vasculature of the brain. The neurocranium has a dome-like roof, the **calvaria** (skullcap), and a floor or **cranial base** (basicranium). The neurocranium is formed by eight bones: four singular bones centered on the midline (*frontal, ethmoid, sphenoid,* and *occipital*) and two sets of bones occurring as bilateral pairs (*temporal* and *parietal*). Most calvarial bones are united by fibrous interlocking *sutures;* however, during childhood, some bones (sphenoid and occipital) are united by hyaline cartilage (*synchondroses*).

The **viscerocranium** (facial skeleton) is made up of the facial bones that mainly develop in the mesenchyme of the embryonic pharyngeal arches (Moore and Persaud, 2003). The viscerocranium forms the anterior part of the cranium and consists of bones surrounding the mouth, nose, and most of the orbits (Fig. 7.1*A*). It consists 15 irregular bones: three singular bones lying in the midline (*mandible, ethmoid,* and *vomer*) and six paired bones occurring bilaterally (*maxilla; inferior nasal concha;* and *zygomatic, palatine, nasal,* and *lacrimal bones*).

Facial Aspect of Cranium

Features of the anterior or **fascial (frontal) aspect of the cranium** (L. *norma facialis* or *frontalis)* are the frontal and zygomatic bones, orbits, nasal region, maxillae, and mandible (Fig. 7.1*A*).

The **frontal bone** forms the skeleton of the forehead, articulating inferiorly with the nasal and zygomatic bones. It also articulates with the lacrimal, ethmoid, and sphenoid bones and forms the roof of the orbit and part of the floor of the anterior part of the cranial cavity. In some

adults, a remnant of the frontal suture, the **metopic suture,** is visible in the midline of the **glabella.** The intersection of the frontal and nasal bones is the **nasion** (L. *nasus,* nose). The **supraorbital margin** of the frontal bone, the angular boundary between the squamous (flat) and the orbital parts, has a **supraorbital foramen,** or **notch** in some crania. Just superior to the supraorbital margin is a ridge, the **superciliary arch.**

The **zygomatic bones** (cheek bones, malar bones), forming the prominences of the cheeks, lie on the inferolateral sides of the orbits and rest on the maxillae. A small **zygomaticofacial foramen** pierces the lateral aspect of each bone. Inferior to the nasal bones is the pear-shaped **piriform aperture,** the anterior nasal opening of the cranium. The bony **nasal septum** can be observed, dividing the nasal cavity into right and left parts. On the lateral wall of each nasal cavity are curved bony plates, the **nasal conchae** (the middle and inferior conchae are shown in Figure 7.1*A*).

The **maxillae** form the upper jaw and are united at the **intermaxillary suture** in the median plane. Their **alveolar processes** include the tooth sockets (alveoli) and constitute the supporting bone for the **maxillary teeth.** The maxillae surround most of the piriform aperture and form the infraorbital margins medially. They have a broad connection with the zygomatic bones laterally and have an **infraorbital foramen** inferior to each orbit.

The **mandible** is the U-shaped bone forming the lower jaw; it has alveolar processes for the **mandibular teeth.** It consists of a horizontal part, the **body,** and a vertical part, the **ramus.** Inferior to the second premolar teeth are **mental foramina.** Forming the prominence of the chin is the **mental protuberance,** a triangular elevation of bone inferior to the **mandibular symphysis** (L. *symphysis menti*), the region where the halves of the infantile mandible fuse.

The bones of the orbit are illustrated and described later in this chapter (Fig. 7.14). Within the orbits are the **superior** and **inferior orbital fissures** and **optic canals.**

Lateral Aspect of Cranium

The **lateral aspect of the cranium** (L. *norma lateralis*) is formed by both the neurocranium and the viscerocranium (Fig. 7.1*B*). The main features of the neurocranial part are the **temporal fossa,** which is bounded superiorly and posteriorly by **superior** and **inferior temporal lines,** anteriorly by the frontal and zygomatic bones, and inferiorly by the zygomatic arch. The **zygomatic arch** is formed by the union of the **temporal process of the zygomatic bone** and the **zygomatic process of the temporal bone.** The *infratemporal fossa* is an irregular space inferior and deep to the zygomatic arch and the mandible and posterior to the maxilla.

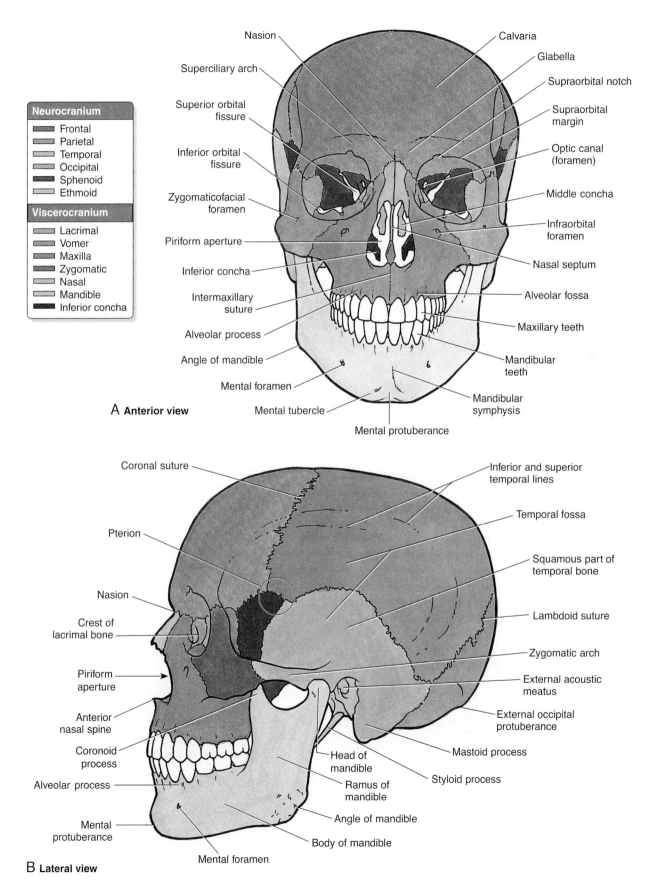

Neurocranium
- Frontal
- Parietal
- Temporal
- Occipital
- Sphenoid
- Ethmoid

Viscerocranium
- Lacrimal
- Vomer
- Maxilla
- Zygomatic
- Nasal
- Mandible
- Inferior concha

Nasion
Superciliary arch
Superior orbital fissure
Inferior orbital fissure
Zygomaticofacial foramen
Piriform aperture
Inferior concha
Intermaxillary suture
Alveolar process
Angle of mandible
Mental foramen
Mental tubercle

Calvaria
Glabella
Supraorbital notch
Supraorbital margin
Optic canal (foramen)
Middle concha
Infraorbital foramen
Nasal septum
Alveolar fossa
Maxillary teeth
Mandibular teeth
Mandibular symphysis

Mental protuberance

A **Anterior view**

Coronal suture
Pterion
Nasion
Crest of lacrimal bone
Piriform aperture
Anterior nasal spine
Coronoid process
Alveolar process
Mental protuberance
Mental foramen

Inferior and superior temporal lines
Temporal fossa
Squamous part of temporal bone
Lambdoid suture
Zygomatic arch
External acoustic meatus
External occipital protuberance
Mastoid process
Styloid process
Head of mandible
Ramus of mandible
Angle of mandible
Body of mandible

B **Lateral view**

Figure 7.1. Adult cranium (skull). In B. observe the pterion, the area of junction of four bones within the temporal fossa.

In the anterior part of the temporal fossa, superior to the midpoint of the zygomatic arch, is the **pterion** (G. *pteron,* wing). It is usually indicated by an H-shaped formation of sutures that unite the frontal, parietal, sphenoid (greater wing), and temporal bones.

The **external acoustic opening** is the entrance to the **external acoustic meatus** (canal), which leads to the tympanic membrane (eardrum). The **mastoid process** of the temporal bone lies posteroinferior to the external acoustic meatus. Anteromedial to the mastoid process is the slender **styloid process** of the temporal bone.

Occipital (Posterior) Aspect of Cranium

The posterior or **occipital aspect of the cranium** is formed by the rounded posterior aspect of the head or **occiput** (L. back of head). The occipital bone, parts of the parietal bones and mastoid parts of the temporal bones form this part of the cranium (Fig. 7.2A). The **external occipital protuberance** is usually an easily palpable elevation in the median plane. The **superior nuchal line**, marking the superior limit of the neck, extends laterally from each side of this

Fractures of Calvaria

The convexity of the calvaria distributes and thereby minimizes the effects of a blow to it. However, hard blows to the head in thin areas of the cranium are likely to produce *depressed fractures,* in which a fragment of bone is depressed inward, compressing and/or injuring the brain (Fig. B7.1). In *comminuted fractures,* the bone is broken into several pieces. *Linear calvarial fractures,* the most frequent type, usually occur at the point of impact, but fracture lines often radiate away from it in two or more directions. If the area of the calvaria is thick at the site of impact, the bone usually bends inward without fracturing; however, a fracture may occur some distance from the site of direct trauma where the calvaria is thinner. In a *contrecoup (counterblow) fracture,* the fracture occurs on the opposite side of the cranium rather than at the point of impact.

Fracture of the pterion can be life-threatening because it overlies the anterior branches of the middle meningeal vessels, which lie in the grooves on the internal aspect of the lateral wall of the calvaria. A hard blow to the side of the head may fracture the thin bones forming the pterion, rupturing the anterior branch of the middle meningeal artery crossing the pterion. The resulting *hematoma* exerts pressure on the underlying cerebral cortex. Untreated *middle meningeal artery hemorrhage* may cause death in a few hours.

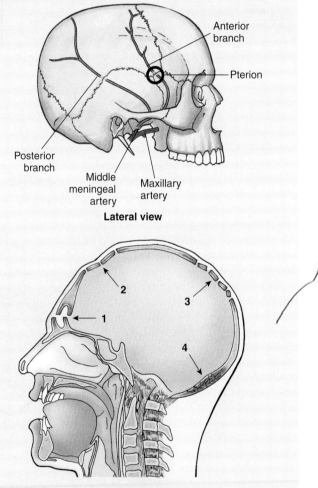

Lateral view

Median section

1. Linear fracture   3. Comminuted fracture
2. Depressed fracture   4. Basilar fracture

Figure B7.1

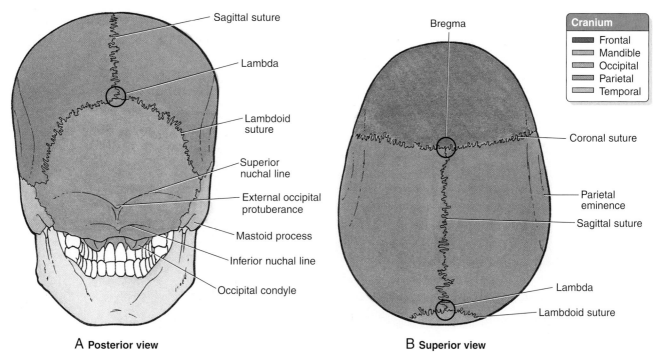

Cranium	
■■■	Frontal
■■■	Mandible
▢▢▢	Occipital
■■■	Parietal
■■■	Temporal

A Posterior view   **B** Superior view

Figure 7.2. Adult cranium. A. The occiput is shown. **B.** Features of the calvaria (skullcap) are defined.

protuberance; the **inferior nuchal line** is less distinct. In the center of the occiput, the **lambda** indicates the junction of the sagittal and lambdoid sutures. The lambda can sometimes be felt as a depression.

Superior Aspect of Cranium

The **superior aspect of the cranium**, usually somewhat oval in form, broadens posterolaterally at the **parietal eminences** (Fig. 7.2*B*). The four bones forming the *calvaria,* the dome-like roof of the neurocranium, are visible from this aspect: the frontal bone anteriorly, the right and left parietal bones laterally, and the occipital bone posteriorly. The **coronal suture** unites the frontal and parietal bones, the **sagittal suture** unites the parietal bones, and the **lambdoid suture** unites the parietal and temporal bones from the occipital bone. The **bregma** is the landmark formed by the intersection of the sagittal and coronal sutures. The *vertex,* the superior (topmost) point of the cranium, is near the midpoint of the sagittal suture.

External Surface of Cranial Base

The **external aspect of the cranial base** or basicranium features the **alveolar arch of the maxillae** (the free border of the **alveolar processes** surrounding and supporting the maxillary teeth); the **palatine processes** of the maxillae; and the palatine, sphenoid, vomer, temporal, and occipital bones (Table 7.1*C*). The *hard palate* (bony palate) is formed

by the **palatine processes of the maxillae** anteriorly and the **horizontal plates of the palatine bones** posteriorly. Posterior to the central incisor teeth is the **incisive fossa.** Posterolaterally are the **greater** and **lesser palatine foramina.** The posterior edge of the palate forms the inferior boundary of the **choanae** (posterior nasal apertures), which are separated from each other by the **vomer.** The vomer is a thin flat bone that forms a major part of the bony **nasal septum** (Fig. 7.1*A*). Wedged between the frontal, temporal, and occipital bones, is the **sphenoid bone,** which consists of a body and three pairs of processes: the **greater** and **lesser wings** and the **pterygoid processes.** The pterygoid processes, consisting of **medial** and **lateral pterygoid plates,** extend inferiorly on each side of the sphenoid from the junction of the body and greater wings. The *groove for the cartilaginous part of the pharyngotympanic (auditory) tube* lies medial to the **spine** of the sphenoid, inferior to the junction of the greater wing of the sphenoid and the **petrous** (L. rock-like) part of the temporal bone. Depressions in the **squamous** (L. flat) **part of the temporal bone,** called the **mandibular fossae,** accommodate the heads of the mandible when the mouth is closed.

The cranial base is formed posteriorly by the **occipital bone,** which articulates with the sphenoid anteriorly. The parts of the occipital bone encircle the large **foramen magnum.** On the lateral parts of the occipital bone are two large protuberances, the **occipital condyles,** by which the cranium articulates with the vertebral column. The large opening between the occipital bone and the petrous part of

Table 7.1 Foramina and Other Apertures of the Cranial Fossae and Contents

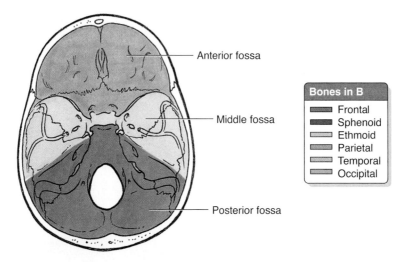

A **Superior view, cranial fossae**

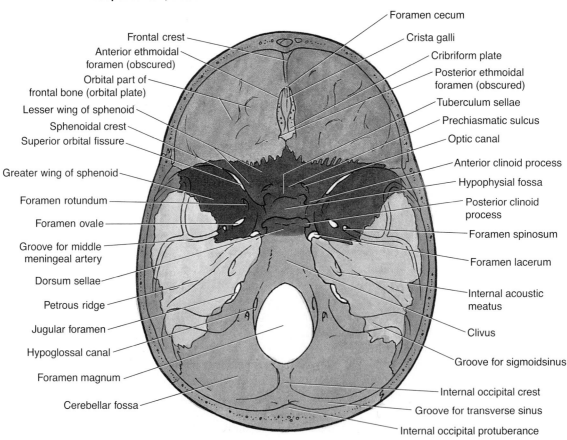

B **Superior view, internal surface of cranial base**

Table 7.1 Foramina and Other Apertures of the Cranial Fossae and Contents (*continued*)

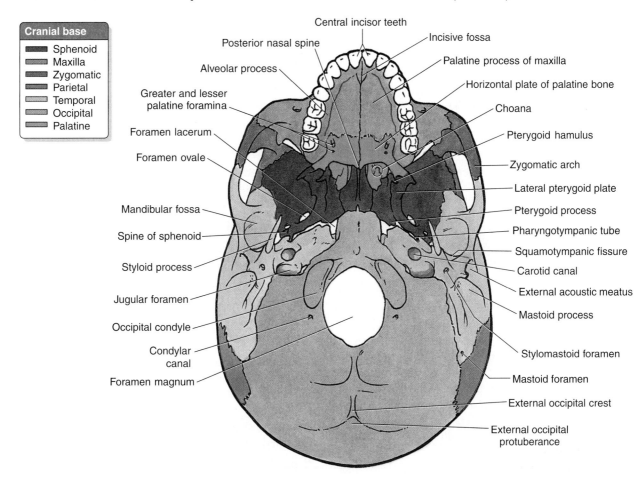

Cranial base
- Sphenoid
- Maxilla
- Zygomatic
- Parietal
- Temporal
- Occipital
- Palatine

Labels: Central incisor teeth, Incisive fossa, Posterior nasal spine, Palatine process of maxilla, Alveolar process, Horizontal plate of palatine bone, Greater and lesser palatine foramina, Choana, Foramen lacerum, Pterygoid hamulus, Foramen ovale, Zygomatic arch, Lateral pterygoid plate, Mandibular fossa, Pterygoid process, Spine of sphenoid, Pharyngotympanic tube, Styloid process, Squamotympanic fissure, Carotid canal, Jugular foramen, External acoustic meatus, Occipital condyle, Mastoid process, Condylar canal, Stylomastoid foramen, Foramen magnum, Mastoid foramen, External occipital crest, External occipital protuberance

C Inferior view, external surface of cranial base

Foramina/Apertures	Contents
Anterior cranial fossa	
Foramen cecum	Nasal emissary vein (1% of population)
Cribriform foramina in cribriform plate	Axons of olfactory cells in olfactory epithelium that form olfactory nerves (CNI)
Anterior and posterior ethmoidal foramina	Vessels and nerves with same names
Middle cranial fossa	
Optic canals	Optic nerves (CN II) and ophthalmic arteries
Superior orbital fissure	Ophthalmic veins; ophthalmic nerve (CN V_1); CN III, IV, and VI; and sympathetic fibers
Foramen rotundum	Maxillary nerve (CN V_2)
Foramen ovale	Mandibular nerve (CN V_3) and accessory meningeal artery
Foramen spinosum	Middle meningeal artery and vein and meningeal branch of CN V_3
Foramen lacerum[a]	Internal carotid artery and its accompanying sympathetic and venous plexuses
Groove or hiatus of greater petrosal nerve	Greater petrosal nerve and petrosal branch of middle meningeal artery
Posterior cranial fossa	
Foramen magnum	Medulla and meninges, vertebral arteries, CN XI, dural veins, anterior and posterior spinal arteries
Jugular foramen	CN IX, X, and XI; superior bulb of internal jugular vein; inferior petrosal and sigmoid sinuses; and meningeal branches of ascending pharyngeal and occipital arteries
Hypoglossal canal	Hypoglossal nerve (CN XII)
Condylar canal	Emissary vein that passes from sigmoid sinus to vertebral veins in neck
Mastoid foramen	Mastoid emissary vein from sigmoid sinus and meningeal branch of occipital artery

[a]Structures actually pass horizontally across (rather than vertically through) the area of the foramen lacerum, an artifact of dry skulls, which is closed by cartilage in life.

the temporal bone is the **jugular foramen.** The entrance to the **carotid canal** for the internal carotid artery is located just anterior to the jugular foramen. The **mastoid processes** provide for muscle attachments. The **stylomastoid foramen** lies posterior to the base of the styloid process.

Internal Surface of Cranial Base

The **internal surface of the cranial base** has three large depressions that lie at different levels: the *anterior, middle,* and *posterior cranial fossae,* which form the bowl-shaped floor of the cranial cavity (Table 7.1*A*). The anterior cranial fossa is at the highest level, and the posterior cranial fossa is at the lowest level.

The **anterior cranial fossa** is formed by the frontal bone anteriorly, the ethmoid bone centrally, and the body and lesser wings of the sphenoid posteriorly (Table 7.1*B*). The greater part of the anterior cranial fossa is formed by ridged **orbital plates of the frontal bone,** which support the frontal lobes of the brain and form the roofs of the orbits. The **frontal crest** is a median bony extension of the frontal bone. At its base is the **foramen cecum of the frontal bone,** which gives passage to vessels during fetal development but is insignificant postnatally. The **crista galli** (L. cock's comb) is a median ridge of bone that projects superiorly from the ethmoid. On each side of the crista galli is the sieve-like **cribriform plate of the ethmoid.**

The butterfly-shaped **middle cranial fossa** has a *central part* composed of the *sella turcica* (Turkish saddle) on the body of the sphenoid and large depressed *lateral parts* on each side. The **sella turcica** is surrounded by the **anterior** and **posterior clinoid processes** (*clinoid* means "bedpost"). The sella turcica is composed of three parts:

- The **tuberculum sellae** (horn of the saddle), the slight elevation anteriorly on the body of the sphenoid.
- The **hypophysial fossa** (pituitary fossa), a saddle-like depression for the pituitary gland (L. *hypophysis*) in the middle.
- The **dorsum sellae** (back of saddle) posteriorly, a square plate of bone on the body of the sphenoid forming the posterior part of the sella turcica, and its prominent superolateral angles make up the **posterior clinoid processes.**

The bones forming the larger, lateral parts of the middle cranial fossa are the greater wings of the sphenoid, squamous parts of the temporal bones laterally, and petrous parts of the temporal bones posteriorly. The lateral parts of the middle cranial fossa support the temporal lobes of the brain. The boundary between the middle and the posterior cranial fossae is formed by the superior border of the petrous part of the temporal bones laterally and the dorsum sellae of the sphenoid medially. The **sphenoidal crests** are the sharp posterior margins of the *lesser*

wings of the sphenoid bones, which overhang the lateral parts of the fossae anteriorly. The *sphenoidal crests* end medially in two sharp bony projections: the *anterior clinoid processes.* The **prechiasmatic sulcus** extends between the right and the left **optic canals.** The **foramen lacerum** lies posterolateral to the hypophysial fossa. In life, it is closed by a cartilage plate. On each side of the body of the sphenoid, four foramina perforate the roots of the greater wings of the sphenoid (Table 7.1):

- **Superior orbital fissure:** an opening between the greater and the lesser wings that communicates with the orbit.
- **Foramen rotundum** (round foramen): located posterior to the medial end of the superior orbital fissure.
- **Foramen ovale** (oval foramen): located posterolateral to the foramen rotundum.
- **Foramen spinosum** (spinous foramen): located posterolateral to the foramen ovale.

The **posterior cranial fossa,** the largest and deepest of the cranial fossae, contains the cerebellum, pons, and medulla oblongata. This fossa is formed mostly by the occipital bone, but parts of the sphenoid and temporal bones make smaller contributions to it. From the dorsum sellae there is a marked incline, the **clivus,** which leads to the **foramen magnum.** Posterior to this large foramen, the **internal occipital crest** is a landmark that divides the posterior part of the fossae into two **cerebellar fossae;** the crest ends superiorly in the **internal occipital protuberance.** Broad grooves in this fossa are formed by the *transverse* and *sigmoid sinuses.* At the base of the petrous ridges of the temporal bones are the **jugular foramina.** Anterosuperior to the jugular foramen is the **internal acoustic meatus.** The **hypoglossal canals** lie superior to the anterolateral margin of the foramen magnum.

Scalp

The **scalp** consists of skin and subcutaneous tissue that covers the neurocranium from the superior nuchal lines on the occipital bone to the supraorbital margins of the frontal bone. Laterally, the scalp extends over the temporal fascia to the zygomatic arches. The neurovascular structures of the scalp are discussed with those of the face.

The scalp consists of five layers, the first three of which are connected intimately, thus moving as a unit (e.g., when wrinkling the forehead). Each letter in the word *scalp* serves as a memory key for one of its five layers that cover the neurocranium (Fig. 7.3*A*):

- **S**kin, thin except in the occipital region, contains many sweat and sebaceous glands and hair follicles; it has an abundant arterial supply and good venous and lymphatic drainage.

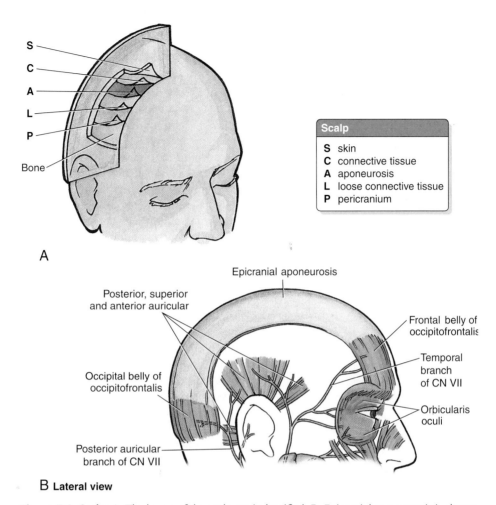

Scalp

S skin
C connective tissue
A aponeurosis
L loose connective tissue
P pericranium

A

Epicranial aponeurosis

Posterior, superior and anterior auricular

Frontal belly of occipitofrontalis

Temporal branch of CN VII

Occipital belly of occipitofrontalis

Orbicularis oculi

Posterior auricular branch of CN VII

B **Lateral view**

Figure 7.3. Scalp. A. The layers of the scalp are indentified. **B.** Epicranial aponeurosis is shown.

- Connective tissue, forming the thick, dense, richly vascularized, subcutaneous layer, is well supplied with cutaneous nerves.
- Aponeurosis (**epicranial aponeurosis**), a strong tendinous sheet that covers the calvaria, serves as the attachment for the frontal and occipital bellies of the occipitofrontalis muscle and the superior auricular muscle (Fig. 7.3 *B*); collectively these structures form the musculoaponeurotic *epicranius.*
- Loose connective tissue, a sponge-like layer, has potential spaces that may distend with fluid as a result of injury or infection; this layer allows free movement of the **scalp proper** (the first three layers) over the underlying calvaria.
- Pericranium, a dense layer of connective tissue, forms the external periosteum of the neurocranium; it is firmly attached but can be stripped fairly easily from the calvaria of living people, except where the pericranium is continuous with the fibrous tissue in the cranial sutures.

Cranial Meninges

The **cranial meninges** are coverings of the brain that lie immediately internal to the cranium. The meninges protect the brain; form the supporting framework for arteries, veins, and venous sinuses; and enclose a fluid-filled cavity, the subarachnoid space. The meninges consist of three membranous connective tissue layers (Fig. 7.4*A*):

- **Dura mater** (dura): tough, thick external fibrous layer.
- **Arachnoid mater** (arachnoid): thin intermediate layer.
- **Pia mater** (pia): delicate internal vascular layer.

The arachnoid and pia are continuous membranes that make up the **leptomeninx**. The arachnoid is separated by the pia by the subarachnoid space, which contains **cerebrospinal fluid** (CSF). Cerebrospinal fluid is a clear liquid similar in constitution to blood; it provides nutrients but has less protein and a different ion concentration. CSF is formed predominantly by the *choroid plexuses* within the four ventricles of the brain (Fig. 7.9*B*). CSF leaves the ven-

Scalp Injuries and Infections

The loose connective tissue layer is the *danger area of the scalp* because pus or blood spreads easily in it. Infection in this layer can also pass into the cranial cavity through *emissary veins,* which pass through parietal foramina in the calvaria and reach intracranial structures such as the meninges (Fig. 7.6C). An infection cannot pass into the neck because the occipital belly of the occipitofrontalis muscle attaches to the occipital bone and mastoid parts of the temporal bones. Neither can a scalp infection spread laterally beyond the zygomatic arches because the epicranial aponeurosis is continuous with the temporal fascia that attaches to these arches. An infection or fluid (e.g., pus or blood) can enter the eyelids and the root of the nose because the frontal belly of the occipitofrontalis muscle inserts into the skin and dense subcutaneous tissue and does not attach to the bone. Consequently, "black eyes" can result from an injury to the scalp or forehead. *Ecchymosis,* or purple patches, develop as a result of extravasation of blood into the subcutaneous tissue and skin of the eyelids and surrounding regions.

tricular system of the brain and enters the subarachnoid space, where it cushions and nourishes the brain.

Dura Mater

The **dura mater** (dura) is adherent to the internal surface of the cranium and is described as a two-layered membrane (Fig. 7.4A):

- An *external periosteal layer,* formed by the periosteum covering the internal surface of the calvaria.
- An *internal meningeal layer,* a strong fibrous membrane that is continuous at the foramen magnum with the dura covering the spinal cord.

DURAL INFOLDINGS OR REFLECTIONS

The internal **meningeal layer of the dura** reflects away from the external periosteal layer of the dura to form **dural infoldings** (reflections), which divide the cranial cavity into compartments and support parts of the brain (Fig. 7.5). The dural infoldings are the *cerebral falx, cerebellar tentorium, cerebellar falx,* and *sellar diaphragm.*

The **cerebral falx** (L. *falx cerebri*), the largest dural infolding, is a sickle-shaped partition that lies in the **longitudinal cerebral fissure** that separates the right and left cerebral hemispheres (Fig. 7.5A). The cerebral falx attaches in the median plane to the internal surface of the calvaria, from the *frontal crest* of the frontal bone and the crista galli of the ethmoid bone anteriorly to the internal occipital protuberance posteriorly. The cerebral falx ends posteriorly by becoming continuous with the cerebellar tentorium.

The **cerebellar tentorium** (L. *tentorium cerebelli*) is a wide crescentic septum that separates the occipital lobes of the cerebral hemispheres from the cerebellum (Fig. 7.5C). The cerebellar tentorium attaches anteriorly to the clinoid processes of the sphenoid bone, anterolaterally to the petrous part of the temporal bone, and posterolaterally to the internal surface of the occipital bone and part of the parietal bone. The cerebral falx attaches to the cerebellar tentorium in the midline and holds it up, giving it a tent-like appearance (L. *tentorium,* tent). The concave anteromedial border of the cerebellar tentorium is free, leaving a gap called the **tentorial notch** through which the brainstem extends from the posterior into the middle cranial fossa (Fig. 7.5A). The cerebellar tentorium divides the cranial cavity into a *supratentorial* and *infratentorial compartments.*

The **cerebellar falx** is a vertical dural infolding that lies inferior to the cerebellar tentorium in the posterior part of the posterior cranial fossa. It partially separates the cerebellar hemispheres.

The **sellar diaphragm,** the smallest dural infolding, is a circular sheet of dura that is suspended between the clinoid processes, forming a partial roof over the hypophysial fossa (Fig. 7.5B). The sellar diaphragm covers the pituitary gland in this fossa and has an aperture for passage of the infundibulum (pituitary stalk) and hypophysial veins.

DURAL VENOUS SINUSES

The **dural venous sinuses** are endothelial-lined spaces between the periosteal and meningeal layers of the dura (Fig. 7.5). They form where dural infoldings attach. Large veins from the surface of the brain empty into these sinuses, and all blood from the brain ultimately drains through them into the internal jugular veins (IJVs).

The **superior sagittal sinus** lies in the convex attached (superior) border of the cerebral falx. It begins at the crista galli and ends near the internal occipital protuberance at the **confluence of sinuses** (Figs. 7.5A and 7.6). The superior sagittal sinus receives the superior cerebral veins and communicates on each side through slit-like openings with the **lateral venous lacunae,** lateral expansions of the superior sagittal sinus (Fig. 7.6A).

Arachnoid granulations (collections of arachnoid villi) are tufted prolongations of the arachnoid that protrude

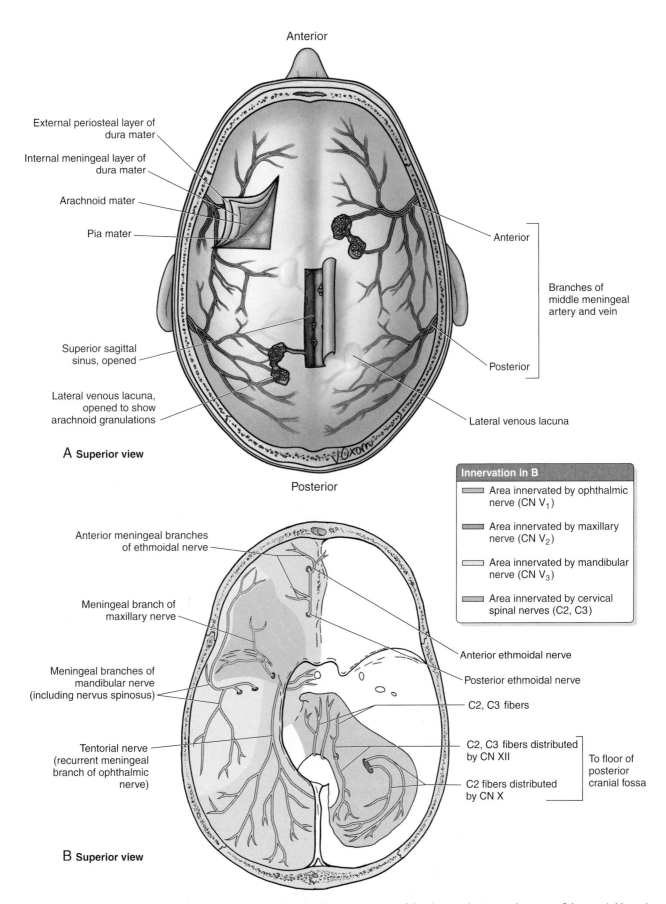

Anterior

External periosteal layer of dura mater

Internal meningeal layer of dura mater

Arachnoid mater

Pia mater

Anterior

Branches of middle meningeal artery and vein

Posterior

Superior sagittal sinus, opened

Lateral venous lacuna, opened to show arachnoid granulations

Lateral venous lacuna

A **Superior view**

Posterior

Innervation in B

Area innervated by ophthalmic nerve (CN V_1)

Area innervated by maxillary nerve (CN V_2)

Area innervated by mandibular nerve (CN V_3)

Area innervated by cervical spinal nerves (C2, C3)

Anterior meningeal branches of ethmoidal nerve

Meningeal branch of maxillary nerve

Meningeal branches of mandibular nerve (including nervus spinosus)

Tentorial nerve (recurrent meningeal branch of ophthalmic nerve)

Anterior ethmoidal nerve

Posterior ethmoidal nerve

C2, C3 fibers

C2, C3 fibers distributed by CN XII

C2 fibers distributed by CN X

To floor of posterior cranial fossa

B **Superior view**

Figure 7.4. Dura mater. A. The meningeal vessels are shown. **B.** The innervation of the dura in the internal aspect of the cranial base is identified.

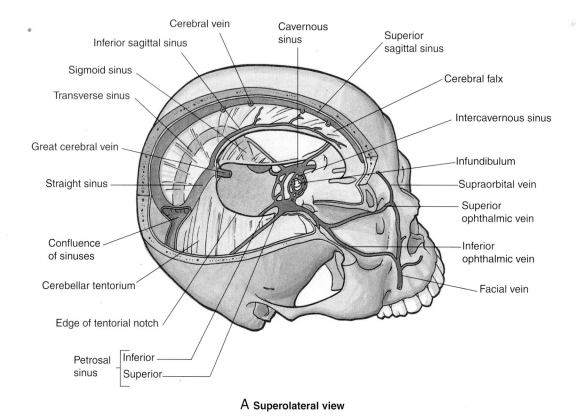

A Superolateral view

B Lateral view

Figure 7.5. Dural infoldings (reflections) and dural venous sinuses. A. The brain and part of the calvaria are removed to demonstrate the sinuses related to the cerebral falx and cerebellar tentorium. **B.** The straight sinus and cerebellar falx are shown.

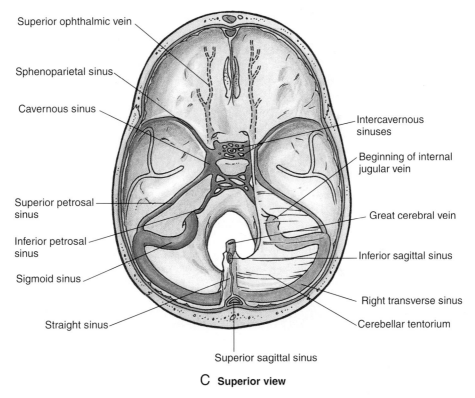

Superior ophthalmic vein

Sphenoparietal sinus

Cavernous sinus

Intercavernous sinuses

Beginning of internal jugular vein

Superior petrosal sinus

Inferior petrosal sinus

Sigmoid sinus

Great cerebral vein

Inferior sagittal sinus

Straight sinus

Right transverse sinus

Cerebellar tentorium

Superior sagittal sinus

C **Superior view**

Figure 7.5. (continued) **C.** This view of the interior of the base of the cranium demonstrates the cavernous sinus and most of its communications.

through the meningeal layer of the dura mater into the dural venous sinuses (Figs. 7.4A and 7.6), and lateral venous lacunae. The archnoid granulations transfer CSF to the venous system.

The **inferior sagittal sinus**, much smaller than the superior sagittal sinus, runs in the inferior, free concave border of the cerebral falx and ends in the straight sinus.

The **straight sinus** is formed by the union of the inferior sagittal sinus with the great cerebral vein. It runs inferoposteriorly along the line of attachment of the cerebral falx to the cerebellar tentorium to join the *confluence of sinuses.*

The **transverse sinuses** pass laterally from the **confluence of sinuses** in the posterior attached margin of the cerebellar tentorium, grooving the occipital bones and the posteroinferior angles of the parietal bones. The transverse sinuses leave the cerebellar tentorium at the posterior aspect of the petrous temporal bone and become the sigmoid sinuses.

The **sigmoid sinuses** follow S-shaped courses in the posterior cranial fossa, forming deep grooves in the temporal and occipital bones (Fig. 7.5C). Each sigmoid sinus turns anteriorly and then continues inferiorly as the internal jugular vein (IJV) after transversing the jugular foramen.

The **occipital sinus** lies in the attached border of the cerebellar falx and ends superiorly in the confluence of sinuses.

The occipital sinus communicates inferiorly with the internal vertebral venous plexus.

The **cavernous sinus** is located bilaterally on each side of the sella turcica on the body of the sphenoid bone (Fig. 7.5C). The cavernous sinus consists of a venous plexus of extremely thin-walled veins that extend from the superior orbital fissure anteriorly to the apex of the petrous part of the temporal bone posteriorly. The cavernous sinus receives blood from the superior and inferior ophthalmic veins, superficial middle cerebral vein, and sphenoparietal sinus. The venous channels in the cavernous sinuses communicate with each other through **intercavernous sinuses** anterior and posterior to the stalk (infundibulum) of the pituitary gland. The cavernous sinuses drain posteroinferiorly through the *superior* and *inferior petrosal sinuses* and via emissary veins to the *pterygoid plexuses* (Fig. 7.12C).

The **internal carotid artery** (Fig. 7.6), surrounded by the carotid plexus of sympathetic nerves, courses through the cavernous sinus and is crossed by the abducent nerve (CN VI). From superior to inferior, the lateral wall of each cavernous sinus contains the oculomotor nerve (CN III), trochlear nerve (CN IV), and CN V_1 and CN V_2 divisions of the trigeminal nerve (Fig. 7.6B).

The **superior petrosal sinuses** run from the posterior ends of the cavernous sinuses to join the transverse

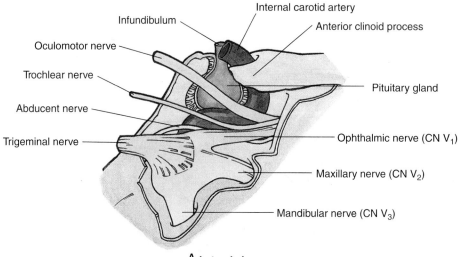

A Lateral view

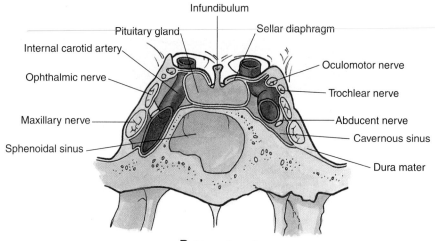

B Coronal section

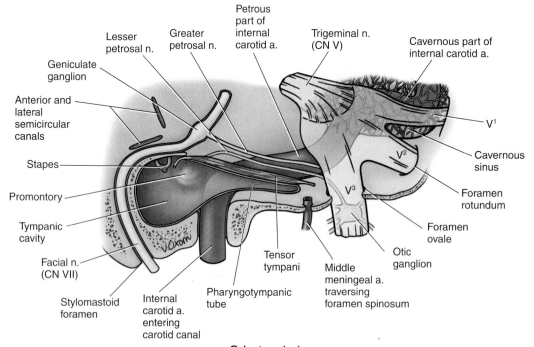

C Lateral view

Figure 7.6. Internal carotid artery and associated structures. A. Observe the relationships of the oculomotor, trochlear, trigeminal, and abducent nerves. **B.** The cavernous sinuses are shown. **C.** The petrous and cavernous parts of the internal carotid artery are detailed.

sinuses, where these sinuses curve inferiorly to form the sigmoid sinuses (Fig. 7.5C). Each superior petrosal sinus lies in the anterolateral attached margin of the cerebellar tentorium, which attaches to the superior border of the petrous part of the temporal bone.

The **inferior petrosal sinuses** commence at the posterior end of the cavernous sinus and drain the cavernous sinuses directly into the origin of the IJVs (Fig. 7.5C). The *basilar plexus* connects the inferior petrosal sinuses and communicates inferiorly with the internal vertebral venous plexus. **Emissary veins** connect the dural venous sinuses with veins outside the cranium (Fig. 7.7C). The size and number of emissary veins vary.

VASCULATURE AND NERVE SUPPLY OF THE DURA MATER

The **arteries of the dura** supply more blood to the calvaria than to the dura. The largest of these vessels, the **middle meningeal artery** (Fig. 7.4A), is a branch of the maxillary artery. The middle meningeal artery enters the middle cranial fossa through the *foramen spinosum,* runs laterally in the fossa, and turns superoanteriorly on the greater wing of the sphenoid, where it divides into anterior and posterior branches. The **anterior branch** runs superiorly to the pterion and then curves posteriorly to ascend toward the vertex of the cranium. The **posterior branch** runs posterosuperiorly and ramifies over the posterior aspect of the cranium. The **veins of the dura** accompany the meningeal arteries (Fig. 7.4A).

The **innervation of the dura** is largely by the three divisions of CN V (Fig. 7.4B). Sensory branches are also conveyed from the vagus (CN X) and hypoglossal (CN XII) nerves, but the fibers probably are peripheral branches from sensory ganglia of the superior three cervical nerves. The sensory endings are more numerous in the dura along each side of the superior sagittal sinus and in the cerebellar tentorium than they are in the floor of the cranium. Pain fibers are most numerous where arteries and veins course in the dura. Pain arising from the dura is generally referred, perceived as a headache arising in cutaneous or mucosal regions supplied by the involved cervical nerve or division of the trigeminal nerve.

Occlusion of Cerebral Veins and Dural Venous Sinuses

Occlusion of cerebral veins and dural venous sinuses may result from thrombi (clots), thrombophlebitis (venous inflammation), or tumors. The facial veins make clinically important connections with the cavernous sinus through the superior ophthalmic veins. Blood from the medial angle of the eye, nose, and lips usually drains inferiorly into the facial vein. However, because the facial vein has no valves, blood may pass superiorly to the superior ophthalmic vein and enter the cavernous sinus. In people with *thrombophlebitis of the facial vein,* pieces of an infected thrombus may extend into the cavernous sinus, producing *thrombophlebitis of the cavernous sinus.*

Metastasis of Tumor Cells to the Dural Sinuses

The basilar and occipital sinuses communicate through the foramen magnum with the internal vertebral venous plexuses. Because these venous channels are valveless, compression of the thorax, abdomen, or pelvis, as occurs during heavy coughing and straining, may force venous blood from these regions into the internal vertebral venous system and subsequently into the dural venous sinuses. As a result, pus in abscesses and tumor cells in these regions may spread to the vertebrae and brain.

Fractures of Cranial Base

In fractures of the cranial base, the internal carotid artery may be torn, producing an *arteriovenous fistula* within the cavernous sinus. Arterial blood rushes into the cavernous sinus, enlarging it and forcing retrograde blood into its venous tributaries, especially the ophthalmic veins. As a result, the eyeball protrudes (*exophthalmos*) and the conjunctiva becomes engorged (*chemosis*). The protruding eyeball pulsates in synchrony with the radial pulse, a phenomenon known as *pulsating exophthalmos.* Because CNs III, IV, V_1, V_2, and VI lie in or close to the lateral wall of the cavernous sinus, they may also be affected when the sinus is injured.

A blow to the head can detach the periosteal layer of dura from the calvaria without fracturing the cranial bones. However, in the cranial base, the two dural layers are firmly attached and difficult to separate from the bones. Consequently, a fracture of the cranial base usually tears the dura and results in leakage of CSF.

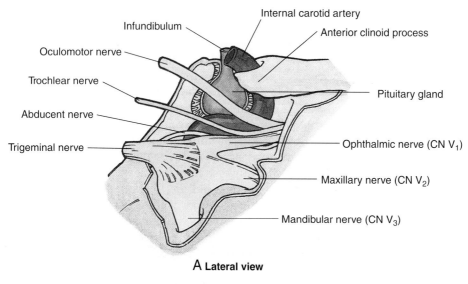

A **Lateral view**

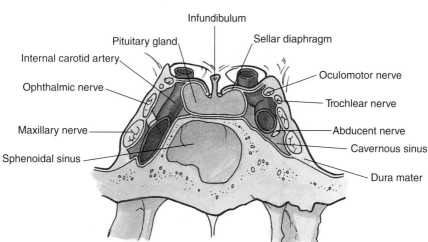

B **Coronal section**

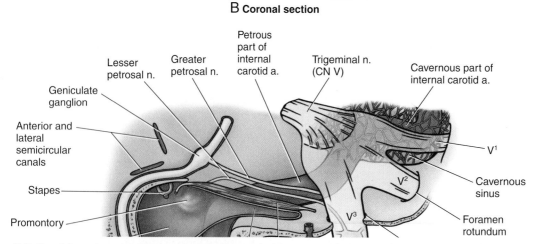

Figure 7.7. Cranial meninges. A. The arachnoid mater and pia mater are shown. **B.** The superior sagittal sinus is cut open to expose the arachnoid granulations. **C.** This section of the cranium and brain shows the superior sagittal sinus and meninges. *CSF,* cerebrospinal fluid.

Leptomeninx (Pia and Arachnoid Mater)

The **arachnoid mater** and **pia mater** (pia-arachnoid) develop from a single layer of mesenchyme surrounding the embryonic brain. CSF-filled spaces form within this layer and coalesce to form the *subarachnoid space* (Fig. 7.7). Web-like **arachnoid trabeculae** pass between the arachnoid and the pia. The avascular arachnoid mater, although closely applied to the meningeal layer of the dura, is held against the inner surface of the dura by the pressure of the CSF. The **pia mater** is a thin membrane that is highly vascularized by a network of fine blood vessels and adheres to the surface of the brain and follows its contours. When the cerebral arteries penetrate the cerebral cortex, the pia follows them for a short distance, forming a pial coat and a periarterial space.

Meningeal Spaces

Of the three meningeal "spaces" commonly mentioned in relation to the cranial meninges, only one exists as a space in the absence of pathology:

- The **dura–cranium interface** (extradural or epidural space) is not a natural space between the cranium and the external periosteal layer of the dura because the dura is attached to the bones. It becomes a space only pathologically—for example, when blood from torn meningeal vessels pushes the periosteum away from the cranium and accumulates.
- The **dura–arachnoid junction** or interface (subdural space) is likewise not a natural space between the dura

and the arachnoid. A space may develop in the dural border cell layer as the result of trauma, such as after a blow to the head (Haines, 2002).

- The **subarachnoid space**, between the arachnoid and pia, is a real space that contains CSF, trabecular cells, arteries, and veins (Fig. 7.7*B*).

Brain

The brain is composed of the *cerebrum, cerebellum,* and *brainstem* (midbrain, pons, and medulla oblongata) (Fig. 7.8). The following brief discussion of the gross structure of the brain shows how the brain relates to the cranium, cranial nerves, meninges, and CSF. Of the 12 crainial nerves, *11 cranial nerves arise from the brain* (Fig. 7.10). They have motor, parasympathetic, and/or sensory functions. Generally, these nerves are surrounded by a dural sheath as they leave the cranium; the dural sheath becomes continuous with the connective tissue of the epineurium. For a summary of the cranial nerves, see Chapter 9.

Head Injuries and Intracranial Hemorrhage

Extradural or epidural hemorrhage is arterial in origin. Blood from torn branches of a middle meningeal artery collects between the external periosteal layer of the dura and the calvaria, usually after a hard blow to the head. This results in the formation of an *extradural* or *epidural hematoma* (Fig. B7.2). Typically, a brief *concussion* (loss of consciousness) occurs, followed by a lucid interval of some hours. Later, drowsiness and coma occur. Compression of the brain occurs as the blood mass increases, necessitating evacuation of the blood and occlusion of the bleeding vessels.

A *dural border hematoma* classically is called a *subdural hematoma;* however, this term is a misnomer because there is no naturally occurring space at the dura–arachnoid junction. Hematomas at this junction are usually caused by extravasated blood that splits open the dural border cell layer (Fig. B7.2). The blood does not collect within a preexisting space but rather creates a space at the dura–arachnoid junction (Haines, 2002). *Dural border hemorrhage* usually follows a blow to the head that jerks the brain inside the cranium and injures it. The precipitating trauma may be trivial or forgotten. Dural border hemorrhage is typically venous in origin and commonly results from tearing of a superior cerebral vein as it enters the superior sagittal sinus.

Subarachnoid hemorrhage is an extravasation (escape) of blood, usually arterial, into the subarachnoid space (Fig. B7.2). Most subarachnoid hemorrhages result from *rupture of a saccular aneurysm* (sac-like dilation on an artery). Some subarachnoid hemorrhages are associated with head trauma involving cranial fractures and cerebral lacerations. Bleeding into the subarachnoid space results in meningeal irritation, a severe headache, stiff neck, and often loss of consciousness.

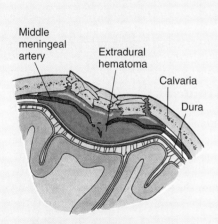

Extradural or epidural hematoma

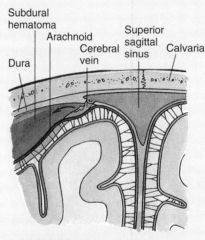

Dural border (subdural) hematoma

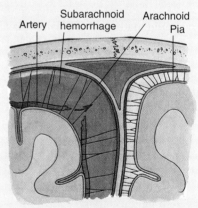

Subarachnoid hemorrhage

Figure B7.2

Parts of Brain

When the calvaria and dura mater are removed, **gyri** (folds), **sulci** (grooves), and **fissures** (clefts) of the cerebral cortex are visible through the delicate arachnoid–pia layer.

- The **cerebrum** includes the cerebral hemispheres. The **cerebral hemispheres** form the largest part of the brain and are separated by the cerebral falx. Each cerebral hemisphere is divided into for lobes: frontal, parietal, temporal, and occipital. The frontal lobes occupy the anterior cranial fossa, the temporal lobes occupy the lateral parts of the middle cranial fossae, and the occipital lobes extend posteriorly over the cerebellar tentorium. (Fig. 7.8).

- The **diencephalon** is composed of the epithalamus, thalamus, and hypothalamus and forms the central core of the brain.

- The **midbrain,** the rostral part of the brainstem, lies at the junction of the middle and posterior cranial fossae. CN III and IV are associated with the midbrain.

- The **pons,** the part of the brainstem between the midbrain rostrally and the medulla oblongata caudally, lies in the anterior part of the posterior cranial fossa. CN V is associated with the pons.

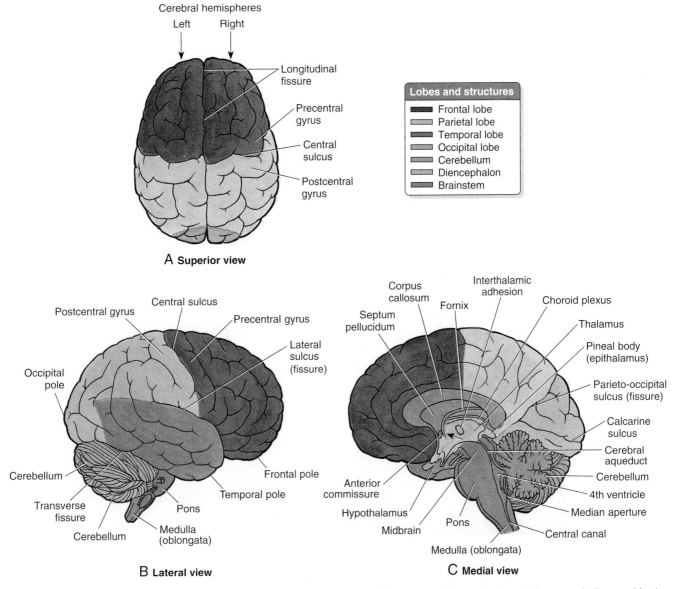

Figure 7.8. Structure of brain. A. The right and left cerebral hemispheres are shown. **B.** Right cerebral hemisphere, cerebellum and brainstem. **C.** The parts of the brain are identified on the medial view of the right cerebral hemisphere. *Arrow*, site of interventricular foramen.

- The **medulla oblongata (medulla)**, the most caudal part of the brainstem, is continuous with the spinal cord and lies in the posterior cranial fossa. CN IX, X, and XII are associated with the medulla, whereas CN VI–VIII are located at the junction of the pons and medulla.
- The **cerebellum** is the large brain mass lying posterior to the pons and medulla and inferior to the posterior part of the cerebrum. It lies beneath the cerebellar tentorium in the posterior cranial fossa and consists of two hemispheres united by a narrow middle part, the **vermis.**

Ventricular System of Brain

The ventricular system of the brain consists of two lateral ventricles and the midline 3rd and 4th ventricles (Fig. 7.9A).

The **lateral ventricles** (1st and 2nd ventricles) open into the 3rd ventricle through the **interventricular foramina** (of Monro). The **3rd ventricle**, a slit-like cavity between the right and the left halves of the diencephalon, is continuous with the **cerebral aqueduct**, a narrow channel in the midbrain connecting the 3rd and 4th ventricles. The **4th ventricle**, lying in the posterior parts of the pons and medulla, extends inferoposteriorly. Inferiorly, it tapers to a narrow channel that continues into the spinal cord as the central canal. CSF drains from the 4th ventricle through a single **median aperture** and paired **lateral apertures** into the subarachnoid space. These apertures are the only means by which CSF enters the subarachnoid space. If they are blocked, the ventricles distend, producing compression of the cerebral hemispheres. At certain areas, mainly at the base of the brain, the arachnoid and

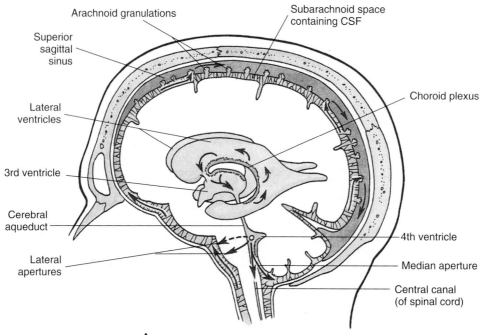

A **Medial view, ventricles viewed from left**

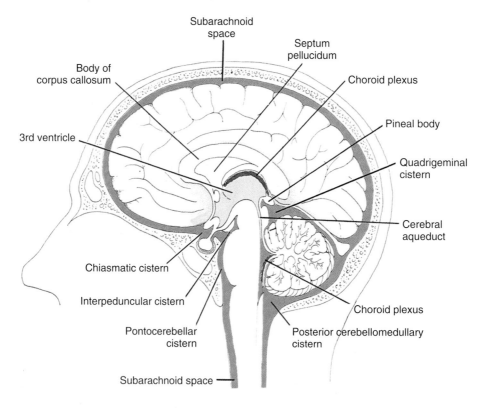

B **Medial view**

Figure 7.9. Ventricular system of brain. A. The ventricles are shown. *Arrows,* direction of cerebrospinal fluid (*CSF*) flow. **B.** The subarachnoid cisterns are identified.

pia mater are widely separated by large pools (cisterns) of CSF (Fig. 7.9*B*). Major **subarachnoid cisterns** include the:

- **Cerebellomedullary cistern**, the largest of the cisterns, located between the cerebellum and the medulla; receives CSF from the apertures of the 4th ventricle; divided into the **posterior cerebellomedullary cistern** (L. *cisterna magna*) and the **lateral cerebellomedullary cistern.**
- **Pontocerebellar cistern** (pontine cistern), an extensive space ventral to the pons and continuous inferiorly with the spinal subarachnoid space.
- **Interpeduncular cistern** (basal cistern), located in the interpeduncular fossa between the cerebral peduncles of the midbrain.
- **Chiasmatic cistern**, inferior and anterior to the optic chiasm.
- **Quadrigeminal cistern** (cistern of the great cerebral vein), located between the posterior part of the corpus callosum and the superior surface of the cerebellum.

CSF is secreted (at the rate of 400–500 mL/day) by choroidal epithelial cells of the **choroid plexuses** in the lateral, 3rd, and 4th ventricles (Fig. 7.9*B*). The choroid plexuses consist of vascular fringes of pia mater (tela choroidea) covered by cuboidal epithelial cells. Some CSF leaves the 4th ventricle to pass inferiorly into the subarachnoid space around the spinal cord and posterosuperiorly over the cerebellum. However, most CSF flows into the interpeduncular and quadrigeminal cisterns. CSF from the various cisterns flows superiorly through the sulci and fissures on the medial and superolateral surfaces of the cerebral hemispheres. CSF also passes into the extensions of the subarachnoid space around the cranial nerves.

The main site of CSF absorption into the venous system is through the **arachnoid granulations**, protrusions of arachnoid villi into the walls of dural venous sinuses, especially the superior sagittal sinus and its lateral venous lacunae (Figs. 7.6*B* and 7.9*A*). Along with the meninges and calvaria, CSF protects the brain by providing a cushion against blows to the head. The CSF in the subarachnoid space provides the buoyancy that prevents the weight of the brain from compressing the cranial nerve roots and blood vessels against the internal surface of the cranium.

Cisternal Puncture

CSF may be obtained, for diagnostic purposes, from the posterior cerebellomedullary cistern, using a procedure known as *cisternal puncture*. The subarachnoid space or the ventricular system may also be entered for measuring or monitoring CSF pressure, injecting antibiotics, or administering contrast media for radiography.

Hydrocephalus

Overproduction of CSF, obstruction of its flow, or interference with its absorption results in an excess of CSF in the ventricles and enlargement of the head, a condition known as *hydrocephalus* (Fig. B7.3). Excess CSF dilates the ventricles; thins the brain; and, in infants, separates the bones of the calvaria because the sutures and fontanelles are still open.

Leakage of Cerebrospinal Fluid

Fractures in the floor of the middle cranial fossa may result in leakage of CSF from the external acoustic meatus (*CSF otorrhea*) if the meninges superior to the middle ear are torn and the tympanic membrane (eardrum) is ruptured. Fractures in the floor of the anterior cranial fossa may involve the cribriform plate of the ethmoid, resulting in leakage of CSF through the nose (*CSF rhinorrhea*). CSF otorrhea and CSF rhinorrhea may be primary indications of a cranial base fracture and increase the risk of *meningitis* because an infection could spread to the meninges from the ear or nose.

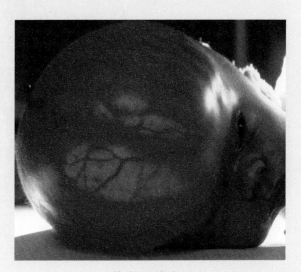

Hydrocephalus

Figure B7.3

Vasculature of Brain

Although it accounts for only about 2.5% of body weight, the brain receives about one sixth of the cardiac output and one fifth of the oxygen consumed by the body at rest. The blood supply to the brain is from the internal carotid and vertebral arteries (Fig. 7.10; Table 7.2).

The **internal carotid arteries** arise in the neck from the common carotid arteries and enter the cranial cavity with the carotid plexus of sympathetic nerves through the carotid canals. The intracranial course of the internal carotid artery can be seen in Figures 7.6C and 7.11. The internal carotid arteries course anteriorly through the cavernous sinuses, with the abducent nerves (CN VI) and in close proximity to the occulomotor (CN III) and trochlear (CN IV) nerves (Fig. 7.6A & B). The terminal branches of the internal carotids are the **anterior** and **middle cerebral arteries.**

The **vertebral arteries** begin in the root of the neck as branches of the first part of the subclavian arteries, pass through the transverse foramina of the first six cervical vertebrae, and perforate the dura and arachnoid to pass through the foramen magnum. The cranial parts of the vertebral arteries unite at the caudal border of the pons to form the **basilar artery** (Fig. 7.10; Table 7.2). The basilar artery runs through the pontocerebellar cistern to the superior border of the pons, where it ends by dividing into the two **posterior cerebral arteries.**

In addition to supplying branches to deeper parts of the brain, the cortical branches of each cerebral artery supply a surface and a pole of the cerebrum. The cortical branches of the:

- *Anterior cerebral artery* supplies most of the medial and superior surfaces and the frontal pole.
- *Middle cerebral arteries* supply the lateral surface and temporal pole.
- *Posterior cerebral arteries* supply the inferior surface and occipital pole.

The **cerebral arterial circle** (of Willis) at the base of the brain is an important anastomosis between the four

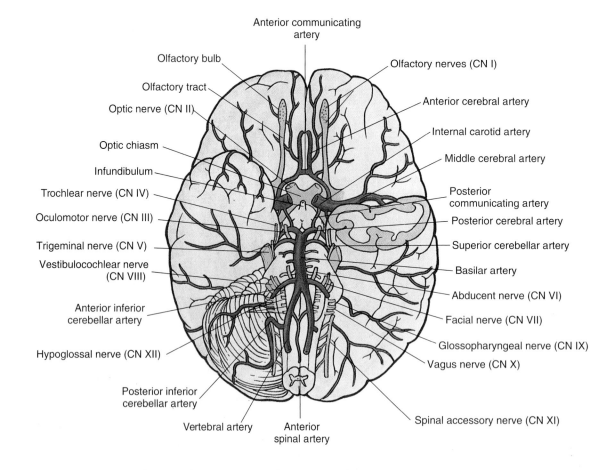

Inferior view

Figure 7.10. Blood supply of brain. The cerebral arterial circle and cranial nerves are identified.

Table 7.2 Arterial Supply of the Cerebral Hemispheres

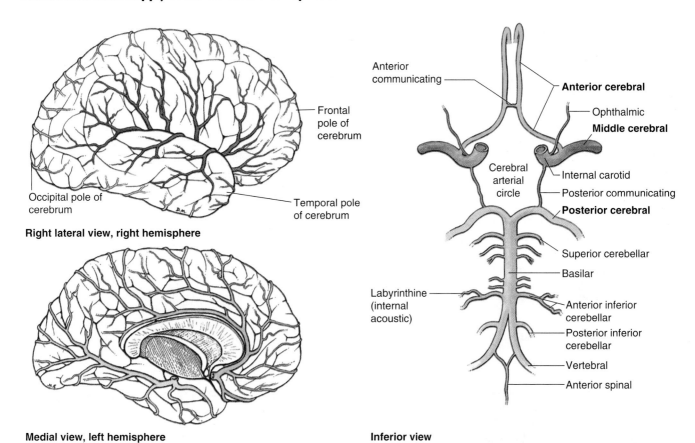

Right lateral view, right hemisphere

Medial view, left hemisphere

Inferior view

Artery	Origin	Distribution
Internal carotid	Common carotid artery at superior border of thyroid cartilage	Gives branches to walls of cavernous sinus, pituitary gland, and trigeminal ganglion; provides primary supply to brain
Anterior cerebral	Internal carotid artery	Cerebral hemispheres, except for occipital lobes
Anterior communicating	Anterior cerebral artery	Cerebral arterial circle (of Willis)
Middle cerebral	Continuation of internal carotid artery distal to anterior cerebral artery	Most of lateral surface of cerebral hemispheres
Vertebral	Subclavian artery	Cranial meninges and cerebellum
Basilar	Formed by union of vertebral arteries	Brainstem, cerebellum, and cerebrum
Posterior cerebral	Terminal branch of basilar artery	Interior aspect of cerebral hemisphere and occipital lobe
Posterior communicating	Posterior cerebral artery	Optic tract, cerebral peduncle, internal capsule, and thalamus

arteries (two vertebral and two internal carotid arteries) that supply the brain (Fig. 7.10). The arterial circle is formed by the *posterior cerebral, posterior communicating, internal carotid, anterior cerebral,* and *anterior communicating arteries.* The various components of the cerebral arterial circle give numerous small branches to the brain. Variations in the origin and size of the vessels forming the cerebral arterial circle are common (e.g., the posterior communicating arteries may be absent, or there may be two anterior communicating arteries). In approximately one in three people, one posterior cerebral artery is a major branch of the internal carotid artery.

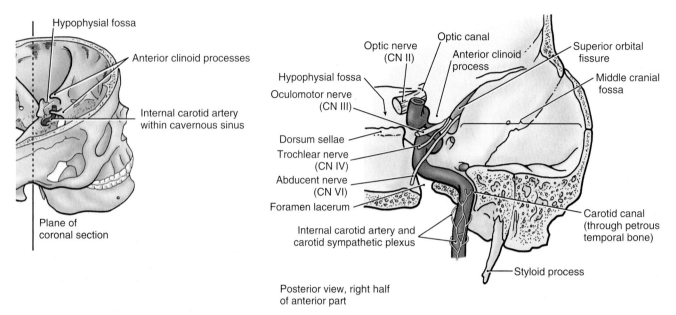

Figure 7.11. Course of internal carotid artery. The cervical part of the artery ascends to the entrance to the carotid canal in the petrous temporal bone. The petrous part of the artery turns horizontally and medially in the carotid canal to emerge superior to the foramen lacerum, entering the cranial cavity. The cavernous part of the artery runs on the lateral side of the sphenoid in the carotid groove as it traverses the cavernous sinus. Inferior to the anterior clinoid process, the artery makes a 180° turn to join the cerebral arterial circle.

The thin-walled, valveless **cerebral veins** draining the brain pierce the arachnoid and meningeal layer of dura to end in the nearest dural venous sinuses. The sinuses drain for the most part into the IJVs. The cerebral veins on the superolateral surface of the brain drain into the superior sagittal sinus; cerebral veins on the posteroinferior aspect drain into the straight, transverse, and superior petrosal sinuses. The **great cerebral vein** (of Galen), a single midline vein, is formed inside the brain by the union of two internal cerebral veins and ends by merging with the inferior sagittal sinus to form the straight sinus (Fig. 7.5*A*).

Face

The face is the anterior aspect of the head from the forehead to the chin and from one ear to the other. The basic shape of the face is determined by the underlying bones, the facial muscles, and the subcutaneous tissue. The skin of the face is thin, pliable, and firmly attached to the underlying cartilages of the external ear and nose.

Muscles of Face

The facial muscles (muscles of facial expression) are in the subcutaneous tissue of the anterior and posterior scalp, face, and neck (Table 7.3). Most of these muscles attach to bone or fascia and produce their effects by pulling the skin. They move the skin and change facial expressions to convey

mood. The *muscles of facial expression* also surround the orifices of the mouth, eyes, and nose and act as sphincters and dilators that close and open the orifices.

The **orbicularis oris** is the sphincter of the mouth and is the first of a series of sphincters associated with the alimentary (digestive) tract. The **buccinator** (L. trumpeter), active in smiling, also keeps the cheek taut, thereby preventing it from folding and being injured during chewing. The orbicularis oris and buccinator work with the tongue to keep food between the teeth during mastication (chewing). The buccinator is also active during sucking, whistling, and blowing (e.g., when playing a wind instrument).

The **orbicularis oculi** closes the eyelids and assists the flow of lacrimal fluid (tears). It has three parts: the *palpebral part,* which gently closes the eyelids; the *lacrimal part,* which passes posterior to the lacrimal sac, aiding drainage of tears; and the *orbital part,* which tightly closes the eyelids to protect the eyeballs against glare and dust.

Nerves of Face

Cutaneous (sensory) innervation of the face is provided primarily by the *trigeminal nerve* (CN V), whereas the motor innervation to the muscles of facial expression is provided by the *facial nerve* (CN VII) and the motor innervation to the muscles of mastication by the *motor root of the trigeminal nerve/the mandibular nerve.*

The cutaneous nerves of the neck overlap those of the face. Cutaneous branches of the cervical nerves from the

Table 7.3 Muscles of Face and Scalp

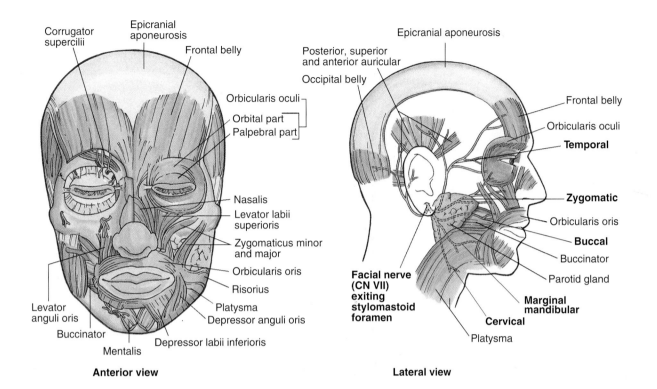

Anterior view

Lateral view

Muscle[a]	Origin	Insertion	Main Action(s)
Occipitofrontalis			
Frontal belly	Epicranial aponeurosis	Skin and subcutaneous tissue of eyebrows and forehead	Elevates eyebrows and wrinkles skin of forehead; protracts scalp (indicating surprise or curiosity)
Occipital belly	Lateral two thirds of superior nuchal line	Epicranial aponeurosis	Retracts scalp; increasing effectiveness of frontal belly
Orbicularis oculi (orbital sphincter)	Medial orbital margin; medial palpebral ligament; lacrimal bone	Skin around margin of orbit; superior and inferior tarsi (tarsal plates)	Closes eyelids: palpebral part does so gently; orbital part tightly (winking)
Orbicularis oris (oral sphincter)	Medial maxilla and mandible; deep surface of perioral skin; angle of mouth	Mucous membrane of lips	Tonus closes mouth; phasic contraction compresses and protrudes lips (kissing) or resists distension (when blowing)
Buccinator (cheek muscle)	Mandible, alveolar processes of maxilla and mandible, pterygomandibular raphe	Angle of mouth (modiolus); orbicularis oris	Presses cheek against molar teeth; works with tongue to keep food between occlusal surfaces and out of oral vestibule; resists distension (when blowing)
Platysma	Subcutaneous tissue of infraclavicular and supraclavicular regions	Base of mandible; skin of cheek and lower lip; angle of mouth; orbicularis oris	Depresses mandible (against resistance); tenses skin of inferior face and neck (conveying tension and stress)

[a]All facial muscles are innervated by the facial nerve (CN VII) via its posterior auricular branch or via the temporal, zygomatic, buccal, marginal mandibular, or cervical branches of the parotid plexus.

Strokes

An *ischemic stroke* denotes the sudden development of neurological deficits that are related to impaired cerebral blood flow. The most common causes of strokes are spontaneous cerebrovascular accidents such as cerebral embolism, cerebral thrombosis, cerebral hemorrhage, and subarachnoid hemorrhage (Rowland, 2000). The cerebral arterial circle is an important means of collateral circulation in the event of gradual obstruction of one of the major arteries forming the circle. Sudden occlusion, even if only partial, results in neurological deficits. In elderly persons, the anastomoses are often inadequate when a large artery (e.g., internal carotid) is occluded, even if the occlusion is gradual (in which case function is impaired at least to some degree).

Hemorrhagic stroke follows the rupture of an artery or a *saccular aneurysm,* a sac-like dilation on a weak part of the arterial wall. The most common type of saccular aneurysm is a *berry aneurysm,* occurring in the vessels of or near the cerebral arterial circle and the medium arteries at the base of the brain (Fig. B7.4). In time, especially in people with hypertension (high blood pressure), the weak part of the arterial wall expands and may rupture, allowing blood to enter the subarachnoid space.

Transient Ischemic Attacks

Transient ischemic attacks (TIAs) refer to neurological symptoms resulting from ischemia (deficient blood supply) of the brain. The symptoms of a TIA may be ambiguous: staggering, dizziness, light-headedness,

fainting, and paresthesias (e.g., tingling in a limb). Most TIAs last a few minutes, but some persist for up to an hour. Individuals with TIAs are at increased risk for myocardial infarction and ischemic stroke (Brust, 2000).

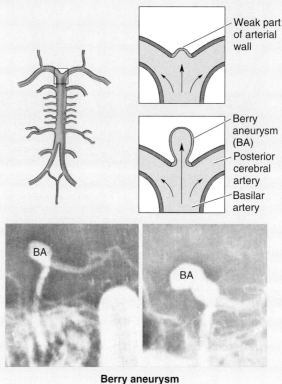

Berry aneurysm

Figure B7.4

Facial Injuries

Because the face does not have a distinct layer of deep fascia and the subcutaneous tissue is loose between the attachments of facial muscles, *facial lacerations* tend to gape (part widely). Consequently, the skin must be sutured carefully to prevent scarring. The looseness of the subcutaneous tissue also enables fluid and blood to accumulate in the loose connective tissue after bruising of the face. Facial inflammation causes considerable swelling.

cervical plexus extend over the ear, the posterior aspect of the neck and scalp. The great auricular nerve innervates the inferior aspect of the auricle and much of the area overlying the angle of the mandible.

The **trigeminal nerve** (CN V) is the sensory nerve for the face and the motor nerve for the muscles of mastication and several small muscles (Table 7.4). Three large groups of peripheral processes from nerve cell bodies of the **trigeminal ganglion**—the large sensory ganglion of CN V—form the **ophthalmic nerve** (CN V_1), the **maxillary nerve** (CN V_2), and the sensory component of the **mandibular nerve** (CN V_3). These nerves are named according to their main regions of termination: the eye, maxilla, and mandible, respectively. The first two divisions (CN V_1 and CN V_2) are wholly sensory. CN V_3 is largely sensory but also

Table 7.4 Cutaneous Nerves of Face and Scalp

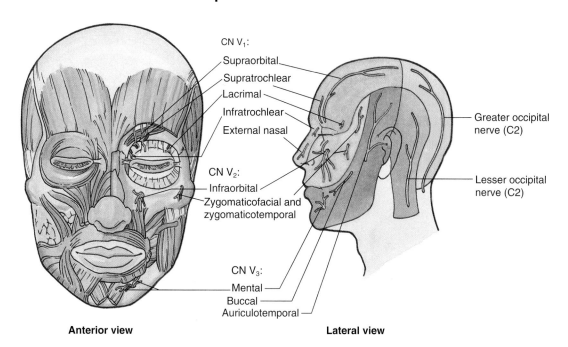

CN V₁:
Supraorbital
Supratrochlear
Lacrimal
Infratrochlear
External nasal

CN V₂:
Infraorbital
Zygomaticofacial and zygomaticotemporal

CN V₃:
Mental
Buccal
Auriculotemporal

Greater occipital nerve (C2)

Lesser occipital nerve (C2)

Anterior view   Lateral view

Nerve	Origin	Course	Distribution
Cutaneous nerves derived from ophthalmic nerve (CN V₁)			
Supraorbital	Branch from bifurcation of *frontal nerve,* approximately in middle of orbital roof	Continues anteriorly along roof of orbit, emerging via supraorbital notch or foramen; ascends forehead, breaking into branches	Mucosa of *frontal sinus;* skin and conjunctiva of middle of *superior eyelid;* skin and pericranium of *anterolateral forehead and scalp* to vertex (interauricular line)
Supratrochlear	Branch from bifurcation of *frontal nerve,* approximately in middle of orbital roof	Continues anteromedially along roof of orbit, passing lateral to trochlea and ascending forehead	Skin and conjunctiva of medial aspect of *superior eyelid;* skin and pericranium of *anteromedial forehead*
Lacrimal	Branch of *CN V₁* proximal to superior	Runs superolaterally through orbit, receiving secretomotor fibers via a communicating branch from the zygomaticotemporal nerve	*Lacrimal gland* (secretomotor fibers); small area of skin and conjunctiva of *lateral part of superior eyelid*
Infratrochlear	Terminal branch (with anterior ethmoidal nerve) of *nasociliary nerve*	Follows medial wall of orbit, passing inferior to trochlea	Skin lateral to *root of nose;* skin and conjunctiva of *eyelids adjacent to medial canthus, lacrimal sac,* and *lacrimal caruncle*
External nasal	Terminal branch of *anterior ethmoidal nerve*	Emerges from nasal cavity by passing between nasal bone and lateral nasal cartilage	Skin of nasal *ala, vestibule,* and *dorsum of nose,* including *apex*
Cutaneous nerves derived from maxillary nerve (CN V₂)			
Infraorbital	Continuation of *CN V₂* distal to its entrance into the orbit via the inferior orbital fissure	Traverses infraorbital groove and canal in orbital floor, giving rise to superior alveolar branches; then emerges via infraorbital foramen, immediately dividing into inferior palpebral, internal and external nasal, and superior labial branches	Mucosa of *maxillary sinus;* premolar, canine, and incisor *maxillary teeth;* skin and conjunctiva of *inferior eyelid;* skin of *cheek, lateral nose,* and anteroinferior *nasal septum;* skin and oral mucosa of *upper lip*
Zygomaticofacial	Smaller terminal branch (with zygomaticotemporal nerve) of *zygomatic nerve*	Traverses zygomaticofacial canal in zygomatic bone at inferolateral angle of orbit	Skin on prominence of *cheek*
Zygomaticotemporal	Larger terminal branch (with zygomaticofacial nerve) of *zygomatic nerve*	Sends communicating branch to lacrimal nerve in orbit; then passes to temporal fossa via zygomaticotemporal canal in zygomatic bone	Skin overlying *anterior part of temporal fossa*

Table 7.4 Cutaneous Nerves of Face and Scalp (continued)

Nerve	Origin	Course	Distribution
Cutaneous nerves derived from mandibular nerve (CN V₃)			
Auriculotemporal	In infratemporal fossa via two roots from *posterior trunk of CN V₃* that encircle middle meningeal artery	Passes posteriorly deep to ramus of mandible and superior deep part of parotid gland, emerging posterior to temporomandibular joint	Skin anterior to auricle and posterior two thirds of *temporal region;* skin of tragus and adjacent helix of *auricle;* skin of roof of *external acoustic meatus;* and skin of superior *tympanic membrane*
Buccal	In infratemporal fossa as sensory branch of *anterior trunk of CN V₃*	Passes between two parts of lateral pterygoid muscle, emerging anteriorly from cover of ramus of mandible and masseter, uniting with buccal branches of facial nerve	Skin and oral mucosa of *cheek* (overlying and deep to anterior part of buccinator); *buccal gingiva* (gums) adjacent to second and third molars
Mental	Terminal branch of *inferior alveolar nerve*	Emerges from mandibular canal via mental foramen in anterolateral aspect of body of mandible	Skin of *chin;* oral mucosa of *lower lip*
Cutaneous nerves derived from anterior rami of cervical spinal nerves			
Great auricular	Spinal nerves C2 and C3 via cervical plexus	Ascends vertically across sternocleidomastoid, posterior to external jugular vein	Skin overlying angle of mandible and inferior lobe of auricle; parotid sheath
Lesser occipital		Follows posterior border of sternocleidomastoid; then ascends posterior to auricle	Scalp posterior to auricle
Cutaneous nerves derived from posterior rami of cervical spinal nerves			
Greater occipital nerve	As medial branch of posterior ramus of spinal nerve C2	Emerges between axis and obliquus capitis inferior; then pierces trapezius	Scalp of occipital region
Third occipital nerve	As lateral branch of posterior ramus of spinal nerve C3	Pierces trapezius	Scalp of lower occipital and suboccipital regions

receives motor fibers (axons) from the motor root of CN V that mainly supply the muscles of mastication (Table 7.4). The major cutaneous branches of the:

- Ophthalmic nerve (CN V₁): lacrimal, supraorbital, supratrochlear, infratrochlear, and external nasal nerves.
- Maxillary nerve (CN V₂): infraorbital, zygomaticotemporal, and zygomaticofacial nerves.
- Mandibular (CN V₃): auriculotemporal, buccal, and mental nerves

The **motor nerves of the face** are the *facial nerve* (CN VII) to the muscles of facial expression and the *mandibular nerve* (CN V₃) to the muscles of mastication (masseter, temporal, medial, and lateral pterygoids) These nerves also supply some more deeply placed muscles (described later in this chapter in relation to the mouth, middle ear, and neck). The **facial nerve** (CN VII) emerges from the cranium via the **stylomastoid foramen** (Tables 7.1 and 7.3). Its extracranial branches (temporal, zygomatic, buccal, mandibular, cervical, and posterior auricular nerves) supply the superficial muscle of the neck and chin (platysma), muscles of facial expression, muscle of the cheek (buccinator), muscles of the ear (auricular), and muscles of the scalp (occipital and frontal bellies of occipitofrontal muscle).

Innervation of the scalp anterior to the auricles is by branches of all three divisions of the **trigeminal nerve** (CN V₁, CN V₂, CN V₃) (Table 7.4). Posterior to the auricles, innervation of the scalp is by spinal cutaneous nerves (C2 and C3).

Superficial Vasculature of Face and Scalp

The face is richly supplied by superficial arteries and external veins, as is evident in blushing and blanching. The terminal branches of both arteries and veins anastomose freely, including anastomoses across the midline with contralateral partners. Most arteries supplying the face are branches of the *external carotid arteries.* Most external facial veins are drained by veins that accompany the arteries of the face. As with most superficial veins, they are subject to many variations and have abundant anastomoses that allow drainage to occur by alternate routes during periods of temporary compression. The alternate routes include both superficial pathways and deep drainage.

The **facial artery** provides the major arterial supply to the

Table 7.5 Superficial Arteries of Face and Scalp

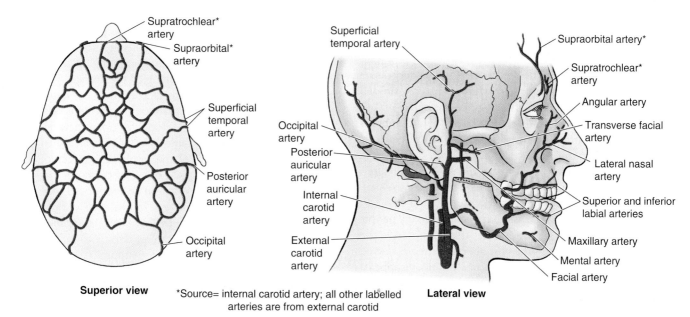

Superior view

*Source= internal carotid artery; all other labelled arteries are from external carotid

Lateral view

Artery	Origin	Course	Distribution
Facial	External carotid artery	Ascends deep to submandibular gland; winds around inferior border of mandible and enters face	Muscles of facial expression and face
Inferior labial	Facial artery near angle of mouth	Runs medially in lower lip	Lower lip
Superior labial		Runs medially in upper lip	Upper lip and ala (side) and septum of nose
Lateral nasal	Facial artery as it ascends alongside nose	Passes to ala of nose	Skin on ala and dorsum of nose
Angular	Terminal branch of facial artery	Passes to medial angle (canthus) of eye	Superior part of cheek and inferior eyelid
Occipital	External carotid artery	Passes medial to posterior belly of digastric and mastoid process; accompanies occipital nerve in occipital region	Scalp of back of head, as far as vertex
Posterior auricular		Passes posteriorly, deep to parotid gland, along styloid process between mastoid process and ear	Auricle and scalp posterior to auricle
Superficial temporal	Smaller terminal branch of external carotid artery	Ascends anterior to ear to temporal region and ends in scalp	Facial muscles and skin of frontal and temporal regions
Transverse facial	Superficial temporal artery within parotid gland	Crosses face superficial to masseter and inferior to zygomatic arch	Parotid gland and duct, muscles and skin of face
Mental	Terminal branch of inferior alveolar artery	Emerges from mental foramen and passes to chin	Facial muscles and skin of chin
Supraorbital	Terminal branch of ophthalmic artery, a branch of internal carotid artery	Passes superiorly from supraorbital foramen	Muscle and skin of forehead and scalp
Supratrochlear		Passes superiorly from supratrochlear notch	Muscles and skin of scalp

Trigeminal Neuralgia

Trigeminal neuralgia (tic douloureux) is a sensory disorder of the sensory root of CN V characterized by sudden attacks of excruciating, lightening-like jabs of facial pain. A *paroxysm* (sudden sharp pain) can last for 15 minutes or more. The maxillary nerve (CN V₂) is most frequently involved; then the mandibular nerve (CN V₃); and, least frequently, the ophthalmic nerve (CN V₁). The pain often is initiated by touching a sensitive *trigger zone* of the skin. The cause of trigeminal neuralgia is unknown; however, some investigators believe that most affected people have an anomalous blood vessel that compresses the sensory root of CN V. When the aberrant artery is moved away from the root, the symptoms usually disappear. Other researchers believe the condition is caused by pathological processes affecting neurons of the trigeminal ganglion. In some cases, it is necessary to section the sensory root for relief of trigeminal neuralgia.

Lesions of Trigeminal Nerve

Lesions of the entire trigeminal nerve cause widespread anesthesia involving the:

- Corresponding anterior half of the scalp.
- Face, except for an area overlying the angle of the mandible.
- Cornea and conjunctiva.
- Mucous membranes of the nose and paranasal sinuses, mouth, and anterior part of the tongue.

Paralysis of the muscles of mastication also occurs.

Bell Palsy

Injury to the facial nerve (CN VII) or its branches produces paralysis of some or all the facial muscles on the affected side (Bell palsy). The affected area sags and facial expression is distorted (Fig. B7.5). The loss of tonus of the orbicularis oculi causes the inferior lid to evert (fall away

from the surface of the eyeball). As a result, the lacrimal fluid is not spread over the cornea, preventing adequate lubrication, hydration, and flushing of the cornea. This makes the cornea vulnerable to ulceration. If the injury weakens or paralyzes the buccinator and orbicularis oris, food will accumulate in the oral vestibule during chewing, usually requiring continual removal with a finger. When the sphincters or dilators of the mouth are affected, displacement of the mouth (drooping of the corner) is produced by gravity and contraction of unopposed contralateral facial muscles, resulting in food and saliva dribbling out of the side of the mouth. Weakened lip muscles affect speech. Affected people cannot whistle or blow a wind instrument effectively. They frequently dab their eyes and mouth with a handkerchief to wipe the fluid (tears and saliva), which runs from the drooping lid and mouth.

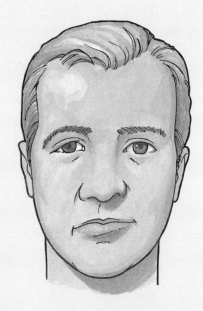

Figure B7.5

face (Fig. 7.12A; Table 7.5). It arises from the external carotid artery and winds its way to the inferior border of the mandible, just anterior to the masseter. It then courses over the face to the medial angle (canthus) of the eye. The facial artery sends branches to the upper and lower lips (**superior** and **inferior labial arteries**) and to the side of the nose (**lateral nasal artery**) and then terminates as the **angular**

artery, which supplies the medial angle of the eye.

The **superficial temporal artery** is the smaller terminal branch of the external carotid artery; the other branch is the *maxillary artery*. The superficial temporal artery emerges on the face between the temporomandibular joint (TMJ) and the auricle and ends in the scalp by dividing into **frontal** and **parietal branches** (Fig. 7.12). The **transverse facial**

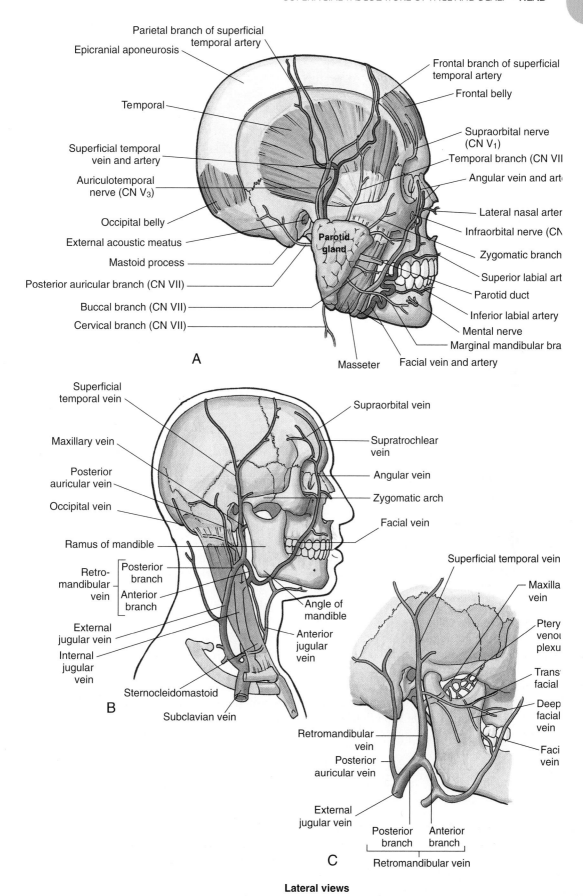

Lateral views

Figure 7.12. Vasculature and nerves of face. The vessels and nerves (**A**), venous drainage (**B**), and veins and pterygoid venous plexus (**C**) are shown.

artery arises from the superficial temporal artery within the parotid gland and crosses the face superficial to the masseter. It divides into numerous branches that supply the parotid gland and duct, the masseter, and the skin of the face. It anastomoses with branches of the facial artery.

The **arteries of the scalp** course within, the subcutaneous connective tissue layer between the skin and the epicranial aponeurosis. They anastomose freely with one another. The arterial walls are firmly attached to the dense connective tissue in which they are embedded, limiting their ability to constrict when cut. Consequently, bleeding from scalp wounds is profuse. The arterial supply is from the *external carotid arteries* through the **occipital, posterior auricular,** and **superficial temporal arteries** and from the *internal carotid arteries* by way of the **supratrochlear** and **supraorbital arteries** (Table 7.5). Arteries of the scalp supply little blood to the cranium, which is supplied primarily by the middle meningeal artery.

The **facial vein** provides the primary superficial venous drainage of the face (Fig. 7.12*B* & *C*). It begins at the medial angle of the eye as the **angular vein.** Among the tributaries of the facial vein is the **deep facial vein,** which drains the *pterygoid venous plexus* of the infratemporal fossa. Inferior to the margin of the mandible, the facial vein is joined by the anterior branch of the retromandibular vein. The facial vein drains directly or indirectly into the **internal jugular vein.** At the medial angle of the eye, the facial vein communicates with the *superior ophthalmic vein,* which drains into the *cavernous sinus.*

The **superficial temporal vein** drains the forehead and scalp and receives tributaries from the veins of the temple and face. Near the auricle, the superficial temporal vein enters the parotid gland (Fig. 7.12*A*). The **retromandibular vein** (Fig. 7.12*B* & *C*), formed by the union of the superficial temporal vein and the maxillary vein, is a deep vein that descends within the parotid gland, superficial to the external carotid artery and deep to the facial nerve. The retromandibular vein divides into an anterior branch, which unites with the facial vein, and a posterior branch, which joins the **posterior auricular vein** to form the **external jugular vein** (EJV). The EJV crosses the superficial surface of the sternocleidomastoid muscle to enter the subclavian vein in the root of the neck.

Venous drainage of the superficial parts of the scalp is through the accompanying veins of the scalp arteries, the **supraorbital** and **supratrochlear veins,** which descend to unite at the medial angle of the eye to form the **angular vein,** which becomes the **facial vein** at the inferior margin of the orbit (Fig. 7.12*B* & *C*). The **superficial temporal veins** and **posterior auricular veins** drain the scalp anterior and posterior to the auricles, respectively. The **occipital veins** drain the occipital region of the scalp. Venous drainage of deep parts of the scalp in the temporal region is through

deep temporal veins, which are tributaries of the pterygoid venous plexus.

There are no lymph nodes in the scalp or face except for the parotid/buccal region. Lymph from the scalp, face, and neck drains into the *superficial ring (pericervical collar) of lymph nodes*—the submental, submandibular, parotid, mastoid, and occipital—located at the junction of the head and neck (Fig. 7.13). Lymph from the superficial ring of nodes drains into the **deep cervical lymph nodes** along the IJV. Lymph from these nodes passes to the jugular lymphatic trunk, which joins the thoracic duct on the left side and the IJV or brachiocephalic vein on the right side. A summary of the lymphatic drainage of the face follows.

- Lymph from the lateral part of the face and scalp drains to the superficial **parotid lymph nodes.**
- Lymph from the deep parotid nodes drains to the **deep cervical lymph nodes.**
- Lymph from the upper lip and lateral parts of the lower lip drains into the **submandibular lymph nodes.**
- Lymph from the chin and central part of the lower lip drains into the **submental lymph nodes.**

Parotid Gland

The parotid gland is the largest of three paired salivary glands. It is enclosed within a tough fascial capsule, the **parotid sheath,** derived from the investing layer of deep cervical fascia. The parotid gland has an irregular shape because the area it occupies, the **parotid bed,** is anteroinferior to the external acoustic meatus, where it is wedged between the ramus of the mandible and the mastoid process (Fig. 7.12*A*). The apex of the parotid gland is posterior to the angle of the mandible, and its base is related to the zygomatic arch. The **parotid duct** passes horizontally from the anterior edge of the gland. At the anterior border of the masseter, the duct turns medially, pierces the buccinator, and enters the oral cavity through a small orifice opposite the second maxillary molar tooth (Fig. 7.12*A*). Embedded within the substance of the parotid gland, from superficial to deep, are the *parotid plexus of the facial nerve* (CN VII) and its branches, the *retromandibular vein* (Fig. 7.12*B*), and the *external carotid artery.* On the parotid sheath and within the gland are *parotid lymph nodes* (Fig. 7.13).

The **great auricular nerve** (C2 and C3), a branch of the cervical plexus, innervates the parotid sheath and the overlying skin (Table 7.4). The **auriculotemporal nerve,** a branch of CN V$_3$, is closely related to the parotid gland and passes superior to it with the superficial temporal vessels (Fig. 7.12*A*). The parasympathetic component of the **glossopharyngeal nerve** (CN IX) supplies secretory fibers to the parotid gland; the postsynaptic fibers are conveyed from the *otic ganglion* to the gland by the auriculotemporal nerve.

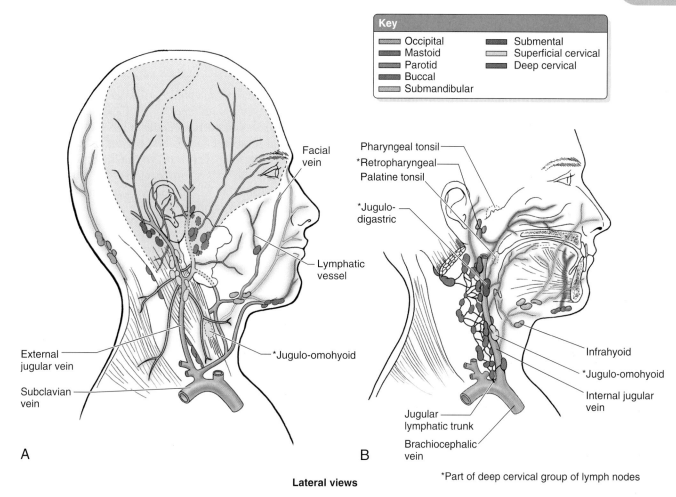

Key

Occipital	Submental
Mastoid	Superficial cervical
Parotid	Deep cervical
Buccal	
Submandibular	

Facial
vein

Pharyngeal tonsil
*Retropharyngeal
Palatine tonsil

*Jugulo-
digastric

Lymphatic
vessel

External
jugular vein

*Jugulo-omohyoid

Subclavian
vein

Infrahyoid

*Jugulo-omohyoid

Internal jugular
vein

Jugular
lymphatic trunk

Brachiocephalic
vein

A

B

Lateral views

*Part of deep cervical group of lymph nodes

Figure 7.13. Lymphatic drainage of head and neck. Superficial (**A**) and deep (**B**) drainage is shown. All lymphatic vessels from the head and neck ultimately drain into the deep cervical nodes, either directly from the tissue or indirectly after passing through an outlying group of nodes.

Pulses of Arteries of the Face

The pulses of the superficial temporal and facial arteries can be used for taking the pulse. For example, anesthesiologists at the head of the operating table often take the *temporal pulse* anterior to the auricle as the artery crosses the zygomatic arch to supply the scalp. The *facial pulse* can be palpated where the facial artery crosses the inferior border of the mandible immediately anterior to the masseter.

Compression of Facial Artery

The facial artery can be occluded by pressure against the mandible where the vessel crosses it. Because of the numerous anastomoses between the branches of the facial artery and other arteries of the face, compression of the facial artery on one side does not stop all bleeding from a lacerated facial artery or one of its branches. In lacerations of the lip, pressure must be applied on both sides of the cut to stop the bleeding. In general, facial wounds bleed freely but heal quickly.

Squamous Cell Carcinoma of Lip

Squamous cell carcinoma (cancer) of the lip usually involves the lower lip. Overexposure to sunshine over many years, is a common factor in these cases. Chronic irritation from pipe smoking is also a contributing cause. Cancer cells from the central part of the lower lip, the floor of the mouth, and apex of the tongue spread to the submental lymph nodes, whereas cancer cells from lateral parts of the lower lip drain to the submandibular lymph nodes.

Stimulation of the parasympathetic fibers produces a thin watery saliva. Sympathetic fibers are derived from the cervical ganglia through the **external carotid nerve plexus** on the external carotid artery. The vasomotor activity of these fibers may reduce secretion from the parotid gland. Sensory nerve fibers pass to the gland and its sheath through the great auricular and auriculotemporal nerves.

Parotidectomy

About 80% of salivary gland tumors occur in the parotid glands. Surgical excision of the parotid gland (*parotidectomy*) is often performed as part of the treatment. Because the parotid plexus of CN VII is embedded in the parotid gland, the plexus and its branches are in jeopardy during surgery. An important step in parotidectomy is the identification, dissection, isolation, and preservation of the facial nerve.

Infection of Parotid Gland

The parotid gland may become infected by infectious agents that pass through the bloodstream, as occurs in *mumps,* an acute communicable viral disease. Infection of the gland causes inflammation (*parotiditis*) and swelling of the gland. Severe pain occurs because the parotid sheath limits swelling. Often the pain is worse during chewing because the enlarged gland is wrapped around the posterior border of the ramus of the mandible and is compressed against the mastoid process of the temporal bone when the mouth is opened. The mumps virus also may cause *inflammation of the parotid duct,* producing redness of the *parotid papilla,* the small projection at the opening of the duct into the superior oral vestibule. Because the pain produced by mumps may be confused with a toothache, redness of the papilla is often an early sign that the disease involves the gland and not a tooth.

Parotid gland disease often causes pain in the auricle, external acoustic meatus, temporal region, and temporomandibular joint (TMJ) because the auriculotemporal nerve, from which the parotid gland receives sensory fibers, also supplies sensory fibers to the skin over the temporal fossa and auricle.

Orbit

The orbits are pyramidal, bony cavities in the facial skeleton with their bases (*orbital openings*) directed anterolaterally and their apices, posteromedially (Fig. 7.14). The orbits contain and protect the *eyeballs* and their muscles, nerves, and vessels, together with most of the lacrimal apparatus. All space in the orbits not occupied by structures is filled with **orbital fat.** The fat forms a matrix in which the structures of the orbit are embedded.

The orbit has a base, four walls, and an apex:

*   The **superior wall** (roof) is approximately horizontal and is formed mainly by the **orbital part of the frontal bone,** which separates the orbital cavity from the anterior cranial fossa. Near the apex of the orbit, the superior wall is formed by the lesser wing of the sphenoid. Anterolaterally the lacrimal gland occupies the **fossa for the lacrimal gland** (lacrimal fossa) in the orbital part of the frontal bone.
*   The **medial wall** is formed by the **ethmoid bone,** along with contributions from the frontal, lacrimal, and sphenoid bones. Anteriorly, the medial wall is indented by the **lacrimal groove** and **fossa for the lacrimal sac.** The bone forming the medial wall is paper thin, and the ethmoid air cells are often visible through the bone of a dried cranium.
*   The **lateral wall** is formed by the **frontal process of the zygomatic bone** and the **greater wing of the sphenoid.** This is the strongest and thickest wall, which is important because it is most exposed and vulnerable to direct trauma. Its posterior part separates the orbit from the temporal lobes of the brain and middle cranial fossae.
*   The **inferior wall** (floor) is formed mainly by the **maxilla** and partly by the **zygomatic** and **palatine bones.** The thin inferior wall is shared by the orbit superiorly and the maxillary sinus inferiorly. It slants inferiorly from the apex to the inferior orbital margin. The inferior wall is demarcated from the lateral wall by the **inferior orbital fissure.**
*   The **apex** of the orbit is at the **optic canal** in the lesser wing of the sphenoid, just medial to the **superior orbital fissure.**

The bones forming the orbit are lined with **periorbita** (periosteum of the orbit). The periorbita is continuous at the *optic canal* and *superior orbital fissure* with the periosteal layer of dura mater. The periorbita is also continuous over the orbital margins and through the *inferior orbital fissure* with the periosteum covering the external surface of the cranium (pericranium) and with the orbital septa at the orbital margins, with the fascial sheaths of the extraocular muscles, and with orbital fascia that forms the fascial sheath of the eyeball.

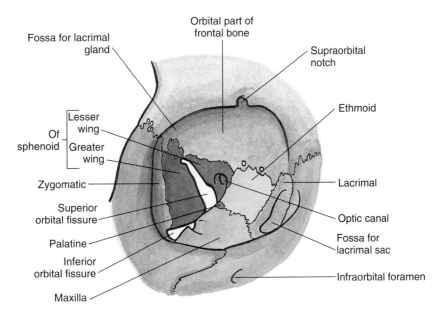

Anterior view

Figure 7.14. **Bones of right orbit.**

Eyelids and Lacrimal Apparatus

The eyelids and lacrimal fluid, secreted by the lacrimal glands, protect the cornea and eyeball from injury and irritation.

EYELIDS

When closed, the **eyelids** (L. *palpebrae*) cover the eyeball anteriorly, thereby protecting it from injury and excessive light (Fig. 7.15). They also keep the cornea moist by spreading the lacrimal fluid. The eyelids are movable folds that are covered externally by thin skin and internally by a transparent mucous membrane, the **palpebral conjunctiva** (Fig. 7.16 B). The palpebral conjunctiva is reflected onto the eyeball, where it is continuous with the **bulbar conjunctiva.** The bulbar conjunctiva is loose and wrinkled over the sclera and contains small blood vessels. The bulbar conjunctiva is adherent to the periphery of the cornea. The lines of

Fractures of the Orbit

When the blows are powerful enough and the impact is directly on the bony rim, the resulting fractures usually occur at the sutures between the bones forming the orbital margin. Because of the thinness of the medial and inferior walls of the orbit, a blow to the eye may fracture the orbital walls while the margin remains intact. Indirect traumatic injury that displaces the orbital walls is called a "blowout" fracture. Fractures of the medial wall may involve the ethmoidal and sphenoidal sinuses, whereas fractures in the inferior wall may involve the maxillary sinus. Although the superior wall is stronger than the medial and inferior walls, it is thin enough to be translucent and may be readily pen-etrated. Thus a sharp object may pass through it into the frontal lobe of the brain. Orbital fractures often result in intraorbital bleeding, which exerts pressure on the eyeball, causing *exophthalmos* (protrusion of the eyeball).

Orbital Tumors

Because of the closeness of the optic nerve to the sphenoidal and posterior ethmoidal sinuses, a malignant tumor in these sinuses may erode the thin bony walls of the orbit and compress the optic nerve and orbital contents. Tumors in the orbit produce exophthalmos. A tumor in the middle cranial fossa may enter the orbital cavity through the superior orbital fissure.

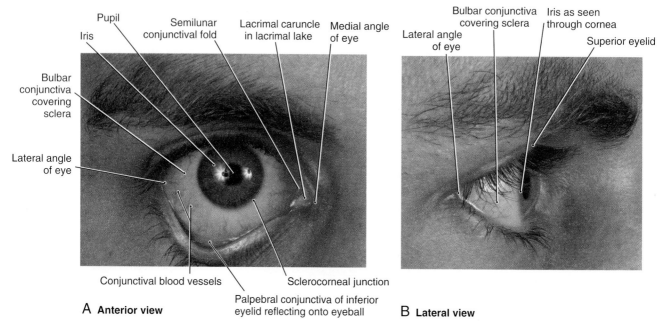

Figure 7.15. Surface anatomy of eyeball and eyelids.

reflection of the palpebral conjunctiva onto the eyeball form deep recesses, the **superior** and **inferior conjunctival fornices.** The **conjunctival sac** is the space bound by the palpebral and bulbar conjunctivae. The conjunctival sac is a specialized form of mucosal "bursa" that enables the eyelids to move freely over the surface of the eyeball as they open and close.

The superior (upper) and inferior (lower) eyelids are strengthened by dense bands of connective tissue, the **superior** and **inferior tarsi** (singular = tarsus). Fibers of the palpebral portion of the *orbicularis oculi* muscle are in the subcutaneous tissue superficial to these tarsi and deep to the skin of the eyelid. Embedded in the tarsal plates are **tarsal glands,** the lipid secretion of which lubricates the edges of the eyelids and prevents them from sticking together when they close (Fig. 7.16B). This secretion also forms a barrier that lacrimal fluid does not cross when produced in normal amounts. When production is excessive, it spills over the barrier onto the cheeks as tears.

The **eyelashes** (L. *cilia*) are in the margins of the eyelids. The large sebaceous glands associated with the eyelashes are the **ciliary glands.** The junctions of the superior and inferior eyelids make up the **medial and lateral palpebral commissures,** defining the **angles of the eyes** (Fig. 7.15). Thus each eye has medial and lateral angles, or *canthi*.

In the **medial angle of the eye,** a reddish shallow reservoir of tears, the **lacrimal lake,** can be observed. Within the lake is the **lacrimal caruncle,** a small mound of moist modified skin (Fig. 7.15A). Lateral to the caruncle is a **semilunar conjunctival fold,** which slightly overlaps the

eyeball. When the edges of the eyelids are everted, a small pit the **lacrimal punctum** is visible at its medial end on the summit of a small elevation, the **lacrimal papilla** (Fig. 7-17).

Between the nose and the medial angle of the eye is the **medial palpebral ligament,** which connects the tarsi to the medial margin of the orbit. The orbicularis oculi originates and inserts onto this ligament (Fig. 7.16C). A similar **lateral palpebral ligament** attaches the tarsi to the lateral margin of the orbit (Fig. 7.16D). The **orbital septum** is a weak membrane that spans from the tarsi to the margins of the orbit, where it becomes continuous with the periosteum. It keeps the orbital fat contained and can limit the spread of infection to and from the orbit.

LACRIMAL APPARATUS

The lacrimal apparatus consists of (Fig. 7.17):

- **Lacrimal glands** secrete lacrimal fluid (tears).
- **Lacrimal ducts** convey lacrimal fluid from the lacrimal glands to the conjunctival sac.
- **Lacrimal canaliculi** (L. small canals), each commencing at a *lacrimal punctum* (opening) on the *lacrimal papilla* near the medial angle of the eye, convey the lacrimal fluid from the *lacrimal lake* to the *lacrimal sac*, the dilated superior part of the nasolacrimal duct
- **Nasolacrimal duct** conveys the lacrimal fluid to the nasal cavity.

The almond-shaped *lacrimal gland* lies in the *fossa for the lacrimal gland* in the superolateral part of each orbit.

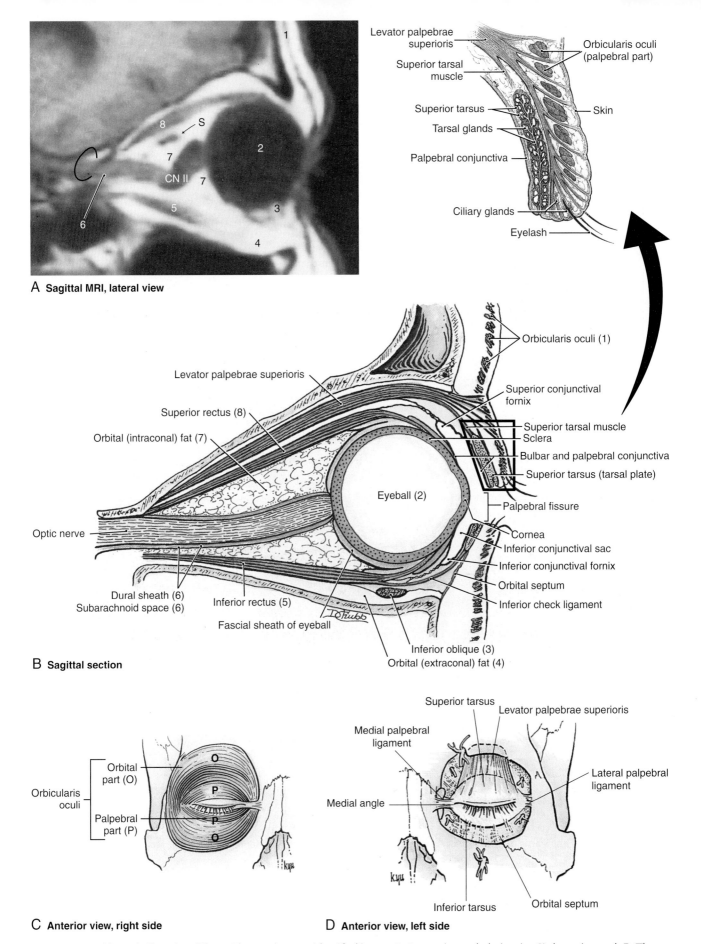

A Sagittal MRI, lateral view

Levator palpebrae superioris
Orbicularis oculi (palpebral part)
Superior tarsal muscle
Skin
Superior tarsus
Tarsal glands
Palpebral conjunctiva
Ciliary glands
Eyelash

Orbicularis oculi (1)
Superior conjunctival fornix
Superior tarsal muscle
Sclera
Bulbar and palpebral conjunctiva
Superior tarsus (tarsal plate)
Palpebral fissure
Cornea
Inferior conjunctival sac
Inferior conjunctival fornix
Orbital septum
Inferior check ligament

Levator palpebrae superioris
Superior rectus (8)
Orbital (intraconal) fat (7)
Optic nerve
Eyeball (2)
Dural sheath (6)
Subarachnoid space (6)
Inferior rectus (5)
Fascial sheath of eyeball
Inferior oblique (3)
Orbital (extraconal) fat (4)

B Sagittal section

Orbicularis oculi
Orbital part (O)
Palpebral part (P)

C Anterior view, right side

Superior tarsus
Levator palpebrae superioris
Medial palpebral ligament
Lateral palpebral ligament
Medial angle
Orbital septum
Inferior tarsus

D Anterior view, left side

Figure 7.16. Orbit, eyeball, and eyelids. A. The numbers are identified in part B. *S,* superior opthalmic vein. *Circle,* optic canal. **B.** The contents of the orbit are identified. *Inset,* the details of the superior eyelid are shown. **C.** The orbicularis oculi is detailed. **D.** The skeleton of the eyelids and orbital septum is shown.

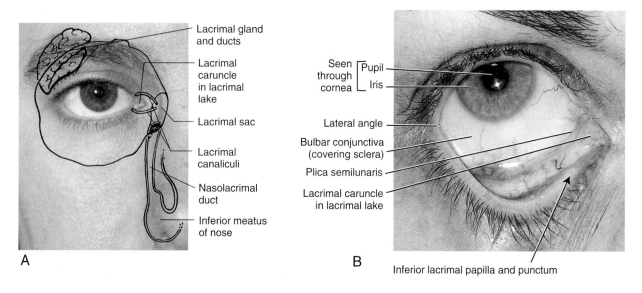

A

Lacrimal gland and ducts

Lacrimal caruncle in lacrimal lake

Lacrimal sac

Lacrimal canaliculi

Nasolacrimal duct

Inferior meatus of nose

B

Seen through cornea — Pupil / Iris

Lateral angle

Bulbar conjunctiva (covering sclera)

Plica semilunaris

Lacrimal caruncle in lacrimal lake

Inferior lacrimal papilla and punctum

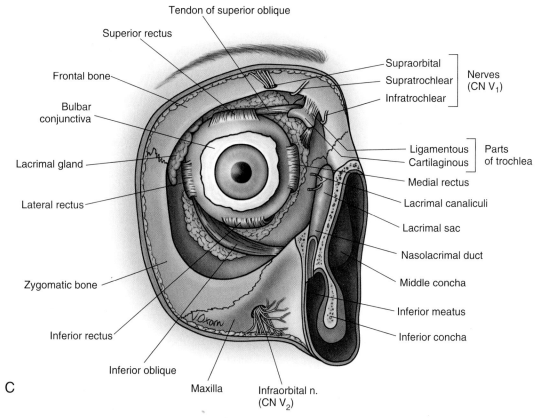

C

Tendon of superior oblique

Superior rectus

Frontal bone

Bulbar conjunctiva

Lacrimal gland

Lateral rectus

Zygomatic bone

Inferior rectus

Inferior oblique

Maxilla

Infraorbital n. (CN V$_2$)

Supraorbital
Supratrochlear — Nerves (CN V$_1$)
Infratrochlear

Ligamentous
Cartilaginous — Parts of trochlea

Medial rectus

Lacrimal canaliculi

Lacrimal sac

Nasolacrimal duct

Middle concha

Inferior meatus

Inferior concha

Anterior views

Figure 7.17. Lacrimal apparatus. A. The surface anatomy of the lacrimal apparatus is identified. **B.** The surface anatomy of the eye, with the inferior eyelid retracted, is shown. **C.** A dissection of the eye and nose is shown.

The production of lacrimal fluid is stimulated by parasympathetic impulses from CN VII. It is secreted through 8–12 **excretory ducts**, which open into the *superior conjunctival fornix* of the conjunctival sac. The fluid flows inferiorly within the sac under the influence of gravity. When the cornea becomes dry, the eyelid blinks. The eyelids come together in a lateral to medial sequence pushing a film of fluid medially over the cornea. The lacrimal fluid containing foreign material such as dust is pushed toward the medial angle of the eye, accumulating in the *lacrimal lake* from which it drains by capillary action through the *lacrimal puncta* and *lacrimal canaliculi* to the *lacrimal sac*. From this sac, the lacrimal fluid passes to the nasal cavity through the *nasolacrimal duct* (Fig. 7.17*C*). Here the fluid flows posteriorly to the nasopharynx and is swallowed.

The **nerve supply of the lacrimal gland** is both sympathetic and parasympathetic. The presynaptic parasympathetic secretomotor fibers are conveyed from the facial nerve by the *greater petrosal nerve* and then by the *nerve of the pterygoid canal* to the *pterygopalatine ganglion,* where they synapse with the cell body of the postsynaptic fiber (Fig. 7.36*B*). Vasoconstrictive, postsynaptic sympathetic fibers—brought from the *superior cervical ganglion* by the *internal carotid plexus* and deep petrosal nerve—join the parasympathetic fibers to form the nerve of the pterygoid canal and traverse the pterygopalatine ganglion. Branches of the *zygomatic nerve* (from the maxillary nerve) then bring both types of fibers to the lacrimal branch of the ophthalmic nerve (CN V$_1$), by which they enter the gland (Fig. 7.36*A*).

Eyeball

The eyeball contains the optical apparatus of the visual system and occupies most of the anterior portion of the orbit. The eyeball proper has three layers; however, there is an additional loose connective tissue layer that surrounds the eyeball, allowing its movement in the orbit. The loose connective tissue layer (fascial sheath) is composed posteriorly of bulbar fascia and anteriorly of the bulbar conjunctiva. The three layers of the eyeball are as follows (Fig. 7.18):

- **Fibrous layer** (outer coat), consisting of the sclera and cornea.
- **Vascular layer** (middle coat), consisting of the choroid, ciliary body, and iris.
- **Inner layer** (inner coat), consisting of the retina, which has both optic and non-visual parts.

The **sclera** is the opaque part of the fibrous layer covering the posterior five sixths of the eyeball. It is the fibrous skeleton of the eyeball, providing shape and resistance as well as attachment for extrinsic (extraocular) and intrinsic muscles of the eye. The anterior part of the sclera is visible through the transparent bulbar conjunctiva as the "white of the eye." The **cornea** is the transparent part of the fibrous

Injury to the Nerves Supplying the Eyelids

Because it supplies the levator palpebrae superioris, a lesion of the occulomotor nerve (CN III) causes paralysis of the muscle, and the superior eyelid droops (*ptosis*). Damage to the facial nerve (CN VII) involves paralysis of the orbicularis oculi, preventing the eyelids from closing fully. Normal rapid protective blinking of the eye is also lost. The loss of tonus of the muscle in the lower eyelid causes the lid to fall away (evert) from the surface of the eye. This leads to drying of the cornea and leaves it unprotected from dust and small particles. Thus irritation of the unprotected eyeball results in excessive but inefficient lacrimation (tear formation).

Inflammation of the Palpebral Glands

Any of the glands in the eyelid may become inflamed and swollen from infection or obstruction of their ducts. If the ducts of the ciliary glands become obstructed, a painful red suppurative (puss-producing) swelling, a *sty*, develops on the eyelid. Cysts of the sebaceous glands of the eyelids, called *chalazia*, may also form.

coat, covering the anterior one sixth of the eyeball.

The vascular layer (also called the **uvea** or **uveal tract**) consists of the choroid, ciliary body, and iris. The **choroid**; a dark reddish brown membrane between the sclera and the retina, forms the largest part of the vascular layer and lines most of the sclera. Engorged with blood in life, this layer is responsible for the "red eye" reflection that occurs in flash photography.

The choroid is continuous anteriorly with the ciliary body. The choroid attaches firmly to the pigment layer of the retina, but it can be stripped easily from the sclera. The **ciliary body**, which is muscular as well as vascular, connects the choroid with the circumference of the iris. The ciliary body provides attachment for the lens; contraction and relaxation of the smooth muscle of the ciliary body controls the thickness (and therefore focus) of the lens. Folds on the internal surface of the ciliary body, the **ciliary processes**, secrete *aqueous humor,* which fills the anterior and posterior chambers of the eye. The **anterior chamber of the eye** is the space between the cornea anteriorly and the iris/pupil posteriorly. The **posterior**

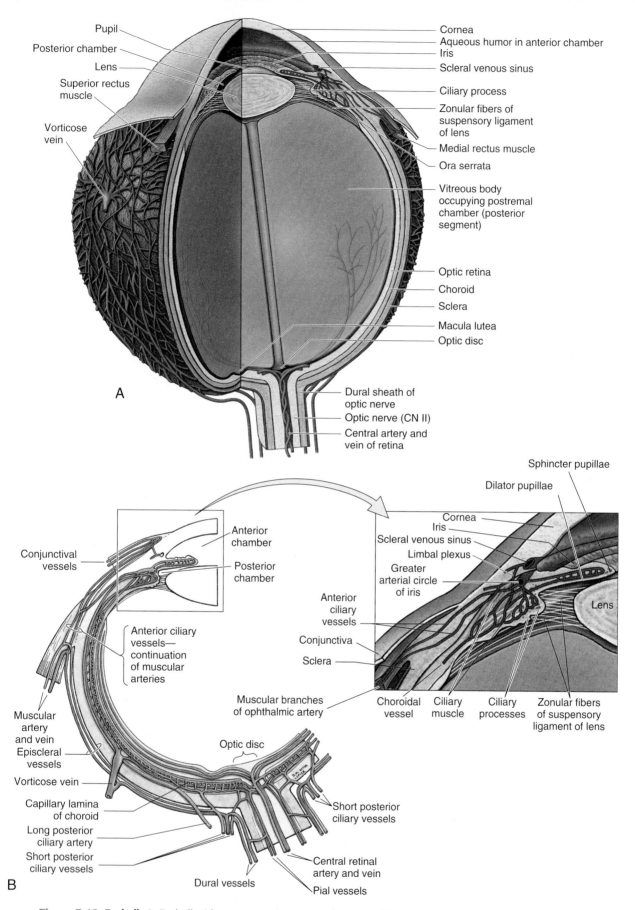

Figure 7.18. Eyeball. A. Eyeball with quarter section removed. **B.** Partial horizontal section of the eyeball is shown.

chamber of the eye is the space between the iris/pupil anteriorly and the lens and ciliary body posteriorly.

The **iris**, which literally lies on the anterior surface of the lens, is a thin contractile diaphragm with a central aperture, the **pupil**, for transmitting light. When a person is awake, the size of the pupil varies continually to regulate the amount of light entering the eye. Two involuntary muscles control the size of the pupil: the parasympathetically stimulated **sphincter pupillae** closes the pupil, and the sympathetically stimulated **dilator pupillae** opens it (Fig. 7.18*B*).

The inner layer of the eyeball is the **retina**. Grossly, the retina consists of two functional parts with distinct locations: the optic part and a nonvisual retina. The **optic part** of the retina is sensitive to visual light rays and has two layers: a neural layer and a pigment cell layer. The *neural layer* is the light receptive. The *pigment cell layer* consists of a single layer of cells that reinforces the light-absorbing property of the choroid in reducing the scattering of light in the eyeball. The **nonvisual retina** is an anterior continuation of the pigment cell layer and a layer of supporting cells over the ciliary body (**ciliary part of the retina**) and the posterior surface of the iris (**iridial part of the retina**), respectively.

The **fundus** is the posterior part of the eyeball. It has a circular distinct area, the **optic disc** (optic papilla) where the sensory fibers and vessels conveyed by the optic nerve enter the eyeball. Because it contains no photoreceptors, the optic disc is insensitive to light. Consequently, this part of the retina is commonly called the *blind spot*. Just lateral to the optic disc is the **macula lutea**. The yellow color of the macula is apparent only when the retina is examined with red-free light. The macula lutea is a small area of the retina with special photoreceptor cones that is specialized for acuity of vision. At the center of the macula lutea is a depression, the *fovea centralis* (L. central pit), the area of most acute vision. The fovea is approximately 1.5 mm in diameter.

The functional optic part of the retina terminates anteriorly along the **ora serrata** (L. serrated edge), an irregular border slightly posterior to the ciliary body. The ora serrata marks the anterior termination of the light-receptive part of the retina. Except for the cones and rods of the neural layer, the retina is supplied by the **central artery of the retina** (Fig. 7.18*A*), a branch of the ophthalmic artery. A corre-

Ophthalmoscopy

Physicians view the fundus (posterior part) of the eye with an *ophthalmoscope*. The retinal arteries and veins radiate over the fundus from the optic disc. The pale, oval optic disc appears on the medial side, with retinal vessels radiating from its center in the ophthalmoscopic view of the retina (Fig. B7.6). Pulsation of the retinal arteries is usually visible. Centrally, at the posterior pole of the eyeball, the macula lutea appears darker than the reddish hue of surrounding areas of the retina.

Detachment of Retina

The layers of the developing retina are separated in the embryo by an intraretinal space. During the early fetal period, the embryonic layers fuse, obliterating this space. Although the pigment cell layer becomes firmly fixed to the choroid, its attachment to the neural layer is not firm. Consequently, detachment of the retina may follow a blow to the eye. A *detached retina* usually results from seepage of fluid between the neural and pigmented layers of the retina, perhaps days or even weeks after trauma to the eye. People with a retinal detachment may complain of flashes of light or specks floating in front of their eye.

Papilledema

An increase in CSF pressure slows venous return from the retina, causing *edema of the retina* (fluid accumulation). The edema is viewed during ophthalmoscopy as swelling of the optic disc, a condition called *papilledema*.

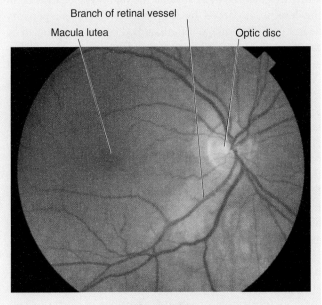

Branch of retinal vessel

Macula lutea

Optic disc

Figure B7.6

sponding system of retinal veins unites to form the **central vein of the retina**. The cones and rods of the outer neural layer receive nutrients from the *capillary lamina of the choroid* (L. *lamina choriocapillaris*). It has the finest vessels of the inner surface of the choroid, against which the retina is pressed.

REFRACTIVE MEDIA OF THE EYEBALL

On their way to the retina, light waves pass through the **refractive media of the eyeball:** cornea, aqueous humor, lens, and vitreous humor (Fig. 7.18*A*). The **cornea** is the circular area of the anterior part of the outer fibrous layer of the eyeball; it is largely responsible for refraction of light that enters the eye. It is transparent, avascular, and sensitive to touch. The cornea is supplied by the ophthalmic nerve (CN V_1). Its nourishment is derived from the capillary beds at its periphery, the aqueous humor, and lacrimal fluid. The latter also provides oxygen absorbed from the air.

The **aqueous humor** in the anterior and posterior chambers of the eye is produced in the posterior chamber by the **ciliary processes** of the ciliary body. This watery solution provides nutrients for the avascular cornea and lens. After passing through the pupil from the posterior chamber into the anterior chamber (Fig. 7.18*B*), the aqueous humor drains into the **scleral venous sinus** (L. *sinus venosus sclerae*, canal of Schlemm) at the **iridocorneal angle.** The humor is removed by the **limbal plexus**, a network of scleral veins close to the limbus, which drain, in turn, into both tributaries of the *vorticose* and *anterior ciliary veins.*

The **lens** is posterior to the iris and anterior to the vitreous humor of the vitreous body. It is a transparent biconvex structure enclosed in a capsule. The highly elastic **capsule of the lens** is anchored by the **zonular fibers** (suspensory ligament of the lens) to the ciliary bodies and is encircled by the ciliary processes. The convexity of the lens, particularly its anterior surface, constantly varies to focus near or distant objects on the retina. Contraction of the **ciliary muscle** in the ciliary body changes the shape of the lens (Fig. 7.18*B*). Stretched within the circle of the relaxed ciliary body, the attachments around its periphery pull the lens relatively flat, enabling far vision. When parasympathetic stimulation causes the smooth muscle of the circular ciliary body to contract, the circle, like a sphincter, becomes smaller in size and the tension on the lens is reduced, allowing the lens to round up. The increased convexity is for near vision. In the absence of parasympathetic stimulation, the ciliary muscles relax again, and the lens is pulled into its flatter, far-vision shape.

The **vitreous humor** is a watery fluid enclosed in the meshes of the **vitreous body**, a transparent jelly-like substance in the posterior four fifths of the eyeball posterior to the lens (**postremal** or **vitreous chamber** or posterior segment). In addition to transmitting light, the vitreous humor holds the retina in place and supports the lens.

Corneal Abrasions and Lacerations

Foreign objects, such as sand or metal filings, produce *corneal abrasions* that cause sudden, stabbing eye pain and tears. Opening and closing the eyelids is also painful. *Corneal lacerations* are caused by sharp objects such as fingernails or the corner of a page of a book.

Corneal Ulcers and Transplants

Damage to the sensory innervation of the cornea from CN V_1 leaves the cornea vulnerable to injury by foreign particles. People with scarred or opaque corneas may receive *corneal transplants* from donors. Corneal implants of non-reactive plastic material are also used.

Presbyopia and Cataracts

As people age, their lenses become harder and more flattened. These changes gradually reduce the focusing power of the lenses, a condition known as *presbyopia.* Some people also experience a loss of transparency (cloudiness) of the lens from areas of opaqueness (*cataracts*). *Cataract extraction* is a common operation.

Glaucoma

When drainage of aqueous humor through the scleral venous sinus into the blood circulation is decreased significantly, pressure builds up in the anterior and posterior chambers of the eye, a condition called glaucoma. Blindness can result from compression of the inner layer of the retina and retinal arteries if aqueous humor production is not reduced to maintain normal intraocular pressure.

Extraocular Muscles of Orbit

The **extraocular muscles of the orbit** are the **levator palpebrae superioris**, four **recti** (superior, inferior, medial, and lateral), and two **obliques** (superior and inferior) (Fig. 7.19). These muscles work together to move the superior eyelids and the eyeballs. The attachments, nerve supply, and main actions of the orbital muscles, beginning from the primary position, are described in Table 7.6. Although the actions of the muscles are described separately, in fact extraocular

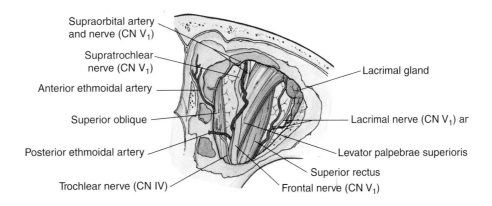

Supraorbital artery and nerve (CN V₁)

Supratrochlear nerve (CN V₁)

Anterior ethmoidal artery

Superior oblique

Posterior ethmoidal artery

Trochlear nerve (CN IV)

Lacrimal gland

Lacrimal nerve (CN V₁) ar

Levator palpebrae superioris

Superior rectus

Frontal nerve (CN V₁)

A **Superior view**

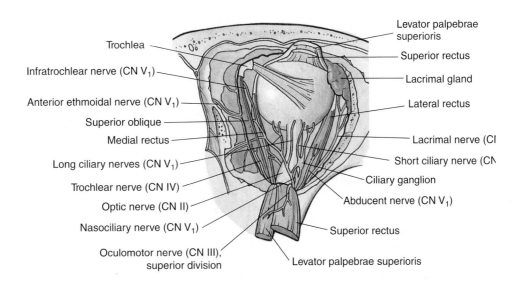

Trochlea

Infratrochlear nerve (CN V₁)

Anterior ethmoidal nerve (CN V₁)

Superior oblique

Medial rectus

Long ciliary nerves (CN V₁)

Trochlear nerve (CN IV)

Optic nerve (CN II)

Nasociliary nerve (CN V₁)

Oculomotor nerve (CN III), superior division

Levator palpebrae superioris

Superior rectus

Lacrimal gland

Lateral rectus

Lacrimal nerve (CI

Short ciliary nerve (CN

Ciliary ganglion

Abducent nerve (CN V₁)

Superior rectus

Levator palpebrae superioris

B **Superior view**

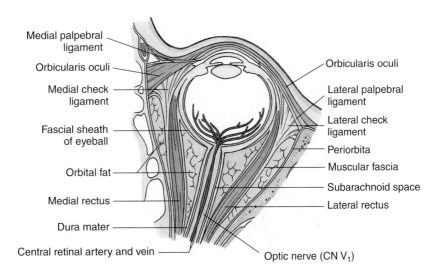

Medial palpebral ligament

Orbicularis oculi

Medial check ligament

Fascial sheath of eyeball

Orbital fat

Medial rectus

Dura mater

Central retinal artery and vein

Orbicularis oculi

Lateral palpebral ligament

Lateral check ligament

Periorbita

Muscular fascia

Subarachnoid space

Lateral rectus

Optic nerve (CN V₁)

C **Horizontal section**

Figure 7.19. Dissections of right orbit. Superficial (**A**) and deep (**B**) dissections show muscles, nerves, and vessels. **C.** Viewed superiorly, this section reveals the fascial sheath of the right eyeball and the check ligaments.

Table 7.6 Muscles of Orbit

Right eyeball

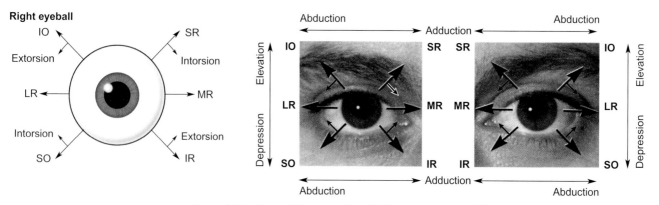

Arrows, direction pupil moves when indicated muscle acts[a]

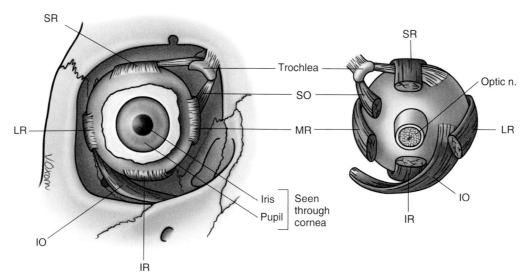

| Anterior view | | | Posterior view |

Muscle	Origin	Insertion	Innervation	Main Action(s)
Levator palpebrae superioris	Lesser wing of sphenoid bone, superior and anterior to optic canal	Superior tarsus and skin of superior eyelid	Oculomotor nerve; deep layer (superior tarsal muscle) supplied by sympathetic fibers	Elevates superior eyelid
Superior oblique (SO)	Body of sphenoid bone	Tendon passes through fibrous ring or trochlea; changes direction and inserts into sclera, deep to superior rectus muscle	Trochlear nerve (CN IV)	Abducts, depresses, and rotates eyeball medially (intorsion)
Inferior oblique (IO)	Anterior part of floor of orbit	Sclera deep to lateral rectus muscle	Oculomotor nerve (CN III)	Abducts, elevates, and rotates eyeball laterally (extorsion)
Superior rectus (SR)	Common tendinous ring	Sclera just posterior to corneoscleral junction		Elevates, adducts, and rotates eyeball medially (intorsion)
Inferior rectus (IR)				Depresses, adducts, and rotates eyeball laterally (extorsion)
Medial rectus (MR)				Adducts eyeball
Lateral rectus (LR)			Abducent nerve (CN VI)	Abducts eyeball

[a]It is essential to appreciate that all muscles are continuously involved in eyeball movements; thus the individual actions are not usually tested clinically. *IO*, inferior oblique (CN III); *IR*, inferior rectus (CN III); *LR*, lateral rectus (CN VI); *MR*, medial rectus (CN III); *SO*, superior oblique (CN IV); *SR*, superior rectus (CN III).

muscles rarely act independently; synergistic and antagonistic activity occurs between the muscles most of the time. Muscles that are synergic for one action may be antagonistic for another.

The four **recti muscles** arise from a fibrous cuff, the **common tendinous ring** (Fig. 7.20A), which surrounds the optic canal and part of the superior orbital fissure. Structures that enter the orbit through this canal and the adjacent part of the fissure lie at first in the cone of recti. The lateral and medial recti lie in the same horizontal plane, and the superior and inferior recti lie in the same vertical plane.

Neither the superior rectus nor the inferior rectus pulls directly parallel to the anteroposterior axis (neutral axis of gaze). As a result, from the primary position both recti tend to move the pupil medially (adduction). This medial pull of the superior and inferior recti normally is balanced by a similar tendency of the **oblique muscles** to move the pupil laterally (abduction). From the primary position, the **inferior oblique** directs the pupil laterally and superiorly; therefore, when the superior rectus and inferior oblique work synergistically, pure elevation of the pupil occurs. Similarly, the **superior oblique** directs the pupil inferiorly and laterally;

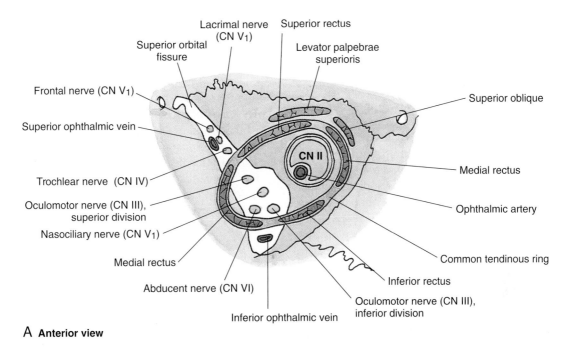

A **Anterior view**

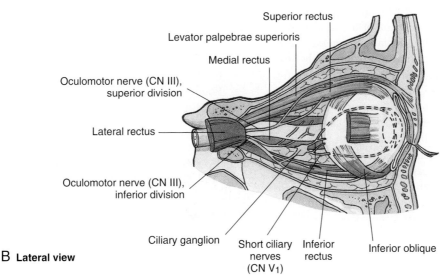

B **Lateral view**

Figure 7.20. Muscles and nerves of orbit. A. The structures in the apex of the right orbit are identified. **B.** The lateral rectus has been reflected to show the ciliary ganglion.

therefore, when the superior oblique works synergistically with the inferior rectus, pure depression results. When the pupil is already in the adducted position (as in the convergence involved in close reading), the oblique muscles are responsible for elevation (inferior oblique) and depression (superior oblique), moving the gaze up or down the page. Elevation and depression in the adducted position are the primary functions of the oblique muscles.

In addition to these four movements around the horizontal and vertical axes, the superior and inferior recti and obliques cause rotation of the eyeball around an anteroposterior axis. Medial movement of the superior pole of the eyeball is **intorsion**; lateral movement of the superior pole is **extorsion**. These movements accommodate changes in the tilt of the head. Absence of these movements resulting from nerve lesions contributes to double vision.

To direct the gaze, coordination of both eyes must be accomplished by the paired action of contralateral *yoke muscles*. For example, in directing the gaze to the right, the right lateral rectus and left medial rectus act as yoke muscles.

The **levator palpebrae superioris** broadens into a wide aponeurosis as it approaches its distal attachments (Fig. 7.19*B*). The superficial lamina attaches to the skin of the superior eyelid and the deep lamina to the superior tarsus. This muscle is opposed most of the time by gravity and is the antagonist of the superior half of the orbicularis oculi, the sphincter of the palpebral fissure. The deep lamina includes smooth muscle fibers, the **superior tarsal muscle**, which produce additional widening of the palpebral fissure during sympathetic response (e.g., fright).

The **fascial sheath of the eyeball** (bulbar sheath, Tenon capsule) envelops the eyeball from the optic nerve nearly to the corneoscleral junction (Fig. 7.19*C*). The facial sheath is pierced by the tendons of the extraocular muscles and is reflected onto each of them as a tubular *muscle sheath*. Triangular expansions from the sheaths of the medial and lateral rectus muscles, called the medial and lateral **check ligaments**, are attached to the lacrimal and zygomatic bones, respectively, limiting abduction and adduction. A blending of the check ligaments with the fascia of the inferior rectus and inferior oblique muscles forms a hammock-like sling, the **suspensory ligament of the eyeball**. A potential **episcleral space** between the eyeball and the fascial sheath allows the eyeball to move inside the cup-like sheath. A similar check ligament from the fascial sheath of the inferior rectus retracts the inferior eyelid when the gaze is directed downward. Because the sheaths of the superior rectus and levator palpebrae superioris are fused, the superior eyelid is elevated when the gaze is directed upward.

Nerves of Orbit

The **nerves of the orbit**, in addition to the *optic nerve* (CN II), are those that enter through the *superior orbital fissure* and supply the ocular muscles (Figs. 7.19 and 7.20):

oculomotor (CN III), trochlear (CN IV), and abducent (CN VI). In summary, all muscles of the orbit are supplied by CN III, except the superior oblique and lateral rectus, which are supplied by CN IV and CN VI, respectively. A memory device is as follows: LR_6, SO_4, AO_3 (lateral rectus, CN VI, superior oblique, CN IV, all others, CN III).

Three branches of the *ophthalmic nerve* (CN V_1) that pass through the superior orbital fissure and supply structures in the orbit are:

* The **lacrimal nerve**, which arises in the lateral wall of the cavernous sinus and passes to the lacrimal gland, giving sensory branches to the conjunctiva and skin of the superior eyelid; its distal part also carries secretomotor fibers conveyed to it from the zygomatic nerve (CN V_2).
* The **frontal nerve**, which enters the orbit through the superior orbital fissure and divides into the supraorbital and supratrochlear nerves, providing sensory innervation to the superior eyelid, scalp, and forehead.
* The **nasociliary nerve**, the sensory nerve to the eyeball, which also supplies several branches to the orbit, face, paranasal sinuses, nasal cavity, and anterior cranial fossa. The **infratrochlear nerve**, a terminal branch of the nasociliary nerve, supplies the eyelids, conjunctiva, skin of the nose, and lacrimal sac. The anterior and posterior **ethmoidal nerves**, also branches of the nasociliary nerve, supply the mucous membrane of the sphenoidal and ethmoidal sinuses and the nasal cavities and dura mater of the anterior cranial fossa. The **long ciliary nerves** are branches of the nasociliary nerve (CN V_1). The **short ciliary nerves** are branches of the ciliary ganglion (Fig. 7.19*B*).

The **ciliary ganglion** is a small group of postsynaptic parasympathetic nerve cell bodies associated with CN V_1. It is located between the optic nerve and the lateral rectus toward the posterior limit of the orbit (Fig. 7.20*B*). The ganglion receives fibers from three sources:

* Sensory fibers from CN V_1 via the communicating branch of the nasociliary nerve.
* Presynaptic parasympathetic fibers from CN III.
* Postsynaptic sympathetic fibers from the internal carotid plexus.

The *short ciliary nerves* consist of postsynaptic parasympathetic fibers originating in the ciliary ganglion, afferent fibers from the nasociliary nerve that pass through the ganglion, and postsynaptic sympathetic fibers that also pass through the ganglion. The *long ciliary nerves* convey postsynaptic sympathetic fibers to the dilator pupillae and afferent fibers from the iris and cornea.

Vasculature of Orbit

The **arteries of the orbit** are mainly from the **ophthalmic artery**, a branch of the internal carotid artery (Table 7.7); the **infraorbital artery**, from the external carotid artery,

Table 7.7 Arteries of Orbit

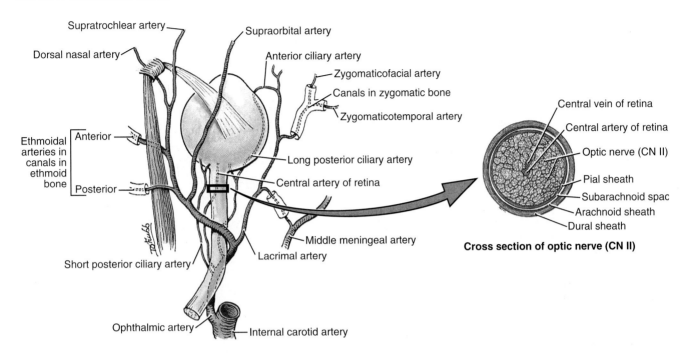

Superior view

Cross section of optic nerve (CN II)

Artery	Origin	Course and Distribution
Ophthalmic	Internal carotid artery	Traverses optic canal to reach orbital cavity
Central artery of retina		Pierces dural sheath and runs in optic nerve to eyeball; branches in center of opticdisc; supplies optic retina (except cones and rods)
Supraorbital		Passes superiorly and posteriorly from supraorbital foramen to supply forehead and scalp
Supratrochlear		Passes from supraorbital margin to forehead and scalp
Lacrimal		Passes along superior border of lateral rectus muscle to supply lacrimal gland, conjunctiva, and eyelids
Dorsal nasal	Ophthalmic artery	Courses along dorsal aspect of nose and supplies its surface
Short posterior ciliaries		Pierces sclera at periphery of optic nerve to supply choroid, which in turn supplies cones and rods of optic retina
Long posterior ciliaries		Pierces sclera to supply ciliary body and iris
Posterior ethmoidal		Passes through posterior ethmoidal foramen to posterior ethmoidal cells
Anterior ethmoidal		Passes through anterior ethmoidal foramen to supply anterior and middle ethmoidal cells, frontal sinus, nasal cavity, and skin on dorsum of nose
Anterior ciliary	Muscular branches of ophthalmic artery	Pierces sclera at attachments of rectus muscles and forms network in iris and ciliary body
Infraorbital	Third part of maxillary artery	Passes along infraorbital groove and foramen to face

Oculomotor and Abducent Nerve Palsy

Complete oculomotor nerve palsy affects most of the ocular muscles, the levator palpebrae superioris, and the sphincter pupillae. The superior eyelid droops (ptosis) and cannot be raised voluntarily because of the unopposed activity of the orbicularis oculi (supplied by the facial nerve). The pupil is also fully dilated and non-reactive because of the unopposed dilator pupillae. The pupil is fully abducted and depressed ("down and out") because of the unopposed activity of the lateral rectus and superior oblique, respectively (Fig. B7.7*A*).

A lesion of the abducent nerve results in loss of lateral gaze to the ipsilateral side because of paralysis of the lateral rectus muscle. On forward gaze, the eye is diverted medially because of the lack of normal resting tone in the lateral rectus, resulting in diplopia (double vision) (Fig. B7.7*B*).

Paralysis of Extraocular Muscles

One or more extraocular muscles may be paralyzed by disease in the brainstem or by head injury; this results in *diplopia* (double vision). Paralysis of a muscle is apparent by limitation of eye movement in the field of action of the muscle and by the production of two images (diplopia) when one attempts to use the muscle.

Horner Syndrome

Horner syndrome results from interruption of a cervical sympathetic trunk and is manifest by the absence of sympathetically stimulated functions on the ipsilateral side of the head. The syndrome includes the following signs: constriction of the pupil (miosis), drooping of the superior eyelid (ptosis), redness and increased temperature of the skin (vasodilatation), and absence of sweating (anhydrosis).

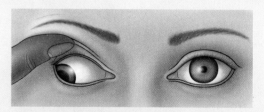

Right eye: Downward and outward gaze, dilated pupil, eyelid manually elevated due to ptosis   Left

Right oculomotor (CN III) nerve palsy

A

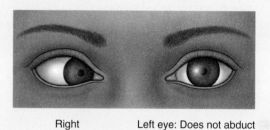

Right   Left eye: Does not abduct

Direction of gaze ⟶

Left abducent (CN VI) nerve palsy

B

Figure B7.7

also contributes to the supply of this region. The **central retinal artery**, a branch of the ophthalmic artery arising inferior to the optic nerve, pierces the dural sheath of the optic nerve and runs within the nerve to the eyeball, emerging at the optic disc (Fig. 7.19*C*). Branches of this artery spread over the internal surface of the retina. The terminal branches of the central retinal artery are *end arteries,* which provide the only blood supply to the internal aspect of the retina.

The external aspect of the retina is also supplied by the **capillary lamina of the choroid** (Fig. 7.18*B*). Of the eight or so posterior ciliary arteries (also branches of the ophthalmic artery), six **short posterior ciliary arteries** directly supply the choroid, which nourishes the outer nonvascular layer of the retina. Two **long posterior ciliary arteries**, one on each side of the eyeball, pass between the sclera and the choroid to anastomose with the **anterior ciliary arteries** (continuations of the **muscular branches of the ophthalmic artery** to the rectus muscles) to supply the ciliary plexus.

Venous drainage of the orbit is through the **superior** and **inferior ophthalmic veins**, which pass through the superior orbital fissure and enter the cavernous sinus (Fig. 7.21). The inferior ophthalmic vein also drains to the pterygoid

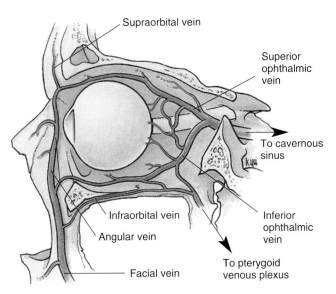

Figure 7.21. **Veins of right orbit.**

Labels on figure: Supraorbital vein; Superior ophthalmic vein; To cavernous sinus; Inferior ophthalmic vein; Infraorbital vein; Angular vein; Facial vein; To pterygoid venous plexus

venous plexus. The **central vein of the retina** usually enters the cavernous sinus directly, but it may join one of the ophthalmic veins (Fig 7.19C). The **vorticose veins** from the vascular layer of the eyeball drain into the inferior ophthalmic vein (Fig. 7.18A). The **scleral venous sinus** is a vascular structure encircling the anterior chamber of the eyeball through which the aqueous humor is returned to the blood circulation (Fig. 7.18B).

Blockage of Central Retinal Artery

Because terminal branches of the central retinal artery are end arteries, obstruction of them by an embolus results in instant and total blindness. Blockage of the artery is usually unilateral and occurs in older people.

Blockage of Central Retinal Vein

Because the central vein of the retina enters the cavernous sinus, *thrombophlebitis* of this sinus may result in passage of a thrombus to the central retinal vein and produce a blockage in one of the small retinal veins. Occlusion of a branch of the central vein of the retina usually results in slow, painless loss of vision.

Temporal Region

The **temporal region** includes the temporal and infratemporal fossae—superior and inferior to the zygomatic arch, respectively (Fig. 7.22).

Temporal Fossa

The **temporal fossa** (Fig. 7.22A & C), in which most of the temporal muscle (L. *temporalis*) is located, is bounded:

- Posteriorly and superiorly by the superior and inferior temporal lines.
- Anteriorly by the frontal and zygomatic bones.
- Laterally by the zygomatic arch.
- Inferiorly by the infratemporal crest.

The *floor of the temporal fossa* is formed by parts of the four bones (frontal, parietal, temporal, and greater wing of the sphenoid) that form the **pterion**. The fan-shaped **temporal muscle** arises from the bony floor and the overlying **temporal fascia**, which makes up the *roof of the temporal fossa* (Fig. 7.24; Table 7.8). The temporal fascia extends from the *superior temporal line* to the zygomatic arch. When the powerful masseter, attached to the inferior border of the arch, contracts and exerts a strong downward pull on the arch, the temporal fascia provides resistance.

Infratemporal Fossa

The **infratemporal fossa** is an irregularly shaped space deep and inferior to the zygomatic arch, deep to the ramus of the mandible, and posterior to the maxilla. The *boundaries of the fossa* are (Fig. 7.22B)

- Laterally: ramus of the mandible.
- Medially: lateral pterygoid plate.
- Anteriorly: posterior aspect of the maxilla.
- Posteriorly: tympanic plate and the mastoid and styloid processes of the temporal bone.
- Superiorly: inferior surface of the greater wing of the sphenoid bone.
- Inferiorly: where the medial pterygoid muscle attaches to the mandible near its angle (Table 7.8).

The *contents of the infratemporal fossa* are (Fig. 7.23)

- Inferior part of the temporal muscle.
- Lateral and medial pterygoid muscles.
- Maxillary artery.
- Pterygoid venous plexus.
- Mandibular, inferior alveolar, lingual, buccal, and chorda tympani nerves, and the otic ganglion.

The **temporal muscle** has a broad proximal attachment to the floor of the temporal fossa and is attached distally to the tip and medial surface of the coronoid process and

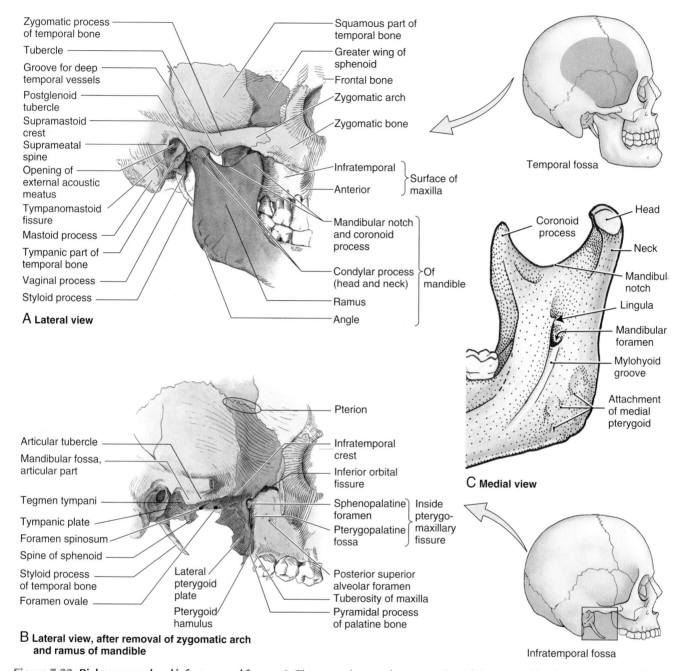

Figure 7.22. Right temporal and infratemporal fossae. A. The space deep to the zygomatic arch is traversed by the temporal muscle and deep temporal nerves and vessels. Through this interval, the temporal fossa communicates freely with the infratemporal fossa. **B.** The bony boundaries of the infratemporal fossa are shown. The mandible and most of the zygomatic arch have been removed. **C.** The ramus of the mandible is detailed.

anterior border of the ramus of the mandible (Fig. 7.23; Table 7.8). It elevates the mandible (closes the lower jaw); its posterior fibers retrude (retract) the protruded mandible.

The two-headed **lateral pterygoid muscle** passes posteriorly. Its upper head attaches to the joint capsule and disc of the TMJ, and the lower head attaches primarily

to the pterygoid fovea at the condylar process of the mandible.

The **medial pterygoid muscle** lies on the medial aspect of the ramus of the mandible. Its two heads embrace the inferior head of the lateral pterygoid and then unite (Fig. 7.23A). The medial pterygoid passes inferoposteriorly and attaches to the medial surface of the mandible near its

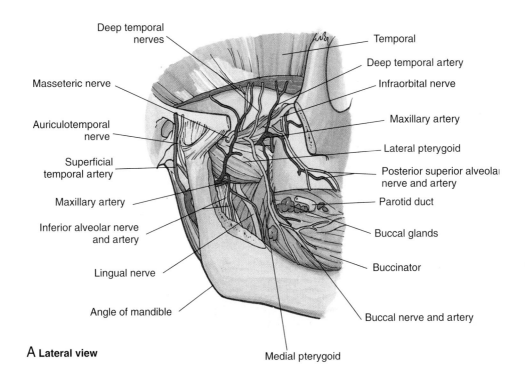

Deep temporal nerves

Masseteric nerve

Auriculotemporal nerve

Superficial temporal artery

Maxillary artery

Inferior alveolar nerve and artery

Lingual nerve

Angle of mandible

Temporal

Deep temporal artery

Infraorbital nerve

Maxillary artery

Lateral pterygoid

Posterior superior alveolar nerve and artery

Parotid duct

Buccal glands

Buccinator

Buccal nerve and artery

A Lateral view

Medial pterygoid

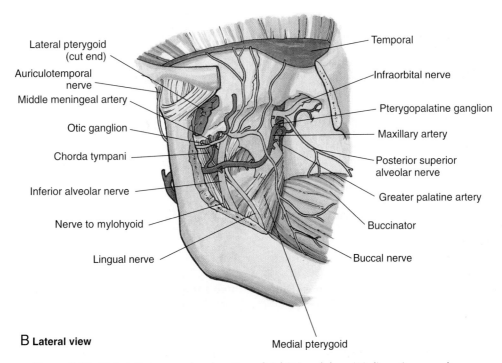

Lateral pterygoid (cut end)

Auriculotemporal nerve

Middle meningeal artery

Otic ganglion

Chorda tympani

Inferior alveolar nerve

Nerve to mylohyoid

Lingual nerve

Temporal

Infraorbital nerve

Pterygopalatine ganglion

Maxillary artery

Posterior superior alveolar nerve

Greater palatine artery

Buccinator

Buccal nerve

B Lateral view

Medial pterygoid

Figure 7.23. Right infratemporal region. Superficial (**A**) and deep (**B**) dissections are shown.

Table 7.8 Muscles of Mastication Acting on the Mandible/Temporomandibular Joint (TMJ)

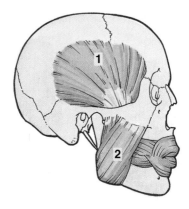 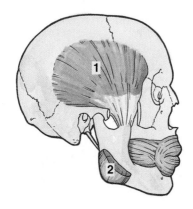 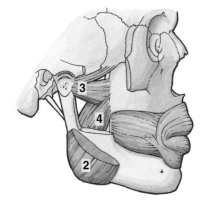

Lateral views

Muscle(s)[a]	Proximal Attachment	Distal Attachment	Innervation		Action on Mandible
Temporal (1)	Triangular muscle with broad attachment to floor of temporal fossa and deep surface of temporal fascia	Narrow attachment to tip and medial surface of coronoid process and anterior border of ramus of mandible		Via deep temporal nerves	Elevates mandible, closing jaws; posterior, more horizontal fibers are retractors of mandible
Masseter (2)	Quadrate muscle attaching to inferior border and medial surface of maxillary process of zygomatic bone and the zygomatic arch	Angle and lateral surface of ramus of mandible		Via masseteric nerve	Elevates mandible; superficial fibers make limited contribution to protrusion of mandible
Lateral pterygoid (3)	Triangular two-headed muscle from (a) infratemporal surface and crest of greater wing of sphenoid and (b) lateral surface of lateral pterygoid plate	Superior head attaches primarily to joint capsule and articular disk of TMJ; inferior head attaches primarily to pterygoid fovea on anteromedial aspect of neck of condyloid process of mandible	Anterior trunk of mandibular nerve (CN V_3)	Via nerves to lateral pterygoid	Acting bilaterally, protracts mandible and depresses chin; acting unilaterally, swings jaw toward contralateral side; alternate unilateral contraction produces larger lateral chewing movements
Medial pterygoid (4)	Quadrangular two-headed muscle from (a) medial surface of lateral pterygoid plate and pyramidal process of palatine bone and (b) tuberosity of maxilla	Medial surface of ramus of mandible, inferior to mandibular foramen; in essence, a "mirror image" of the ipsilateral masseter, the two muscles flanking the ramus		Via nerve to medial pterygoid	Acts synergistically with masseter to elevate mandible; contributes to protrusion; alternate unilateral activity produces smaller grinding movements

[a] Numbers refer to the figures

angle. The attachments, nerve supply, and actions of the pterygoid muscles are described in Table 7.8.

The **maxillary artery,** *the larger of the two terminal branches of the external carotid artery,* arises posterior to the neck of the mandible, courses anteriorly deep to the neck of the mandibular condyle, and then passes superficial or deep to the lateral pterygoid (Figs. 7.23 and 7.24A). The artery passes medially from the infratemporal fossa through the **pterygomaxillary fissure** to enter the **pterygopalatine fossa** (Fig. 7.25). The maxillary artery is thus divided into three parts by its relation to the lateral pterygoid muscle (Figs. 7.24A and 7.25B).

Branches of the first, or retromandibular, part of the maxillary artery are the:

- *Deep auricular artery,* supplying the external acoustic meatus.
- *Anterior tympanic artery,* supplying the tympanic membrane.
- *Middle meningeal artery,* supplying the dura mater and calvaria.

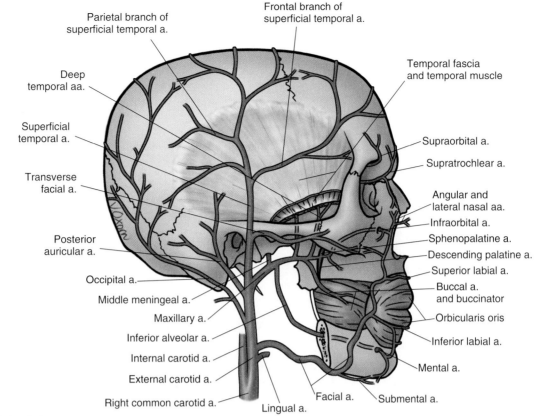

A **Lateral view**

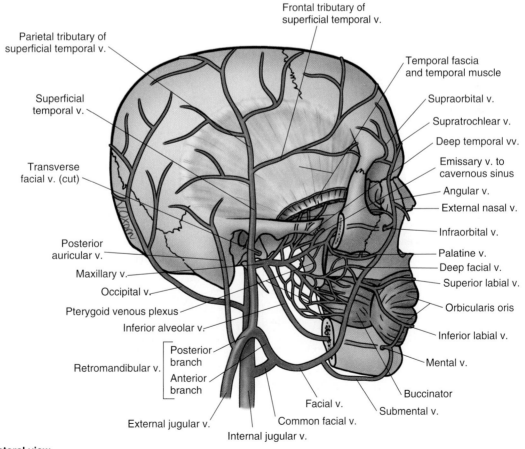

B **Lateral view**

Figure 7.24. Vasculature of head. A. The external carotid artery and its branches are identified. **B.** The venous drainage of the face, scalp and infratemporal fossa is shown.

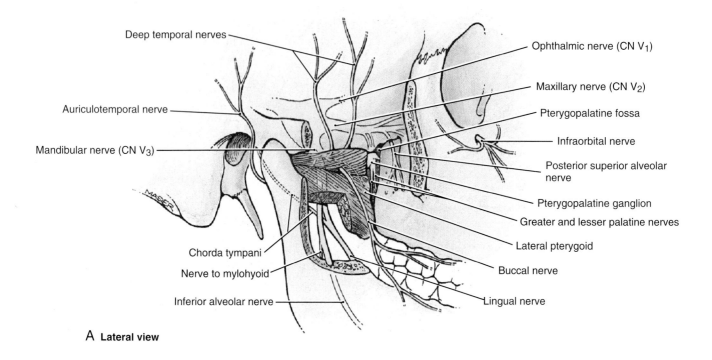

Deep temporal nerves

Ophthalmic nerve (CN V₁)

Maxillary nerve (CN V₂)

Auriculotemporal nerve

Pterygopalatine fossa

Infraorbital nerve

Mandibular nerve (CN V₃)

Posterior superior alveolar nerve

Pterygopalatine ganglion

Greater and lesser palatine nerves

Lateral pterygoid

Chorda tympani

Buccal nerve

Nerve to mylohyoid

Inferior alveolar nerve

Lingual nerve

A Lateral view

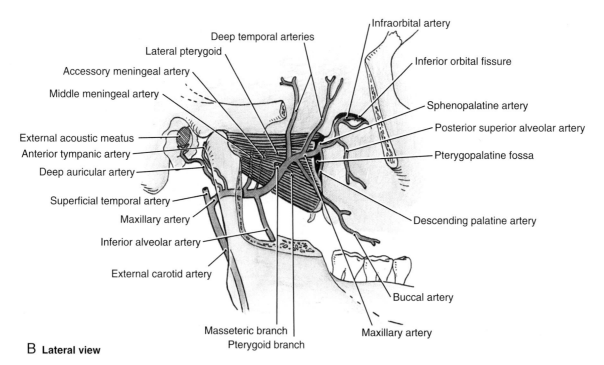

Deep temporal arteries

Infraorbital artery

Lateral pterygoid

Inferior orbital fissure

Accessory meningeal artery

Middle meningeal artery

Sphenopalatine artery

External acoustic meatus

Posterior superior alveolar artery

Anterior tympanic artery

Pterygopalatine fossa

Deep auricular artery

Superficial temporal artery

Maxillary artery

Descending palatine artery

Inferior alveolar artery

External carotid artery

Buccal artery

Masseteric branch

Maxillary artery

Pterygoid branch

B Lateral view

Figure 7.25. Mandibular division of trigeminal nerve and maxillary artery. A. The innervation of the mandible is shown. **B.** The branches of the maxillary artery are identified.

- *Accessory meningeal arteries,* supplying the cranial cavity.
- *Inferior alveolar artery,* which supplies the mandible, gingivae (gums), teeth, and floor of the mouth.

Branches of the second, or pterygoid part, of the maxillary artery are the:

- *Deep temporal arteries,* anterior and posterior, which ascend to supply the temporal muscle.
- *Pterygoid arteries,* which supply the pterygoid muscles.
- *Masseteric artery,* which passes laterally through the mandibular notch to supply the masseter muscle.
- *Buccal artery,* which supplies the buccinator muscle and mucosa of the cheek.

Branches of the third, or pterygopalatine, part of the maxillary artery are the:

- *Posterior superior alveolar artery,* supplying the maxillary molar and premolar teeth, the buccal gingiva, and the lining of the maxillary sinus.
- *Infraorbital artery,* supplying the inferior eyelid, lacrimal sac, infraorbital region of the face, side of the nose, and the upper lip.
- *Descending palatine artery,* supplying the mucous membrane and glands of the palate (roof of the mouth) and palatine gingiva.
- *Artery of pterygoid canal,* supplying the superior part of the pharynx, the pharyngotympanic (auditory) tube, and the tympanic cavity.
- *Pharyngeal artery,* supplying the roof of the pharynx, the sphenoidal sinus, and the inferior part of the pharyngotympanic tube.
- *Sphenopalatine artery,* the termination of the maxillary artery, which supplies the lateral nasal wall, the nasal septum, and the adjacent paranasal sinuses.

The **pterygoid venous plexus** occupies most of the infratemporal fossa (Fig. 7.24*B*). It is located partly between the temporal and pterygoid muscles. The plexus drains anteriorly to the facial vein via the deep facial vein but mainly drains posteriorly via the maxillary and then the retromandibular veins.

The **mandibular nerve** (CN V$_3$) receives the motor root of the trigeminal nerve (CN V) and descends through the foramen ovale to enter the infratemporal fossa, dividing into anterior and posterior trunks (Fig. 7.23*B*). The branches of the large posterior trunk are the auriculotemporal, inferior alveolar, and lingual nerves (Figs. 7.23 and 7.25*A*). The smaller anterior division gives rise to the **buccal nerve** and branches to the four muscles of mastication (temporal, masseter, and medial and lateral pterygoids) but not the buccinator, which is supplied by the facial nerve (CN VII).

The **otic ganglion** (parasympathetic) is in the infratemporal fossa (Fig. 7.23*B*), just inferior to the foramen ovale, medial to the mandibular nerve, and posterior to the lateral pterygoid muscle. Presynaptic parasympathetic fibers, derived mainly from the glossopharyngeal nerve (CN IX), synapse in the otic ganglion. Postsynaptic parasympathetic fibers, which are secretory to the parotid gland, pass from the ganglion to this gland through the auriculotemporal nerve.

The **auriculotemporal nerve** arises via two roots that encircle the middle meningeal artery and then unite into a single trunk (Figs. 7.23 and 7.25). The trunk divides into numerous branches, the largest of which passes posteriorly, medial to the neck of the mandible and supplies sensory fibers to the auricle and temporal region. The auriculotemporal nerve also sends articular fibers to the TMJ and parasympathetic secretomotor fibers to the parotid gland.

The **inferior alveolar nerve** enters the mandibular foramen and passes through the mandibular canal, forming the **inferior dental plexus**, which sends branches to all mandibular teeth on that side. The *nerve to mylohyoid*, a small branch of the inferior alveolar nerve, is given off just before the nerve enters the mandibular foramen (Fig. 7.25*A*). A branch of the inferior dental plexus, the **mental**

Mandibular Nerve Block

To perform a mandibular nerve block, an anesthetic agent is injected near the mandibular nerve where it enters the infratemporal fossa. This block usually anesthetizes the auriculotemporal, inferior alveolar, lingual, and buccal branches of the mandibular nerve.

Inferior Alveolar Nerve Block

An perform alveolar nerve block—commonly used by dentists when repairing mandibular teeth—anesthetizes the inferior alveolar nerve, a branch of CN V$_3$. The anesthetic agent is injected around the **mandibular foramen,** the opening into the **mandibular canal** on the medial aspect of the ramus of the mandible. This canal gives passage to the inferior alveolar nerve, artery, and vein (Fig. 7.28). When this nerve block is successful, all mandibular teeth are anesthetized to the median plane. The skin and mucous membrane of the lower lip, the labial alveolar mucosa and gingiva, and the skin of the chin are also anesthetized because they are supplied by the mental branch of this nerve.

nerve, passes through the mental foramen and supplies the skin and mucous membrane of the lower lip, the skin of the chin, and the vestibular gingiva of the mandibular incisor teeth (see Fig. 7.29*A*).

The **lingual nerve** lies anterior to the inferior alveolar nerve (Figs. 7.23 and 7.25). It is sensory to the anterior two thirds of the tongue, the floor of the mouth, and the lingual gingivae. It enters the mouth between the medial pterygoid and the ramus of the mandible and passes anteriorly under cover of the oral mucosa, just inferior to the 3rd molar tooth.

The **chorda tympani nerve**, a branch of CN VII (Fig. 7.25*A*), carries taste fibers from the anterior two thirds of the tongue and presynaptic parasympathetic secretomotor fibers for the submandibular and sublingual salivary glands. The chorda tympani joins the lingual nerve in the infratemporal fossa.

Temporomandibular Joint

The **temporomandibular joint (TMJ)** is a modified hinge-type of synovial joint, permitting movement in three planes. The articular surfaces involved are the **head of the mandible**, the **articular tubercle** of the temporal bone, and the **mandibular fossa** (Fig. 7.26*A* & *B*). The articular surfaces of the TMJ are covered by fibrocartilage rather than hyaline cartilage as in a typical synovial joint. An **articular disc** divides the joint cavity into two separate synovial compartments. The **joint capsule** of the TMJ is loose. The fibrous layer of the capsule attaches to the margins of the articular area on the temporal bone and around the neck of the mandible. The thick part of the joint capsule forms the intrinsic **lateral ligament** (temporomandibular ligament), which strengthens the TMJ laterally and, with the **postglenoid tubercle**, acts to prevent posterior dislocation of the joint (Fig. 7.26*C*).

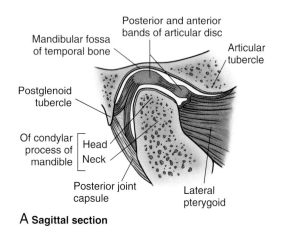

A Sagittal section

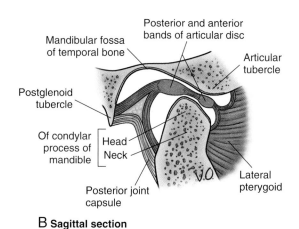

B Sagittal section

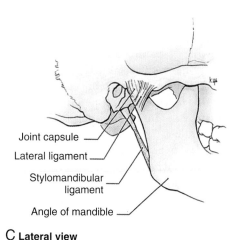

C Lateral view

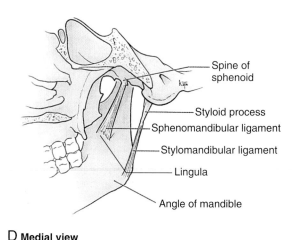

D Medial view

Figure 7.26. Right temporomandibular joint. The joint is shown with the mouth closed (**A**) and open (**B**). **C and D.** The ligaments of the joint are identified.

Two extrinsic ligaments and the lateral ligament connect the mandible to the cranium. The **stylomandibular ligament**, a thickening of the fibrous capsule of the parotid gland, runs from the styloid process to the angle of the mandible (Fig. 7.26*D*). It does not contribute significantly to the strength of the TMJ. The **sphenomandibular ligament** runs from the spine of the sphenoid to the lingula of the mandible.

To enable more than a small amount of depression of the mandible—that is, to open the mouth wider than just separating the upper and lower teeth (Fig. 7.26*B*), the head of the mandible and articular disc must move anteriorly on the articular surface until the head lies inferior to the articular tubercle (a movement referred to as *translation* by dentists). If this anterior gliding occurs unilaterally, the head of the mandible on the retracted side rotates (pivots) on the inferior surface of the articular disc, permitting simple side-to-side chewing or grinding movements over a small range. During protrusion and retrusion of the mandible, the mandibular head and articular disc slide anteriorly and posteriorly on the articular surface of the temporal bone, with both sides moving together. TMJ movements are produced chiefly by the muscles of mastication. The attachments, nerve supply, and actions of these muscles are described in Tables 7.8 and 7.9.

Oral Region

The **oral region** includes the oral cavity (mouth), teeth, gingivae (gums), tongue, palate, and the region of the palatine tonsils. The oral cavity is where food is ingested and prepared for digestion in the stomach and small intestine. When food is chewed, the teeth and saliva from the salivary glands facilitate the formation of a manageable *food bolus* (L. lump).

Dislocation of TMJ

Sometimes during yawning or taking a large bite, excessive contraction of the lateral pterygoids may cause the heads of the mandibles to dislocate anteriorly (pass anterior to the articular tubercles). In this position, the mandible remains depressed and the person may not be able to close their mouth. Most commonly, a sideways blow to the chin when the mouth is open dislocates the TMJ on the side that received the blow. *Fracture(s) of the mandible* may be accompanied by dislocation of the TMJ. Because of the close relationship of the facial and auriculotemporal nerves to the TMJ, care must be taken during surgical procedures to preserve both the branches of the facial nerve overlying it and the articular branches of the auriculotemporal nerve that enter the posterior part of the joint. Injury to articular branches of the auriculotemporal nerve supplying the TMJ—associated with traumatic dislocation and rupture of the joint capsule and lateral ligament—leads to laxity and instability of the TMJ.

Oral Cavity

The **oral cavity** consists of two parts: the *oral vestibule* and the *oral cavity proper* (Fig. 7.27). The oral vestibule communicates with the exterior through the mouth. The size of the **oral fissure** opening (L. *rima oris*) is controlled by muscles such as the orbicularis oris (the sphincter of the oral fissure). The **oral cavity proper** is the space posterior and medial to the upper and lower **dental arches.** It is limited laterally and anteriorly by the maxillary and mandibular alveolar arches housing the teeth. The *roof of the oral cavity* is formed by the palate. Posteriorly, the oral cavity communicates with the **oropharynx,** the oral part of the pharynx. When the mouth is closed and at rest, the oral cavity is fully occupied by the tongue.

Oral Vestibule

The **oral vestibule** is the slit-like space between the lips and cheeks superficially and the teeth and gingivae deeply. The **lips,** the mobile, fleshy muscular folds surrounding

Table 7.9 Movements at the Temporomandibular Joint

Movements of Mandible	Muscles
Elevation (close mouth)	Temporal, masseter, and medial pterygoid
Depression (open mouth)	Lateral pterygoid and suprahyoid and infrahyoid muscles[a]
Protrusion (protrude chin)	Lateral pterygoid, masseter, and medial pterygoid[b]
Retrusion (retrude chin)	Temporal (posterior oblique and near horizontal fibers) and masseter
Lateral movements (grinding and chewing)	Temporal of same side, pterygoids of opposite side, and masseter

[a] The prime mover is normally gravity; these muscles are mainly active against resistance.
[b] The lateral pterygoid is the prime mover here, with minor secondary roles played by the masseter and medial pterygoid.

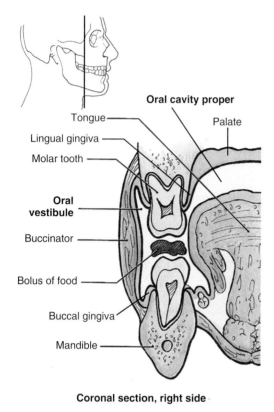

Oral cavity proper

Tongue

Palate

Lingual gingiva

Molar tooth

**Oral
vestibule**

Buccinator

Bolus of food

Buccal gingiva

Mandible

Coronal section, right side

Figure 7.27. Oral cavity.

the mouth, contain the orbicularis oris and superior and inferior labial muscles, vessels, and nerves. They are covered externally by skin and internally by mucous membrane. The upper lip has a vertical groove, the **philtrum** (Fig. 7.28). As the skin of the lips approaches the mouth, it changes color abruptly to red; this red margin of the lips is the **vermillion border**, a transitional zone between the skin and mucous membrane. The skin of the **transitional**

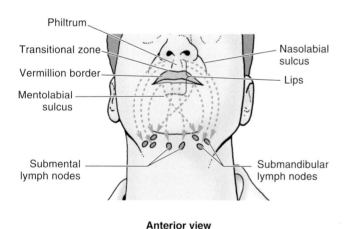

Philtrum

Transitional zone

Vermillion border

Mentolabial
sulcus

Nasolabial
sulcus

Lips

Submental
lymph nodes

Submandibular
lymph nodes

Anterior view

Figure 7.28. Surface anatomy and lymphatic drainage of cheeks, lips, and chin.

zone of the lips is hairless and so thin that it appears red because of the underlying capillary bed. The upper lip is supplied by superior labial branches of the **facial** and **infraorbital arteries**. The lower lip is supplied by inferior labial branches of the **facial** and **mental arteries**. The upper lip is supplied by the superior labial branches of the **infraorbital nerves** (CN V_2), and the lower lip is supplied by the inferior labial branches of the mental nerves (CN V_3).

Lymph from the upper lip and lateral parts of the lower lip passes primarily to the **submandibular lymph nodes** (Fig. 7.28), whereas lymph from the medial part of the lower lip passes initially to the **submental lymph nodes**.

The **cheeks** (L. *buccae*) include the lateral distensible walls of the oral cavity and the facial prominences over the zygomatic bones. The cheeks have essentially the same structure as the lips, with which they are continuous. The principal muscles of the cheeks are the **buccinators** (Fig. 7.27). The lips and cheeks function as an oral sphincter that pushes food from the oral vestibule into the oral cavity proper. The tongue and buccinators work together to keep the food between the occlusal surfaces of the molar teeth during chewing. The labial and **buccal glands** are small mucous glands between the mucous membrane and the underlying orbicularis oris and buccinator muscles (Fig. 7.23A).

The **gingivae** (gums) are composed of fibrous tissue covered with mucous membrane, which is firmly attached to the alveolar processes of the mandible and maxilla and the necks of the teeth. The **buccal gingivae** of the mandibular molar teeth are supplied by the **buccal nerve**, a branch of the mandibular nerve (Fig. 7.25B). The **lingual gingivae** of all mandibular teeth are supplied by the lingual nerve. The **palatine gingivae** of the maxillary premolar and molar teeth are supplied by the **greater palatine nerve**; and the palatine gingivae of the incisors, by the **nasopalatine nerve** (Fig. 7.31B). The labial and buccal aspects of the maxillary gingivae are supplied by the anterior, middle, and posterior **superior alveolar nerves** (Fig. 7.29A).

Teeth

The **teeth** are hard conical structures set in the **dental alveoli** (tooth sockets) of the upper and lower jaws and are used in mastication (chewing) and assisting in articulation. Children have *20 deciduous (primary) teeth*. The first tooth usually erupts at 6–8 months of age and the last tooth by 20–24 months of age. Eruption of the *permanent (secondary) teeth*, normally 16 in each jaw (3 molars, 2 premolars, 1 canine, and 2 incisors on each side), usually is complete by the midteens (Fig. 7.29C), except for the third molars ("wisdom teeth"), which usually erupt during the late teens or early 20s.

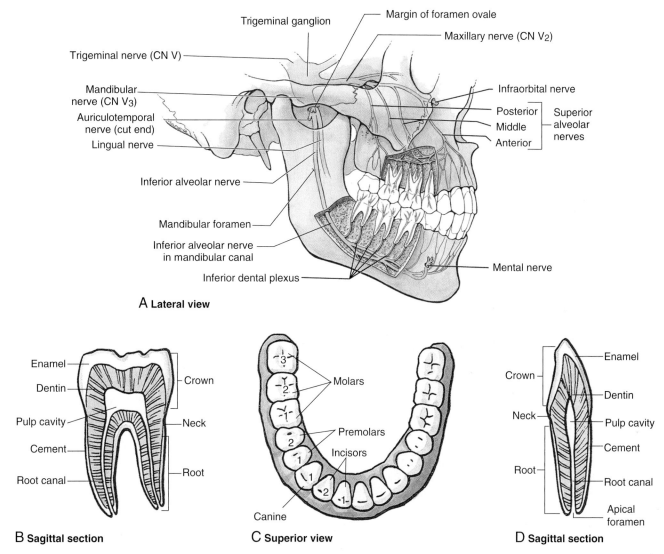

Figure 7.29. Teeth. A. The alveolar nerves and innervation of the teeth are shown. **B.** A typical molar tooth is detailed. **C.** The adult mandibular dentition is shown. **D.** An incisor tooth is detailed.

A tooth has a crown, neck, and root. Each type of tooth has a characteristic appearance (Fig. 7.29B & D). The **crown** projects from the gingiva. The **neck** is the part of the tooth between the crown and the root. The **root** is fixed in the alveolus (tooth socket) by the fibrous *periodontium* (periodontal membrane). Most of the tooth is composed of **dentin** (L. *dentinium*), which is covered by **enamel** over the crown and **cement** (L. *cementum*) over the root. The **pulp cavity** contains connective tissue, blood vessels, and nerves. The **root canal** (pulp canal) transmits the nerves and vessels to and from the pulp cavity through the **apical foramen**.

The **superior** and **inferior alveolar arteries**, branches of the **maxillary artery**, supply the maxillary (upper) and the mandibular (lower) teeth, respectively (Fig. 7.25B). **Veins** with the same names and distribution accompany the arteries (Fig. 7.24B). **Lymphatic vessels** from the teeth and gingivae pass mainly to the **submandibular lymph nodes** (Fig. 7.28). The superior and inferior **alveolar nerves**, branches of CN V_2 and CN V_3, respectively, form superior and inferior dental plexuses that supply the maxillary and mandibular teeth (Fig. 7.29A).

Palate

The palate forms the arched roof of the oral cavity proper and the floor of the nasal cavities (Fig. 7.30). The palate consists of hard and soft parts: the hard palate anteriorly and the soft palate posteriorly. The hard palate separates the anterior part of the oral cavity from the nasal cavities, and the soft palate separates the posterior part of the oral cavity from the nasopharynx superior to it.

Dental Caries, Pulpitis and Toothache

Decay of the hard tissues of a tooth results in the formation of *dental caries* (cavities). Invasion of the pulp of the tooth by a carious lesion (cavity) results in infection and irritation of the tissues in the pulp cavity. This condition causes an inflammatory process (*pulpitis*). Because the pulp cavity is a rigid space, the swollen pulpal tissues cause pain (*toothache*).

Gingivitis and Periodontitis

Improper oral hygiene results in food deposits in tooth and gingival crevices, which may cause inflammation of the gingivae (*gingivitis*). If untreated, the disease spreads to other supporting structures (including the alveolar bone), producing *periodontitis*. Periodontitis results in inflammation of the gingivae and may result in absorption of alveolar bone and gingival recession. Gingival recession exposes the sensitive cement of the teeth.

The **hard palate** is the anterior vaulted (concave) part; this space is filled with the tongue when it is at rest. The hard palate (covered by a mucous membrane) is formed by the palatine processes of the maxillae and the horizontal plates of the palatine bones (Fig. 7.31*A*). Three foramina open on the oral aspect of the hard palate: the incisive fossa and the greater and lesser palatine foramina. The **incisive fossa** is a slight depression posterior to the central incisor teeth. The **nasopalatine nerves** pass from the nose through a variable number of incisive canals and foramina that open into the incisive fossa (Fig. 7.31*B*). Medial to the third molar tooth, the **greater palatine foramen** pierces the lateral border of the bony palate. The *greater palatine vessels and nerve* emerge from this foramen and run anteriorly on the palate. The **lesser palatine foramina** transmit the *lesser palatine nerves and vessels* to the soft palate and adjacent structures.

The **soft palate** is the movable third of the palate, which is suspended from the posterior border of the hard palate (Fig. 7.31*B* & *C*). The soft palate extends posteroinferiorly as a curved free margin from which hangs a conical process, the **uvula**. The soft palate is strengthened by the **palatine aponeurosis**, formed by the expanded tendon of the **tensor veli palatini** (Fig. 7.31*B*). The aponeurosis, attached to the posterior margin of the hard palate, is thick anteriorly and thin posteriorly. The anterior part of the soft palate is formed mainly by the palatine aponeurosis, whereas its posterior part is muscular.

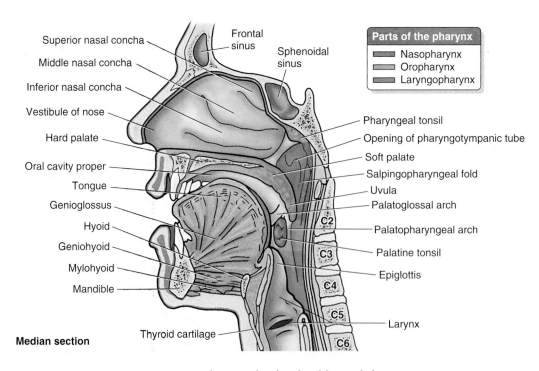

Parts of the pharynx
- Nasopharynx
- Oropharynx
- Laryngopharynx

Superior nasal concha
Middle nasal concha
Inferior nasal concha
Vestibule of nose
Hard palate
Oral cavity proper
Tongue
Genioglossus
Hyoid
Geniohyoid
Mylohyoid
Mandible
Median section
Thyroid cartilage

Frontal sinus
Sphenoidal sinus
Pharyngeal tonsil
Opening of pharyngotympanic tube
Soft palate
Salpingopharyngeal fold
Uvula
Palatoglossal arch
Palatopharyngeal arch
Palatine tonsil
Epiglottis
Larynx

C2
C3
C4
C5
C6

Figure 7.30. Palate, nasal and oral cavities, and pharynx.

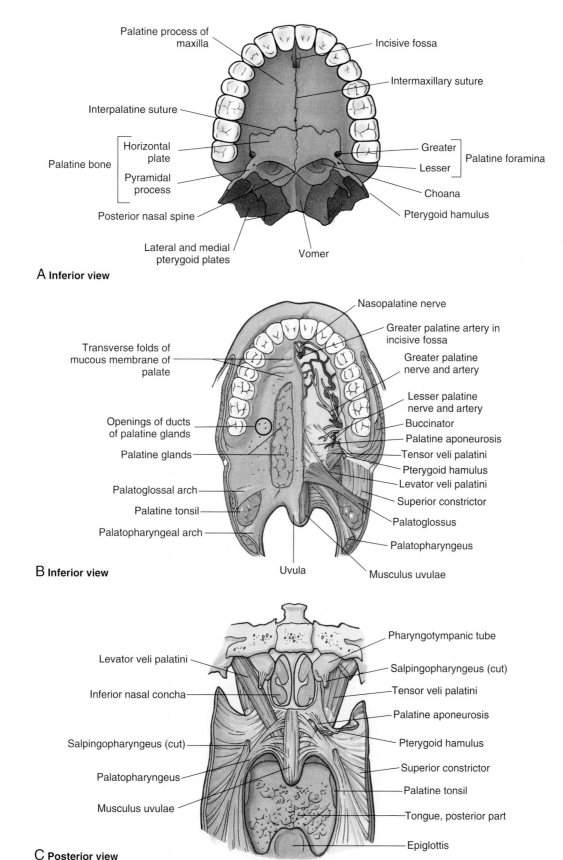

A Inferior view

- Palatine process of maxilla
- Incisive fossa
- Intermaxillary suture
- Interpalatine suture
- Palatine bone
  - Horizontal plate
  - Pyramidal process
- Greater
- Lesser
- Palatine foramina
- Choana
- Pterygoid hamulus
- Posterior nasal spine
- Lateral and medial pterygoid plates
- Vomer

B Inferior view

- Nasopalatine nerve
- Greater palatine artery in incisive fossa
- Transverse folds of mucous membrane of palate
- Greater palatine nerve and artery
- Lesser palatine nerve and artery
- Buccinator
- Openings of ducts of palatine glands
- Palatine aponeurosis
- Tensor veli palatini
- Palatine glands
- Pterygoid hamulus
- Levator veli palatini
- Palatoglossal arch
- Superior constrictor
- Palatine tonsil
- Palatoglossus
- Palatopharyngeal arch
- Palatopharyngeus
- Musculus uvulae
- Uvula

C Posterior view

- Pharyngotympanic tube
- Levator veli palatini
- Salpingopharyngeus (cut)
- Inferior nasal concha
- Tensor veli palatini
- Palatine aponeurosis
- Salpingopharyngeus (cut)
- Pterygoid hamulus
- Palatopharyngeus
- Superior constrictor
- Palatine tonsil
- Musculus uvulae
- Tongue, posterior part
- Epiglottis

Figure 7.31. Palate. A. The bones forming the hard palate are shown. **B.** Part of the right side has been dissected to show the palatine glands. The left side has been dissected to show the muscles of the soft palate and palatine arteries and nerves. **C.** This dissection of the soft palate shows the muscles and their relationship to the posterior part of the tongue.

When a person swallows, the soft palate is initially tensed to allow the tongue to press against it, squeezing the bolus of food to the back of the oral cavity proper. The soft palate is then elevated posteriorly and superiorly against the wall of the pharynx, thereby preventing passage of food into the nasal cavity. Laterally, the soft palate is continuous with the wall of the pharynx and is joined to the tongue and pharynx by the **palatoglossal** and **palatopharyngeal arches** (Figs. 7.31C and 7.32A), respectively. The **palatine tonsils**, often referred to as "the tonsils," are masses of lymphoid tissue, one on each side of the oropharynx (Fig. 7.32). Each tonsil lies in a *tonsillar sinus* (fossa), bounded by the palatoglossal and palatopharyngeal arches and the tongue.

The **muscles of the soft palate** arise from the cranial base and descend to the palate (Fig. 7.31B & C). The soft palate may be elevated so that it is in contact with the posterior wall of the pharynx, sealing off the oral passage from the nasopharynx (e.g., when swallowing or breathing through the mouth). The soft palate can also be drawn inferiorly so that it is in contact with the posterior part of the tongue, sealing off the oral cavity from the nasal passage (e.g., when breathing exclusively through the nose, even with the

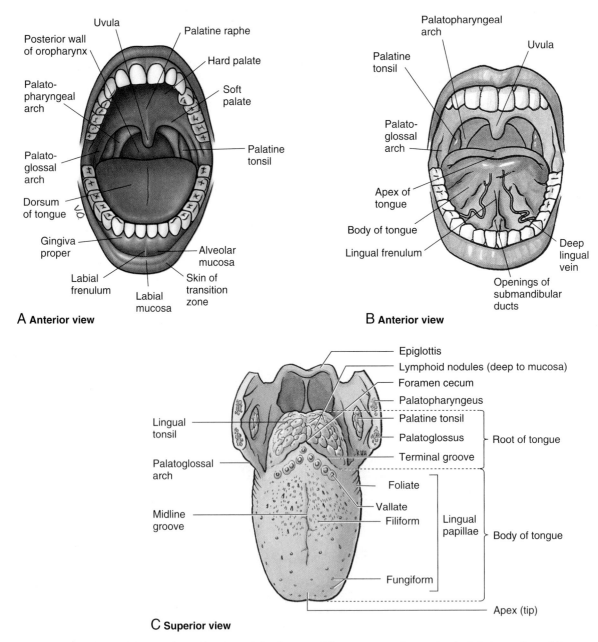

Figure 7.32. Tongue and oral cavity. A. The oral cavity and the dorsum of the tongue are shown. **B.** The inferior surface of the tongue is detailed. **C.** Features of the dorsum of the tongue are identified.

Table 7.10 Muscles of Soft Palate

Muscle	Origin	Insertion	Innervation	Main Action(s)
Tensor veli palatini	Scaphoid fossa at root of posterior border of medial pterygoid plate, spine of sphenoid bone, and cartilage of pharyngotympanic tube	Palatine aponeurosis (Fig. 7.31 B & C)	Nerve to medial pterygoid (a branch of CN V_3) via otic ganglion	Tenses soft palate and opens mouth of pharyngotympanic tube during swallowing and yawning
Levator veli palatini	Cartilage of pharyngotympanic tube and petrous part of temporal bone			Elevates soft palate during swallowing and yawning
Palatoglossus	Palatine aponeurosis	Side of tongue	Pharyngeal branch of CN via pharyngeal plexus	Elevates posterior part of tongue and draws soft palate onto tongue
Palatopharyngeus	Hard palate and palatine aponeurosis	Lateral wall of pharynx		Tenses soft palate and pulls walls of pharynx superiorly, anteriorly, and medially during swallowing
Musculus uvulae	Posterior nasal spine and palatine aponeurosis	Mucosa of uvula		Shortens uvula and pulls it superiorly

mouth open). For attachments, nerve supply, and actions of the five muscles of the soft palate, see Table 7.10.

- The **levator veli palatini** (lifter of the soft palate) is a cylindrical muscle that runs inferoanteriorly, spreading out in the soft palate where it attaches to the superior surface of the palatine aponeurosis.
- The **tensor veli palatini** (tensor of the soft palate) is a muscle with a triangular belly that passes inferiorly; the tendon formed at its apex hooks around the **pterygoid hamulus**—the hook-shaped inferior projection of the medial pterygoid plate—before spreading out as the palatine aponeurosis.
- The **palatoglossus** is a slender slip of muscle that is covered with a mucous membrane; it forms the *palatoglossal arch.* Unlike the other muscles ending in *-glossus,* the palatoglossus is a palatine muscle (in function and innervation) rather than a tongue muscle.
- The **palatopharyngeus** is a thin, flat muscle also covered with a mucous membrane; it forms the *palatopharyngeal arch* and blends inferiorly with the longitudinal muscle of the pharynx.
- The **musculus uvulae** inserts into the mucosa of the uvula.

VASCULATURE AND INNERVATION OF THE PALATE

The palate has a rich blood supply, chiefly from the right and left **greater palatine arteries,** branches of the descending palatine arteries (Fig. 7.31*B*). The **lesser palatine artery,** a smaller branch of the descending palatine artery, enters the palate through the **lesser palatine foramen** and anastomoses with the ascending palatine artery, a branch of the

facial artery. **Venous drainage of the palate,** corresponding and accompanying the branches of the maxillary artery, are tributaries of the **pterygoid venous plexus** (Fig. 7.24*B*).

The *sensory nerves of the palate* pass through the **pterygopalatine ganglion** and are considered branches of the maxillary nerve (Fig. 7.25*A*). The **greater palatine nerve** supplies the gingivae, mucous membrane, and glands of most of the hard palate (Fig. 7.31*B*). The **nasopalatine nerve** supplies the mucous membrane of the anterior part of the hard palate. The **lesser palatine nerves** supply the soft palate. The palatine nerves accompany the arteries through the greater and lesser palatine foramina, respectively. Except for the tensor veli palatini supplied by CN V_3, all muscles of the soft palate are supplied through the *pharyngeal plexus of nerves* (see Chapter 8), derived from pharyngeal branches of the vagus nerve (CN X).

Tongue

The **tongue** (L. *lingua;* G. *glossa*) is a mobile muscular organ that can assume a variety of shapes and positions. The tongue is partly in the oral cavity proper and partly in the oropharynx (Fig. 7.30). At rest, it occupies essentially all the oral cavity proper. The tongue—mainly composed of muscles and covered by mucous membrane—assists with mastication (chewing), taste, deglutition (swallowing), articulation (speech), and oral cleansing. The tongue has a root, a body, an apex, a curved dorsal surface (dorsum), and an inferior surface. A V-shaped groove, the **terminal groove** (L. *sulcus terminalis*) of the tongue (Fig. 7.32*C*), marks the separation between the *anterior (presulcal) part* and the *posterior (postsulcal) part.*

Nasopalatine Nerve Block

The nasopalatine nerves can be anesthetized by injecting anesthetic into the mouth of the *incisive fossa* in the hard palate. The needle is inserted posterior to the *incisive papilla*, a slight elevation of the mucosa that covers the incisive fossa. The affected tissues are the palatal mucosa, the lingual gingivae, and the alveolar bone of the six anterior maxillary teeth and the hard palate.

Greater Palatine Nerve Block

The greater palatine nerve can be anesthetized by injecting anesthetic into the greater palatine foramen. The nerve emerges between the second and the third molar teeth. This nerve block anesthetizes, on the side concerned, all the palatal mucosa and lingual gingivae posterior to the maxillary canine teeth and the underlying bone of the palate.

The **root of the tongue** (base) is the posterior third that rests on the floor of the mouth. The anterior two thirds of the tongue form the **body of the tongue**. The pointed anterior part of the body is the **apex (tip) of the tongue.** The body and apex are extremely mobile. The **dorsum (dorsal surface) of the tongue** is the posterosuperior surface of the tongue, which includes the **terminal groove**. At the apex of this groove is the **foramen cecum**, a small pit that is the non-functional remnant of the proximal part of the embryonic thyroglossal duct from which the thyroid gland developed. The mucous membrane on the anterior part of the tongue is rough because of the presence of numerous **lingual papillae** (Fig. 7.32C):

- **Vallate papillae** are large and flat topped; they lie directly anterior to the terminal groove and are surrounded by deep moat-like trenches, the walls of which are studded by *taste buds;* the ducts of serous *lingual glands* (of von Ebner) open into these trenches.
- **Foliate papillae** are small lateral folds of lingual mucosa; they are poorly developed in humans.
- **Filiform papillae** are long, numerous, thread-like and scaly; they contain afferent nerve endings that are sensitive to touch.
- **Fungiform papillae** are mushroom-shaped and appear as pink or red spots; they are scattered among the filiform papillae but are most numerous at the apex and sides (margins) of the tongue.

The vallate, foliate, and most of the fungiform papillae contain taste receptors in the **taste buds.** A few taste buds are also in the epithelium covering the oral surface of the soft palate, the posterior wall of the oropharynx, and the epiglottis.

The mucous membrane of the dorsum of the tongue is thin over the anterior part of the tongue and is closely attached to the underlying muscle. A depression on the dorsal surface, the **midline groove of the tongue** (median sulcus), divides the tongue into right and left halves (Fig. 7.32C); it also indicates the site of fusion of the embryonic distal tongue buds. Deep to the midline groove is a fibrous **lingual septum**, which forms a vertical partition.

The **root** of the tongue lies within the oropharynx; posterior to the *terminal groove* and the *palatoglossal arches* (Fig. 7.32C). Its mucous membrane is thick and freely movable. It has no lingual papillae, but the underlying **lymphoid nodules**, known collectively as the lingual tonsil, give this part of the tongue its cobblestone appearance.

The **inferior surface of the tongue** (sublingual surface) is covered with a thin, transparent mucous membrane through which one can see the underlying **deep lingual veins.** With the tongue raised, observe the **lingual frenulum** (Fig. 7.32B), a large midline fold of mucosa that passes from the gingiva covering the lingual aspect of the anterior alveolar ridge to the posteroinferior surface of the tongue. The frenulum connects the tongue to the floor of the mouth while allowing the anterior part of the tongue to move freely. At the base of the frenulum are the *openings of the submandibular ducts* from the submandibular salivary glands.

MUSCLES OF TONGUE

The tongue is essentially a mass of muscles that is mostly covered by mucous membrane. Although it is traditional to do so, providing descriptions of the actions of tongue muscles by ascribing a single action to a specific muscle—or implying that a particular movement is the consequence of a single muscle—greatly oversimplifies the actions of the tongue and is misleading. The muscles of the tongue do not act in isolation, and some muscles perform multiple actions with parts of one muscle capable of acting independently, producing different—even antagonistic—actions. *In general, however, extrinsic muscles alter the position of the tongue and intrinsic muscles alter its shape.*

The four intrinsic and four extrinsic muscles in each half of the tongue are separated by the fibrous lingual septum (Table 7.11B). The **intrinsic muscles of tongue** (superior and inferior longitudinal, transverse, and vertical) are confined to the tongue and are not attached to bone. The **extrinsic muscles of the tongue** (genioglossus, hyoglossus, styloglossus, and palatoglossus) originate outside the

Table 7.11 Muscles of Tongue

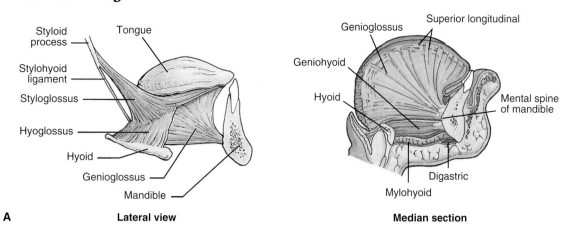

A   Lateral view   Median section

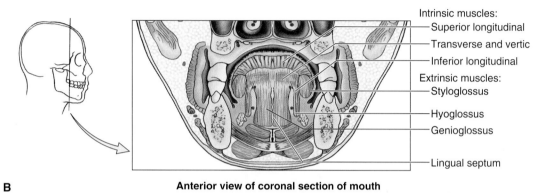

B   Anterior view of coronal section of mouth

Muscle	Shape and Position	Proximal Attachment	Distal Attachment	Main Action(s)
Extrinsic muscles of tongue				
Genioglossus	Fan-shaped muscle; constitutes bulk of tongue	Via a short tendon from superior part of mental spine of mandible	Entire dorsum of tongue; inferiormost and posterior most fibers attach to body of hyoid	Bilateral activity depresses tongue, especially central part, creating a longitudinal furrow; posterior part pulls tongue anteriorly for protrusion;[a] most anterior part retracts apex of protruded tongue; unilateral contraction deviates ("wags") tongue to contralateral side
Hyoglossus	Thin, quadrilateral muscle	Body and greater horn of hyoid	Inferior aspects of lateral part of tongue	Depresses tongue, especially pulling its sides inferiorly; helps shorten (retrude) tongue
Styloglossus	Short triangular muscle	Anterior border of distal styloid process; stylohyoid ligament	Sides of tongue posteriorly, interdigitating with hyoglossus	Retrudes tongue and curls (elevates) its sides, working with genioglossus to form a central trough during swallowing
Palatoglossus	Narrow crescent-shaped palatine muscle; forms posterior column of isthmus of fauces	Palatine aponeurosis of soft palate	Enters posterolateral tongue transversely, blending with intrinsic transverse muscles	Capable of elevating posterior tongue or depressing soft palate; most commonly acts to constrict isthmus of fauces (L. the throat)
Intrinsic muscles of tongue				
Superior longitudinal	Thin layer deep to mucous membrane of dorsum	Submucosal fibrous layer and median fibrous septum	Margins of tongue and mucous membrane	Curls tongue longitudinally upward, elevating apex and sides of tongue; shortens (retrudes) tongue
Inferior longitudinal	Narrow band close to inferior surface	Root of tongue and body of hyoid	Apex of tongue	Curls tongue longitudinally downward, depressing apex; shortens (retrudes) tongue
Transverse	Deep to superior longitudinal muscle	Median fibrous septum	Fibrous tissue at lateral lingual margins	Narrows and elongates (protrudes) tongue[a]
Vertical	Fibers intersect transverse muscle	Submucosal fibrous layer of dorsum of tongue	Inferior surface of borders of tongue	Flattens and broadens tongue[a]

[a] Act simultaneously to protrude tongue.

tongue and attach to it. They mainly move the tongue but they can alter its shape as well.

INNERVATION OF THE TONGUE

All the muscles of the tongue are supplied by the CN XII, the **hypoglossal nerve** (Figs. 7.33A and 7.34A), except for the palatoglossus (actually a palatine muscle supplied by the *pharyngeal plexus,* the plexus of nerves which includes motor branches of CNX). For general sensation (touch and temperature), the mucosa of the anterior two thirds of the tongue is

supplied by the **lingual nerve**, a branch of CN V$_3$. For special sensation (taste), this part of the tongue, except for the vallate papillae, is supplied through the **chorda tympani nerve**, a branch of CN VII. The chorda tympani joins the lingual nerve and runs anteriorly in its sheath (Fig. 7.33A).

The mucous membrane of the posterior third of the tongue and the vallate papillae are supplied by the lingual branch of the **glossopharyngeal nerve** (CN IX) for both general and special sensation (taste). Twigs of the **internal laryngeal nerve**, a branch of the vagus nerve (CN X), supply mostly general but some special sensation to a small area of

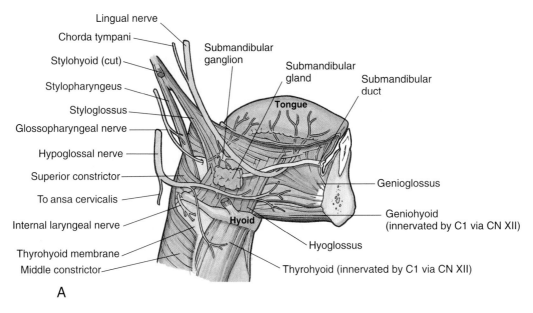

A

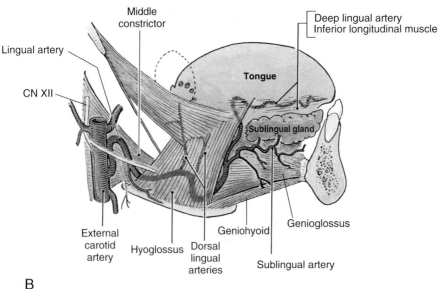

B

Lateral views

Figure 7.33. Muscles, nerves, and arteries of the tongue. A. Nerves and muscles **B.** Lingual artery.

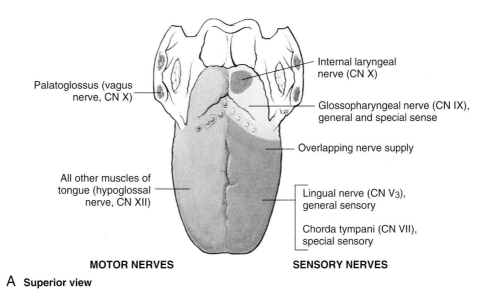

Figure 7.34. Innervation and lymphatic drainage of tongue. A. The innervation of the tongue is shown. **B.** The lymphatic drainage in the dorsum of the tongue is shown. **C.** The lymphatic drainage to the deep cervical lymph nodes is demonstrated.

the tongue just anterior to the epiglottis. These mostly sensory nerves also carry **parasympathetic secretomotor fibers** to serous glands in the tongue. These nerve fibers probably synapse in the **submandibular ganglion** suspended from the lingual nerve (Fig. 7.33A).

There are four basic taste sensations: sweet, salty, sour, and bitter. Sweetness is detected at the apex, saltiness at the lateral margin, and sourness and bitterness at the posterior part of the tongue. All other "tastes" expressed by gourmets are olfactory (smell and aroma).

VASCULATURE OF THE TONGUE

The **arteries of the tongue** derive from the **lingual artery**, which arises from the *external carotid artery* (Fig. 7.33 B). On entering the tongue, the lingual artery passes deep to the hyoglossus muscle. The *main branches of the lingual artery* are the:

- **Dorsal lingual arteries**, which supply the posterior part (root) of the tongue and send a tonsillar branch to the palatine tonsil.
- **Deep lingual artery**, which supplies the anterior part of the tongue; the dorsal and deep arteries communicate with each other near the apex of the tongue.
- **Sublingual artery**, which supplies the sublingual gland and the floor of the mouth.

The *veins of the tongue* are the:

- *Dorsal lingual veins,* which accompany the lingual artery.
- *Deep lingual veins* (Fig. 7.32 B), which begin at the apex of the tongue and run posteriorly beside the lingual frenulum to join the *sublingual vein.*

All lingual veins terminate, directly or indirectly, in the IJV.

Lymphatic drainage of the tongue takes the following routes (Fig. 7.34 B & C):

- Lymph from the posterior third drains to the *superior deep cervical lymph nodes* on both sides.
- Lymph from the *medial part of the anterior two thirds* drains to the *inferior deep cervical lymph nodes.*
- Lymph from *lateral parts of the anterior two thirds* drains to the *submandibular lymph nodes.*
- Lymph from the *apex of the tongue and frenulum* drains to the *submental lymph nodes.*
- Lymph from the *posterior third* and the area near the midline groove drain bilaterally.

Salivary Glands

The **salivary glands** include the parotid, submandibular, and sublingual glands (Fig. 7.35 A). Saliva, the clear, tasteless, odorless viscid fluid secreted by these glands and the mucous glands of the oral cavity:

- Keeps the mucous membrane of the mouth moist.
- Lubricates the food during mastication.
- Begins digestion of starches.

Gag Reflex

One may touch the anterior part of the tongue without feeling discomfort; however, when the posterior part is touched, one usually gags. CN IX and CN X are responsible for the muscular contraction of each side of the pharynx. Glossopharyngeal branches (CN IX) provide the afferent limb of the gag reflex.

Paralysis of Genioglossus

When the genioglossus is paralyzed, the tongue mass has a tendency to shift posteriorly, obstructing the airway and presenting the risk of suffocation. Total relaxation of the genioglossus muscles occurs during general anesthesia; therefore, the tongue of an anesthetized patient must be prevented from relapsing by inserting an airway.

Injury to Hypoglossal Nerve

Trauma, such as a fractured mandible, may injure the hypoglossal nerve (CN XII), resulting in paralysis and eventual atrophy of one side of the tongue. The tongue deviates to the paralyzed side during protrusion because of the action of the unaffected genioglossus on the other side.

Sublingual Absorption of Drugs

For quick transmucosal absorption of a drug—for instance, when nitroglycerin is used as a vasodilator in angina pectoris (chest pain)—the pill (or spray) is put under the tongue where the thin mucosa allows the absorbed drug to enter the deep lingual veins in less than a minute.

Lingual Carcinoma

Malignant tumors in the posterior part of the tongue metastasize to the superior deep cervical lymph nodes on both sides. In contrast, tumors in the apex and anterolateral parts usually do not metastasize to the inferior deep cervical nodes until late in the disease. Because the deep nodes are closely related to the IJVs, metastases from the carcinoma may spread to the submental and submandibular regions and along the IJVs into the neck.

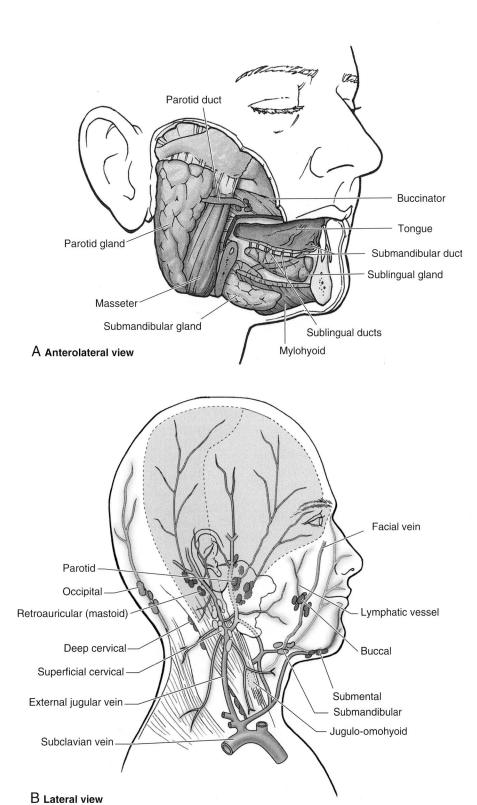

Parotid duct

Buccinator

Tongue

Submandibular duct

Sublingual gland

Parotid gland

Masseter

Submandibular gland

Sublingual ducts

Mylohyoid

A **Anterolateral view**

Facial vein

Parotid

Occipital

Retroauricular (mastoid)

Deep cervical

Superficial cervical

External jugular vein

Subclavian vein

Lymphatic vessel

Buccal

Submental

Submandibular

Jugulo-omohyoid

B **Lateral view**

Figure 7.35. Face and salivary glands. A. This dissection of the right side of the face shows the location of glands and ducts. **B.** Lymphatic drainage of the face and glands is shown.

- Serves as an intrinsic "mouthwash."
- Plays a significant role in the prevention of tooth decay and in the ability to taste.

In addition to the three major salivary glands, small *accessory salivary glands* are scattered over the palate, lips, cheeks, tonsils, and tongue.

The **parotid glands** are the largest of the major salivary glands. Each parotid gland has an irregular shape because it occupies the gap between the ramus of the mandible and the styloid and mastoid processes of the temporal bone. The purely serous secretion of the gland passes through the **parotid duct** and empties into the vestibule of the oral cavity opposite the second maxillary molar tooth (Fig. 7.35A). In addition to its digestive function, it washes food particles into the mouth proper. The **arterial supply** of the parotid gland and duct is from branches of the *external carotid* and *superficial temporal arteries*. The **veins** from the parotid gland drain into the *retromandibular veins* (Fig. 7.24B). The **lymphatic vessels** from the parotid gland end in the **superficial and deep cervical lymph nodes** (Fig. 7.35B). The parotid gland was discussed earlier in this chapter, when its innervation was described.

The **submandibular glands** lie along the body of the mandible, partly superior and partly inferior to the posterior half of the mandible and partly superficial and partly deep to the mylohyoid muscle (Fig. 7.35A). The **submandibular duct** arises from the part of the gland that lies between the mylohyoid and the hyoglossus. Passing from lateral to medial, the **lingual nerve** loops under the duct as it runs anteriorly to open via one to three orifices on a small, fleshy *sublingual papilla* on each side of the lingual frenulum (Figs. 7.32B and 7.33A). The orifices of the submandibular ducts are visible, and saliva often sprays from it when the tongue is elevated and retracted (as when yawning).

The **arterial supply of the submandibular glands** is from the **submental arteries** (Fig. 7.24A). The **veins** accompany the arteries. The submandibular gland is supplied by presynaptic parasympathetic secretomotor fibers conveyed from the facial nerve to the lingual nerve by the *chorda tympani nerve* (Fig. 33A), which synapse with postsynaptic neurons in the *submandibular ganglion*. The latter fibers accompany arteries to reach the gland, along with vasoconstrictive postsynaptic sympathetic fibers from the superior cervical ganglion. The **lymphatic vessels** of the submandibular gland drain into the *deep cervical lymph nodes,* particularly the *jugulo-omohyoid lymph node* (Fig. 7.35B).

The **sublingual glands** are the smallest and most deeply situated (Fig. 7.35A). Each almond-shaped gland lies in the floor of the mouth between the mandible and the genioglossus muscle. The glands from each side unite to form a horseshoe-shaped mass around the lingual frenulum. Numerous small **sublingual ducts** open into the floor of the mouth alongside the lingual folds.

Excision of the Submandibular Gland

Excision of a submandibular gland because of a *calculus* (stone) in its duct or a tumor in the gland is not uncommon. Risks to the mandibular branch of the facial nerve may be avoided by making the skin incision at least 2.5 cm inferior to the angle of the mandible.

Sialography

The parotid and submandibular salivary glands may be examined radiographically after the injection of a contrast medium into their ducts. This special type of radiograph (*sialogram*) demonstrates the salivary ducts and some secretory units. Because of the small size and number of sublingual ducts of the sublingual glands, one cannot usually inject contrast medium into them.

The **arterial supply of the sublingual glands** is from the *sublingual* and *submental arteries*—branches of the lingual and facial arteries, respectively (Figs. 7.24A and 7.33B). The **innervation** of the sublingual glands is the same as that described for the submandibular gland.

Pterygopalatine Fossa

The **pterygopalatine fossa** is a small pyramidal space inferior to the apex of the orbit. It lies between the pterygoid process of the sphenoid and the posterior aspect of the maxilla anteriorly (Fig. 7.36A). The fragile perpendicular plate of the palatine bone forms its medial wall. The incomplete *roof of the pterygopalatine fossa* is formed by the *greater wing of the sphenoid*. The *floor of the pterygopalatine fossa* is formed by the *pyramidal process of the palatine bone*. Its superior, larger end opens into the *inferior orbital fissure;* its inferior end is closed except for the palatine foramina. The pterygopalatine fossa communicates (Fig. 7.36A & B)

- Laterally with the *infratemporal fossa* through the *pterygomaxillary fissure*.
- Medially with the *nasal cavity* through the *sphenopalatine foramen*.
- Anterosuperiorly with the *orbit* through the *inferior orbital fissure*.

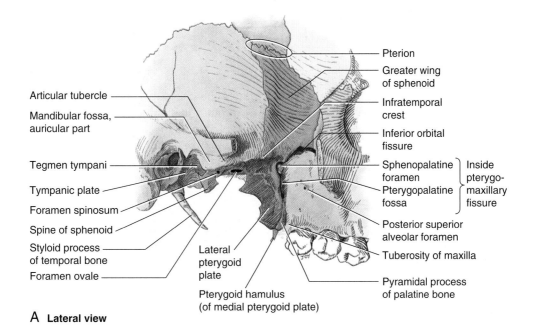

A **Lateral view**

Articular tubercle

Mandibular fossa, auricular part

Tegmen tympani

Tympanic plate

Foramen spinosum

Spine of sphenoid

Styloid process of temporal bone

Foramen ovale

Lateral pterygoid plate

Pterygoid hamulus (of medial pterygoid plate)

Pterion

Greater wing of sphenoid

Infratemporal crest

Inferior orbital fissure

Sphenopalatine foramen
Pterygopalatine fossa
Inside pterygo-maxillary fissure

Posterior superior alveolar foramen

Tuberosity of maxilla

Pyramidal process of palatine bone

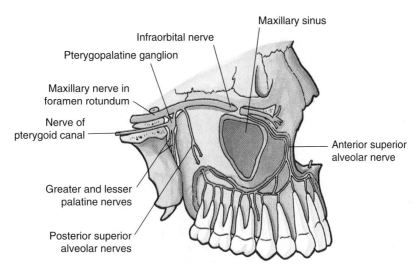

B **Lateral view**

Pterygopalatine ganglion

Maxillary nerve in foramen rotundum

Nerve of pterygoid canal

Greater and lesser palatine nerves

Posterior superior alveolar nerves

Infraorbital nerve

Maxillary sinus

Anterior superior alveolar nerve

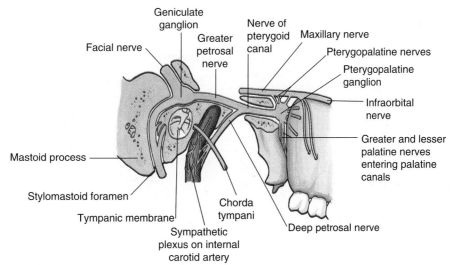

C **Lateral view**

Geniculate ganglion

Facial nerve

Greater petrosal nerve

Nerve of pterygoid canal

Maxillary nerve

Pterygopalatine nerves

Pterygopalatine ganglion

Infraorbital nerve

Greater and lesser palatine nerves entering palatine canals

Mastoid process

Stylomastoid foramen

Tympanic membrane

Chorda tympani

Sympathetic plexus on internal carotid artery

Deep petrosal nerve

Figure 7.36. Pterygopalatine fossa. A. The bony walls are identified. **B.** The infraorbital and superior alveolar nerves are shown. **C.** The course of the presynaptic parasympathetic nerves to the pterygopalatine ganglion is demonstrated.

- Posterosuperiorly with the *middle cranial fossa* through the *foramen rotundum* and *pterygoid canal*.

The contents of the pterygopalatine fossa are the (Figs. 7.36 and 7.37):

- Terminal (third) part of the maxillary artery and its branches.
- Maxillary nerve (CN V$_2$), with which are associated the nerve of the pterygoid canal and the pterygopalatine ganglion.

The **maxillary nerve** (CN V$_2$) enters the pterygopalatine fossa posterosuperiorly through the foramen rotundum and runs anterolaterally in the fossa (Fig. 7.36*A* & *B*). Within the fossa, the maxillary nerve gives off the *zygomatic nerve,* which divides into the *zygomaticofacial* and *zygomaticotemporal nerves* (Fig. 7.37*A*). These nerves emerge from the zygomatic bone through the cranial foramina of the same name and supply the lateral region of the cheek and the temple. The *zygomaticotemporal nerve* also gives rise to a communicating branch, which conveys parasympathetic secretomotor fibers to the lacrimal gland by way of the lacrimal nerve from CN V$_1$.

While in the pterygopalatine fossa, the maxillary nerve also gives off the two *pterygopalatine nerves,* which suspend the parasympathetic *pterygopalatine ganglion* in the superior part of the pterygopalatine fossa (Figs. 7.36*C* and 7.37*A*). The pterygopalatine nerves convey general sensory fibers of the maxillary nerve, which pass through the pterygopalatine ganglion without synapsing and supply the nose, palate, tonsil, and gingivae. The maxillary nerve leaves the pterygopalatine fossa through the inferior orbital fissure, after which it is known as the *infraorbital nerve* (Figs. 7.36*B* and 7.37*A*).

The **parasympathetic fibers to the pterygopalatine ganglion** come from the facial nerve by way of its first branch, the *greater petrosal nerve* (Fig. 7.36*B* & *C*). This nerve joins the *deep petrosal nerve* as it passes through the foramen lacerum to form the **nerve of the pterygoid canal.** This nerve passes anteriorly through the pterygoid canal to the **pterygopalatine fossa.** The parasympathetic fibers of the greater petrosal nerve synapse in the pterygopalatine ganglion.

The **deep petrosal nerve** is a sympathetic nerve arising from the *internal carotid plexus.* It conveys postsynaptic fibers from nerve cell bodies in the superior cervical sympathetic ganglion (Fig. 7.36*C*). Thus these fibers do not synapse in the pterygopalatine ganglion but pass directly to join the branches of the ganglion (maxillary nerve). The postsynaptic parasympathetic and sympathetic fibers pass to the lacrimal gland and the glands of the nasal cavity, palate, and superior pharynx (Fig. 7.37*A*).

The **maxillary artery,** a terminal branch of the external carotid artery, passes anteriorly and traverses the infratemporal fossa. It passes over the lateral pterygoid muscle and enters the pterygopalatine fossa. The **pterygopalatine part of the maxillary artery,** its third part, passes through the *pterygomaxillary fissure* and enters the pterygopalatine fossa (Fig. 7.25*B*). The artery gives rise to branches that accompany all nerves in the fossa with the same names. The *branches of the third, or pterygopalatine, part of the maxillary artery* are the (Fig. 7.37*B*):

- Posterior superior alveolar artery.
- Descending palatine artery, which divides into greater and lesser palatine arteries.
- Artery of the pterygoid canal.
- Sphenopalatine artery, which divides into posterior lateral nasal branches to the lateral wall of the nasal cavity and its associated paranasal sinuses, and the posterior septal branches.
- Infraorbital artery, which gives rise to the anterior superior alveolar artery and terminates as branches to the inferior eyelid, nose, and upper lip.

Nose

The **nose** is the part of the respiratory tract superior to the hard palate and contains the peripheral organ of smell. It includes the external nose and nasal cavities, which are divided into right and left cavities by the *nasal septum.* Each nasal cavity is divisible into an *olfactory area* and a *respiratory area.* The functions of the nose and nasal cavities are:

- Olfaction (smelling).
- Respiration (breathing).
- Filtration of dust.
- Humidification of inspired air.
- Reception and elimination of secretions from the nasal mucosa, paranasal sinuses, and nasolacrimal ducts.

External Nose

The **external nose** varies considerably in size and shape, mainly because of differences in the nasal cartilages. The **dorsum of the nose** extends from its superior angle, the **root** (Fig. 7.38*A*), to the **apex** (tip) of the nose. The inferior surface of the nose is pierced by two piriform (L. pearshaped) openings, the **nares** (nostrils, anterior nasal apertures), which are bound laterally by the **alae** (wings) of the nose and separated from each other by the **nasal septum.** The external nose consists of bony and cartilaginous parts (Fig. 7.38*B*).

The **bony part of the nose** consists of the:

- Nasal bones.
- Frontal processes of the maxillae.
- Nasal part of the frontal bone and its nasal spine.
- Bony part of the nasal septum.

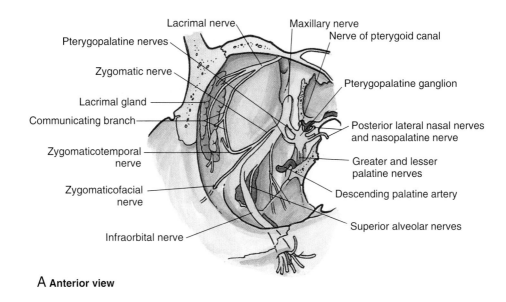

A Anterior view

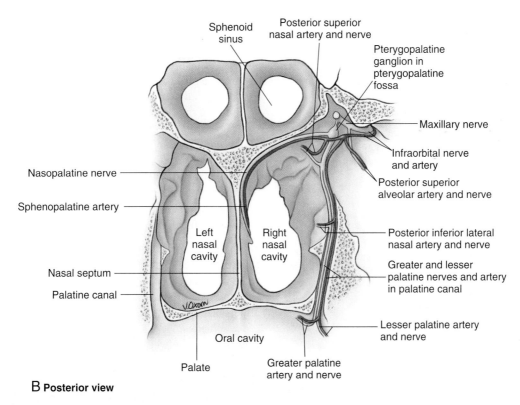

B Posterior view

Figure 7.37. Nerves of pterygopalatine fossa. A. The fossa is viewed through the floor of the orbit to show the maxillary nerve (CN V$_2$) and its branches. **B.** In this coronal section, the nasopalatine and greater and lesser palatine nerves can be seen.

The **cartilaginous part of the nose** consists of five main cartilages: two **lateral cartilages**, two **alar cartilages**, and a **septal cartilage**. The U-shaped alar cartilages are free and movable; they dilate or constrict the nares when the muscles acting on the nose contract. (Fig. 7.39A).

Nasal Cavities

The nasal cavities, entered through the nares, open posteriorly into the nasopharynx through the *choanae*. Mucosa lines the nasal cavities, except the *nasal vestibule*, which is lined with skin (Fig. 7.40A). The **nasal mucosa** is firmly

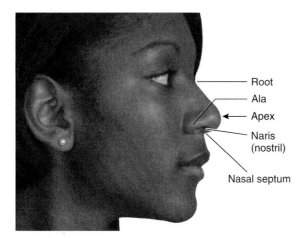

A Lateral view

Root
Ala
Apex
Naris
(nostril)
Nasal septum

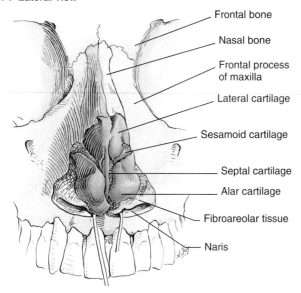

Frontal bone
Nasal bone
Frontal process
of maxilla
Lateral cartilage
Sesamoid cartilage
Septal cartilage
Alar cartilage
Fibroareolar tissue
Naris

B Anterior view

Figure 7.38. External nose. A. The surface anatomy of the nose is shown. **B.** The nasal bones and cartilages (pulled inferiorly) are identified.

Nasal Fractures

Deformity of the external nose usually is present with a fracture, particularly when a lateral force is applied by someone's elbow, for example. When the injury results from a direct blow (e.g., from a hockey stick), the cribriform plate of the ethmoid bone may fracture, resulting in CSF rhinorrhea.

bound to the periosteum and perichondrium of the supporting bones and cartilages of the nose. The mucosa is continuous with the lining of all the chambers with which the nasal cavities communicate: the nasopharynx posteriorly, the paranasal sinuses superiorly and laterally, and the lacrimal sac and conjunctiva superiorly. The inferior two thirds of the nasal mucosa is the **respiratory area**, and the superior one third is the *olfactory area*. Air passing over the respiratory area is warmed and moistened before it passes through the rest of the upper respiratory tract to the lungs. The **olfactory area** is specialized mucosa containing the peripheral organ of smell; sniffing draws air to the area (Fig. 7.39C). The central processes of the olfactory receptor neurons in the olfactory epithelium unite to form nerve bundles that pass through the cribriform plate and enter the **olfactory bulb.**

The *boundaries of the nasal cavity* are (Fig. 7.39A) as follows:

- The *roof of the nasal cavity* is curved and narrow, except at the posterior end; the roof is divided into three parts (frontonasal, ethmoidal, and sphenoidal), which are named from the bones that form each part.
- The *floor of the nasal cavity* is wider than the roof and is formed by the *palatine process of the maxilla* and the *horizontal plate of the palatine bone.*
- The *medial wall of the nasal cavity* is formed by the nasal septum, the the main components of which are the *perpendicular plate of the ethmoid, vomer, septal cartilage,* and the *nasal crests of the maxillary and palatine bones.*
- The *lateral wall of the nasal cavity* is uneven because of the **nasal conchae (superior, middle,** and **inferior)** three elevations that project inferiorly like scrolls. The conchae curve inferomedially, each forming a roof for a **meatus,** or recess.

The **nasal conchae** (L. shells) divide the nasal cavity into four passages (Figs. 7.39A and 7.40A): sphenoethmoidal recess, superior nasal meatus, middle nasal meatus, and inferior nasal meatus. The **sphenoethmoidal recess,** lying superoposterior to the superior concha, receives the *opening of the sphenoidal sinus.* The **superior nasal meatus** is a narrow passage between the superior and the middle nasal conchae (parts of the ethmoid bone) into which the posterior ethmoidal sinuses open by one or more orifices. The **middle nasal meatus** is longer and deeper than the superior one. The anterosuperior part of this passage leads into the *ethmoidal infundibulum,* an opening through which it communicates with the frontal sinus, via the **frontonasal duct.** The **semilunar hiatus** (L. *hiatus semilunaris*) is a semicircular groove into which the frontonasal duct opens. The **ethmoidal bulla** (L. bubble), a rounded elevation located superior to the semilunar hiatus, is visible when the middle concha is removed. The bulla is formed by *middle ethmoidal cells,* which constitute the *ethmoidal sinuses* (Fig. 7.40). The

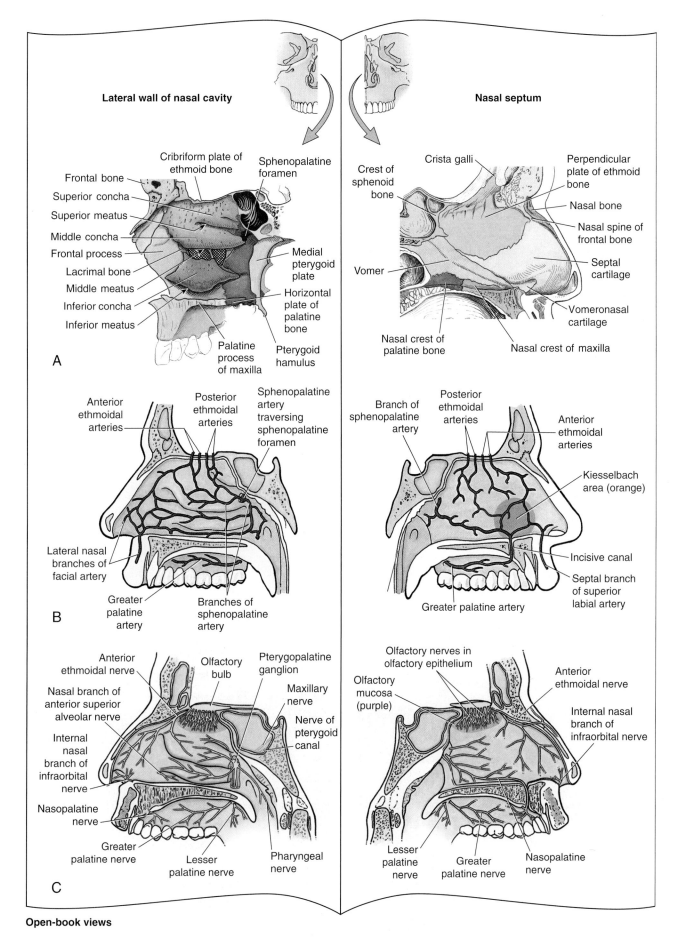

Lateral wall of nasal cavity

Nasal septum

A

Frontal bone
Superior concha
Superior meatus
Middle concha
Frontal process
Lacrimal bone
Middle meatus
Inferior concha
Inferior meatus

Cribriform plate of ethmoid bone
Sphenopalatine foramen

Medial pterygoid plate
Horizontal plate of palatine bone
Pterygoid hamulus
Palatine process of maxilla

Crest of sphenoid bone
Crista galli
Perpendicular plate of ethmoid bone
Nasal bone
Nasal spine of frontal bone
Septal cartilage
Vomer
Vomeronasal cartilage
Nasal crest of palatine bone
Nasal crest of maxilla

B

Anterior ethmoidal arteries
Posterior ethmoidal arteries
Sphenopalatine artery traversing sphenopalatine foramen

Lateral nasal branches of facial artery
Greater palatine artery
Branches of sphenopalatine artery

Branch of sphenopalatine artery
Posterior ethmoidal arteries
Anterior ethmoidal arteries
Kiesselbach area (orange)
Incisive canal
Septal branch of superior labial artery
Greater palatine artery

C

Anterior ethmoidal nerve
Olfactory bulb
Pterygopalatine ganglion
Nasal branch of anterior superior alveolar nerve
Maxillary nerve
Nerve of pterygoid canal
Internal nasal branch of infraorbital nerve
Nasopalatine nerve
Greater palatine nerve
Lesser palatine nerve
Pharyngeal nerve

Olfactory nerves in olfactory epithelium
Olfactory mucosa (purple)
Anterior ethmoidal nerve
Internal nasal branch of infraorbital nerve
Lesser palatine nerve
Greater palatine nerve
Nasopalatine nerve

Open-book views

Figure 7.39. Bones, arteries and nerves of lateral wall of nose and nasal septum.

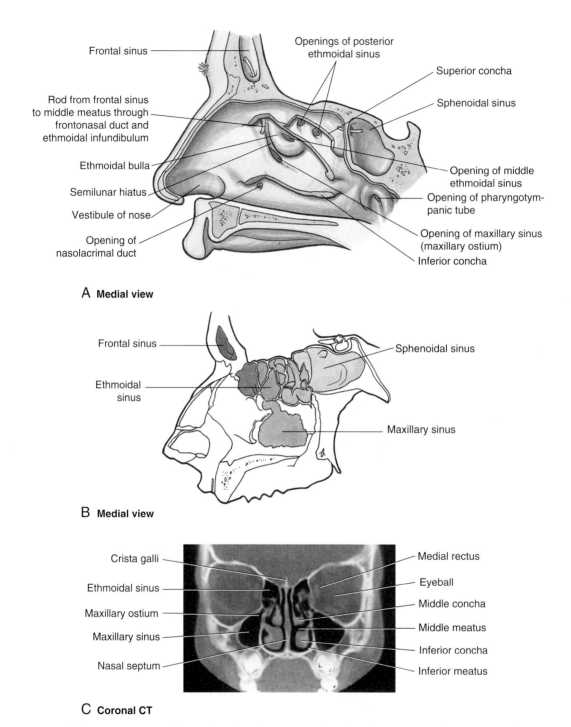

Figure 7.40. Paranasal sinuses. A. Parts of the conchae have been removed to show the openings of sinuses and other structures. **B.** The right paranasal sinuses are identified. **C.** The paranasal sinuses are shown.

maxillary sinus also opens into the posterior end of the semilunar hiatus. The **inferior nasal meatus** is a horizontal passage, inferolateral to the inferior nasal concha (an independent, paired bone). The **nasolacrimal duct** from the lacrimal sac opens into the anterior part of this meatus.

The *arterial supply of the medial and lateral walls of the nasal cavity* is from branches of the **sphenopalatine artery, anterior and posterior ethmoidal arteries, greater palatine artery, superior labial artery,** and the **lateral nasal branches of the facial artery** (Fig. 7.39A). On the anterior part of the nasal septum is an area rich in capillaries (Kiesselbach area) where all five arteries supplying the septum anastomose.

This area is often where profuse bleeding from the nose occurs. A rich *plexus of veins* drains deep to the nasal mucosa into the sphenopalatine, facial, and ophthalmic veins.

The *nerve supply of the posteroinferior half to two thirds of the nasal mucosa* is chiefly from CN V_2 by way of the **nasopalatine nerve** to the nasal septum and posterior lateral nasal branches of the **greater palatine nerve** to the lateral wall (Fig. 7.39C). The anterosuperior part of the nasal mucosa (both the septum and lateral wall) is supplied by the **anterior ethmoidal nerves**, branches of CN V_1.

Paranasal Sinuses

The **paranasal sinuses** are air-filled extensions of the respiratory part of the nasal cavity into the following cranial bones: frontal, ethmoid, sphenoid, and maxilla (Fig. 7.40). They are named according to the bones in which they are located.

The **frontal sinuses** are between the outer and the inner tables of the frontal bone, posterior to the superciliary arches and the root of the nose. Each sinus drains through a **frontonasal duct** into the *ethmoidal infundibulum,* which opens into the *semilunar hiatus* of the middle meatus. The frontal sinuses are innervated by branches of the *supraorbital nerves* (CN V_1).

The **ethmoidal cells (sinuses)** include several cavities that are located in the lateral mass of the ethmoid between the nasal cavity and the orbit. The **anterior ethmoidal cells** drain directly or indirectly into the middle meatus through the infundibulum. The **middle ethmoidal cells** open directly into the middle meatus. The **posterior ethmoidal cells**, which form the **ethmoidal bulla**, open directly into the superior meatus. The ethmoidal sinuses are supplied by the anterior and posterior ethmoidal branches of the *nasociliary nerves* (CN V_1) (Fig. 7.39C).

The **sphenoidal sinuses**, unevenly divided and separated by a bony septum, occupy the body of the sphenoid bone; they may extend into the wings of this bone in the elderly. Because of these sinuses, the body of the sphenoid is fragile. Only thin plates of bone separate the sinuses from several important structures: the optic nerves and optic chiasm, the pituitary gland, the internal carotid arteries, and the cavernous sinuses. The *posterior ethmoidal artery* and *nerve* supply the sphenoidal sinuses (Fig. 7.40).

The **maxillary sinuses** are the largest of the paranasal sinuses (Fig. 7.40B & C). These large pyramidal cavities occupy the bodies of the maxillae. The **apex** of the maxillary sinus extends toward and often into the zygomatic bone. The **base** of the maxillary sinus forms the inferior part of the lateral wall of the nasal cavity. The **roof** of the maxillary sinus is formed by the floor of the orbit. The **floor** of the maxillary sinus is formed by the alveolar part of the maxilla. The roots of the maxillary teeth, particularly the first two molars, often produce conical elevations in the floor of the maxillary sinus. Each sinus drains by an opening, the **maxillary ostium** (Fig. 7.40A), into the middle meatus of the nasal cavity by way of the semilunar hiatus. Because of the superior location of this opening, it is impossible for the sinus to drain when the head is erect until the sinus is full.

Epistaxis

Epistaxis (nose bleeding) is relatively common because of the rich blood supply to the nasal mucosa. In most cases, the cause is trauma, and the bleeding is from an area in the anterior third of the nose (Kiesselbach area). Recall that this area is supplied by the anastomosing of branches from five different arterial sources (Fig. 7.39B). Spurting of blood from the nose results from rupture of these arteries. Mild epistaxis may also result from nose picking, which tears veins in the vestibule of the nose.

CSF Rhinorrhea

Although nasal discharges are commonly associated with upper respiratory tract infections, a nasal discharge after a head injury may be cerebrospinal fluid. CSF rhinorrhea results from fracture of the cribriform plate, tearing of the cranial meninges, and leakage of CSF from the nose.

Rhinitis

The nasal mucosa becomes swollen and inflamed (*rhinitis*) during upper respiratory infections and allergic reactions (e.g., hayfever). Swelling of this mucous membrane occurs readily because of its vascularity and abundant mucosal glands. *Infections of the nasal cavities may spread to the:*

- Anterior cranial fossa through the cribriform plate.
- Nasopharynx and retropharyngeal soft tissues.
- Middle ear through the pharyngotympanic (auditory) tube.
- Paranasal sinuses.
- Lacrimal apparatus and conjunctiva.

Infection of Ethmoidal Cells

If nasal drainage is blocked, infections of the ethmoidal cells of the ethmoidal sinuses may break through the fragile medial wall of the orbit. Severe infections from this source may cause blindness because some posterior ethmoidal cells lie close to the optic canal, which gives passage to the optic nerve and ophthalmic artery. Spread of infection from these cells could also affect the dural sheath of the optic nerve, causing *optic neuritis*.

Infection of Maxillary Sinuses

The maxillary sinuses are the most commonly infected, probably because their ostia are small and located high on their superomedial walls (Fig. 7.40*A* and *B*), a poor location for natural drainage of the sinus. When the mucous membrane of the sinus is congested, the maxillary ostia often are obstructed. The maxillary sinus can be cannulated and drained by passing a cannula from the nares through the maxillary ostium into the sinus.

The proximity of the molar teeth to the floor of the maxillary sinus poses potentially serious problems. During removal of a maxillary molar tooth, a fracture of a root may occur. If proper retrieval methods are not used, a piece of the root may be driven superiorly into the maxillary sinus. As a result a communication may be created between the oral cavity and the maxillary sinus.

The arterial supply of the maxillary sinus is mainly from superior alveolar branches of the *maxillary artery;* however, branches of the *greater palatine artery* supply the floor of the sinus (Fig. 7.39*B*). Innervation of the maxillary sinus is from the anterior, middle, and posterior *superior alveolar nerves* (Fig. 7.29*A*), branches of CN V$_2$.

Ear

The **ear** is divided into *external, middle,* and *internal parts* (Fig. 7.41). The external and middle parts are mainly concerned with the transference of sound to the internal ear, which contains the organ for equilibrium (the condition of being evenly balanced) as well as for hearing. The *tympanic membrane* (eardrum) separates the external ear from the middle ear. The *pharyngotympanic (auditory) tube* joins the middle ear to the nasopharynx.

External Ear

The **external ear** is composed of the *auricle* (pinna), which collects sound, and the *external acoustic meatus (canal),* which conducts sound to the tympanic membrane (Fig. 7.41*A* and *C*).

The **auricle** (L. *auris*) is composed of elastic cartilage covered by thin skin. The auricle has several depressions and elevations. The **concha** is the deepest depression, and the elevated margin of the auricle is the **helix.** The noncartilaginous **lobule** (earlobe) consists of fibrous tissue, fat, and blood vessels. It is easily pierced for taking small blood samples and inserting earrings. The **tragus** is a tongue-like projection overlapping the opening of the external acoustic meatus. The **arterial supply** to the auricle is derived mainly from the *posterior auricular* and *superficial temporal arteries* (Table 7.5). The main **nerves to the skin of the auricle** are the *great auricular* and *auriculotemporal nerves* (Table 7.4), with minor contributions from the facial (CN VII) and vagus (CN X) nerves.

Lymphatic drainage from the lateral surface of the superior half of the auricle is to the *superficial parotid lymph nodes.* Lymph from the cranial surface of the superior half of the auricle drains to the *mastoid* and *deep cervical lymph nodes* (Fig. 7.35*B*). Lymph from the remainder of the auricle, including the lobule, drains to the *superficial cervical lymph nodes.*

The **external acoustic meatus** is a canal that leads inward through the tympanic part of the temporal bone from the auricle to the tympanic membrane, a distance of 2–3 cm in adults (Fig. 7.41*C*). The lateral third of this slightly S-shaped canal is cartilaginous and lined with skin, which is continuous with the skin of the auricle. Its medial two thirds is bony and lined with thin skin that is continuous with the external layer of the tympanic membrane. The ceruminous and sebaceous glands produce *cerumen* (earwax).

The **tympanic membrane**, approximately 1 cm in diameter, is a thin, oval, semitransparent membrane at the medial end of the external acoustic meatus. It forms a partition between the meatus and the *tympanic cavity* of the middle ear (Fig.7.41*C*). The tympanic membrane is covered with thin skin externally and the mucous membrane of the middle ear internally.

Viewed through an otoscope (an instrument used for examining the tympanic membrane), the tympanic membrane is normally translucent and pearly gray. It has a concavity toward the external acoustic meatus with a shallow, cone-like central depression, the peak of which is the **umbo** (Fig. 7.42). The handle of the malleus (one of the small ear bones, or auditory ossicles, of the middle ear) is usually visible near the umbo. From the inferior end of

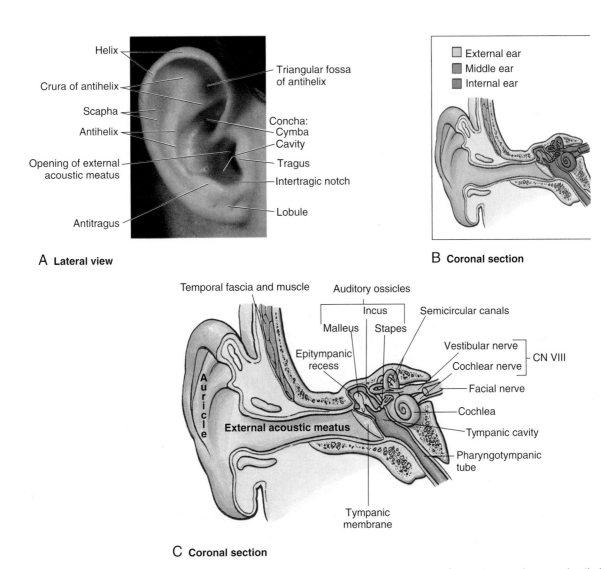

Figure 7.41. Ear. A. The surface anatomy of the ear is shown. B and C. The external, middle, and internal ear are detailed.

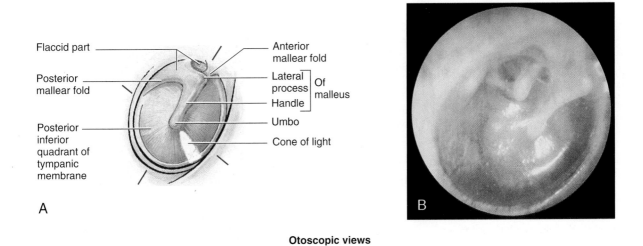

Otoscopic views

Figure 7.42. Right tympanic membrane.

the handle of the malleus, a bright **cone of light** is reflected from the otoscope's illuminator. This light reflex is visible, radiating anteroinferiorly in a healthy ear. Superior to the attachment of the lateral process of the malleus, the membrane is thin and is called the **flaccid part** (L. *pars flaccida*). It lacks the radial and circular fibers present in the remainder of the tympanic membrane, called the **tense part** (L. *pars tensa*).

The tympanic membrane moves in response to air vibrations that pass to it through the external acoustic meatus. Movements of the membrane are transmitted by the **auditory ossicles** (malleus, incus, and stapes) through the middle ear to the internal ear (Fig. 7.43). The external surface of the tympanic membrane is supplied mainly by the *auriculotemporal nerve,* a branch of CN V$_3$. Some innervation is supplied by a small *auricular branch of the vagus nerve* (CN

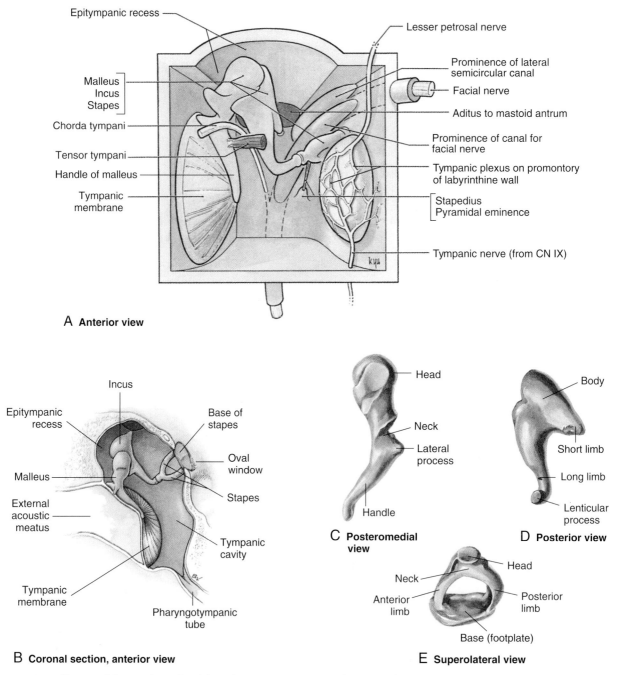

Figure 7.43. Auditory ossicles. A. The walls of the right tympanic cavity are shown. **B.** This view of the tympanic cavity shows the ossicles in situ. The features of the malleus (**C**), incus (**D**), and stapes (**E**) are shown.

X). The internal surface of the tympanic membrane is supplied by the *glossopharyngeal nerve* (CN IX).

Middle Ear

The **cavity of the middle ear** or **tympanic cavity,** is the narrow air-filled chamber in the petrous part of the temporal bone. The cavity has two parts: the **tympanic cavity proper,** the space directly internal to the tympanic membrane, and the **epitympanic recess,** the space superior to the membrane (Fig. 7.43*A* & *B*). The tympanic cavity is connected anteromedially with the nasopharynx by the **pharyngotympanic tube** and posterosuperiorly with the **mastoid antrum.** The tympanic cavity is lined with mucous membrane, which is continuous with the lining of the pharyngotympanic tube, mastoid cells, and mastoid antrum.

The contents of the middle ear are the:

- Auditory ossicles: malleus, incus, and stapes.
- Stapedius and tensor tympani muscles.
- Chorda tympani nerve, a branch of CN VII.
- Tympanic plexus of nerves.

WALLS OF THE TYMPANIC CAVITY

The middle ear, shaped like a narrow box with concave sides, has six walls (Figs. 7.43 and 7.44).

- The **tegmental wall (roof)** is formed by a thin plate of temporal bone, the *tegmen tympani,* which separates the tympanic cavity from the dura mater on the floor of the middle cranial fossa.
- The **jugular wall (floor)** is formed by a layer of bone that separates the tympanic cavity from the superior bulb of the IJV.
- The **membranous wall (lateral wall)** is formed almost entirely by the peaked convexity of the *tympanic membrane;* superiorly, it is formed by the lateral bony wall of the *epitympanic recess.* The handle of the malleus is attached to the tympanic membrane, and its head extends into the epitympanic recess.
- The **labyrinthine wall (medial wall)** separates the tympanic cavity from the internal ear. It also features the *promontory of the labyrinthine wall,* formed by the initial part (basal turn) of the cochlea, and the *oval* and *round windows.*
- The **carotid wall (anterior wall)** separates the tympanic cavity from the carotid canal, which contains the internal carotid artery; superiorly it has the **opening of the pharyngotympanic tube** and the **canal for the tensor tympani muscle.**
- The **mastoid wall (posterior wall)** has an opening in its superior part, the **aditus** (L. access) **to the mastoid antrum,** connecting the tympanic cavity to the mastoid cells; the canal for the facial nerve descends between the posterior wall and the antrum, medial to the aditus. The

tendon of the **stapedius muscle** emerges from the apex of the **pyramidal eminence,** a hollow, bony cone enclosing the stapedius muscle.

The **mastoid antrum** is a cavity in the mastoid process of the temporal bone (Fig. 7.44). The mastoid antrum is separated from the middle cranial fossa by the thin plate of temporal bone, called the **tegmen tympani.** The tegmen tympani forms part of the *tegmental wall* of the tympanic cavity and part of the floor of the middle cranial fossa lateral. The mastoid antrum is the common cavity into which the mastoid air cells open. The antrum and mastoid air cells are lined by mucous membrane, which is continuous with the lining of the middle ear. Anteroinferiorly, the mastoid antrum is related to the canal for the facial nerve.

AUDITORY OSSICLES

The **auditory ossicles** (malleus, incus, and stapes) form a mobile chain of small bones across the tympanic cavity from the tympanic membrane to the **oval window** (L. *fenestra vestibuli*), an oval opening on the labyrinthine wall of the tympanic cavity leading to the vestibule of the bony labyrinth (Fig. 7.43*B*). The ossicles are covered with the mucous membrane lining the tympanic cavity; but unlike other bones of the body, they are not directly covered with a layer of periosteum.

The **malleus** (L. hammer) is attached to the tympanic membrane (Fig. 7.43*C*). The rounded superior **head** of the malleus, lies in the epitympanic recess. The **neck** lies against the flaccid part of the tympanic membrane and the **handle** is embedded in the tympanic membrane with its tip at the umbo. The head of the malleus articulates with the incus; the tendon of the tensor tympani inserts into the handle of the malleus. The *chorda tympani nerve* crosses the medial surface of the neck of the malleus.

The **incus** (L. anvil) is located between the malleus and the stapes and articulates with them (Fig. 7.43*B* and *D*). The **body** of the incus lies in the epitympanic recess where it articulates with the head of the malleus. The **long limb** lies parallel to the handle of the malleus, and its inferior end articulates with the stapes by way of the **lenticular process.** The **short limb** is connected by a ligament to the posterior wall of the tympanic cavity. The **base of the stapes** fits into the oval window on the medial wall of the tympanic cavity.

The **stapes** (L. a stirrup) is the smallest ossicle (Fig. 7.43*E*). The **base** (footplate) of the stapes is attached to the margins of the oval window. The base is considerably smaller than the tympanic membrane; as a result, the vibratory force of the stapes is increased approximately 10 times over that of the tympanic membrane. Consequently, the auditory ossicles increase the force but decrease the amplitude of the vibrations transmitted from the tympanic membrane.

Two muscles dampen or resist movements of the auditory ossicles; one also dampens movements (vibrations) of the

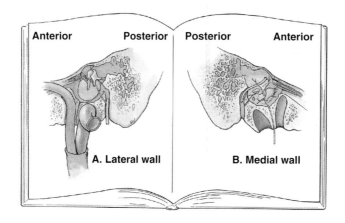

Anterior Posterior   Posterior Anterior

A. Lateral wall   B. Medial wall

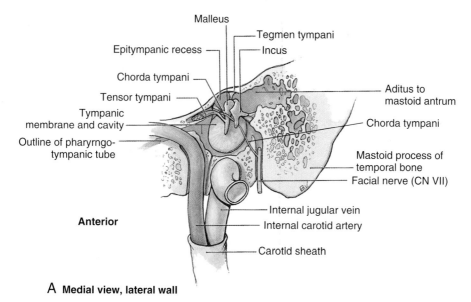

Malleus

Tegmen tympani

Epitympanic recess — Incus

Chorda tympani

Tensor tympani

Tympanic membrane and cavity

Outline of pharyrngo-tympanic tube

Aditus to mastoid antrum

Chorda tympani

Mastoid process of temporal bone

Facial nerve (CN VII)

Internal jugular vein

Internal carotid artery

Anterior

Carotld sheath

A **Medial view, lateral wall**

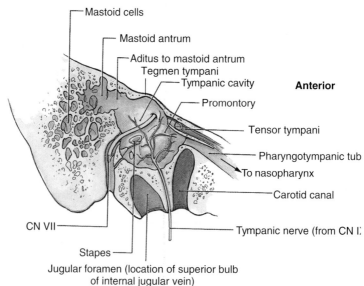

Mastoid cells

Mastoid antrum

Aditus to mastoid antrum
Tegmen tympani

Tympanic cavity **Anterior**

Promontory

Tensor tympani

Pharyngotympanic tub

To nasopharynx

Carotid canal

CN VII

Tympanic nerve (from CN I.

Stapes

Jugular foramen (location of superior bulb of internal jugular vein)

B **Lateral view, medial wall**

Figure 7.44. Dissections of right middle ear.

tympanic membrane. The **tensor tympani** is a short muscle that arises from the superior surface of the cartilaginous part of the pharyngotympanic tube, the greater wing of the sphenoid, and the petrous part of temporal bone (Figs. 7.43*A* and 7.44). The tensor tympani inserts into the handle of the malleus. The tensor tympani, supplied by CN V$_3$, pulls the handle of the malleus medially, tensing the tympanic membrane and reducing the amplitude of its oscillations. This action tends to prevent damage to the internal ear when one is exposed to loud sounds. The **stapedius** is a tiny muscle inside the **pyramidal eminence** (pyramid), a hollow, cone-shape prominence on the posterior wall of the tympanic cavity (Fig. 7.43*A*). Its tendon enters the tympanic cavity by emerging from a small foramen in the apex of the pyramidal eminence and inserts on the neck of the stapes. The nerve to the stapedius arises from CN VII. The stapedius pulls the stapes posteriorly and tilts its base in the *oval window,* thereby tightening the anular ligament and reducing the oscillatory range. It also prevents excessive movement of the stapes.

PHARYNGOTYMPANIC TUBE

The **pharyngotympanic tube** connects the tympanic cavity to the nasopharynx (Figs. 7.44*B* and 7.45), where it opens posterior to the inferior nasal meatus. The posterolateral third of the tube is bony and the remainder is cartilaginous. The

pharyngotympanic tube is lined by mucous membrane, which is continuous posteriorly with the lining of the tympanic cavity and anteriorly with the lining of the nasopharynx. The function of the pharyngotympanic tube is to equalize pressure in the middle ear with the atmospheric pressure, thereby allowing free movement of the tympanic membrane. By allowing air to enter and leave the tympanic cavity, this tube balances the pressure on both sides of the membrane. Because the walls of the cartilaginous part of the tube are normally in apposition, the tube must be actively opened. The tube is opened by the expanding girth of the belly of the *levator veli palatini* as it contracts longitudinally, pushing against one wall while the *tensor veli palatini* pulls on the other (Fig. 7.45). Because these are muscles of the soft palate, equalizing pressure (popping the eardrums) is commonly associated with activities such as yawning and swallowing.

The **arteries** of the pharyngotympanic tube are derived from the *ascending pharyngeal artery,* a branch of the external carotid artery, the *middle meningeal artery,* and the *artery of the pterygoid canal,* branches of the maxillary artery (Fig. 7.25). The **veins** of the pharyngotympanic tube drain into the *pterygoid venous plexus.* The **nerves** of the pharyngotympanic tube arise from the *tympanic plexus* (Fig. 7.43), which is formed by fibers of CN IX. The anterior part of the tube also receives nerve fibers from the *pterygopalatine ganglion.*

Internal Ear

The **internal ear** contains the **vestibulocochlear organ** concerned with the reception of sound and the maintenance of balance. Buried in the petrous part of the temporal bone (Fig. 7.46*A*), the internal ear consists of the sacs and ducts of the membranous labyrinth. The *membranous labyrinth,* containing *endolymph,* is suspended within the perilymph-filled *bony labyrinth,* either by delicate filaments similar to the filaments of arachnoid mater that traverse the subarachnoid space or by the spiral ligament (Figs. 7.46*C* and 7.47). These fluids are involved in stimulating the end organs for balance and hearing, respectively.

BONY LABYRINTH

The **bony labyrinth** is a series of cavities (cochlea, vestibule, and semicircular canals) contained within the otic capsule of the petrous part of the temporal bone. The **otic capsule** is made of bone that is denser than the remainder of the petrous temporal bone and can be isolated from it using a dental drill. The otic capsule is often erroneously illustrated and identified as being the bony labyrinth. However, the bony labyrinth is the *fluid-filled space,* which is surrounded by the otic capsule and is most accurately represented by a cast of the otic capsule after removal of the surrounding bone (Fig. 7.46*C*).

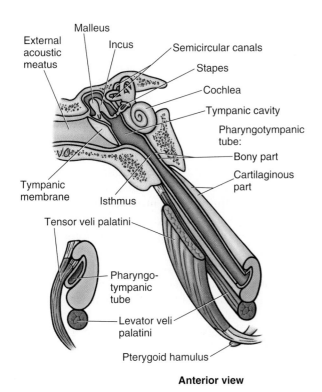

Anterior view

Figure 7.45. Right pharyngotympanic (auditory) tube. The tube is open throughout its length by removing its membranous wall and the lateral part of its bony wall.

Paralysis of the Stapedius

The tympanic muscles have a protective action in that they dampen large vibrations of the tympanic membrane resulting from loud noises. Paralysis of the stapedius muscle (e.g., resulting from a lesion of the facial nerve) is associated with excessive acuteness of hearing called *hyperacusis* or hyperacusia. This condition results from uninhibited movements of the stapes.

Blockage of Pharyngotympanic Tube

The pharyngotympanic tube forms a route for infections to pass from the nasopharynx to the tympanic cavity. This tube is blocked easily by swelling of its mucous membrane, even as a result of mild infections, because the walls of its cartilaginous part are normally already in apposition. When the pharyngotympanic tube is occluded, residual air in the tympanic cavity is usually absorbed into the mucosal blood vessels, resulting in lower pressure in the tympanic cavity, retraction of the tympanic membrane, and interference with its free movement. Finally, hearing is affected.

The **cochlea** is the shell-shaped part of the bony labyrinth that contains the **cochlear duct**, the part of the internal ear concerned with hearing (Fig. 7.46C). The **spiral canal** of the cochlea begins at the vestibule and makes 2.5 turns around a bony core, the **modiolus**. The modiolus contains canals for blood vessels and for the distribution of the branches of the cochlear nerve (Fig. 7.47). The large basal turn of the cochlea produces the *promontory of the labyrinthine wall* of the tympanic cavity (Fig. 7.43). At the basal turn, the bony labyrinth communicates with the subarachnoid space superior to the jugular foramen through the **cochlear aqueduct**. It also features the **round window**, closed by the **secondary tympanic membrane**.

The **vestibule of the bony labyrinth** is a small oval chamber (approximately 5 mm long) that contains the **utricle** and **saccule** and parts of the balancing apparatus (vestibular labyrinth) (Fig. 7.46). The vestibule features the *oval window* on its lateral wall, occupied by the base of the stapes. The vestibule is continuous with the bony cochlea anteriorly, the semicircular canals posteriorly, and the posterior cranial fossa by the **aqueduct of the vestibule**. The aqueduct extends to the posterior surface of the petrous part of the temporal bone, where it opens posterolateral to the *internal acoustic meatus*. The vestibular aqueduct transmits the **endolymphatic duct** and two small blood vessels.

The **semicircular canals** (anterior, posterior, and lateral) communicate with the vestibule of the bony labyrinth. The canals lie posterosuperior to the vestibule into which they open and are set at right angles to each other. They occupy three planes in space (Fig. 7.47B). Each semicircular canal forms about two thirds of a circle and is about 1.5 mm in diameter, except at one end where there is a swelling, the **bony ampulla**. The canals have only five openings into the vestibule because the anterior and posterior canals share a common limb to both. Lodged within the canals are the *semicircular ducts* of the membranous labyrinth.

MEMBRANOUS LABYRINTH

The **membranous labyrinth** consists of a series of communicating sacs and ducts that are suspended in the bony labyrinth (Fig. 7.46). The membranous labyrinth contains **endolymph**, a watery fluid similar in composition to intracellular fluid, thus differing in composition from the surrounding **perilymph** (which is like extracellular fluid), which fills the remainder of the bony labyrinth. The membranous labyrinth is composed of two divisions, the *vestibular labyrinth* and the *cochlear labyrinth,* and consists of more parts than does the bony labyrinth:

- **Vestibular labyrinth**—utricle and saccule, two small communicating sacs in the vestibule of the bony labyrinth.
- Three **semicircular ducts** in the semicircular canals.
- **Cochlear labyrinth**—cochlear duct in the cochlea.

The **spiral ligament**, a spiral thickening of the periosteal lining of the cochlear canal, *secures the cochlear duct* to the spiral canal of the cochlea (Fig. 7.47).

The **semicircular ducts** open into the *utricle* through five openings, reflecting the way the surrounding semicircular canals open into the vestibule. The utricle communicates with the saccule through the **utriculosaccular duct**, from which the *endolymphatic duct* arises (Fig. 7.46C). The *saccule* is continuous with the cochlear duct through the **ductus reunions**, a uniting duct (Fig. 7.46B). The utricle and saccule have specialized areas of sensory epithelium called *maculae*. The **macula of the utricle** (L. *macula utriculi*) is in the floor of the utricle, parallel to the base of the cranium (Fig. 7.46B); whereas the **macula of the saccule** (L. *macula sacculi*) is vertically placed on the medial wall of the saccule. The **hair cells in the maculae** are innervated by fibers of the vestibular division of the **vestibulocochlear nerve** (CN VIII). The cell bodies of the sensory neurons are in the **vestibular ganglia**, which are in the internal acoustic meatus (Fig. 7.46A).

The *endolymphatic duct* traverses the vestibular aqueduct and emerges through the bone of the posterior cranial fossa,

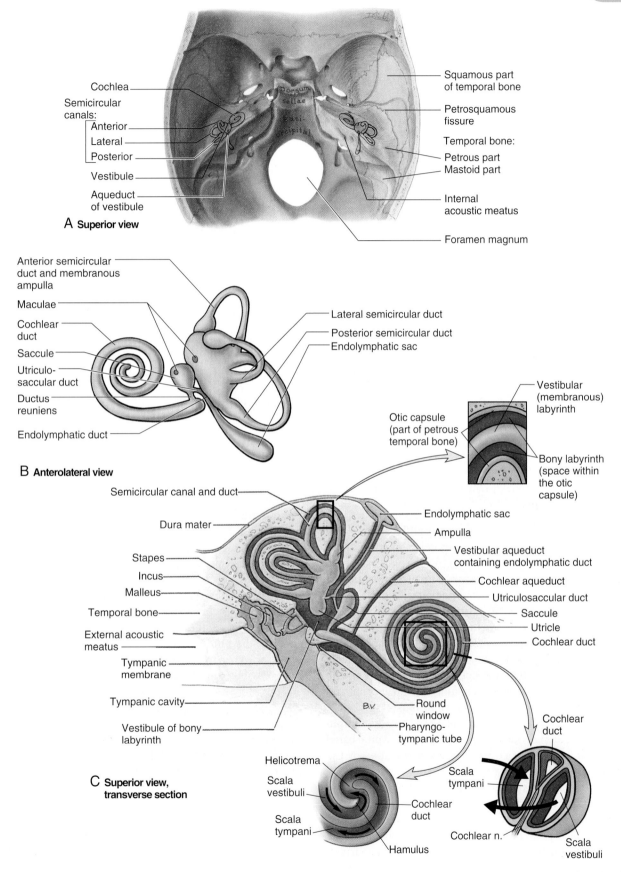

Figure 7.46. Internal ear. A. Parts of the temporal bone and bony labyrinth are shown in situ. **B.** The left vestibular labyrinth is detailed. **C.** Note the relationships of the structures of the middle and inner ear. Observe that the membranous labyrinth is suspended in the bony labyrinth.

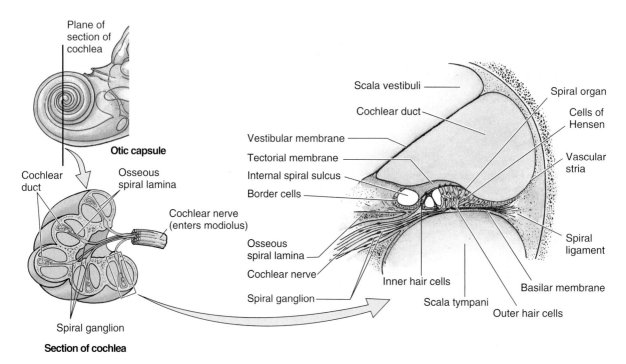

Plane of section of cochlea

Otic capsule

Cochlear duct

Osseous spiral lamina

Cochlear nerve (enters modiolus)

Spiral ganglion

Section of cochlea

Scala vestibuli

Cochlear duct

Vestibular membrane

Tectorial membrane

Internal spiral sulcus

Border cells

Osseous spiral lamina

Cochlear nerve

Spiral ganglion

Spiral organ

Cells of Hensen

Vascular stria

Spiral ligament

Inner hair cells

Scala tympani

Basilar membrane

Outer hair cells

Figure 7.47. Structure of cochlea and spiral organ.

where it expands into a blind pouch called the **endolymphatic sac.** It is located under the dura on the posterior surface of the petrous part of the temporal bone (Fig. 7.46A & C). The endolymphatic sac is a storage reservoir for excess endolymph formed by the blood capillaries in the membranous labyrinth.

Each **semicircular duct** has an **ampulla** at one end containing a sensory area, the **ampullary crest** (L. *crista ampullaris*). The crests are sensors for recording movements of the endolymph in the ampulla, resulting from rotation of the head in the plane of the duct. The hair cells of the crest, like those of the maculae, stimulate primary sensory neurons whose cell bodies are in the *vestibular ganglia.*

The **cochlear duct** is a spiral, blind tube, closed at one end and triangular in cross-section (Fig. 7.46C). The duct is firmly suspended across the cochlear canal between the *spiral ligament* on the external wall of the cochlear canal and the **osseous spiral lamina** of the modiolus (Fig. 7.47). Spanning the spiral canal in this manner, the endolymph-filled cochlear duct divides the perilymph-filled spiral canal into two channels that communicate at the apex of the cochlea at the **helicotrema** (Fig. 7.46C).

Waves of hydraulic pressure created in the perilymph of the vestibule by the vibrations of the base of the stapes ascend to the apex of the cochlea by one channel, the **scala vestibule.** The pressure waves then pass through the helicotrema and then descend back to the basal turn of the cochlea by the other channel, the **scala tympani.** There the pressure waves again become vibrations, this time of the *secondary tympanic membrane,* which occupies the

round window. Here the energy initially received by the (primary) tympanic membrane is finally dissipated into the air of the tympanic cavity.

The roof of the cochlear duct is formed by the **vestibular membrane** (Fig. 7.47). The floor of the duct is formed by part of the duct, the **basilar membrane,** plus the outer edge of the osseous spiral lamina. The receptor of auditory stimuli is the **spiral organ** (of Corti), situated on the basilar membrane. It is overlaid by the gelatinous **tectorial membrane.** The spiral organ contains hair cells, the tips of which are embedded in the tectorial membrane. The spiral organ is stimulated to respond by deformation of the cochlear duct induced by hydraulic pressure waves in the perilymph, which ascend and descend in the surrounding scala vestibuli and tympani.

INTERNAL ACOUSTIC MEATUS

The **internal acoustic meatus** is a narrow canal that runs laterally for approximately 1 cm within the petrous part of the temporal bone (Fig. 7.46A). The **internal acoustic opening** of the meatus is in the posteromedial part of this bone, in line with the external acoustic meatus. The internal acoustic meatus is closed laterally by a thin, perforated plate of bone that separates it from the internal ear. Through this plate pass the facial nerve (CN VII), the vestibulocochlear nerve (CN VIII) and blood vessels. The vestibulocochlear nerve divides near the lateral end of the internal acoustic meatus into two parts: a cochlear nerve

Otoscopic Examination

Examination of the external acoustic meatus and tympanic membrane begins by straightening the meatus. In adults, the helix is grasped and pulled posterosuperiorly (up, out, and back). These movements reduce the curvature of the external acoustic meatus, facilitating insertion of the *otoscope*. The external acoustic meatus is relatively short in infants; therefore, extra care must be taken to prevent damage to the tympanic membrane.

Otitis Media

An earache and bulging red tympanic membrane may indicate pus or fluid in the middle ear, a sign of **otitis media.** Infection of the middle ear often is secondary to upper respiratory infections. Inflammation and swelling of the mucous membrane lining the tympanic cavity may cause partial or complete *blockage of the pharyngotympanic tube.* The tympanic membrane becomes red and bulges and the person may complain of "ear popping" (Fig. B7.8A). If untreated, otitis media may produce impaired hearing as the result of scarring of the auditory ossicles, limiting the ability of these bones to move in response to sound.

Perforation of Tympanic Membrane

Perforation of the tympanic membrane (ruptured eardrum) may result from *otitis media.* Perforation may also result from foreign bodies in the external acoustic meatus, trauma, or excessive pressure (e.g., during scuba diving). Because the superior half of the tympanic membrane is much more vascular than the inferior half, incisions (e.g., to release pus from a middle ear abscess) are made posteroinferiorly through the membrane. This incision also avoids injury to the chorda tympani nerve and auditory ossicles.

Mastoiditis

Infections of the mastoid antrum and mastoid cells (**mastoiditis**) result from middle ear infections that cause inflammation of the mastoid process (Fig. B7.8B). Infections may spread superiorly into the middle cranial fossa through the petrosquamous fissure in children or may cause *osteomyelitis* (bone infection) of the tegmen tympani. Since the advent of antibiotics, mastoiditis is uncommon. During operations for mastoiditis, surgeons are conscious of the course of the facial nerve so that it will not be injured. One point of access to the tympanic cavity is through the mastoid antrum. In children, only a thin plate of bone must be removed from the lateral wall of the mastoid antrum to expose the tympanic cavity. In adults, bone must be penetrated for 15 mm or more. At present, most *mastoidectomies* are endaural (i.e., performed through the posterior wall of the external acoustic meatus).

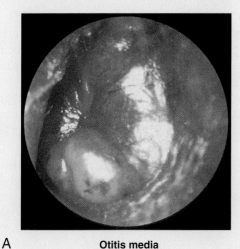

A   **Otitis media**

Figure B7.8A

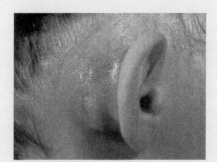

B   **Mastoiditis (ruptured retroauricular abscess)**

Figure B7.8B

Motion Sickness

The maculae of the membranous labyrinth are primarily static organs, which have small dense particles (otoliths) embedded among the hair cells. Under the influence of gravity, the *otoliths* cause bending of the hair cells, which stimulate the vestibular nerve and provide awareness of the position of the head in space; the hairs also respond to quick tilting movements and to linear acceleration and deceleration. *Motion sickness* results mainly from discordance between vestibular and visual stimuli.

High-Tone Deafness

Persistent exposure to excessively loud sounds causes degenerative changes in the spiral organ, resulting in *high-tone deafness*. This type of hearing loss commonly occurs in workers who are exposed to loud noises and do not wear protective earmuffs (e.g., people working for long periods around jet engines).

Otic Barotrauma

Injury caused to the ear by an imbalance in pressure between the ambient (surrounding) air and the air in the middle ear is called *otic barotrauma*. This type of injury occurs in fliers and divers.

Medical Imaging of Head

Radiography, although replaced by newer imaging modalities in many specific cases, is often used for cranial examinations. Because crania vary considerably in shape, one must examine radiographs carefully for abnormalities (Fig. 7.48). To visualize the arteries of the brain, a radiopaque contrast medium is injected into the carotid or vertebral artery and radiographs are taken, producing arteriograms. This type of radiograph is used for detecting cerebral aneurysms and arteriovenous malformations.

CT is the premier imaging method for neurodiagnosis (Fig. 7.49) and is more informative than plain cranial radiographs. For reasons of cost, speed, and availability, CT is widely used for evaluation of head injury. It is especially useful for people who are neuro-logically or medically unstable, uncooperative, or claustrophobic and for patients with pacemakers or other metallic implants.

MRI is slower and more expensive than CT but shows much more detail in the soft tissues than does CT (Fig. 7.50). MRI is the gold standard for detecting and delineating intracranial and spinal lesions because it provides good soft tissue contrast of normal and pathological structures. It also permits multiplanar capability, which provides three-dimensional information and relationships that are not so readily available with CT. MRI can also demonstrate blood and CSF flow. Magnetic resonance angiography (MRA) is useful for determining the patency of vessels of the cerebral arterial circle. ●

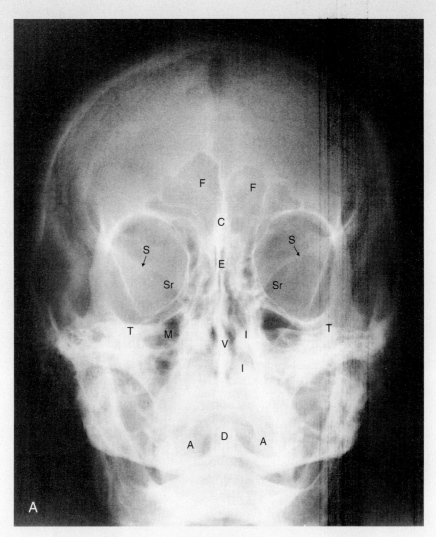

Anteroposterior view

Figure 7.48. Radiographs of cranium (skull). A. Observe the superior orbital fissure (*Sr*), the lesser wings of the sphenoid (*S*), and the superior surface of the petrous part of the temporal bone (*T*). Also observe that the nasal septum is formed by the perpendicular plate of the ethmoid (*E*) and the vomer (*V*). Examine the inferior and middle conchae (*I*) of the lateral wall of the nose, the crista galli (*C*), the frontal sinus (*F*), and the maxillary sinus (*M*). Superimposed on the facial skeleton (viscerocranium) is the dens of the axis (*D*) and the lateral masses of the atlas (*A*).

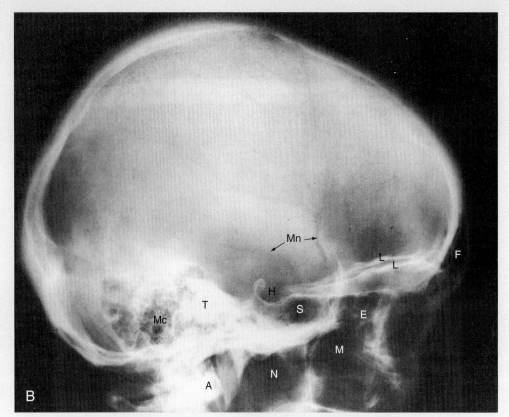

Lateral view

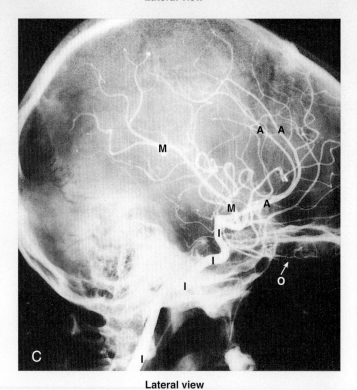

Lateral view

Figure 7.48. *(continued)* **B.** Observe the paranasal sinuses: frontal (*F*), ethmoidal (*E*), sphenoidal (*S*), and maxillary (*M*). Also observe the hypophysial fossa (*H*) for the pituitary gland, the great density of the petrous part of the temporal bone (*T*), and the mastoid cells (*Mc*). Note that the right and left orbital parts of the frontal bone are not superimposed; thus the floor of the anterior cranial fossa appears as two lines (*L*). Observe the bony grooves for the branches of the middle meningeal vessels (*Mn*), the anterior arch of the atlas (*A*), and the nasopharynx (*N*). (Courtesy of Dr. E. Becker, Associate Professor of Diagnostic Imaging, University of Toronto, Toronto, Ontario, Canada.) **C.** In this carotid arteriogram, observe the internal carotid artery (*I*), anterior cerebral artery (*A*), middle cerebral artery (*M*), and ophthalmic artery (*O*).

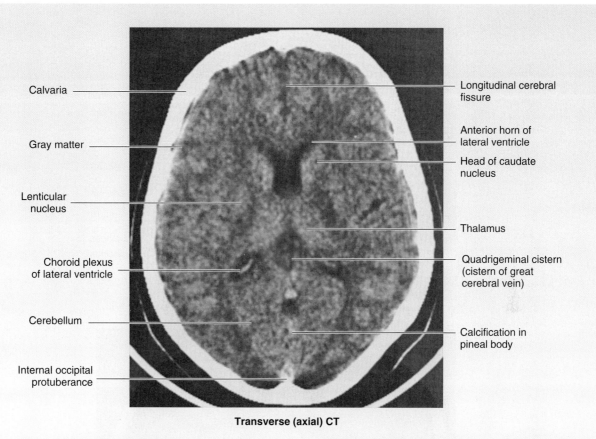

Calvaria

Gray matter

Lenticular
nucleus

Choroid plexus
of lateral ventricle

Cerebellum

Internal occipital
protuberance

Longitudinal cerebral
fissure

Anterior horn of
lateral ventricle

Head of caudate
nucleus

Thalamus

Quadrigeminal cistern
(cistern of great
cerebral vein)

Calcification in
pineal body

Transverse (axial) CT

Figure 7.49. CT scan of brain. Observe the ventricles, various parts of the brain, and the choroid plexus of the lateral ventricle.

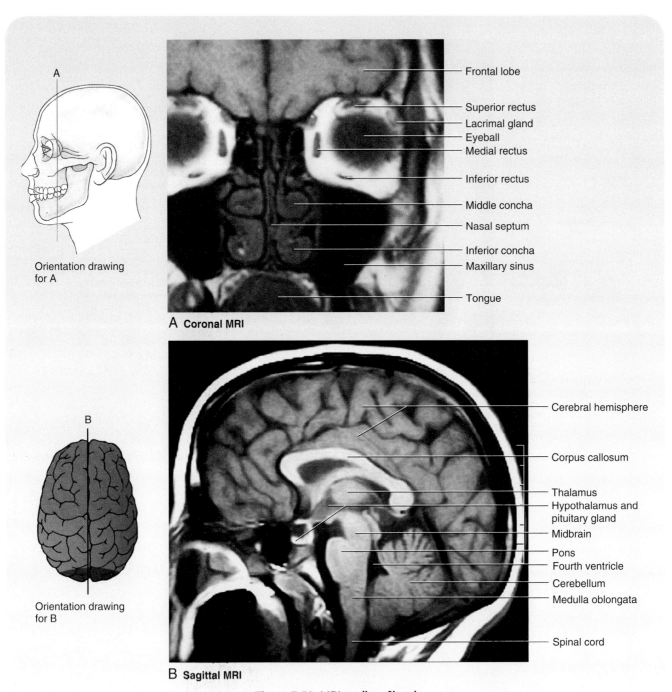

A **Orientation drawing for A**

Frontal lobe

Superior rectus
Lacrimal gland
Eyeball
Medial rectus

Inferior rectus

Middle concha

Nasal septum

Inferior concha
Maxillary sinus

Tongue

A **Coronal MRI**

B **Orientation drawing for B**

Cerebral hemisphere

Corpus callosum

Thalamus
Hypothalamus and pituitary gland
Midbrain
Pons
Fourth ventricle
Cerebellum
Medulla oblongata

Spinal cord

B **Sagittal MRI**

Figure 7.50. MRI studies of head.

8 Neck

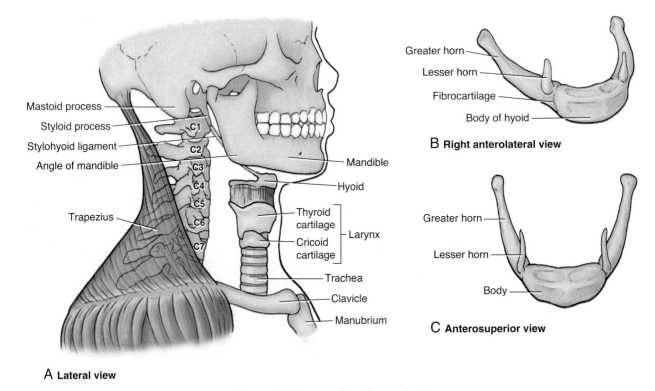

Figure 8.1. Bones and cartilages of neck.

The **neck** (L. *collum, cervix*) joins the head to the trunk and limbs and serves as a major conduit for structures passing between them. In addition, several important organs with unique functions are located here: the larynx and the thyroid and parathyroid glands, for example.

The *skeleton of the neck* is formed by the seven cervical vertebrae, hyoid bone (referred to as the *hyoid* in common usage), manubrium of the sternum, and clavicles (Fig. 8.1*A*). The mobile hyoid lies in the anterior part of the neck at the level of the C3 vertebra in the angle between the mandible and thyroid cartilage. The hyoid does not articulate with any other bone and functionally serves as an attachment for anterior neck muscles and a prop to keep the airway open (Fig. 8.1*B* & *C*).

Fascia of Neck

Structures in the neck are surrounded by a layer of fatty subcutaneous tissue (superficial fascia) and are compartmentalized by layers of deep cervical fascia. The fascial planes determine the direction in which an infection in the neck may spread.

Cervical Subcutaneous Tissue and Platysma

The **subcutaneous tissue of the neck** (superficial cervical fascia) is usually a thin layer of connective tissue that lies between the dermis of the skin and the investing layer of deep cervical fascia (Fig. 8.2). It contains cutaneous nerves, blood and lymphatic vessels, superficial lymph nodes, and variable amounts of fat; anterolaterally, it contains the platysma. The **platysma**, a muscle of facial expression, arises in fascia covering the superior parts of the deltoid and pectoralis major muscles and sweeps superomedially over the clavicle to the inferior border of the mandible (Table 8.2).

Deep Cervical Fascia

The **deep cervical fascia** consists of three fascial layers (Fig. 8.2): *investing, pretracheal,* and *prevertebral.* These layers support the viscera (e.g., thyroid gland), muscles, vessels, and deep lymph nodes. These fascial layers provide the slipperiness that allows structures in the neck to move and pass over one another without difficulty, e.g., when swallowing and turning the head and neck. These fascial layers form natural cleavage planes, allowing separation of tissues during surgery.

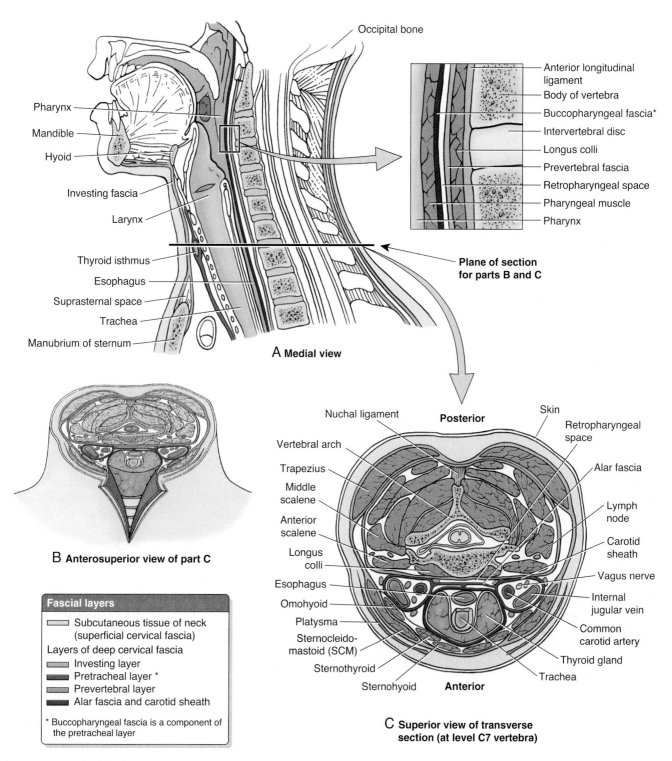

Occipital bone

Pharynx

Mandible

Hyoid

Investing fascia

Larynx

Thyroid isthmus

Esophagus

Suprasternal space

Trachea

Manubrium of sternum

A Medial view

Anterior longitudinal ligament
Body of vertebra
Buccopharyngeal fascia*
Intervertebral disc
Longus colli
Prevertebral fascia
Retropharyngeal space
Pharyngeal muscle
Pharynx

Plane of section for parts B and C

B Anterosuperior view of part C

Fascial layers

Subcutaneous tissue of neck (superficial cervical fascia)

Layers of deep cervical fascia
Investing layer
Pretracheal layer *
Prevertebral layer
Alar fascia and carotid sheath

* Buccopharyngeal fascia is a component of the pretracheal layer

Nuchal ligament
Vertebral arch
Trapezius
Middle scalene
Anterior scalene
Longus colli
Esophagus
Omohyoid
Platysma
Sternocleido-mastoid (SCM)
Sternothyroid
Sternohyoid

Posterior

Skin
Retropharyngeal space
Alar fascia
Lymph node
Carotid sheath
Vagus nerve
Internal jugular vein
Common carotid artery
Thyroid gland
Trachea

Anterior

C Superior view of transverse section (at level C7 vertebra)

Figure 8.2. Cervical fascia. A. *Inset,* note the fascia in the retropharyngeal region. **B.** This view of the fascial compartments of the neck demonstrates an anterior midline approach to the thyroid gland. **C.** This section of the neck passes through the isthmus of the thyroid gland.

INVESTING LAYER OF DEEP CERVICAL FASCIA

The **investing layer of deep cervical fascia**, the most superficial deep fascial layer, surrounds the entire neck deep to the skin and subcutaneous tissue (Fig. 8.2). At the "four corners" of the neck, the investing layer splits into superficial and deep layers of fascia to enclose (invest) the *sternocleidomastoid* (SCM) and *trapezius muscles*. Superiorly, the investing layer of fascia attaches to the superior nuchal line of the occipital bone, mastoid processes of the temporal bones, zygomatic arches, inferior border of the mandible, hyoid, and spinous processes of the cervical vertebrae. Just inferior to its attachment to the mandible, the investing layer of fascia splits to enclose the submandibular gland; posterior to the mandible, it splits to form the fibrous capsule of the parotid gland.

Inferiorly, the investing layer of fascia attaches to the manubrium of the sternum, clavicles, acromions, and spines of the scapulae. The investing layer is continuous posteriorly with the periosteum covering the C7 spinous process and the **nuchal ligament** (L. *ligamentum nuchae*) (Fig.8.2*B*). Just superior to the manubrium, the fascia remains divided into the two layers that enclose the SCM; one layer attaches to the anterior and the other to the posterior surface of the manubrium. A **suprasternal space** lies between these layers and encloses the inferior ends of the anterior jugular veins, the jugular venous arch, fat, and a few deep lymph nodes (Fig. 8.2*A*).

PRETRACHEAL LAYER OF DEEP CERVICAL FASCIA

The thin **pretracheal layer of deep cervical fascia** is limited to the anterior part of the neck (Fig. 8.2). It extends inferiorly from the hyoid into the thorax, where it blends with the fibrous pericardium covering the heart. The pretracheal layer includes a thin *muscular part,* which encloses the infrahyoid muscles, and a *visceral part,* which encloses the thyroid gland, trachea, and esophagus and is continuous posteriorly and superiorly with the *buccopharyngeal fascia* (Fig. 8.2). The pretracheal layer blends laterally with the *carotid sheaths*.

The **carotid sheath** is a tubular fascial investment that extends from the cranial base to the root of the neck. This sheath blends anteriorly with the investing and pretracheal layers of fascia and posteriorly with the prevertebral layer of deep cervical fascia. The carotid sheath contains (Fig. 8.2*B* & *C*):

- The common and internal carotid arteries.
- The internal jugular vein (IJV).
- The vagus nerve (CN X).
- Some deep cervical lymph nodes.
- The carotid sinus nerve.
- Sympathetic nerve fibers (carotid periarterial plexuses).

The carotid sheath communicates with the mediastinum of the thorax inferiorly and the cranial cavity superiorly.

These communications represent potential pathways for the spread of infection and extravasated blood.

PREVERTEBRAL LAYER OF DEEP CERVICAL FASCIA

The **prevertebral layer of deep cervical fascia** forms a tubular sheath for the vertebral column and the muscles associated with it, such as the *longus colli* and *longus capitis* anteriorly, the *scalenes* laterally, and the *deep cervical muscles* posteriorly (Fig. 8.2). This layer of fascia is fixed to the cranial base superiorly and inferiorly and fuses with the *anterior longitudinal ligament* centrally at approximately T3 vertebra. The prevertebral layer extends laterally as the *axillary sheath* (see Chapter 6), which surrounds the axillary vessels and brachial plexus.

RETROPHARYNGEAL SPACE

The **retropharyngeal space** is the largest and most important interfascial space in the neck because it is the major pathway for the spread of infection (Fig.8.2*A*). It is a potential space that consists of loose connective tissue between the visceral part of the prevertebral layer of deep cervical fascia and *the buccopharyngeal fascia* surrounding the pharynx superficially. Inferiorly, the buccopharyngeal fascia is continuous with the pretracheal layer of deep cervical fascia. The *alar fascia* forms a further subdivision of the retropharyngeal space. This thin layer is attached along the midline of the buccopharyngeal fascia from the cranium to the level of the C7 vertebra and extends laterally to blend with the carotid sheath. The retropharyngeal space is closed superiorly by the base of the cranium and on each side by the carotid sheath. This space permits movement of the pharynx, esophagus, larynx, and trachea relative to the vertebral column during swallowing.

Superficial Structures of Neck: Cervical Regions

To allow clear communications regarding the location of structures, injuries, or pathologies, the neck is divided into regions (Table 8.1). The four major regions are the (1) sternocleidomastoid region, (2) posterior cervical region, (3) lateral cervical region, and (4) anterior cervical region.

Sternocleidomastoid Region

The **sternocleidomastoid** (SCM) visibly divides each side of the neck into *anterior* and *lateral cervical triangles* (Table 8.1). The region between these triangular regions, corresponding to the area of this broad, strap-like muscle, is the **sternoclei-**

Table 8.1 Cervical Regions/Triangles and Contents[a]

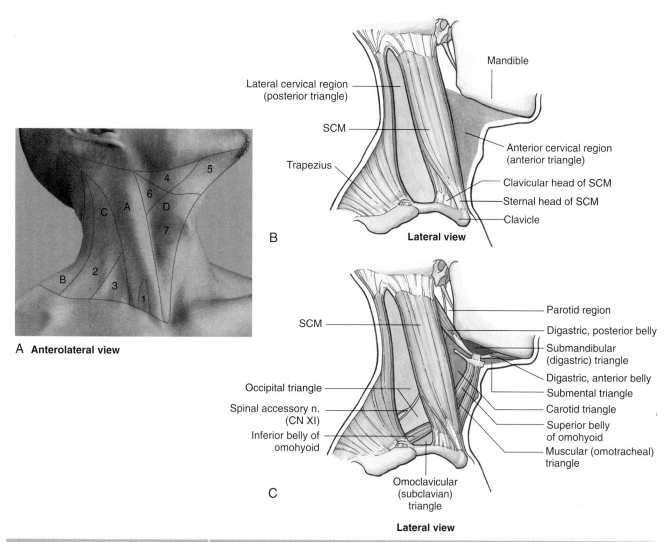

A Anterolateral view

B Lateral view

Lateral cervical region (posterior triangle)
SCM
Trapezius
Mandible
Anterior cervical region (anterior triangle)
Clavicular head of SCM
Sternal head of SCM
Clavicle

C Lateral view

SCM
Occipital triangle
Spinal accessory n. (CN XI)
Inferior belly of omohyoid
Omoclavicular (subclavian) triangle
Parotid region
Digastric, posterior belly
Submandibular (digastric) triangle
Digastric, anterior belly
Submental triangle
Carotid triangle
Superior belly of omohyoid
Muscular (omotracheal) triangle

Region	Main Contents and Underlying Structures
Sternocleidomastoid region (A)	Sternocleidomastoid (SCM) muscle; superior part of the external jugular vein; greater auricular nerve; transverse cervical nerve
Lesser supraclavicular fossa (1)	Inferior part of internal jugular vein
Posterior cervical region (B)	Trapezius muscle; cutaneous branches of posterior rami of cervical spinal nerves; suboccipital region or triangle (E) lies deep to superior part of this region
Lateral cervical region (posterior triangle of neck) (C)	
Occipital triangle (2)	Part of external jugular vein; posterior branches of cervical plexus of nerves; spinal accessory nerve; trunks of brachial plexus; transverse cervical artery; cervical lymph nodes
Omoclavicular (subclavian) triangle (3)	Subclavian artery (third part); part of subclavian vein (sometimes); suprascapular artery; supraclavicular lymph nodes
Anterior cervical region (anterior triangle of neck) (D)	
Submandibular (digastric) triangle (4)	Submandibular gland almost fills triangle; submandibular lymph nodes; hypoglossal nerve; mylohyoid nerve; parts of facial artery and vein
Submental triangle (5)	Submental lymph nodes and small veins that unite to form anterior jugular vein
Carotid triangle (6)	Common carotid artery and its branches; internal jugular vein and its tributaries; vagus nerve; external carotid artery and some of its branches; hypoglossal nerve and superior root of ansa cervicalis; spinal accessory nerve; thyroid gland, larynx; pharynx; deep cervical lymph nodes; branches of cervical plexus
Muscular (omotracheal) triangle (7)	Sternothyroid and sternohyoid muscles; thyroid and parathyroid glands

[a]Letters and numbers in parentheses refer to the figure A.

Spread of Infection in the Neck

The investing layer of deep cervical fascia helps prevent the spread of abscesses caused by tissue destruction. If an infection occurs between the investing layer of deep cervical fascia and the muscular part of the pretracheal fascia surrounding the infrahyoid muscles, the infection usually will not spread beyond the superior edge of the manubrium. If, however, the infection occurs between the investing fascia and the visceral part of the pretracheal fascia, it can spread into the thoracic cavity anterior to the pericardium. Pus from an abscess posterior to the prevertebral layer of deep cervical fascia may extend laterally in the neck and form a swelling posterior to the SCM. The pus may perforate the prevertebral layer of deep cervical fascia and enter the retropharyngeal space, producing a bulge in the pharynx (*retropharyngeal abscess*). This swelling may cause difficulty in swallowing (*dysphagia*) and speaking (*dysarthria*). Similarly, air from a ruptured trachea, bronchus, or esophagus (*pneumomediastinum*) can pass superiorly in the neck.

Torticollis

Torticollis is a contraction of the cervical muscles that produces twisting of the neck and slanting of the head (Fig. B8.1). The most common type of *congenital torticollis* (wry neck) results from a fibrous tissue tumor (L. *fibromatosis colli*) that develops in the SCM before or shortly after birth. Occasionally, the SCM is injured when an infant's head is pulled excessively during a difficult birth, tearing its fibers (*muscular torticollis*). A hematoma occurs that may develop into a fibrous mass that entraps a branch of the spinal accessory nerve (CN XI), thus denervating part of the SCM. Surgical release of a partially fibrotic SCM from its distal attachments to the manubrium and clavicle may be necessary to enable the person to tilt and rotate the head normally.

Cervical dystonia (abnormal tonicity of the cervical muscles), commonly known as *spasmodic torticollis,* usually begins in adulthood. It may involve any bilateral combination of lateral neck muscles, especially the SCM and trapezius.

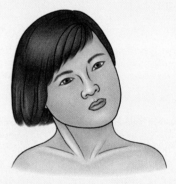

Figure B8.1.

domastoid region of the neck. The SCM has two heads: the rounded tendon of the **sternal head** attaches to the manubrium, and the thick fleshy **clavicular head** attaches to the superior surface of the medial third of the clavicle. The two heads are separated inferiorly by a space, the **lesser supraclavicular fossa.** The heads join superiorly as they pass obliquely upward to attach to the mastoid process of the temporal bone and the superior nuchal line of the occipital bone. The attachments, innervation, and actions of the SCM are summarized in Table 8.2.

Posterior Cervical Region

The region posterior to the anterior border of the trapezius is the **posterior cervical region** (Table 8.1). The *suboccipital region* is deep to the superior part of this region. The **trapezius** is a large, flat triangular muscle that covers the posterolateral aspect of the neck and thorax. It is a superficial muscle of the back, a muscle of the pectoral girdle, and a cervical muscle. The trapezius attaches the pectoral girdle to the cranium and vertebral column and assists in suspending it. Its attachments, nerve supply, and main actions are described in Table 8.2.

Lateral Cervical Region

The **lateral cervical region** (posterior triangle of the neck) is bounded (Table 8.1)

- Anteriorly by the posterior border of the SCM.
- Posteriorly by the anterior border of the trapezius.
- Inferiorly by the middle third of the clavicle between the trapezius and the SCM.
- By an *apex,* where the SCM and trapezius meet on the superior nuchal line of the occipital bone.
- By a *roof,* formed by the investing layer of deep cervical fascia.

Table 8.2 Cutaneous and Superficial Muscles of the Neck

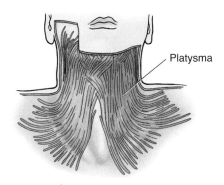

Platysma

A **Anterior view**

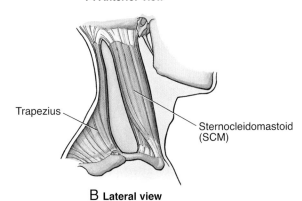

Trapezius

Sternocleidomastoid (SCM)

B **Lateral view**

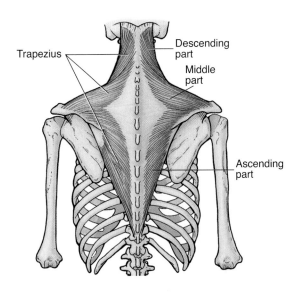

Trapezius

Descending part

Middle part

Ascending part

C **Posterior view**

Muscle	Superior Attachment	Inferior Attachment	Innervation	Main Action(s)
Platysma	Inferior border of mandible, skin, and subcutaneous tissues of lower face	Fascia covering superior parts of pectoralis major and deltoid muscles	Cervical branch of facial nerve (CN VII)	Draws corners of mouth inferiorly and widens it as in expressions of sadness and fright; draws skin of neck superiorly when teeth are clenched
Sternocleidomastoid	Lateral surface of mastoid process of temporal bone and lateral half of superior nuchal line	*Sternal head:* anterior surface of manubrium of sternum *Clavicular head:* superior surface of medial third of clavicle	Spinal accessory nerve (CN XI; motor); C2 and C3 nerves (pain and proprioception)	*Unilateral contraction:* tilts head to same side (i.e., laterally flexes neck) and rotates it so face is turned superiorly toward opposite side *Bilateral contraction:* (1) extends neck at atlanto-occipital joints, (2) flexes cervical vertebrae so that chin approaches manubrium, or (3) extends superior cervical vertebrae while flexing inferior vertebrae so chin is thrust forward with head kept level With cervical vertebrae fixed, may elevate manubrium and medial end of clavicles, assisting pump-handle action of deep respiration
Trapezius	Medial third of superior nuchal line, external occipital protuberance, nuchal ligament, spinous processes of C7–T12 vertebrae, and lumbar and sacral spinous processes	Lateral third of clavicle, acromion and spine of scapula	Spinal accessory nerve (CN XI; motor); C2 and C3 nerves (pain and proprioception)	Elevates, retracts, and rotates scapula *Descending (superior) part:* elevate pectoral girdle, maintain level of shoulders against gravity or resistance *Middle part:* retract scapula *Ascending (inferior) part:* depress shoulders *Descending and ascending parts:* rotate scapula upward With shoulders fixed, bilateral contraction extends neck; unilateral contraction produces lateral flexion to same side

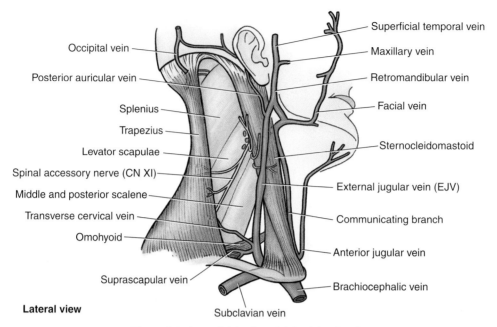

Lateral view

Figure 8.3. Superficial veins of right side of neck.

- By a *floor,* formed by muscles covered by the prevertebral layer of deep cervical fascia.

The lateral cervical region wraps around the lateral surface of the neck like a spiral and is covered by skin and subcutaneous tissue containing the platysma.

MUSCLES IN THE LATERAL CERVICAL REGION

The floor of the lateral cervical region is usually formed by the prevertebral fascia overlying four muscles (Figs. 8.3 and 8.4): splenius capitis, levator scapulae, middle scalene (L. *scalenus medius*), and posterior scalene (L. *scalenus posterior*). Sometimes part of the inferior part of the anterior scalene (L. *scalenus anterior*) appears in the inferomedial angle of the lateral cervical region.

For more precise localization of structures, the lateral cervical region is divided into a larger occipital triangle superiorly and a small omoclavicular triangle inferiorly by the *inferior belly of the omohyoid* (Table 8.1).

The important nerve crossing the **occipital triangle** is the *spinal accessory nerve* (CN XI). The small **omoclavicular** (subclavian) **triangle** is indicated on the superior surface of the neck by the *supraclavicular fossa.* The inferior part of the external jugular vein (EJV) crosses this triangle superficially (Figs 8.3 and 8.4A); the *subclavian artery* lies deep in the triangle.

ARTERIES IN THE LATERAL CERVICAL REGION

The arteries in the lateral cervical region are the transverse cervical and suprascapular arteries, the third part of the subclavian artery, and part of the occipital artery (Fig. 8.4C).

The **transverse cervical artery** originates from the *thyrocervical trunk,* a branch of the subclavian artery. The transverse cervical artery runs superficially and laterally across the phrenic nerve and anterior scalene muscle, 2–3 cm superior to the clavicle. It then crosses (passes through) the *trunks of the brachial plexus,* supplying branches to their *vasa nervorum* (blood vessels of nerves) and passing deep to the trapezius. The *superficial branch* of the transverse cervical artery accompanies CN XI along the anterior (deep) surface of the trapezius. The *deep branch* runs anterior to the rhomboid muscles as the *dorsal scapular artery,* accompanying the dorsal scapular nerve. The dorsal scapular artery may arise independently, directly from the subclavian artery.

The **suprascapular artery,** also a branch of the thyrocervical trunk, passes inferolaterally across the anterior scalene muscle and phrenic nerve. It then crosses the subclavian artery (third part) and the cords of the brachial plexus. It then passes posterior to the clavicle to supply muscles on the posterior aspect of the scapula. The suprascapular artery may arise directly from the subclavian artery.

The **occipital artery,** a branch of the external carotid artery (Fig. 8.5A), enters the lateral cervical region at its superior apex and ascends over the head to supply the posterior half of the scalp.

The **third part of the subclavian artery** supplies blood to the upper limb. It begins approximately a finger's breadth superior to the clavicle, opposite the lateral border of the anterior scalene muscle. It lies posterosuperior to the subclavian vein in the inferior part of the lateral cervical region (Fig. 8.4C). The pulsations of the artery can be felt on deep pressure in the omoclavicular triangle (Table 8.1).

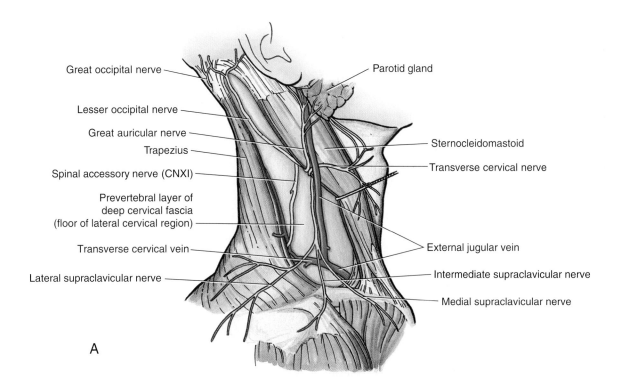

Great occipital nerve

Lesser occipital nerve

Great auricular nerve

Trapezius

Spinal accessory nerve (CNXI)

Prevertebral layer of
deep cervical fascia
(floor of lateral cervical region)

Transverse cervical vein

Lateral supraclavicular nerve

Parotid gland

Sternocleidomastoid

Transverse cervical nerve

External jugular vein

Intermediate supraclavicular nerve

Medial supraclavicular nerve

A

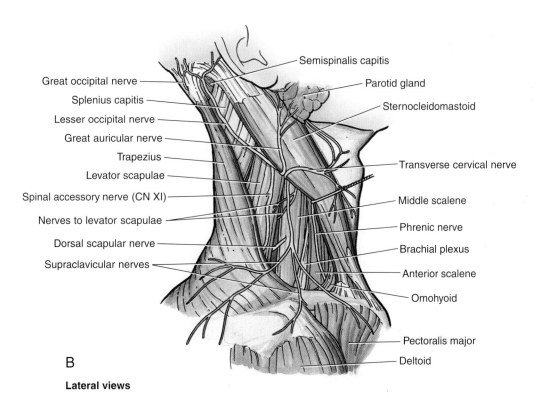

Semispinalis capitis

Great occipital nerve

Splenius capitis

Lesser occipital nerve

Great auricular nerve

Trapezius

Levator scapulae

Spinal accessory nerve (CN XI)

Nerves to levator scapulae

Dorsal scapular nerve

Supraclavicular nerves

Parotid gland

Sternocleidomastoid

Transverse cervical nerve

Middle scalene

Phrenic nerve

Brachial plexus

Anterior scalene

Omohyoid

Pectoralis major

Deltoid

B

Lateral views

Figure 8.4. Dissections of lateral cervical region. Superficial (**A**) and deep (**B**) dissections of the cervical plexus and muscles are shown.

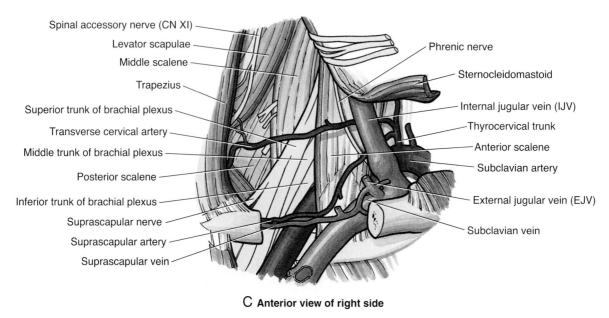

C **Anterior view of right side**

Figure 8.4. (continued) C. A deeper dissection of the inferior part of the lateral cervical region is shown.

The artery is in contact with the 1st rib as it passes posterior to the anterior scalene muscle; consequently, compression of the artery against this rib can control bleeding in the upper limb.

VEINS IN THE LATERAL CERVICAL REGION

The **external jugular vein** begins near the angle of the mandible (just inferior to the auricle of the external ear) by the union of the posterior division of the *retromandibular vein* with the *posterior auricular vein* (Fig. 8.3). The EJV crosses the SCM obliquely, deep to the platysma, and then pierces the investing layer of deep cervical fascia, which forms the roof of this region, at the posterior border of the SCM. The EJV descends to the inferior part of the lateral cervical region and terminates in the subclavian vein.

The major venous channel draining the upper limb, the **subclavian vein,** courses through the inferior part of the lateral cervical region, passing anterior to the anterior scalene muscle and phrenic nerve (Fig. 8.4C). The subclavian vein joins the IJV to form the **brachiocephalic vein** posterior to the medial end of the clavicle (Figs. 8.3 and 8.4C). Just superior to the clavicle, the EJV receives the *transverse cervical, suprascapular,* and *anterior jugular veins.*

NERVES OF THE LATERAL CERVICAL REGION

The **spinal accessory nerve** passes deep to the SCM, supplying it before entering the lateral cervical region at or inferior to the junction of the superior and middle thirds of the posterior border of the SCM (Fig. 8.4B). It passes posteroinferiorly, within or deep to the investing layer of deep cervical fascia, running on the levator scapulae from

which it is separated by the prevertebral layer of fascia. CN XI then disappears deep to the anterior border of the trapezius at the junction of its superior two thirds with its inferior one third.

The **roots of brachial plexus** (anterior rami of C5–C8 and T1) appear between the anterior and the middle scalene muscles. Five rami unite to form the *three trunks of the brachial plexus* (Fig. 8.4C), which descend inferolaterally through the lateral cervical region. The plexus then passes between the 1st rib, clavicle, and superior border of the scapula (the *cervicoaxillary canal*) to enter the axilla, providing innervation for most of the upper limb (see Chapter 6).

The **suprascapular nerve,** which arises from the superior trunk of the brachial plexus, runs laterally across the lateral cervical region to supply the supraspinatus and infraspinatus muscles on the posterior aspect of the scapula. It also sends articular branches to the glenohumeral joint (Fig. 8.4C).

The anterior rami of C1–C4 make up the roots of the **cervical plexus,** which consists of nerve loops. The plexus lies anteromedial to the levator scapulae and middle scalene muscle and deep to the SCM. The superficial branches of the plexus that initially pass posteriorly are cutaneous branches (Fig. 8.4A & B). The deep branches passing anteromedially are motor branches, including the roots of the phrenic nerve and the **ansa cervicalis** (Fig. 8.5B).

Cutaneous branches of the cervical plexus emerge around the middle of the posterior border of the SCM, often called the **nerve point of the neck,** and supply the skin of the neck, superolateral thoracic wall, and the scalp between the

Subclavian Vein Puncture

The right or left subclavian vein is often the point of entry to the venous system for *central line placement* (Fig. B8.2). Central lines are inserted to administer parenteral (venous nutritional) fluids and medications and to measure central venous pressure. The pleura and/or the subclavian artery are in danger of puncture during this procedure.

Prominence of External Jugular Vein

The EJV and may serve as an "internal barometer." When venous pressure is in the normal range, the EJV is usually visible superior to the clavicle for only a short distance. However, when venous pressure rises (e.g., as in heart failure) the vein is prominent throughout its course along the side of the neck. Consequently, routine observation for distention of the EJVs during physical examinations may reveal diagnostic signs of heart failure, obstruction of the superior vena cava, enlarged supraclavicular lymph nodes, or increased intrathoracic pressure.

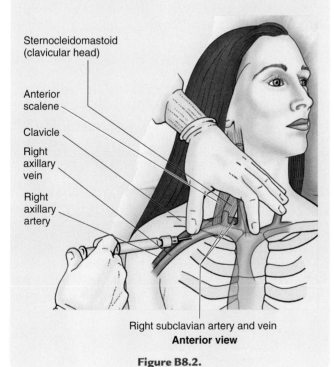

Sternocleidomastoid
(clavicular head)

Anterior
scalene

Clavicle

Right
axillary
vein

Right
axillary
artery

Right subclavian artery and vein

Anterior view

Figure B8.2.

Lesions of the Spinal Accessory Nerve (CN XI)

Lesions of the spinal accessory nerve are uncommon; however, the nerve may be damaged by penetrating trauma, surgical procedures, tumors, and fractures of the jugular foramen. A unilateral lesion usually does not produce an abnormal position of the head; however, weakness can occur in turning the head to one side against resistance. Lesions of CN XI produce weakness and atrophy of the trapezius. *Drooping of the shoulder* is an obvious sign of injury to CN XI. *Unilateral paralysis of the trapezius* is evident by the patient's inability to elevate and retract the shoulder and by difficulty in elevating the arm superior to the horizontal level.

auricle and the external occipital protuberance. Close to their origin, the roots of the cervical plexus receive communicating branches (L. *rami communicantes*), most of which descend from the *superior cervical ganglion* in the superior part of the neck.

The branches of the cervical plexus arising from the nerve loop between the anterior rami of C2 and C3 are the (Fig. 8.4*A* & *B*):

- **Lesser occipital nerve** (C2), supplying the skin of the neck and scalp posterosuperior to the auricle.
- **Great auricular nerve** (C2 and C3), ascending vertically across the SCM onto the parotid gland, where it divides and supplies skin over the gland, posterior aspect of the auricle, and the area of skin extending from the angle of the mandible to the mastoid process.
- **Transverse cervical nerve** (C2 and C3), supplying the skin covering the anterior cervical region; the nerve curves around the middle of the posterior border of the SCM and passes anteriorly and horizontally across it deep to the the EJV and platysma.

Branches of the cervical plexus arising from the loop formed between the anterior rami of C3 and C4 are the **supraclavicular nerves** (C3 and C4), which emerge as a common trunk under cover of the SCM and send small branches to the skin of the neck and cross the clavicle to supply the skin over the shoulder (Fig. 8.4*A*).

In addition to the ansa cervicalis and phrenic nerves, arising from loops of the cervical plexus, deep motor branches include branches arising from the anterior rami of cervical nerves that supply the rhomboids—dorsal scapular nerve (C4 and C5), serratus anterior, long thoracic nerve (C5, **C6**, and C7)—and nearby prevertebral muscles.

The **phrenic nerves** originate chiefly from the 4th cervical nerve (C4) but receive contributions from the C3 and C5 nerves. The phrenic nerves contain motor, sensory, and sympathetic nerve fibers. These nerves provide the sole motor supply to the diaphragm as well as sensation to its central part. In the thorax, the nerves supply the mediastinal pleura and the pericardium. Receiving variable communicating fibers in the neck and fibers from the cervical sympathetic ganglia or their branches, each phrenic nerve forms at the superior part of the lateral border of the anterior scalene muscle at the level of the superior border of the thyroid cartilage. The phrenic nerves descend obliquely with the IJVs across the anterior scalene, deep to the prevertebral layer of the deep cervical fascia and the transverse cervical and suprascapular arteries (Fig. 8.4C). *On the left,* the phrenic nerve crosses anterior to the first part of the subclavian artery; *on the right,* it lies anterior on the anterior scalene muscle and crosses anterior to the second part of the subclavian artery. On both sides, the phrenic nerve runs posterior to the subclavian vein and anterior to the internal thoracic artery as it enters the thorax. The contribution from C5 to the phrenic nerve may derive from an **accessory phrenic nerve,** which is frequently a branch of the nerve to the subclavius. If present, the accessory phrenic nerve lies lateral to the main nerve and descends posterior and sometimes anterior to the subclavian vein. The accessory phrenic nerve joins the phrenic nerve either in the root of the neck or in the thorax.

Anterior Cervical Region

The **anterior cervical region (anterior triangle of the neck)** has a/an:

- *Anterior boundary:* formed by the median line of the neck.
- *Posterior boundary:* formed by the anterior border of the SCM.
- *Superior boundary:* formed by the inferior border of the mandible.
- *Apex:* located at the jugular notch in the manubrium of the sternum.
- *Roof:* formed by subcutaneous tissue containing the platysma.
- *Floor:* formed by the pharynx, larynx, and thyroid gland.

The anterior cervical region is subdivided into four smaller triangles (the unpaired submental triangle and three small paired triangles: submandibular, carotid, and muscular) by the digastric and omohyoid muscles. The contents of the triangles of the neck are listed in Table 8.1.

Severance of the Phrenic Nerve and Phrenic Nerve Block

Severance of a phrenic nerve results in paralysis of the corresponding half of the diaphragm. A phrenic nerve block produces a short period of paralysis of the diaphragm on one side (e.g., for a lung operation). The anesthetic agent is injected around the nerve where it lies on the anterior surface of the anterior scalene muscle.

Nerve Blocks in the Lateral Cervical Region

Regional anesthesia is often used for surgical procedures in the neck region or upper limb. In a **cervical plexus block,** an anesthetic agent is injected at several points along the posterior border of the SCM, mainly at the junction of its superior and middle thirds, the nerve point of the neck (Fig. B8.3). For anesthesia of the upper limb, the anesthetic agent in a *supraclavicular brachial plexus block* is injected around the supraclavicular part of the brachial plexus. The main injection site is superior to the midpoint of the clavicle.

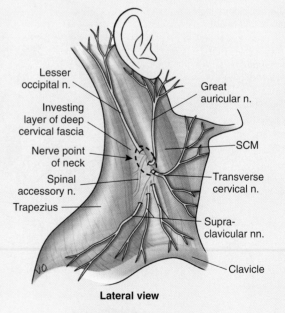

Lateral view

Figure B8.3.

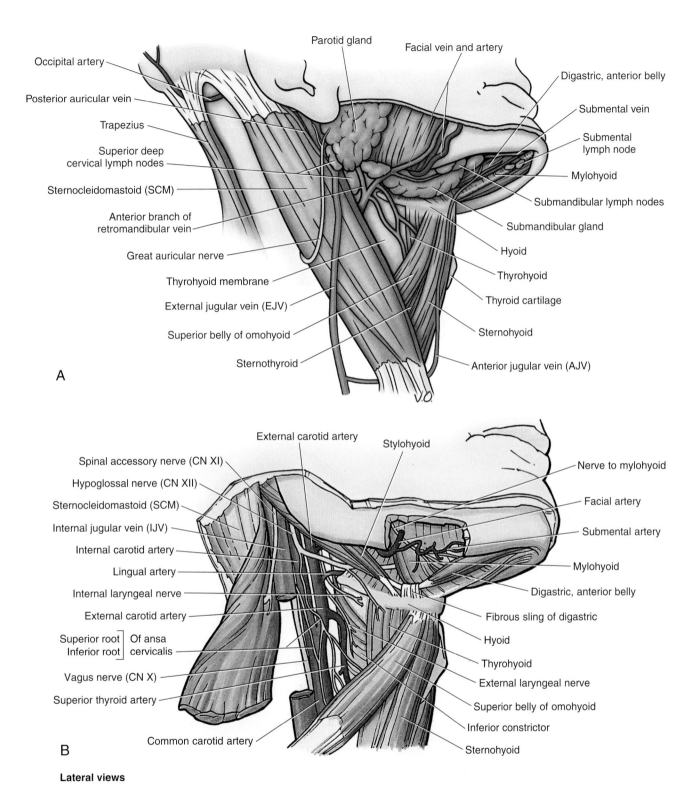

Occipital artery

Posterior auricular vein

Trapezius

Superior deep cervical lymph nodes

Sternocleidomastoid (SCM)

Anterior branch of retromandibular vein

Great auricular nerve

Thyrohyoid membrane

External jugular vein (EJV)

Superior belly of omohyoid

Sternothyroid

Parotid gland

Facial vein and artery

Digastric, anterior belly

Submental vein

Submental lymph node

Mylohyoid

Submandibular lymph nodes

Submandibular gland

Hyoid

Thyrohyoid

Thyroid cartilage

Sternohyoid

Anterior jugular vein (AJV)

A

Spinal accessory nerve (CN XI)

Hypoglossal nerve (CN XII)

Sternocleidomastoid (SCM)

Internal jugular vein (IJV)

Internal carotid artery

Lingual artery

Internal laryngeal nerve

External carotid artery

Superior root / Inferior root | Of ansa cervicalis

Vagus nerve (CN X)

Superior thyroid artery

Common carotid artery

External carotid artery

Stylohyoid

Nerve to mylohyoid

Facial artery

Submental artery

Mylohyoid

Digastric, anterior belly

Fibrous sling of digastric

Hyoid

Thyrohyoid

External laryngeal nerve

Superior belly of omohyoid

Inferior constrictor

Sternohyoid

B

Lateral views

Figure 8.5. Anterior cervical region and suprahyoid region. Superficial (**A**) and deep (**B**) dissections are shown.

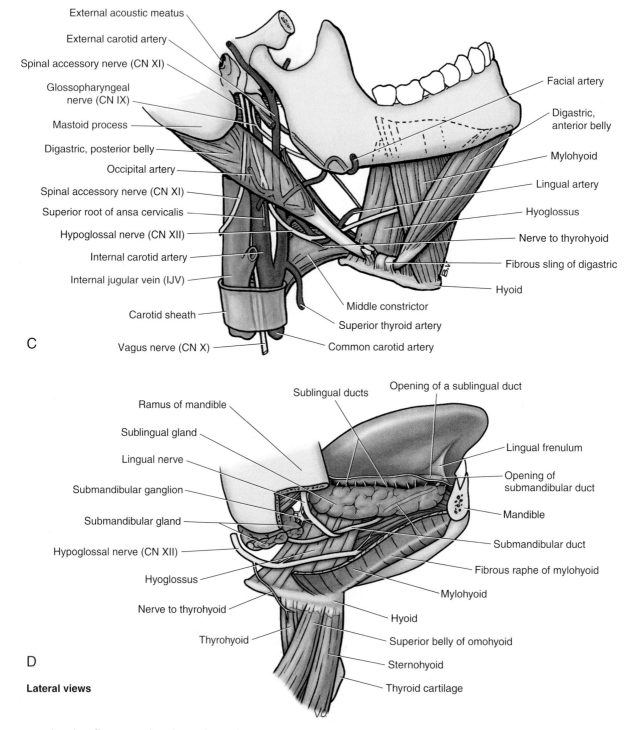

C. Note the relationships of the nerves and vessels to the suprahyoid muscles. **D.** The right half of the mandible and the superior half of the mylohyoid muscle have been removed to show the suprahyoid region.

Figure 8.5. (continued) C. Note the relationships of the nerves and vessels to the suprahyoid muscles. **D.** The right half of the mandible and the superior half of the mylohyoid muscle have been removed to show the suprahyoid region.

The **submental triangle** is inferior to the chin. The apex of the triangle is at the **mandibular symphysis**, the site of union of the halves of the mandible during infancy, and the base of the triangle is formed by the hyoid. Laterally, it is bounded by the right and left anterior bellies of the digastric muscles. The floor of the submental triangle is formed by the two mylohyoid muscles, which meet in a median **fibrous raphe** (Fig. 8.5D). This triangle contains several small **submental lymph nodes** and small veins that unite to form the *anterior jugular vein*.

The **submandibular triangle** is a glandular area between the inferior border of the mandible and the anterior and posterior bellies of the digastric muscle (Fig. 8.5). The floor of the submandibular triangle is formed by the mylohyoid and hyoglossus muscles, and the middle constrictor muscle of the pharynx (Fig. 8.5). The **submandibular gland** nearly fills this triangle. **Submandibular lymph nodes** lie on each side of the submandibular gland and along the inferior border of the mandible. The *hypoglossal nerve* (CN XII) provides motor innervation to the muscles of the tongue. It passes into the submandibular triangle, as do the *nerve to the mylohyoid muscle,* parts of the *facial artery* and *vein,* and the *submental artery,* a branch of the facial artery (Fig. 8.5*C*).

The **carotid triangle** is a vascular area bounded by the superior belly of the omohyoid, the posterior belly of the digastric, and the anterior border of the SCM (Fig. 8.5*A*). The **common carotid artery** ascends into the carotid triangle. Its pulse can be auscultated or palpated by compressing it lightly against the transverse processes of the cervical vertebrae. At the level of the superior border of the thyroid cartilage (C4 vertebral level), the common carotid artery divides into the **internal** and **external carotid arteries** (Fig. 8.6*A*). At this bifurcation, there is a slight dilation of the proximal part of the internal carotid artery—the **carotid sinus** (Fig. 8.6*B*). Innervated principally by the glossopharyngeal nerve (CN IX) through the **carotid sinus nerve,** as well as the vagus nerve, the carotid sinus is a *baroreceptor* (pressoreceptor) that reacts to changes in arterial blood pressure.

The **carotid body,** an ovoid mass of tissue, lies on the medial (deep) side of the bifurcation of the common carotid artery in close relation to the carotid sinus (Fig. 8.6*C*). Supplied mainly by the carotid sinus nerve (CN IX) and by CN X, the carotid body is a *chemoreceptor* that monitors the level of oxygen in the blood. It is stimulated by low levels of oxygen and initiates a reflex that increases the rate and depth of respiration, cardiac rate, and blood pressure.

The **muscular triangle** is bounded by the superior belly of the omohyoid muscle, the anterior border of SCM, and the median plane of the neck (Fig. 8.5*A* & *B*). This triangle contains the *infrahyoid muscles* and viscera, such as the thyroid and parathyroid glands.

MUSCLES IN THE ANTERIOR CERVICAL REGION

In the anterolateral part of the neck, the *hyoid* provides attachments for the suprahyoid muscles superior to it and the infrahyoid muscles inferior to it (Fig. 8.5). These **hyoid muscles** steady or move the hyoid bone and larynx. The attachments, innervation, and main actions of the suprahyoid and infrahyoid muscles are presented in Table 8.3.

The **suprahyoid muscles** are superior to the hyoid bone and connect it to the cranium. The suprahyoid muscle group includes the mylohyoid, geniohyoid, stylohyoid, and digastric muscles. As a group, these muscles constitute the

substance of the floor of the mouth, supporting the hyoid in providing a base from which the tongue functions and elevating the hyoid and larynx in relation to swallowing and tone production. Each **digastric muscle** has two bellies joined by an **intermediate tendon,** that descends toward the hyoid. A **fibrous sling** allows the tendon to slide anteriorly and posteriorly as it connects this tendon to the body and greater horn of the hyoid bone (Fig. 8.5*B* & *C*).

The **infrahyoid muscles** (strap muscles) are inferior to the hyoid. These four muscles anchor the hyoid, sternum, clavicle, and scapula and depress the hyoid and larynx during swallowing and speaking (Table 8.3). They also work with the suprahyoid muscles to steady the hyoid, providing a firm base for the tongue. The infrahyoid group of muscles are arranged in two planes: a *superficial plane* made up of the sternohyoid and omohyoid, and a *deep plane* composed of the sternothyroid and thyrohyoid. The **omohyoid** has two bellies united by an intermediate tendon that is connected to the clavicle by a fascial sling. The **sternothyroid** is wider than the **sternohyoid,** under which it lies. The sternothyroid covers the lateral lobe of the thyroid gland, attaching to the oblique line of the lamina of the thyroid cartilage immediately superior to the gland. This muscle limits superior expansion of an enlarged thyroid gland. The **thyrohyoid,** running superiorly from the oblique line of the thyroid cartilage to the hyoid bone, appears to be a continuation of the sternothyroid muscle.

ARTERIES IN THE ANTERIOR CERVICAL REGION

The anterior cervical region contains the **carotid system of arteries,** consisting of the common carotid artery and its terminal branches, the internal and external carotid arteries (Figs. 8.5*C* and 8.6*C*). It also contains the IJV and its tributaries and the anterior jugular veins (AJVs). The common carotid artery and one of its terminal branches, the *external carotid artery,* are the main arterial vessels in the carotid triangle. Each *common carotid artery* ascends within the *carotid sheath* with the IJV and vagus nerve to the level of the superior border of the thyroid cartilage. Here, each common carotid artery terminates by dividing into the internal and external carotid arteries. The **right common carotid artery** begins at the bifurcation of the brachiocephalic trunk. In contrast, the **left common carotid artery** arises from the arch of the aorta and ascends in the neck.

The **internal carotid arteries,** the direct continuation of the common carotid arteries, have no branches in the neck. They enter the cranium through the carotid canals and become the main arteries of the brain and structures in the orbits. The proximal part of each internal carotid artery is the site of the *carotid sinus* (discussed earlier). The *carotid body* is located in the cleft between the internal and external carotid arteries (Fig. 8.6*C*).

The **external carotid arteries** supply most structures external to the cranium; the orbit and part of the forehead and

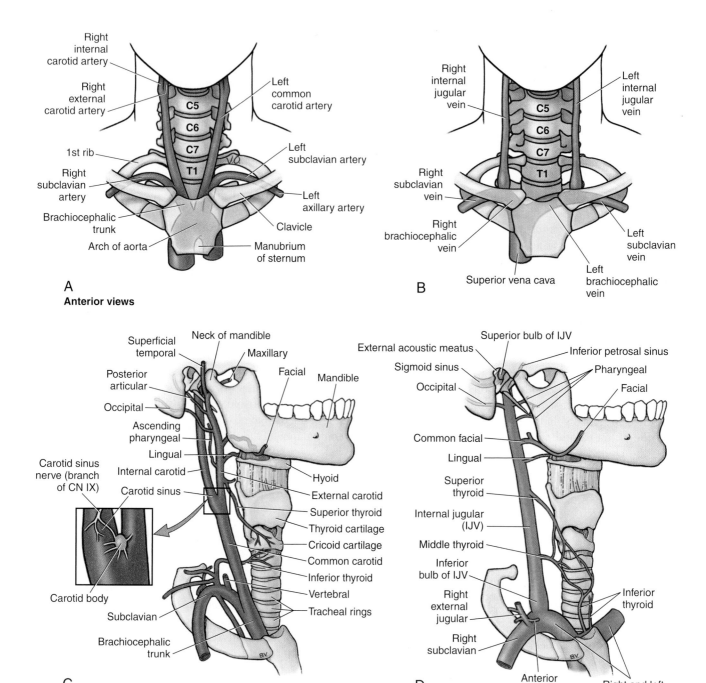

Figure 8.6. Arteries and veins in neck. A. The subclavian and carotid arteries are shown. **B.** The internal jugular and subclavian veins are identified. **C.** Branches of the subclavian and external carotid arteries are detailed. **D.** The internal jugular vein is shown.

scalp supplied by the supraorbital artery are the major exceptions (Figs. 8.5 *B* and 8.6 *C*). Each external carotid artery runs posterosuperiorly to the region between the neck of the mandible and the lobule of the auricle, where it is embedded in the parotid gland. Here it divides into two terminal branches: the *maxillary* and *superficial temporal arteries* (Fig. 8.6 *C*). Before these terminal branches, six arteries arise from the external carotid artery (Figs. 8.5 and 8.6 *C*):

- **Ascending pharyngeal artery** arises as the first or second branch of the external carotid artery and is its only medial branch; ascends on the pharynx and sends branches to the pharynx, prevertebral muscles, middle ear, and cranial meninges.
- **Occipital artery** arises from the posterior aspect of the external carotid artery, superior to the origin of the facial artery; passes posteriorly, immediately medial and par-

allel to the attachment of the posterior belly of the digastric muscle, ending in the posterior part of the scalp. During its course, it passes superficial to the internal carotid artery and CN IX–CN XI.

- **Posterior auricular artery**, a small posterior branch of the external carotid artery, ascends posteriorly between the external acoustic meatus and the mastoid process and contributes to the blood supply of adjacent muscles, parotid gland, facial nerve, structures in the temporal bone, auricle, and scalp.
- **Superior thyroid artery**, the most inferior of the three anterior branches of the external carotid artery, runs anteroinferiorly deep to the infrahyoid muscles to reach the thyroid gland. In addition to supplying this gland, it gives off branches to the infrahyoid muscles and the SCM and gives rise to the *superior laryngeal artery*, supplying the larynx.

- **Lingual artery** arises from the anterior aspect of the external carotid artery, where it lies on the middle constrictor muscle of the pharynx; arches superoanteriorly and passes deep to CN XII, the stylohyoid muscle, and the posterior belly of the digastric muscle; and disappears deep to the hyoglossus muscle, giving branches to the posterior tongue. It then turns superiorly at the anterior border of this muscle, bifurcating into the deep lingual and sublingual arteries.
- **Facial artery** arises anteriorly from the external carotid artery, either in common with the lingual artery or immediately superior to it; after giving rise to the *ascending palatine artery* and a *tonsillar branch,* passes superiorly under cover of the digastric and stylohyoid muscles and the angle of the mandible. It loops anteriorly and enters a deep groove in and supplies the submandibular gland and then gives rise to the submental

Ligation of the External Carotid Artery

Sometimes *ligation of an external carotid artery* is necessary to control bleeding from one of its relatively inaccessible branches. This procedure decreases blood flow through the artery and its branches but does not eliminate it. Blood flows in a retrograde (backward) direction into the artery from the external carotid artery on the other side through communications between its branches (e.g., those in the face and scalp) and across the midline. When the external carotid or subclavian arteries are ligated, the descending branch of the occipital artery provides the main collateral circulation, anastomosing with the vertebral and deep cervical arteries.

Surgical Dissection of Carotid Triangle

The carotid triangle provides an important surgical approach to the carotid system of arteries, the IJV, the vagus and hypoglossal nerves, and the cervical sympathetic trunk. Damage or compression of the vagus and/or recurrent laryngeal nerves during surgical dissection of the triangle may produce an alteration in the voice because these nerves supply laryngeal muscles.

Carotid Pulse

The carotid pulse (neck pulse) is easily felt by palpating the common carotid artery in the side of the neck, where it lies in a groove between the trachea and the infrahyoid muscles. It is usually easily palpated just deep to the anterior border of the SCM at the level of the superior border of the thyroid cartilage. It is routinely checked during *cardiopulmonary resuscitation (CPR)*. Absence of a carotid pulse indicates cardiac arrest.

Carotid Occlusion and Endarterectomy

Atherosclerotic thickening of the intima (innermost coat) of the internal carotid artery may obstruct blood flow. Symptoms resulting from this obstruction depend on the degree of obstruction and the amount of collateral blood flow to the brain from other arteries. A partial occlusion may cause a *transient ischemic attack (TIA)*, a sudden focal loss of neurological function (e.g., dizziness and disorientation) that disappears within 24 hr. Arterial occlusion may also cause a *stroke*.

Carotid occlusion, causing stenosis (narrowing), can be relieved by opening the artery at its origin and stripping off the atherosclerotic plaque with the intima. This procedure is called *carotid endarterectomy*. Because of the relations of the internal carotid artery, there is risk of cranial nerve injury during the procedure involving one or more of the following nerves: CN IX, CN X (or its branch, the superior laryngeal nerve), CN XI, or CN XII.

artery to the floor of the mouth and hooks around the middle of the inferior border of the mandible to enter the face.

VEINS IN THE ANTERIOR CERVICAL REGION

Most veins in the anterior cervical region are tributaries of the IJV, usually the largest vein in the neck (Fig. 8.6*B* & *D*). The *IJV* drains blood from the brain, anterior face, cervical viscera, and deep muscles of the neck. The IJV commences at the jugular foramen in the posterior cranial fossa as the direct continuation of the sigmoid sinus (see Chapter 7). From the dilation at its origin, the **superior bulb of the IJV**, the vein runs inferiorly through the neck in the *carotid sheath* with the internal carotid artery superior to the carotid bifurcation and the common carotid artery and CN X inferiorly. The vein lies laterally within the sheath, with the nerve located posteriorly (Fig. 8.2*C*). The *cervical sympathetic trunk* lies posterior to the carotid sheath and is embedded in the prevertebral layer of deep cervical fascia. The IJV leaves the anterior cervical region by passing deep to the SCM. Posterior to the sternal end of the clavicle, the IJV unites with the subclavian vein to form the *brachiocephalic vein*. The inferior end of the IJV dilates to form the **inferior bulb of the IJV**. This bulb has a bicuspid valve that permits blood to flow toward the heart while preventing backflow into the vein. The tributaries of the IJV are the inferior petrosal sinus and the facial, lingual, pharyngeal, and superior and middle thyroid veins. The **occipital vein** usually drains into the *suboccipital venous plexus,* drained by the deep cervical vein and the vertebral vein but may drain into the IJV.

NERVES IN THE ANTERIOR CERVICAL REGION

The **transverse cervical nerve** (C2 and C3) supplies the skin covering the anterior cervical region. The **hypoglossal nerve** (CN XII), the motor nerve of the tongue, enters the submandibular triangle deep to the posterior belly of the digastric muscle to supply the muscles of the tongue (Fig. 8.5*C* & *D*). Branches of the **glossopharyngeal** and **vagus nerves** are located in the submandibular and carotid triangles.

Internal Jugular Pulse

Pulsations of the IJV can provide information about heart activity corresponding to electrocardiogram (ECG) recordings and right atrial pressure. The vein's pulsations are transmitted through the surrounding tissues and may be observed deep to the SCM superior to the medial end of the clavicle. Because there are no valves in the brachiocephalic vein or the superior vena cava, a wave of contraction passes up these vessels to the IJV. The pulsations are especially visible when the person's head is inferior to the feet (the *Trendelenburg position*). The internal jugular pulse increases considerably in conditions such as mitral valve disease, which increases pressure in the pulmonary circulation and the right side of the heart.

Internal Jugular Vein Puncture

A needle and catheter may be inserted into the IJV for diagnostic or therapeutic purposes. The right internal jugular vein is preferable because it is usually larger and straighter. During this procedure, the clinician palpates the common carotid artery and inserts the needle into the IJV just lateral to it at a 30° angle, aiming at the apex of the triangle between the sternal and the clavicular heads of the SCM. The needle is then directed inferolaterally toward the ipsilateral nipple (Fig. B8.4).

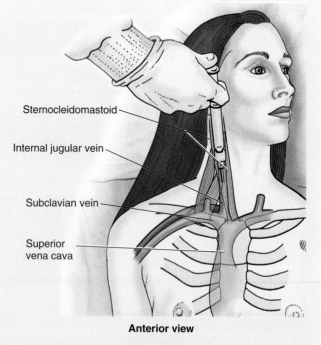

Sternocleidomastoid

Internal jugular vein

Subclavian vein

Superior vena cava

Anterior view

Figure B8.4.

Table 8.3 Muscles of the Anterior Cervical Region (Extrinsic Muscles of the Larynx)

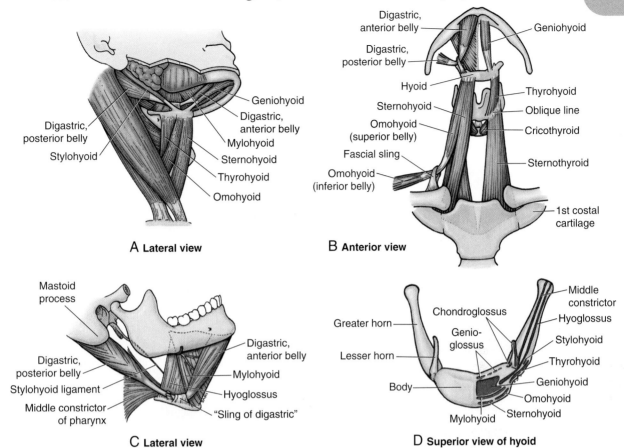

A **Lateral view**

B **Anterior view**

C **Lateral view**

D **Superior view of hyoid**

Muscle	Origin	Insertion	Innervation	Main Action(s)
Suprahyoid muscles				
Mylohyoid	Mylohyoid line of mandible	Mylohyoid raphe and body of hyoid	Nerve to mylohyoid, a branch of inferior alveolar nerve (from mandibular nerve, CN V₃)	Elevates hyoid, floor of mouth, and tongue during swallowing and speaking
Geniohyoid	Inferior mental spine of mandible	Body of hyoid	C1 via hypoglossal nerve (CN XII)	Pulls hyoid anterosuperiorly; shortens floor of mouth; widens pharynx
Stylohyoid	Styloid process of temporal bone	Body of hyoid	Stylohyoid branch of facial nerve (CN VII)	Elevates and retracts hyoid, thus elongating floor of mouth
Digastric	*Anterior belly:* digastric fossa of mandible *Posterior belly:* mastoid notch of temporal bone	Intermediate tendon to body and greater horn of hyoid	*Anterior belly:* Nerve to mylohyoid, a branch of inferior alveolar nerve *Posterior belly:* Digastric branch of facial nerve (CN VII)	Working with infrahyoid muscles, depresses mandible against resistance; elevates and steadies hyoid during swallowing and speaking
Infrahyoid muscles				
Sternohyoid	Manubrium of sternum and medial end of clavicle	Body of hyoid	C1–C3 by a branch of ansa cervicalis	Depresses hyoid after elevation during swallowing
Omohyoid	Superior border of scapula near suprascapular notch	Inferior border of hyoid	C1–C3 by a branch of ansa cervicalis	Depresses, retracts, and steadies hyoid
Sternothyroid	Posterior surface of manubrium of sternum	Oblique line of thyroid cartilage	C2 and C3 by a branch of ansa cervicalis	Depresses hyoid and larynx
Thyrohyoid	Oblique line of thyroid cartilage	Inferior border of body and greater horn of hyoid	C1 via hypoglossal nerve	Depresses hyoid and elevates larynx

Surface Anatomy of Cervical Regions and Triangles of Neck

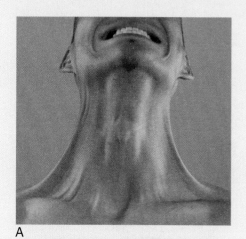

A

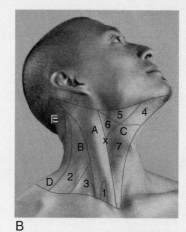

B

A Sternocleidomastoid region
B Lateral cervical region
C Anterior cervical region
D Posterior cervical region
E Suboccipital region
1 Lesser supraclavicular fossa
2 Occipital triangle
3 Omoclavicular triangle
4 Submental triangle
5 Submandibular triangle
6 Carotid triangle
7 Muscular triangle
X Carotid bifurcation
(take pulse inferior to this point)

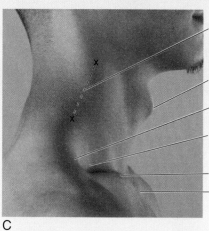

C

Approximated course of spinal accessory nerve (CN XI)

Laryngeal prominence

Anterior border of trapezius

Greater supraclavicular fossa

Clavicle

Jugular notch

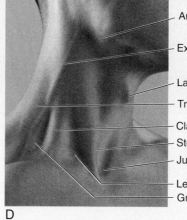

D

Angle of mandible

External jugular vein

Laryngeal prominence

Trapezius

Clavicular ⎱ Heads of
Sternal ⎰ sternocleidomastoid

Jugular notch

Lesser ⎱ Supraclavicular fossae
Greater ⎰

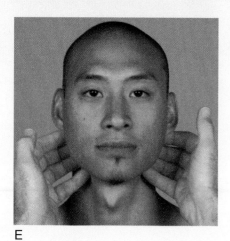

E

Figure SA8.1.

continued >

The cervical regions and triangles are outlined in Figure SA8.1*B*. Some of the important structures found in the regions and triangles are discussed below.

The **skin of the neck** is thin and pliable. The subcutaneous connective tissue contains the **platysma**, a thin sheet of striated muscle that ascends to the face (Fig. SA8.1*A*).

The broad **SCM** is the key muscular landmark of the neck. It defines the **sternocleidomastoid region** and divides the neck into anterior and lateral cervical regions (Fig. SA8.1*D*). It is easy to observe and palpate throughout its length as it passes superolaterally from the clavicle and manubrium to the mastoid process of the temporal bone. The SCM can be made to stand out by asking the person to rotate the face toward the contralateral side and elevate the chin.

The EJV runs vertically across the SCM toward the angle of the mandible (Fig. SA8.1*D*). This vein may be prominent, especially if distended by asking the person to take a deep breath (*Valsalva maneuver*). The **jugular notch** in the manubrium is the fossa between the sternal heads of the SCM. The lesser supraclavicular fossa, between the sternal and the clavicular heads of the SCM, overlies the inferior end of the IJV. Deep to the superior half of the SCM is the cervical plexus, and deep to the inferior half of the SCM are the IJV, common carotid artery, and vagus nerve in the carotid sheath.

The **trapezius**, which defines the posterior cervical region, can be observed and palpated by asking the person to shrug the shoulders against resistance (Fig. SA8.1*C*).

Just inferior to the belly of the omohyoid is the greater supraclavicular fossa (Fig. SA8.1*D*), the depression overlying the omoclavicular triangle. The subclavian arterial pulsations can be palpated here in most people.

The **occipital triangle** contains the **spinal accessory nerve** (CN XI). Because of its vulnerability and frequency of iatrogenic injury (damage resulting from medical treatment), it is important to be able to estimate the location of the nerve (Fig. SA8.1*C*). Its course can be approximated by a line that intersects the junction of the superior and middle thirds of the posterior border of the SCM and the junction of the middle and lower thirds of the anterior border of the trapezius.

The **submandibular gland** nearly fills the submandibular triangle. The **submandibular lymph nodes** lie superficial to the gland and, if enlarged, can be palpated by moving the fingers from the angle of the mandible along its inferior border (Fig. SA8.1*E*). If continued until the fingers meet under the chin, enlarged **submental lymph nodes** can be palpated in the **submental triangle**.

The carotid arterial system is located in the **carotid triangle**. The **carotid sheath** can be mapped out by a line joining the sternoclavicular joint to a point midway between the mastoid process and the angle of the mandible (Fig. SA8.1*B*). The **carotid pulse** can be palpated by placing the index and 3rd fingers on the thyroid cartilage and pointing them posterolaterally between the trachea and SCM. The pulse is palpable just medial to the SCM. ●

Deep Structures of Neck

The **deep structures of the neck** are the prevertebral muscles, located posterior to the cervical viscera and anterolateral to the vertebral column, and structures located on the cervical side of the superior thoracic aperture, the *root of the neck*.

Prevertebral Muscles

The **anterior vertebral muscles**, consisting of the longus colli and capitis and rectus capitis anterior and the anterior scalene muscles, lie directly posterior to the retropharyngeal space (Fig. 8.2). The **lateral vertebral muscles**, consisting of the rectus capitis lateralis, splenius capitis, levator scapulae, and middle and posterior scalene muscles, lie posterior to the neurovascular plane of the cervical and brachial plexuses and subclavian artery, except the rectus capitis lateralis, which lies in the floor of the lateral cervical region. The muscles are illustrated and described in Table 8.4.

Root of Neck

The **root of the neck** is the junctional area between the thorax and the neck (Fig. 8.7). The inferior boundary of the root of the neck is formed laterally by the 1st pair of ribs and their costal cartilages, anteriorly by the manubrium of the sternum, and posteriorly by the body of the T1 vertebra. Only the neurovascular elements of the root of the neck are described here; the visceral structures are discussed later in this chapter.

Table 8.4 Prevertebral Muscles

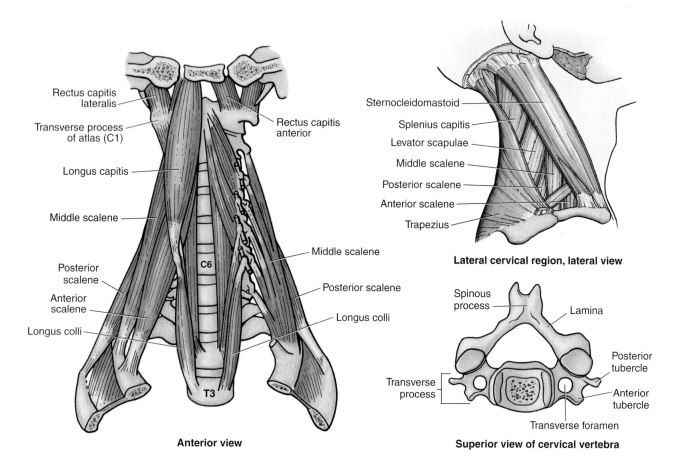

Anterior view

Lateral cervical region, lateral view

Superior view of cervical vertebra

Muscle	Superior Attachment	Inferior Attachment	Innervation	Main Action(s)
Anterior vertebral muscles				
Longus colli	Anterior tubercle of C1 vertebra (atlas); bodies of C1–C3 and transverse processes of C3–C6 vertebrae	Bodies of C5–T3 vertebrae; transverse processes of C3–C5 vertebrae	Anterior rami of C2–C6 spinal nerves	Flexes neck with rotation (torsion) to opposite side if acting unilaterally[a]
Longus capitis	Basilar part of occipital bone	Anterior tubercles of C3–C6 transverse processes	Anterior rami of C1–C3 spinal nerves	Flexes head[b]
Rectus capitis anterior	Base of cranium, just anterior to occipital condyle	Anterior surface of lateral mass of atlas (C1 vertebra)	Branches from loop between C1 and C2 spinal nerves	Flexes head[b]
Anterior scalene	Transverse processes of C4–C6 vertebrae	1st rib	Cervical spinal nerves C4–C6	

Table 8.4 Prevertebral Muscles *(continued)*

Muscle	Superior Attachment	Inferior Attachment	Innervation	Main Action(s)
Lateral vertebral muscles				
Rectus capitis lateralis	Jugular process of occipital bone	Transverse process of atlas (C1 vertebra)	Branches from loop between C1 and C2 spinal nerves	Flexes head and helps stabilize it[b]
Splenius capitis	Inferior half of nuchal ligament and spinous processes of superior six thoracic vertebrae	Lateral aspect of mastoid process and lateral third of superior nuchal line	Posterior rami of middle cervical spinal nerves	Laterally flexes and rotates head and neck to same side; acting bilaterally, extend head and neck[c]
Levator scapulae	Posterior tubercles of transverse processes of C1–C4 vertebrae	Superior part of medial border of scapula	Dorsal scapular nerve C5 and cervical spinal nerves C3 and C4	Elevates scapula and tilts its glenoid cavity inferiorly by rotating scapula
Middle scalene	Posterior tubercles of transverse processes of C4–C6 vertebrae	Superior surface of 1st rib; posterior groove for subclavian artery	Anterior rami of cervical spinal nerves	Flexes neck laterally; elevates 1st rib during forced inspiration[a]
Posterior scalene		External border of 2nd rib	Anterior rami of cervical spinal nerves C7 and C8	Flexes neck laterally; elevates 2nd rib during forced inspiration[a]

[a]Flexion of neck = anterior (or lateral) bending of cervical vertebrae C2–C7.
[b]Flexion of head = anterior (or lateral) bending of the head relative to the vertebral column at the atlanto-occipital joints.
[c]Rotation of the head occurs at the atlantoaxial joints.

ARTERIES IN ROOT OF NECK

The **brachiocephalic trunk**, covered anteriorly by the sternohyoid and sternothyroid muscles, is the largest branch of the arch of the aorta. It arises in the midline, posterior to the manubrium, passes superolaterally to the right, and divides into the right common carotid and right subclavian arteries posterior to the right sternoclavicular (SC) joint (Fig. 8.7A).

The **subclavian arteries** supply the upper limbs and send branches to the neck and brain. The **right subclavian artery** arises from the brachiocephalic trunk, and the **left subclavian artery** arises from the arch of the aorta (Figs. 8.6A and 8.7). Their courses in the neck begin posterior to the respective SC joints as they ascend through the superior thoracic aperture. The arteries arch superolaterally, extending between their origin and the medial margin of the anterior scalene muscle. As the arteries begin to descend, they travel deep to the middle of the clavicles and cross the outer margin of the 1st ribs, where their name changes to the axillary arteries.

For purposes of description, the anterior scalene muscle divides each subclavian artery into three parts: the first part is medial to the muscle, the second is posterior to it, and the third is lateral to it (Fig. 8.7C). The cervical pleurae, apex of lung, and sympathetic trunk lie posterior to this part of the arteries. The **branches of the subclavian artery** are the (Fig. 8.7):

- *Vertebral artery, internal thoracic artery,* and *thyrocervical trunk* from the first part of the subclavian artery.

- *Costocervical trunk* from the second part of the subclavian artery.

- *Dorsal scapular artery,* often arising from the third part of the subclavian artery.

The **cervical part of the vertebral artery** arises from the first part of the subclavian artery and ascends in the pyramidal space formed between the scalene and the longus muscles. The artery then passes through the foramina of the transverse processes of vertebrae C1–C6. This **vertebral part of the vertebral artery** may enter a foramen more superior than the C6 vertebra. The **suboccipital part of the vertebral artery** courses in a groove on the posterior arch of the atlas before it enters the cranial cavity through the foramen magnum, demarcating the beginning of the **cranial part of the vertebral artery.**

The **internal thoracic artery** arises from the anteroinferior aspect of the subclavian artery and passes inferomedially into the thorax (Fig. 8.7C). The internal thoracic artery has no branches in the neck; its thoracic distribution is described in Chapter 1.

The **thyrocervical trunk** arises from the anterosuperior aspect of the first part of the subclavian artery, near the medial border of the anterior scalene muscle. It has three branches, the largest and most important of which is the **inferior thyroid artery,** the primary visceral artery of the neck (Fig. 8.9). Often arising from the thyrocervical trunk are the *suprascapular artery,* supplying muscles on the posterior scapula, and the *transverse cervical artery,* sending branches to muscles in the lateral cervical region, the trapezius, and medial scapular muscles. The ascending cervical arteries, branches of the inferior thyroid arteries, supply the lateral muscles of the upper neck.

The **costocervical trunk** arises posteriorly from the second part of the subclavian artery (posterior to the anterior scalene muscle on the right side and usually just medial to this muscle on the left side). The trunk passes posterosuperiorly and divides into the superior intercostal and deep cervical arteries, which supply the first two intercostal spaces and the posterior deep cervical muscles, respectively (Fig. 8.7C).

The **dorsal scapular artery** often arises as the deep descending branch of the transverse cervical artery (Fig. 8.7C), but it may be an independent branch of the second or third part of the subclavian artery. It runs deep to supply the levator scapulae and rhomboid muscles, supplying both and participating in the arterial anastomoses around the scapula (see Chapter 6).

VEINS IN ROOT OF NECK

Two large veins terminate in the root of the neck: the **external jugular vein**, draining blood received mostly from the scalp and face, and the variable **anterior jugular vein** (Fig. 8.3). The AJV typically arises near the hyoid bone from the confluence of superficial submandibular veins. At the root of the neck, the vein turns laterally, posterior to the SCM, and opens into the termination of the EJV or into the subclavian vein. Superior to the manubrium, the right and left AJVs commonly unite across the midline to form the **jugular venous arch** in the suprasternal space.

The *subclavian vein,* the continuation of the axillary vein, begins at the lateral border of the 1st rib and ends when it unites with the IJV posterior to the medial end of the clavicle, to form the **brachiocephalic vein** (Fig. 8.7A). This union is commonly referred to as the **venous angle** and is the site where the *thoracic duct* (left side) and the *right lymphatic trunk* (right side) drain lymph collected throughout the body into the venous circulation. Throughout its course, the IJV is enclosed by the *carotid sheath.*

NERVES IN ROOT OF NECK

There are three pairs of major nerves in the root of the neck: (1) the vagus nerves, (2) the phrenic nerves, and (3) the sympathetic trunks (Fig. 8.7A).

Vagus Nerves.   After their exit from the jugular foramen, each **vagus nerve** passes inferiorly in the neck within the posterior part of the **carotid sheath** in the angle between the IJV and the common carotid artery (Fig. 8.2B). The **right vagus nerve** passes anterior to the first part of the subclavian artery and posterior to the brachiocephalic vein and SC

joint to enter the thorax. The **left vagus nerve** descends between the left common carotid and the left subclavian arteries and posterior to the SC joint to enter the thorax.

The **recurrent laryngeal nerves** arise from the vagus nerves in the inferior part of the neck. The nerves of the two sides have essentially the same distribution; however, they arise and recur (loop around) different structures and at different levels on the two sides. The **right recurrent laryngeal nerve** loops inferior to the right subclavian artery (Fig. 8.7), and the **left recurrent laryngeal nerve** loops inferior to the arch of the aorta (Fig. 8.9D). After looping, both recurrent laryngeal nerves ascend superiorly to the posteromedial aspect of the thyroid gland, where they ascend in the **tracheoesophageal groove** (Fig. 8.9A), supplying both the trachea and esophagus and all the intrinsic muscles of the larynx except the cricothyroid.

The **cardiac branches of CN X** originate in the neck as well as in the thorax and convey presynaptic parasympathetic and visceral afferent fibers to the cardiac plexus of nerves.

Phrenic Nerves.   The **phrenic nerves** are formed at the lateral borders of the anterior scalene muscles (Fig. 8.7), mainly from the C4 nerve with contributions from C3 and C5. The phrenic nerves descend anterior to the anterior scalene muscles under cover of the SCMs and IJVs. They pass deep to the prevertebral layer of deep cervical fascia, between the subclavian arteries and veins and proceed through the thorax on each side of the mediastinum, supplying the diaphragm (see Chapter 1). In addition to their sensory distribution, they provide the sole motor supply to their own half of the diaphragm.

Sympathetic trunks.   The **cervical portion of the sympathetic trunks** lie anterolateral to the vertebral column, extending superiorly to the level of the C1 vertebra or the cranial base (Fig. 8.7A & B). The sympathetic trunks receive no white communicating branches (L. *rami communicantes*) in the neck. The cervical portion of the trunks contains three **cervical sympathetic ganglia**: superior, middle, and inferior. These ganglia receive presynaptic fibers conveyed to the sympathetic trunk by the superior thoracic spinal nerves and their associated white communicating branches, which then ascend through the sympathetic trunk to the ganglia. After synapsing with the postsynaptic neuron in the cervical sympathetic ganglia, postsynaptic neurons send fibers to the:

- Cervical spinal nerves via *gray communicating branches.*
- Thoracic viscera via *cardiopulmonary splanchnic nerves.*
- Head and viscera of the neck via *cephalic arterial branches,* which accompany arteries (especially the vertebral and internal and external carotid arteries) as the *sympathetic periarterial plexuses.*

The **inferior cervical ganglion** usually fuses with the 1st thoracic ganglion to form the large **cervicothoracic ganglion (stellate ganglion)**. This star-shaped (L. *stella,* a star)

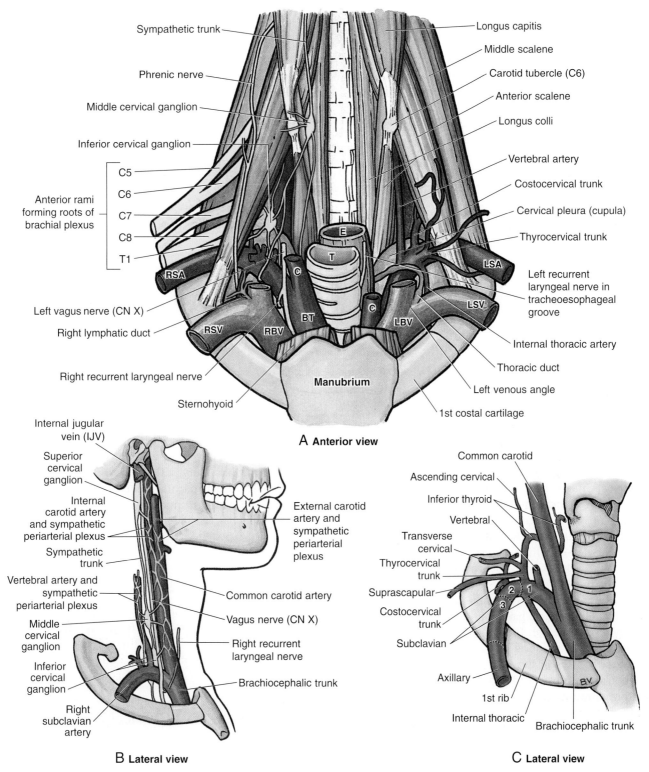

Figure 8.7. Root of neck and prevertebral region. A. A dissection of the root of the neck is shown. *BT,* brachiocephalic trunk; *C,* left and right common carotid arteries; *E,* esophagus; *LBV,* left brachiocephalic vein; *LSA,* left subclavian artery; *LSV,* left subclavian vein; *RBV,* right brachiocephalic vein; *RSA,* right subclavian artery; *RSV,* right subclavian vein; *T,* trachea. **B.** The nerves in the neck are identified. **C.** The branches of the subclavian artery are demonstrated.

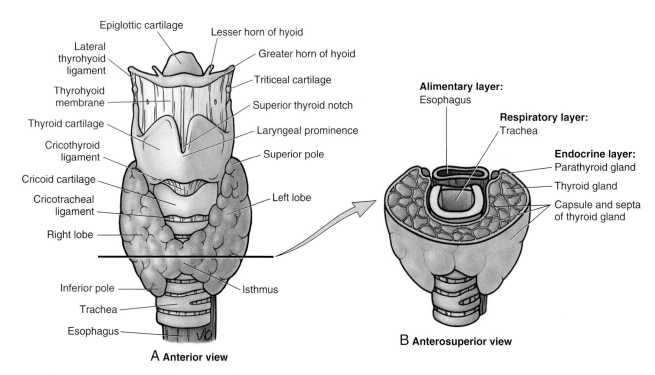

Figure 8.8. Relationships of thyroid gland.

ganglion lies anterior to the transverse process of the C7 vertebra, just superior to the neck of the 1st rib on each side and posterior to the origin of the vertebral artery. Some postsynaptic fibers from the ganglion pass via gray communicating branches to the anterior rami of the C7 and C8 spinal nerves. Other fibers pass to the heart via the **inferior cervical cardiac nerve** (a cardiopulmonary splanchnic nerve), which passes along the trachea to the deep *cardiac plexus.* Other fibers pass via arterial branches to contribute to the sympathetic periarterial nerve plexus around the vertebral artery running into the cranial cavity.

The **middle cervical ganglion,** usually small and occasionally absent, lies on the anterior aspect of the inferior thyroid artery at the level of the cricoid cartilage and the transverse process of the C6 vertebra, just anterior to the vertebral artery. Postsynaptic fibers pass from the ganglion via gray communicating branches to the anterior rami of the C5 and C6 spinal nerves, via a **middle cervical cardiac** (cardiopulmonary splanchnic) **nerve** to the heart and via arterial branches to form periarterial plexuses to the thyroid gland.

The **superior cervical ganglion** is at the level of the C1 and C2 vertebrae. Because of its large size, it forms a good landmark for locating the sympathetic trunk. Postsynaptic fibers pass from it by means of cephalic arterial branches to form the internal carotid sympathetic plexus and enter the cranial cavity (Fig. 8.7 *B*). This ganglion also sends ar-

terial branches to the external carotid artery and gray communicating branches to the anterior rami of the superior four cervical spinal nerves. Other postsynaptic fibers pass from it to the cardiac plexus of nerves via a **superior cervical cardiac** (cardiopulmonary splanchnic) **nerve** (see Chapter 1).

Viscera of Neck

The cervical viscera are organized in three layers, named for their primary function (Fig. 8.8). Superficial to deep, they are the *endocrine layer* (thyroid and parathyroid glands), the *respiratory layer* (larynx and trachea), and the *alimentary layer* (pharynx and esophagus).

Endocrine Layer of Cervical Viscera

The cervical organs in the **endocrine layer** are part of the body's endocrine system of ductless, hormone-secreting glands. The thyroid gland produces *thyroid hormone,* which controls the rate of metabolism, and *calcitonin,* a hormone controlling calcium metabolism. The parathyroid glands produce *parathormone* (PTH), which controls the metabolism of phosphorus and calcium in the blood.

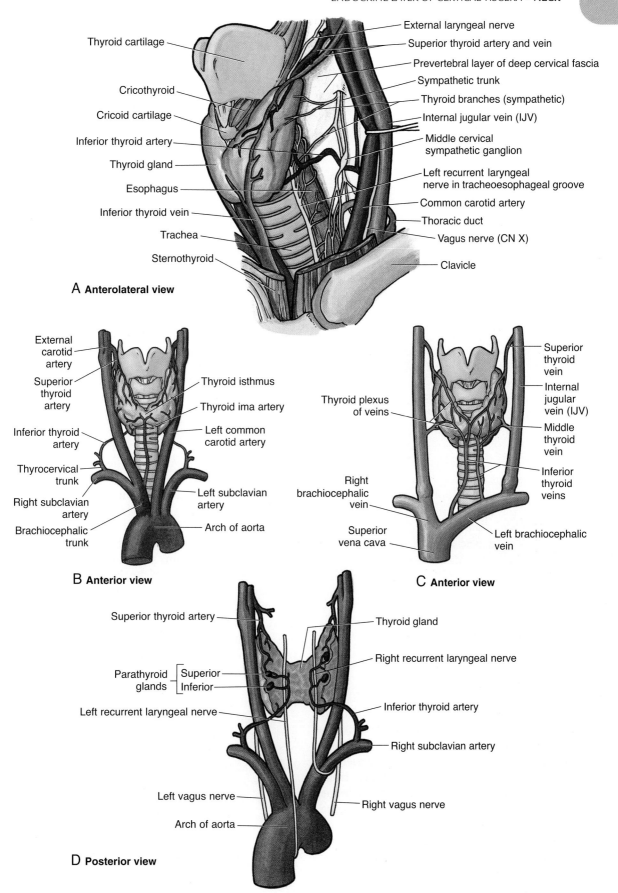

A **Anterolateral view**

Thyroid cartilage
Cricothyroid
Cricoid cartilage
Inferior thyroid artery
Thyroid gland
Esophagus
Inferior thyroid vein
Trachea
Sternothyroid

External laryngeal nerve
Superior thyroid artery and vein
Prevertebral layer of deep cervical fascia
Sympathetic trunk
Thyroid branches (sympathetic)
Internal jugular vein (IJV)
Middle cervical sympathetic ganglion
Left recurrent laryngeal nerve in tracheoesophageal groove
Common carotid artery
Thoracic duct
Vagus nerve (CN X)
Clavicle

B **Anterior view**

External carotid artery
Superior thyroid artery
Inferior thyroid artery
Thyrocervical trunk
Right subclavian artery
Brachiocephalic trunk

Thyroid isthmus
Thyroid ima artery
Left common carotid artery
Left subclavian artery
Arch of aorta

C **Anterior view**

Thyroid plexus of veins
Right brachiocephalic vein
Superior vena cava

Superior thyroid vein
Internal jugular vein (IJV)
Middle thyroid vein
Inferior thyroid veins
Left brachiocephalic vein

D **Posterior view**

Superior thyroid artery
Parathyroid glands { Superior / Inferior }
Left recurrent laryngeal nerve
Left vagus nerve
Arch of aorta

Thyroid gland
Right recurrent laryngeal nerve
Inferior thyroid artery
Right subclavian artery
Right vagus nerve

Figure 8.9. Thyroid and parathyroid glands. A. The vasculature and innervation of the root of the neck is shown. The arterial supply (**B**) and venous drainage (**C**) are detailed. **D.** This dissection of the posterior surface of the thyroid gland shows the blood supply of the parathyroid glands.

Cervicothoracic Ganglion Block

Anesthetic injected around the cervicothoracic (stellate) ganglion blocks transmission of stimuli through the cervical and superior thoracic ganglia. This ganglion block may relieve vascular spasms involving the brain and upper limb. It is also useful when deciding if surgical resection of the ganglion would be beneficial to a person with excess vaso-constriction of the ipsilateral limb.

Lesion of Cervical Sympathetic Trunk

A lesion of a sympathetic trunk in the neck results in a sympathetic disturbance called *Horner syndrome*, which is characterized by:

- Pupillary constriction, resulting from paralysis of the dilator pupillae muscle.
- Ptosis (drooping of the superior eyelid), resulting from paralysis of the smooth (tarsal) muscle in-termingled with striated muscle of the levator palpebrae superioris.
- Sinking in of the eyeball (enophthalmos), possi-bly caused by paralysis of smooth (orbitalis) muscle in the floor of the orbit.
- Vasodilation and absence of sweating on the face and neck (anhydrosis), caused by a lack of sympathetic (vasoconstrictive) nerve supply to the blood vessels and sweat glands.

THYROID GLAND

The **thyroid gland** is located anteriorly in the neck. It lies deep to the sternothyroid and sternohyoid muscles from the level of the C5–T1 vertebrae (Fig. 8.2*B*). It consists pri-marily of right and left **lobes**, anterolateral to the larynx and trachea. A relatively thin **isthmus** unites the lobes over the trachea, usually anterior to the 2nd and 3rd tracheal rings (Fig. 8.8). The thyroid gland is surrounded by a thin **fibrous capsule**, which sends septa deeply into the gland. Dense connective tissue attaches the fibrous capsule to the cricoid cartilage and superior tracheal rings. External to the cap-sule is a loose *fascial sheath* formed by the visceral portion of the pretracheal layer of deep cervical fascia.

The rich blood supply of the thyroid gland is from the paired **superior** and **inferior thyroid arteries** (Fig. 8.9*A* & *B*). These vessels lie between the fibrous capsule and the loose fascial sheath. Usually, the first branches of the exter-nal carotid artery, the *superior thyroid arteries,* descend to the superior poles of the gland, pierce the pretracheal layer of deep cervical fascia, and divide into anterior and posterior branches. The *inferior thyroid arteries,* the largest branches of the thyrocervical trunks, arising from the subclavian ar-teries (Fig. 8.9*B*), run superomedially posterior to the carotid sheaths to reach the posterior aspect of the thyroid gland. The right and left superior and inferior thyroid ar-teries anastomose extensively within the gland, ensuring its supply while providing potential collateral circulation be-tween the subclavian and the external carotid arteries.

In approximately 10% of people, a **thyroid ima artery** (L. *arteria thyroidea ima*) arises from the brachiocephalic trunk, the arch of the aorta, or from the right common carotid, subclavian, or internal thoracic arteries (Fig. 8.9*B*). This small artery ascends on the anterior surface of the trachea, which it supplies, and continues to the isthmus of the thy-roid gland. The possible presence of this lowest artery (L. *ima*) must be considered when performing procedures in the midline of the neck inferior to the isthmus because it is a potential source of bleeding.

Three pairs of thyroid veins usually drain the **thyroid plexus of veins** on the anterior surface of the thyroid gland and trachea (Fig. 8.9*A* & *C*). The **superior thyroid veins** accompany the superior thyroid arteries and drain the su-perior poles of the gland. The **middle thyroid veins** drain the middle of the lobes, and the **inferior thyroid veins** drain the inferior poles. The superior and middle thyroid veins drain into the IJVs, and the inferior thyroid veins drain into the brachiocephalic veins posterior to the manubrium.

The **lymphatic vessels of the thyroid gland** communicate with a capsular network of lymphatic vessels. From this network, the vessels pass initially to **prelaryngeal, pretra-cheal,** and **paratracheal lymph nodes,** which drain in turn to the **superior** and **inferior deep cervical nodes** (Fig. 8.10). Inferior to the thyroid gland, the lymphatic vessels pass directly to the **inferior deep cervical lymph nodes.** Some lymphatic vessels may drain into *brachiocephalic lymph nodes* or the *thoracic duct.*

The **nerves of the thyroid gland** are derived from the su-perior, middle, and inferior *cervical sympathetic ganglia* (Fig. 8.7*B*). They reach the gland through the *cardiac and supe-rior and inferior thyroid periarterial plexuses* that accompany the thyroid arteries. These fibers are vasomotor, causing constriction of blood vessels. Endocrine secretion from the thyroid gland is hormonally regulated by the pituitary gland.

PARATHYROID GLANDS

The small flattened, oval **parathyroid glands** lie external to the fibrous capsule on the medial half of the posterior surface of each lobe of the thyroid gland (Fig. 8.9*D*). Most

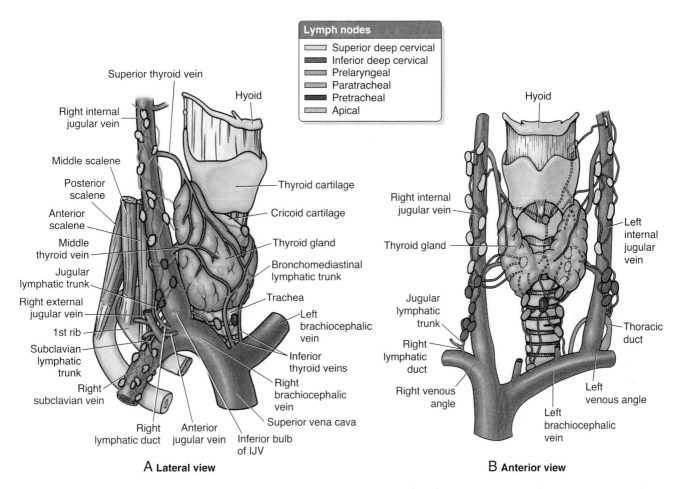

Figure 8.10. Lymphatic drainage of thyroid gland, larynx, and trachea. *IJV,* internal jugular vein.

people have four parathyroid glands. Approximately 5% of people have more; some have only two glands. The two **superior parathyroid glands** are usually at the level of the inferior border of the cricoid cartilage. The **inferior parathyroid glands** are usually near the inferior poles of the thyroid gland, but they may lie in a variety of positions.

The **inferior thyroid arteries** supply both the superior and the inferior parathyroid glands; however, these glands may also be supplied by branches from the superior thyroid arteries, the thyroid ima artery, or the laryngeal, tracheal, and esophageal arteries. The **parathyroid veins** drain into the *thyroid plexus of veins* of the thyroid gland and trachea (Fig. 8.9*C*). The **lymphatic vessels from the parathyroid glands** drain with those of the thyroid gland into the deep cervical and paratracheal lymph nodes (Fig. 8.10).

The **nerves of the parathyroid glands** are derived from thyroid branches of the *cervical sympathetic ganglia* (Fig. 8.9*A*). The nerves are vasomotor but not secretomotor because these glands are hormonally regulated.

Respiratory Layer of Cervical Viscera

The viscera of the **respiratory layer**, the larynx and trachea, contribute to the respiratory functions of the body (Fig. 8.8). The main functions of the cervical respiratory viscera are

- Routing air and food into the respiratory tract and esophagus, respectively.
- Providing a patent airway and a means of sealing it off temporarily.
- Producing voice.

LARYNX

The **larynx**, the complex organ of voice production, lies in the anterior part of the neck at the level of the bodies of the C3–C6 vertebrae (Fig. 8.1). It connects the inferior part of the pharynx (oropharynx) with the trachea. Although most commonly known for its role as the phonating mechanism for voice production, its most vital function is to guard the air passages, especially during swallowing when it serves as a sphincter or valve of the lower respiratory tract, thus maintaining a patent airway.

Pyramidal Lobe of the Thyroid Gland

Approximately 50% of thyroid glands have a small prominence, the *pyramidal lobe,* on the superior surface of the isthmus of the thyroid gland, usually to the left of the median plane. A band of connective tissue, often containing accessory thyroid tissue, may continue from the apex of the pyramidal lobe to the hyoid bone.

Thyroidectomy

During a total thyroidectomy (e.g., excision of a malignant thyroid gland), the parathyroid glands are in danger of being inadvertently damaged or removed. These glands are safe during *subtotal thyroidectomy* because the most posterior part of the thyroid gland usually is preserved. Variability in the position of the parathyroid glands, especially the inferior ones, puts them in danger of being removed during surgery on the thyroid gland. If the parathyroid glands are inadvertently removed during surgery, the patient suffers from *tetany,* a severe convulsive disorder. The generalized convulsive muscle spasms result from a fall in blood calcium levels.

Accessory Thyroid Glandular Tissue

Accessory thyroid tissue may develop in the neck lateral to the thyroid cartilage (Fig. B8.5); usually, the accessory thyroid gland lies on the thyrohyoid muscle. The pyramidal lobe and its connective tissue continuation may also contain thyroid tissue. Accessory thyroid tissue, like that of a pyramidal lobe, originates from remnants of the *thyroglossal duct*—a transitory endodermal tube extending from the posterior tongue region of the embryo carrying the thyroid-forming tissue at its descending distal end. Although the accessory tissue may be functional, it is usually too small to maintain normal function if the thyroid gland is removed.

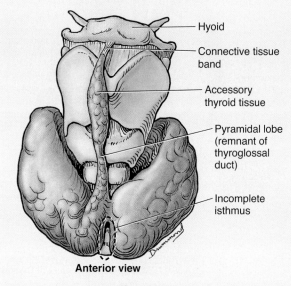

Labels: Hyoid; Connective tissue band; Accessory thyroid tissue; Pyramidal lobe (remnant of thyroglossal duct); Incomplete isthmus

Anterior view

Figure B8.5.

Laryngeal Skeleton The **laryngeal skeleton** consists of nine cartilages joined by ligaments and membranes (Fig. 8.11). Three cartilages are single (thyroid, cricoid, and epiglottic) and three are paired (arytenoid, corniculate, and cuneiform).

The **thyroid cartilage** is the largest of the cartilages. Its superior border lies opposite the C4 vertebra. The inferior two thirds of its two plate-like **laminae** are fused anteriorly in the median plane to form the **laryngeal prominence** ("Adam's apple"). Superior to this prominence, the laminae diverge to form the V-shaped **superior thyroid notch** (Fig. 8.8). The small **inferior thyroid notch** is a shallow indentation in the middle of the inferior border of the cartilage. The posterior border of each lamina projects superiorly as the **superior horn** and inferiorly as the **inferior horn** (Fig. 8.11A). The superior border and superior horns attach to the hyoid by the **thyrohyoid** membrane. The thick median part of this membrane is the **median thyrohyoid ligament**, and its lateral parts are the **lateral thyrohyoid ligaments**. The inferior horns of the thyroid cartilages articulate with the lateral surfaces of the cricoid cartilage at the **cricothyroid joints** (Fig. 8.11B). The main movements at these joints are rotation and gliding of the thyroid cartilage, which result in changes in the length of the vocal folds.

The **cricoid cartilage** forms a complete ring around the airway, the only laryngeal cartilage to do so. It is shaped like a signet ring with its band facing anteriorly (Fig. 8.11). The ring-like opening of the cartilage fits an average finger. The posterior (signet) part of the cricoid cartilage is the *lamina;* the anterior (band) part is the *arch.* The cricoid cartilage is smaller but thicker and stronger than the thyroid cartilage. The cricoid cartilage is attached to the inferior margin of the thyroid cartilage by the **median cricothyroid ligament**

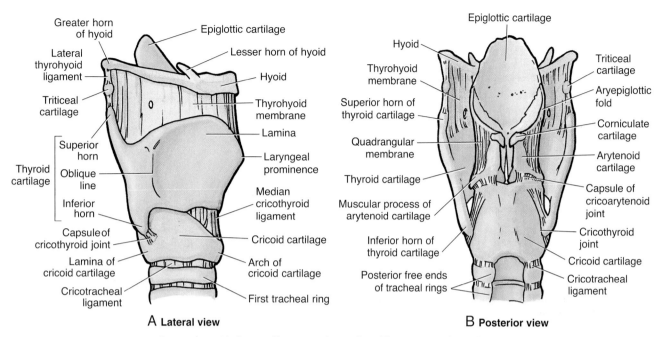

Figure 8.11. Skeleton of larynx and associated ligaments and membranes.

and to the first tracheal ring by the **cricotracheal ligament.** Where the larynx is closest to the skin and most accessible, the median cricothyroid ligament may be felt as a soft spot during palpation inferior to the thyroid cartilage.

The **arytenoid cartilages** are paired, three-sided pyramidal cartilages that articulate with lateral parts of the superior border of the cricoid cartilage lamina. Each cartilage has an apex superiorly, a vocal process anteriorly, and a large muscular process that projects laterally from its base (Figs. 8.11*B* and 8.12*A*). The **apex** of each arytenoid cartilage bears the corniculate cartilage and attaches to the aryepiglottic fold. The **vocal process** provides the posterior attachment for the vocal ligament, and the **muscular process** serves as a lever to which the posterior and lateral cricoarytenoid muscles are attached.

The **cricoarytenoid joints,** located between the bases of the arytenoid cartilages and the superolateral surfaces of the lamina of the cricoid cartilage (Fig. 8.11*B*), permit the arytenoid cartilages to slide toward or away from one another, to tilt anteriorly and posteriorly, and to rotate. These movements are important in approximating, tensing, and relaxing the vocal folds. The elastic **vocal ligaments** extend from the junction of the laminae of the thyroid cartilage anteriorly to the vocal process of the arytenoid cartilage posteriorly (Fig. 8.12*A*). The vocal ligaments form the submucosal skeleton of the vocal folds. The vocal ligaments are the thickened, free superior border of the **conus elasticus** or **cricovocal membrane** (Fig. 8.13*A*). The parts of the membrane extending laterally between the vocal folds and the superior border of the cricoid are the **lateral**

cricothyroid ligaments. The fibroelastic conus elasticus blends anteriorly with the *median cricothyroid ligament.* The **conus elasticus** and overlying mucosa close the tracheal inlet, except for the central **rima glottidis** (opening between the vocal folds).

The **epiglottic cartilage,** consisting of elastic cartilage, gives flexibility to the **epiglottis** (Figs. 8.11 and 8.12). It is a heart-shaped cartilage covered with mucous membrane. Situated posterior to the root of the tongue and the hyoid and anterior to the **laryngeal inlet,** the epiglottic cartilage forms the superior part of the anterior wall and the superior margin of the inlet. Its broad superior end is free; its tapered inferior end, the **stalk of the epiglottis,** is attached to the angle formed by the thyroid laminae and the **thyroepiglottic ligament** (Fig. 8.13*A*).

The **hyoepiglottic ligament** attaches the anterior surface of the epiglottic cartilage to the hyoid. A thin submucosal sheet of connective tissue, the **quadrangular membrane,** extends between the lateral aspects of the arytenoid and epiglottic cartilages (Fig. 8.12*A*). Its free inferior margin constitutes the **vestibular ligament,** which is covered loosely by mucosa to form the **vestibular fold** (Fig. 8.12). This fold lies superior to the vocal fold and extends from thyroid cartilage to the arytenoid cartilage. The free superior margin of the quadrangular membrane forms the **aryepiglottic ligament,** which is covered with mucosa to form the **aryepiglottic fold.**

The **corniculate and cuneiform cartilages** appear as small nodules in the posterior part of the aryepiglottic folds (Figs. 8.11 and 8.12). The corniculate cartilages attach to

Surface Anatomy of Larynx

The U-shaped **hyoid** lies superior to the **thyroid cartilage** at the level of the C4 and C5 vertebrae (Fig. SA8.2). The **laryngeal prominence** is produced by the fused *laminae of the thyroid cartilage*, which meet in the median plane. The **cricoid cartilage** can be felt inferior to the laryngeal prominence. It lies at the level of the C6 vertebra. The cartilaginous **tracheal rings** are palpable in the inferior part of the neck. The 2nd–4th rings cannot be felt because the **isthmus** of the thyroid, connecting its right and left lobes, covers them. The first tracheal ring is just superior to the isthmus. ●

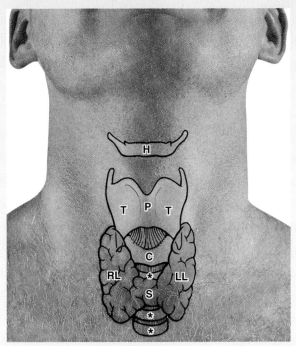

Anterior view

Key			
C	Cricoid cartilage	**RL**	Right lobe of thyroid gland
H	Hyoid	**S**	Isthmus
LL	Left lobe of thyroid gland	**T**	Thyroid cartilage
P	Laryngeal prominence	★	Tracheal rings

Figure SA8.2.

the apices of the arytenoid cartilages; the cuneiform cartilages do not directly attach to other cartilages.

Interior of the Larynx   The **laryngeal cavity** extends from the *laryngeal inlet,* through which it communicates with the *laryngopharynx,* to the level of the inferior border of the cricoid cartilage. Here, the laryngeal cavity is continuous with the lumen of the trachea. The laryngeal cavity includes the (Fig. 8.12 *B*):

- **Laryngeal vestibule,** between the laryngeal inlet and the vestibular folds.
- **Middle part of laryngeal cavity,** the central cavity (airway) between the vestibular and vocal folds.
- **Laryngeal ventricle,** recesses extending laterally from the middle part of the laryngeal cavity between vestibular and vocal folds. The **laryngeal saccule** is a blind pocket opening into each ventricle that is lined with mucosal glands.
- **Infraglottic cavity,** the inferior cavity of the larynx between the vocal folds and the inferior border of the cricoid cartilage, where it is continuous with the lumen of the trachea.

The **vocal folds** (true vocal cords) control sound production. The apex of each wedge-shaped fold projects medially into the laryngeal cavity (Figs. 8.12 and 8.13). Each fold contains a:

- *Vocal ligament,* consisting of thickened elastic tissue that is the medial free edge of the conus elasticus.
- *Vocalis muscle,* composed of exceptionally fine muscle fibers immediately lateral to and terminating at intervals relative to the length of the vocal ligaments (Table 8.5).

The **vocal folds** are the source of sounds (tone) that come from the larynx (Fig. 8.13). The vocal folds produce audible vibrations when their free margins are closely (but not tightly) apposed during phonation and air is forcibly expired intermittently. The vocal folds also serve as the main inspiratory sphincter of the larynx when they are tightly closed. Complete adduction of the folds forms an effective sphincter that prevents entry of air.

The **glottis** (vocal apparatus of the larynx) makes up the vocal folds and processes, together with the *rima glottidis,* the aperture between the vocal folds. The shape of the rima (L. slit) varies according to the position of the vocal folds. During ordinary breathing, the rima is narrow and wedge shaped (Fig. 8.13 *B*); during forced respiration it is wide and kite shaped. The rima glottidis is slit-like when the vocal folds are closely approximated during phonation (Fig. 8.13 *C*). Variation in the tension and length of the vocal folds, in the width of the rima glottidis, and the intensity of the expiratory effort produces changes in the pitch of the voice. The lower range of pitch of the voice of postpubertal males results from the greater length of the vocal folds.

The *vestibular folds* (false vocal cords), extending between the thyroid and the arytenoid cartilages (Fig. 8.12), play little or no part in voice production. They are protective in function. They consist of two thick folds of mucous membrane enclosing the *vestibular ligaments.* The space between these ligaments is the **rima vestibuli.** The lateral recesses between the vocal and the vestibular folds are the *laryngeal ventricles.*

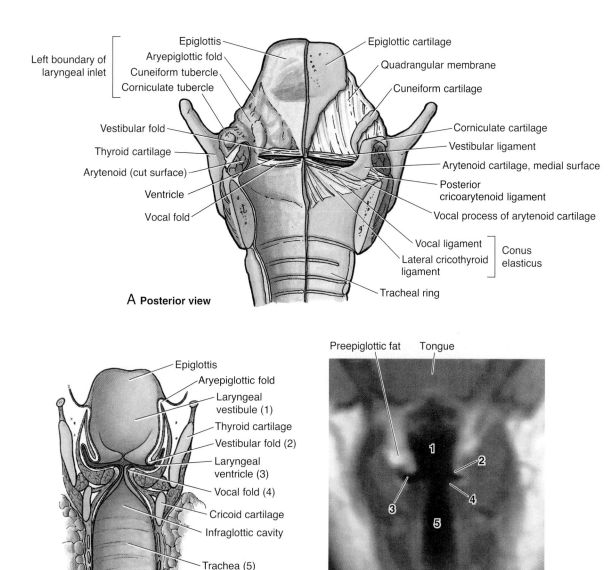

Figure 8.12. Interior and compartments of larynx.

Muscles of the Larynx. The laryngeal muscles are divided into extrinsic and intrinsic groups:

- The **extrinsic laryngeal muscles** move the larynx as a whole (Table 8.5). The *infrahyoid muscles* are depressors of the hyoid and larynx, whereas the *suprahyoid* and *stylopharyngeus muscles* are elevators of the hyoid and larynx.
- The **intrinsic laryngeal muscles** move the laryngeal parts, making alterations in the length and tension of the vocal folds and in the size and shape of the rima glottidis. All but one of the intrinsic muscles of the larynx are supplied by the *recurrent laryngeal nerve* (Fig. 8.14), a branch of CN X. The cricothyroid muscle is supplied by the external laryngeal nerve, one of the two terminal branches of the *su-*

perior laryngeal nerve. The actions of the intrinsic laryngeal muscles are described in Table 8.5.

Vessels of the Larynx. The laryngeal arteries, branches of the superior and inferior thyroid arteries, supply the larynx (Fig. 8.14*B*). The **superior laryngeal artery** accompanies the internal branch of the superior laryngeal nerve through the thyrohyoid membrane and branches to supply the internal surface of the larynx. The **inferior laryngeal artery**, a branch of the inferior thyroid artery, accompanies the *inferior laryngeal nerve* (terminal part of the recurrent laryngeal nerve) and supplies the mucous membrane and muscles in the inferior part of the larynx.

The laryngeal veins accompany the laryngeal arteries. The **superior laryngeal vein** usually joins the superior thyroid

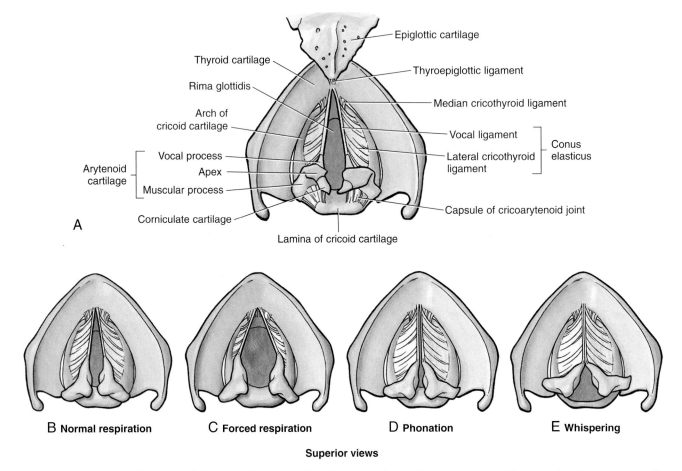

Figure 8.13. Rima glottidis. A. The skeleton and ligaments of the larynx are shown. **B–E.** The shape of the rima glottidis varies according to the position of the vocal folds.

vein and through it drains into the IJV. The **inferior laryngeal vein** joins the inferior thyroid vein or the thyroid plexus of veins on the anterior aspect of the trachea, which empties into the left brachiocephalic vein.

The **lymphatic vessels of the larynx** superior to the vocal folds accompany the superior laryngeal artery through the thyrohyoid membrane and drain into the **superior deep cervical lymph nodes** (Fig. 8.10). The lymphatic vessels inferior to the vocal folds drain into the *pretracheal* or *paratracheal lymph nodes,* which drain into the **inferior deep cervical lymph nodes.**

Nerves of the Larynx.   The nerves of the larynx are the superior and inferior laryngeal branches of the vagus nerve (Fig. 8.14). The **superior laryngeal nerve** arises from the **inferior vagal ganglion** and divides into two terminal branches within the carotid sheath: the internal laryngeal nerve (sensory and autonomic) and the external laryngeal nerve (motor).

The **internal laryngeal nerve**, the larger terminal branch of the superior laryngeal nerve, pierces the thyrohyoid membrane with the superior laryngeal artery, supplying sensory fibers to the laryngeal mucous membrane of the laryngeal vestibule and middle laryngeal cavity, including the superior surface of the vocal folds.

The **external laryngeal nerve** descends posterior to the sternothyroid muscle in company with the superior thyroid artery. At first the nerve lies on the inferior constrictor muscle of the pharynx; it then pierces the muscle, contributing to its innervation (with the pharyngeal plexus), and continues to supply the cricothyroid muscle.

The **inferior laryngeal nerve**, the continuation of the recurrent laryngeal nerve (a branch of the vagus) supplies all intrinsic muscles of the larynx except the cricothyroid, which is supplied by the external laryngeal nerve. It also supplies sensory fibers to the mucosa of the infraglottic cavity. The inferior laryngeal nerve, enters the larynx by passing deep to the inferior border of the inferior constrictor muscle of the pharynx. It divides into anterior and posterior branches that accompany the inferior laryngeal artery into the larynx.

TRACHEA

The **trachea**, extending from the inferior end of the larynx into the thorax, terminates at the sternal angle, where it

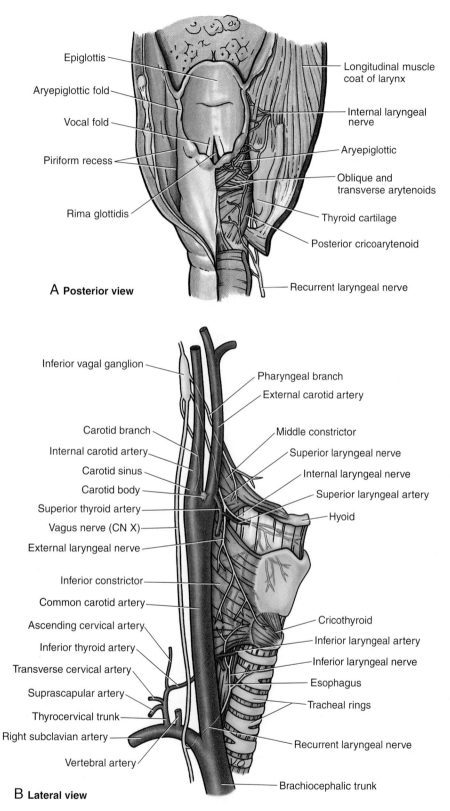

A Posterior view

Epiglottis
Aryepiglottic fold
Vocal fold
Piriform recess
Rima glottidis

Longitudinal muscle coat of larynx
Internal laryngeal nerve
Aryepiglottic
Oblique and transverse arytenoids
Thyroid cartilage
Posterior cricoarytenoid
Recurrent laryngeal nerve

Inferior vagal ganglion
Carotid branch
Internal carotid artery
Carotid sinus
Carotid body
Superior thyroid artery
Vagus nerve (CN X)
External laryngeal nerve
Inferior constrictor
Common carotid artery
Ascending cervical artery
Inferior thyroid artery
Transverse cervical artery
Suprascapular artery
Thyrocervical trunk
Right subclavian artery
Vertebral artery

Pharyngeal branch
External carotid artery
Middle constrictor
Superior laryngeal nerve
Internal laryngeal nerve
Superior laryngeal artery
Hyoid
Cricothyroid
Inferior laryngeal artery
Inferior laryngeal nerve
Esophagus
Tracheal rings
Recurrent laryngeal nerve
Brachiocephalic trunk

B Lateral view

Figure 8.14. Muscles, vessels, and nerves of larynx. A. The muscles and nerves are shown. *Pink,* mucosa. **B.** The vessels and nerves are identified.

Table 8.5 Muscles of the Larynx

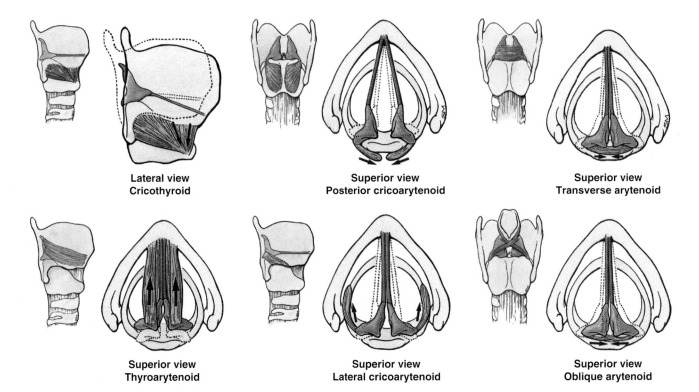

Lateral view
Cricothyroid

Superior view
Posterior cricoarytenoid

Superior view
Transverse arytenoid

Superior view
Thyroarytenoid

Superior view
Lateral cricoarytenoid

Superior view
Oblique arytenoid

Muscle	Origin	Insertion	Innervation	Main Action(s)
Cricothyroid	Anterolateral part of cricoid cartilage	Inferior margin and inferior horn of thyroid cartilage	External laryngeal nerve (from CN X)	Stretches and tenses vocal ligament
Thyroarytenoid[a]	Lower half of posterior aspect of angle of thyroid laminae and cricothyroid ligament	Anterolateral arytenoid surface	Inferior laryngeal nerve (terminal part of recurrent laryngeal nerve, from CN X)	Relaxes vocal ligament
Posterior cricoarytenoid	Posterior surface of lamina of cricoid cartilage	Vocal process of arytenoid cartilage		Abducts vocal folds
Lateral cricoarytenoid	Arch of cricoid cartilage			Adducts vocal folds (interligamentous portion)
Transverse and oblique arytenoids[b]	One arytenoid cartilage	Contralateral arytenoid cartilage		Adduct arytenoid cartilages (adducting intercartilaginous portion of vocal folds, closing posterior rima glottidis)
Vocalis[c]	Lateral surface of vocal process of arytenoid cartilage	Ipsilateral vocal ligament		Relaxes posterior vocal ligament while maintaining (or increasing) tension of anterior part

[a]Superior fibers of the thyroarytenoid muscles pass into the aryepiglottic fold, and some of them reach the epiglottic cartilage; these fibers constitute the thyroepiglottic muscle, which widens the laryngeal inlet.
[b]Some fibers of the oblique arytenoid muscles continue as aryepiglottic muscles.
[c]This slender muscle slip lies medial to and is composed of fibers finer than those of the thyroarytenoid muscle.

Injury to the Laryngeal Nerves

The inferior laryngeal nerves are vulnerable to injury during thyroidectomy and other surgical operations in the anterior triangles of the neck. Because the inferior laryngeal nerve innervates the muscles moving the vocal fold, injury results in *paralysis of the vocal fold*. The voice is initially poor because the paralyzed fold cannot adduct to meet the normal vocal fold. When bilateral paralysis of the vocal folds occurs, the voice is almost absent because the vocal folds are motionless in a position that is slightly narrower than the usual neutral respiratory position. They cannot be adducted for phonation, nor can they be abducted for increased respiration, resulting in stridor (high-pitched, noisy respiration) often accompanied by anxiety. Injury to the external branch of the superior laryngeal nerve results in a voice that is monotonous in character because the paralyzed cricothyroid muscle supplied by it is unable to vary the length and tension of the vocal fold.

Hoarseness is the most common symptom of serious disorders of the larynx, such as carcinoma of the vocal folds.

Fractures of the Laryngeal Skeleton

Laryngeal fractures may result from blows received in sports such as kick boxing and hockey or from compression by a shoulder strap during an automobile accident. Laryngeal fractures produce submucous hemorrhage and edema, respiratory obstruction, hoarseness, and sometimes a temporary inability to speak. The thyroid, cricoid, and most of the arytenoid cartilages often ossify as age advances, commencing at approximately 25 years of age in the thyroid cartilage.

Laryngoscopy

Laryngoscopy is the procedure used to examine the interior of the larynx. The larynx may be examined visually by *indirect laryngoscopy* using a laryngeal mirror or it may be viewed by *direct laryngoscopy* using a tubular endoscopic instrument, a *laryngoscope*. The vestibular and vocal folds can be observed in Figure B8.6.

Aspiration of Foreign Bodies

A foreign object, such as a piece of steak, may accidentally *aspirate* through the laryngeal inlet into the vestibule of the larynx, where it becomes trapped superior to the vestibular folds. When a foreign object enters the vestibule, the laryngeal muscles go into spasm, tensing the vocal folds. The rima glottidis closes and no air enters the trachea. Asphyxiation occurs, and the person will die in approximately 5 min from lack of oxygen if the obstruction is not removed. Emergency therapy must be given to open the airway. The procedure used depends on the condition of the patient, the facilities available, and the experience of the person giving first aid. Because the lungs still contain air, sudden compression of the abdomen (Heimlich maneuver) causes the diaphragm to elevate and compress the lungs, expelling air from the trachea into the larynx (Fig. B8.7). This maneuver usually dislodges the food or other material from the larynx.

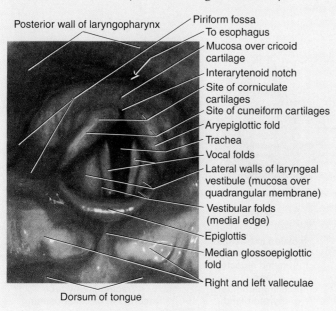

Posterior wall of laryngopharynx
Piriform fossa
To esophagus
Mucosa over cricoid cartilage
Interarytenoid notch
Site of corniculate cartilages
Site of cuneiform cartilages
Aryepiglottic fold
Trachea
Vocal folds
Lateral walls of laryngeal vestibule (mucosa over quadrangular membrane)
Vestibular folds (medial edge)
Epiglottis
Median glossoepiglottic fold
Right and left valleculae
Dorsum of tongue

Laryngoscopic examination

Figure B8.6.

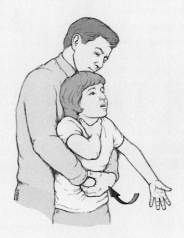

Heimlich maneuver

Figure B8.7.

divides into the right and left main bronchi (Fig. 8.9A). Deviation of the trachea from the midline, often signals the presence of a pathological process. In adults, the trachea is approximately 2.5 cm in diameter, whereas in infants it is the diameter of a pencil.

The trachea is a fibrocartilaginous tube, supported by incomplete cartilaginous **tracheal rings**. They are deficient posteriorly where the trachea is adjacent to the esophagus (Fig. 8.8). The rings keep the trachea patent. The posterior gap in the tracheal rings is spanned by the involuntary **trachealis muscle**, smooth muscle connecting the ends of the tracheal rings.

Lateral to the trachea are the common carotid arteries and thyroid lobes (Fig. 8.14B). Inferior to the isthmus of the thyroid gland are the jugular venous arch and the inferior thyroid veins.

Alimentary Layer of Cervical Viscera

In the **alimentary layer**, cervical viscera take part in the digestive functions of the body. Although the pharynx conducts air to the larynx, trachea, and lungs, its constrictor muscles direct (and the epiglottis deflects) food to the esophagus. The esophagus, also involved in food

Tracheotomy and Tracheostomy

A transverse incision through the skin of the neck and anterior wall of the trachea (*tracheostomy*) establishes an airway in patients with upper airway obstruction or respiratory failure. The infrahyoid muscles are retracted laterally, and the isthmus of the thyroid gland is either divided or retracted superiorly. An opening is made in the trachea between the 1st and 2nd tracheal rings or through the 2nd through 4th rings. A *tracheostomy tube* is then inserted into the trachea and secured (Fig. B8.8). To avoid complications during a tracheostomy, the following anatomical relationships are important:

- The *inferior thyroid veins* arise from a venous plexus on the thyroid gland and descend anterior to the trachea.

- A small *thyroid ima artery* is present in approximately 10% of people; it ascends from the brachiocephalic trunk or the arch of the aorta to the isthmus of the thyroid gland.
- The *left brachiocephalic vein*, jugular venous arch, and pleurae may be encountered, particularly in infants and children.
- The *thymus* covers the inferior part of the trachea in infants and children.
- The trachea is small, mobile, and soft in infants, making it easy to cut through its posterior wall and damage the esophagus.

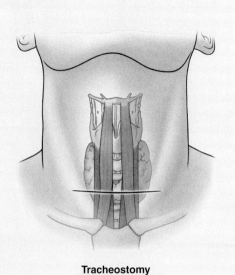

Tracheostomy

Anterior views

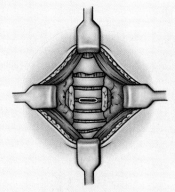

Incision in trachea after retracting infrahyoid muscles and incising isthmus of thyroid gland

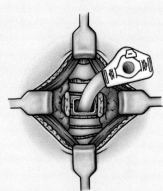

Tracheostomy tube inserted in tracheal opening

Figure B8.8.

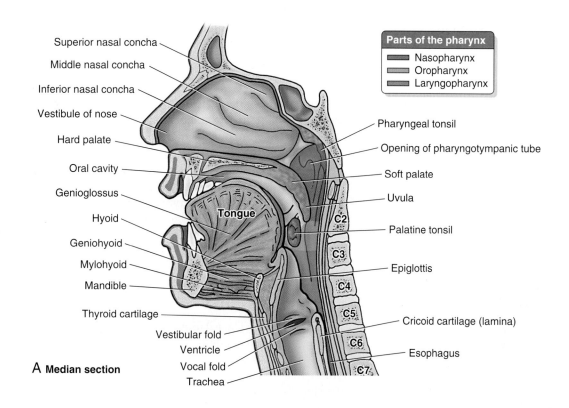

Parts of the pharynx
- Nasopharynx
- Oropharynx
- Laryngopharynx

Superior nasal concha
Middle nasal concha
Inferior nasal concha
Vestibule of nose
Hard palate
Oral cavity
Genioglossus
Hyoid
Geniohyoid
Mylohyoid
Mandible
Thyroid cartilage

A Median section

Vestibular fold
Ventricle
Vocal fold
Trachea

Pharyngeal tonsil
Opening of pharyngotympanic tube
Soft palate
Uvula
Palatine tonsil
Epiglottis
Cricoid cartilage (lamina)
Esophagus

C2
C3
C4
C5
C6
C7

Tongue

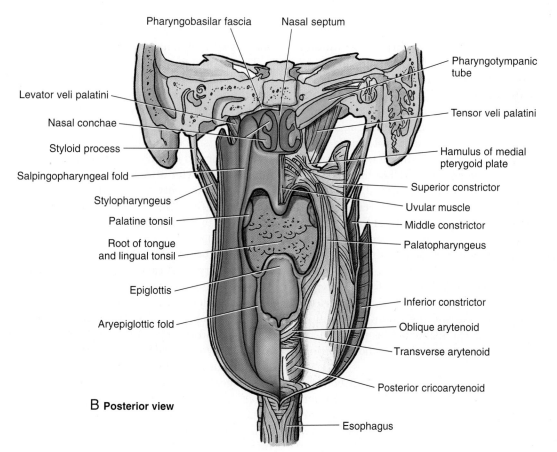

Pharyngobasilar fascia   Nasal septum

Levator veli palatini
Nasal conchae
Styloid process
Salpingopharyngeal fold
Stylopharyngeus
Palatine tonsil
Root of tongue
and lingual tonsil
Epiglottis
Aryepiglottic fold

Pharyngotympanic
tube
Tensor veli palatini
Hamulus of medial
pterygoid plate
Superior constrictor
Uvular muscle
Middle constrictor
Palatopharyngeus
Inferior constrictor
Oblique arytenoid
Transverse arytenoid
Posterior cricoarytenoid

B Posterior view

Esophagus

Figure 8.15. Nasopharynx, oropharynx, and laryngopharynx. A. Structures of the head and neck are shown. **B.** The posterior wall of the pharynx has been cut in the midline and reflected laterally, and the mucous membrane has been removed from the right side.

propulsion, is the beginning of the *alimentary canal* (digestive tract).

PHARYNX

The **pharynx** is the superior expanded part of the alimentary system posterior to the nasal and oral cavities, extending inferiorly past the larynx (Fig. 8.15*A*). The pharynx extends from the cranial base to the inferior border of the cricoid cartilage anteriorly and the inferior border of C6 vertebra posteriorly. The pharynx is widest opposite the hyoid and narrowest at its inferior end, where it is continuous with the esophagus. The flat posterior wall of the pharynx lies against the prevertebral layer of deep cervical fascia (Fig. 8.2*A*).

Interior of the Pharynx. The pharynx is divided into three parts:

- *Nasopharynx,* posterior to the nose and superior to the soft palate.
- *Oropharynx,* posterior to the mouth.
- *Laryngopharynx,* posterior to the larynx.

The **nasopharynx** has a respiratory function. It lies superior to the *soft palate* and is the posterior extension of the nasal cavities (Fig. 8.15*A*). The nose opens into the nasopharynx through two **choanae** (paired openings between the nasal cavity and nasopharynx). The roof and posterior wall of the nasopharynx form a continuous surface that lies inferior to the body of the sphenoid bone and the basilar part of the occipital bone.

The lymphoid tissue in the pharynx forms an incomplete *tonsillar ring* around the superior part of the pharynx. The lymphoid tissue is aggregated in certain regions to form masses called *tonsils.* The **pharyngeal tonsils** (commonly called adenoids when enlarged), are in the mucous membrane of the roof and posterior wall of the nasopharynx. Extending inferiorly from the medial end of the pharyngotympanic tube (auditory tube) is a vertical fold of mucous membrane, the **salpingopharyngeal fold.** It covers the salpingopharyngeus muscle, which opens the pharyngeal orifice of the pharyngotympanic tube during swallowing. The collection of lymphoid tissue in the submucosa of the pharynx near the pharyngeal orifice of the pharyngotympanic tube is the **tubal tonsil.** Posterior to the **torus of the pharyngotympanic tube** and the salpingopharyngeal fold is a slit-like lateral extension of the pharynx, the **pharyngeal recess,** which extends laterally and posteriorly (Fig. 8.15*B*).

The **oropharynx** has a digestive function. It is bounded by the soft palate superiorly, the base of the tongue inferiorly, and the palatoglossal and palatopharyngeal arches laterally (Figs. 8.15 and 8.16). It extends from the soft palate to the superior border of the epiglottis. **Deglutition** (swallowing) is the process that transfers a food bolus from the mouth through the pharynx and esophagus into the stomach. Solid food is masticated (chewed) and mixed with saliva to form a soft bolus that is easier to swallow. Deglutition occurs in three stages (Fig. 8.17):

- **Stage 1:** voluntary; the bolus is compressed against the palate and pushed from the mouth into the oropharynx, mainly by movements of the muscles of the tongue and soft palate.
- **Stage 2:** involuntary and rapid; the soft palate is elevated, sealing off the nasopharynx from the oropharynx and laryngopharynx. The pharynx widens and shortens to receive the bolus of food as the suprahyoid muscles and longitudinal pharyngeal muscles contract, elevating the larynx.
- **Stage 3:** involuntary; sequential contraction of all three pharyngeal constrictor muscles forces the food bolus inferiorly into the esophagus.

The **palatine tonsils** are collections of lymphoid tissue on each side of the oropharynx that lie in the **tonsillar sinus** (also called the tonsillar fossa or bed). The tonsillar sinus is between the **palatoglossal** and the **palatopharyngeal arches** (Fig. 8.16). The tonsillar bed is formed by the superior constrictor of the pharynx and the thin sheet of **pharyngobasilar fascia** (Fig. 8.18*A*). This fascia blends with the periosteum of the cranial base and defines the limits of the pharyngeal wall in its superior part.

The **laryngopharynx** (hypopharynx) lies posterior to the larynx, extending from the superior border of the epiglottis and the pharyngoepiglottic folds to the inferior border of the cricoid cartilage, where it narrows and becomes continuous with the esophagus (Fig. 8.15). Posteriorly, the laryngopharynx is related to the bodies of the C4–C6 vertebrae. Its posterior and lateral walls are formed by the **middle and inferior constrictor muscles** (Fig. 8.18). Internally, the wall is formed by the *palatopharyngeus* and *stylopharyngeus muscles* (Fig. 8.16*C*). The laryngopharynx communicates with the larynx through the *laryngeal inlet* on its anterior wall (Fig. 8.12*B*).

The **piriform fossa** (recess) is a small depression of the laryngopharyngeal cavity on each side of the inlet (Fig. 8.14*A*). This mucosa-lined fossa is separated from the laryngeal inlet by the *aryepiglottic fold.* Laterally, the piriform fossa is bounded by the medial surfaces of the thyroid cartilage and the *thyrohyoid membrane.* Branches of the internal laryngeal and recurrent laryngeal nerves lie deep to the mucous membrane of the piriform fossa.

Pharyngeal Muscles. The wall of the pharynx has a muscular layer composed entirely of voluntary muscle arranged mainly into an external circular and an internal longitudinal layer. In most of the **alimentary canal,** the muscular layer consists of smooth muscle. The external layer consists of three **pharyngeal constrictors: superior,**

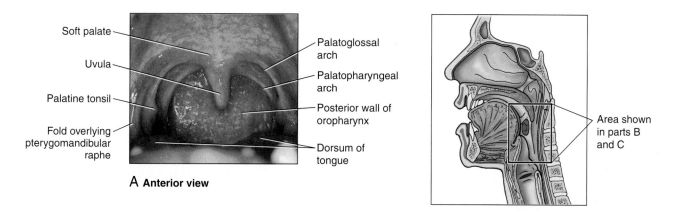

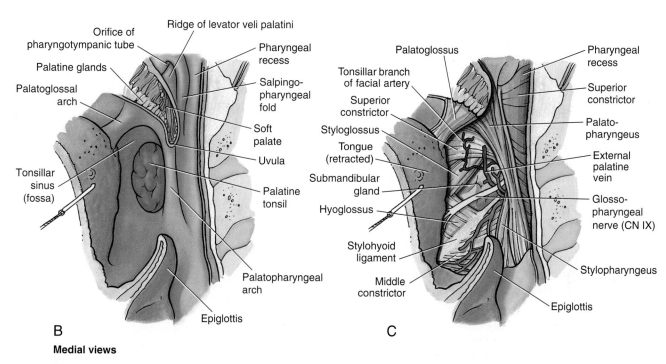

Figure 8.16. Oral cavity and tonsils. A. The structures of the oral cavity are shown in an adult male whose mouth is wide open with the tongue protruded. (Courtesy of Dr. B. Liebgott, Professor, Division of Anatomy, Department of Surgery, University of Toronto, Ontario, Canada.) **B.** The internal aspect of the lateral wall of the pharynx is shown. **C.** This deep dissection reveals the tonsillar bed.

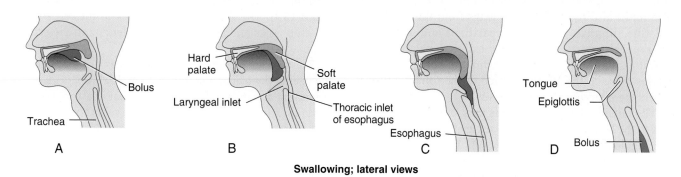

Swallowing; lateral views

Figure 8.17. Swallowing. A. The bolus of food is squeezed to the back of the oral cavity by pushing the tongue against the palate. **B.** The nasopharynx is sealed off and the larynx is elevated, enlarging the pharynx to receive food. **C.** The pharyngeal sphincters contract sequentially, squeezing food into the esophagus. **D.** The bolus of food moves down the esophagus by peristaltic contractions.

middle, and **inferior** (Figs. 8.15 and 8.18). The internal, mainly longitudinal, layer of muscles consists of the **palatopharyngeus, stylopharyngeus,** and **salpingopharyngeus.** These muscles elevate the larynx and shorten the pharynx during swallowing and speaking. The attachments, nerve supply, and actions of the pharyngeal muscles are described in Table 8.6.

The pharyngeal constrictors have a strong internal fascial lining, the *pharyngobasilar fascia,* and a thin external fascial lining, the *buccopharyngeal fascia.* The pharyngeal constrictors contract involuntarily so that contraction takes place sequentially from the superior to the inferior end of the pharynx, propelling food into the esophagus. All three constrictors are supplied by the *pharyngeal plexus of nerves* that lies on the lateral wall of the pharynx, mainly on the middle constrictor (Fig. 8.18). The overlapping of the constrictor muscles leaves four gaps in the musculature for structures to enter or leave the pharynx (Fig. 8.18):

- Superior to the superior constrictor, the levator veli palatini, pharyngotympanic tube, and ascending palatine artery pass through the *gap between the superior constrictor and the cranium.* It is here that the pharyngobasilar fascia blends with the buccopharyngeal fascia to form, with the mucous membrane, the thin wall of the pharyngeal recess (Fig. 8.20*B*).
- A *gap between the superior and the middle constrictors* forms a passageway that allows the stylopharyngeus, glossopharyngeal nerve, and stylohyoid ligament to pass to the internal aspect of the pharyngeal wall.
- A *gap between the middle and the inferior constrictors* allows the internal laryngeal nerve and superior laryngeal artery and vein to pass to the larynx.
- A *gap inferior to the inferior constrictor* allows the recurrent laryngeal nerve and inferior laryngeal artery to pass superiorly into the larynx.

Vessels of the Pharynx. The **tonsillar artery,** a branch of the facial artery (Fig. 8.16*C*), passes through the superior constrictor muscle and enters the inferior pole of the tonsil. The tonsil also receives arterial twigs from the ascending palatine, lingual, descending palatine, and ascending pharyngeal arteries. The large **external palatine vein** (paratonsillar vein) descends from the soft palate and passes close to the lateral surface of the tonsil before it enters the pharyngeal venous plexus.

The **tonsillar lymphatic vessels** pass laterally and inferiorly to the lymph nodes near the angle of the mandible and the **jugulodigastric node** (Fig. 8.19). The jugulodigastric node is referred to as the *tonsillar node* because of its frequent enlargement when the tonsil is inflamed *(tonsillitis).* The palatine, lingual, and pharyngeal tonsils form the pharyngeal **tonsillar ring** (of Waldeyer), an incomplete circular band of lymphoid tissue around the superior part of the pharynx. The anteroinferior part of the ring is formed by the **lingual tonsil,** a collection of lymphoid tissue in the posterior part of the tongue (Fig. 8.15*B*). Lateral parts of the ring are formed by the palatine and tubal tonsils, and posterior and superior parts are formed by the pharyngeal tonsil.

Pharyngeal Nerves. The **nerve supply to the pharynx** (motor and most of sensory) derives from the **pharyngeal plexus of nerves** (Fig. 8.18*B* & *C*). Motor fibers in the plexus are derived from the vagus nerve (CN X) via its pharyngeal branch(es). They supply all the muscles of the pharynx and soft palate, except the stylopharyngeus (supplied by CN IX) and the tensor veli palatini (supplied by CN V₃). The inferior pharyngeal constrictor also receives some motor fibers from the external and recurrent laryngeal branches of the vagus. Sensory fibers in the plexus are derived from CN IX. They supply most of the mucosa of all three parts of the pharynx. The sensory nerve supply of the mucous membrane of the anterior and superior nasopharynx is mainly from the maxillary nerve (CN V₂). The **tonsillar nerves** are derived from the *tonsillar plexus of nerves* formed by branches of CN IX and CN X and the pharyngeal plexus of nerves.

ESOPHAGUS

The **esophagus,** a muscular tube, extends from the laryngopharynx at the **pharyngoesophageal junction** to the stomach at the cardial orifice. The esophagus consists of striated (voluntary) muscle in its upper third, smooth (involuntary) muscle in its lower third, and a mixture of striated and smooth muscle in between. Its first part, the *cervical esophagus,* begins at the inferior border of the cricoid cartilage (the level of the C6 vertebra) in the median plane. Externally, the pharyngoesophageal junction appears as a constriction produced by the **cricopharyngeal part of the inferior constrictor muscle** (the superior esophageal sphincter). The cervical esophagus lies between the trachea and the cervical vertebral bodies and is in contact with the cervical pleura at the root of the neck (Figs. 8.7*A* and 8.15*A*). The thoracic duct adheres to the left side of the esophagus and lies between the pleura and the esophagus.

The **arteries** of the cervical esophagus are branches of the *inferior thyroid arteries* (Fig. 8.14*B*). Each artery gives off ascending and descending branches that anastomose with each other and across the midline. The **veins** are tributaries of the *inferior thyroid veins.* **Lymphatic vessels** of the cervical esophagus drain into the *paratracheal lymph nodes* and *inferior deep cervical lymph nodes* (Fig. 8.10).

The **nerve supply** of the esophagus is somatic, motor, and sensory to the superior half and parasympathetic (vagal), sympathetic, and visceral sensory to the inferior half.

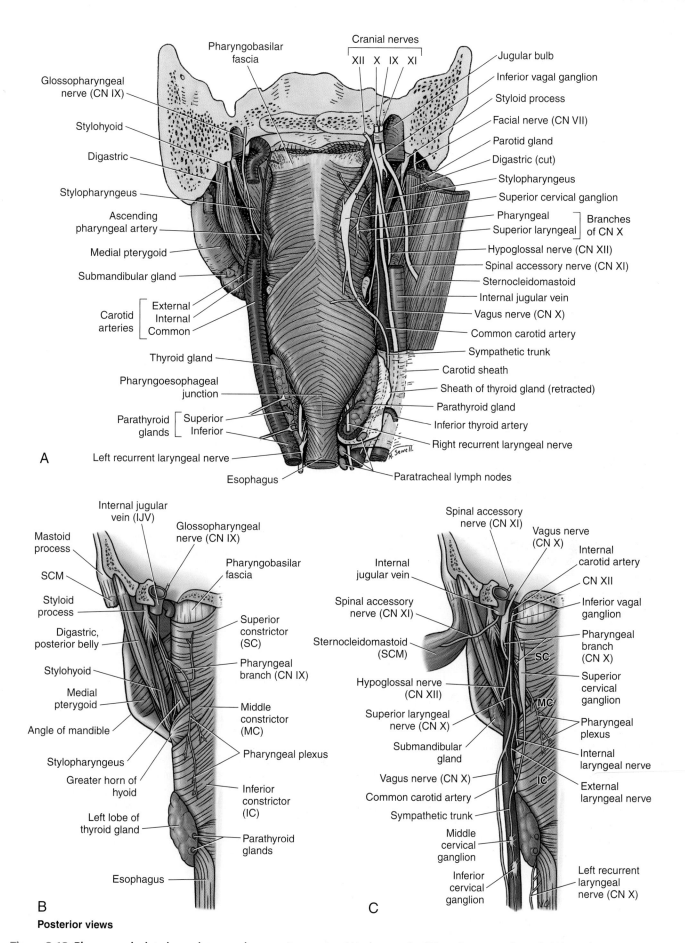

Figure 8.18. Pharynx and related vasculature and nerves. An overview (**A**), the muscles (**B**), and nerves and vessels (**C**) are shown. *SCM,* sternocleidomastoid.

Table 8.6 Muscles of the Pharynx

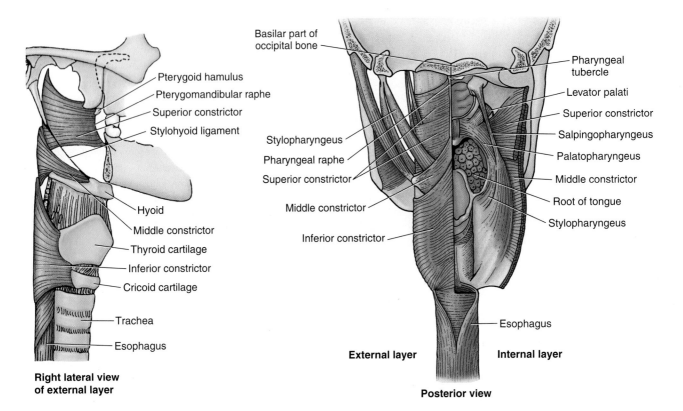

Right lateral view of external layer

Posterior view

Muscle	Origin	Insertion	Innervation	Main Action(s)
External layer				
Superior constrictor	Pterygoid hamulus, pterygo-mandibular raphe; posterior end of mylohyoid line of mandible and side of tongue	Pharyngeal tubercle on basilar part of occipital bone	Pharyngeal branch of vagus (CN X) and pharyngeal plexus	Constrict walls of pharynx during swallowing
Middle constrictor	Stylohyoid ligament and greater and lesser horns of hyoid	(Median) pharyngeal raphe	Pharyngeal branch of vagus (CN X) and pharyngeal plexus, plus branches of external and recurrent laryngeal nerves of vagus	
Inferior constrictor	Oblique line of thyroid cartilage and side of cricoid cartilage	Cricopharyngeal part encircles pharyngo-esophageal junction without forming a raphe		
Internal layer				
Palatopharyngeus	Hard palate and palatine aponeurosis	Posterior border of lamina of thyroid cartilage and side of pharynx and esophagus	Pharyngeal branch of vagus (CN X) and pharyngeal plexus	Elevate (shorten and widen) pharynx and larynx during swallowing and speaking
Salpingopharyngeus	Cartilaginous part of pharyngotympanic tube	Blends with palatopharyngeus		
Stylopharyngeus	Styloid process of temporal bone	Posterior and superior borders of thyroid cartilage with palatopharyngeus	Glossopharyngeal nerve (CN IX)	

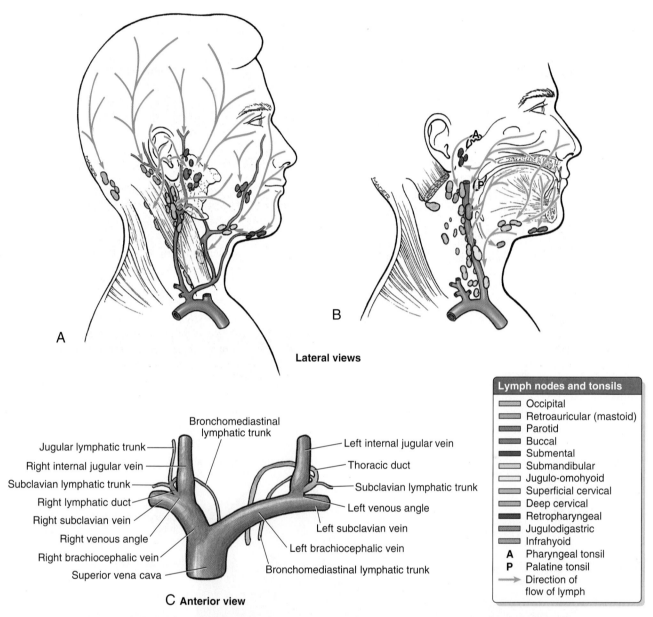

Lateral views

C Anterior view

Bronchomediastinal lymphatic trunk

Jugular lymphatic trunk

Right internal jugular vein

Subclavian lymphatic trunk

Right lymphatic duct

Right subclavian vein

Right venous angle

Right brachiocephalic vein

Superior vena cava

Left internal jugular vein

Thoracic duct

Subclavian lymphatic trunk

Left venous angle

Left subclavian vein

Left brachiocephalic vein

Bronchomediastinal lymphatic trunk

Lymph nodes and tonsils

Occipital
Retroauricular (mastoid)
Parotid
Buccal
Submental
Submandibular
Jugulo-omohyoid
Superficial cervical
Deep cervical
Retropharyngeal
Jugulodigastric
Infrahyoid
A Pharyngeal tonsil
P Palatine tonsil
→ Direction of flow of lymph

Figure 8.19. Lymphatic drainage of head and neck. The superficial (**A**) and deep (**B**) lymph nodes are identified. **C.** The termination of the thoracic and right lymphatic ducts at the venous angles is shown.

The cervical esophagus receives the somatic fibers via branches from the *recurrent laryngeal nerves* and vasomotor fibers from the *cervical sympathetic trunks* through the plexus around the inferior thyroid artery (Fig. 8.9A).

Lymphatics in Neck

Most superficial tissues of the neck are drained by lymphatic vessels that enter the *superficial cervical lymph nodes,* which are located along the course of the EJV (Fig. 8.19A). Lymph from these nodes drains into *inferior deep cervical lymph nodes* (Figs. 8.10 and 8.19B). The specific group of inferior deep cervical nodes involved here descends across the lateral cervical region with the spinal accessory nerve (CN XI). Most lymph from the six to eight nodes then drains into the *supraclavicular lymph nodes,* which accompany the transverse cervical artery. The main group of deep cervical nodes forms a chain along the IJV, mostly under cover of the SCM. Other deep cervical nodes

Tonsillectomy

Tonsillectomy (removal of the tonsils) is performed by dissecting the palatine tonsil from the tonsillar sinus (bed) or by a guillotine or snare operation. Each procedure involves removal of the tonsil and the fascial sheet covering the tonsillar sinus. Because of the rich blood supply of the tonsil, bleeding commonly arises from the large *external palatine vein* or less commonly from the tonsillar artery or other arterial twigs (Fig. 8.16C). The glossopharyngeal nerve accompanies the tonsillar artery on the lateral wall of the pharynx and is vulnerable to injury because this wall is thin. The internal carotid artery is especially vulnerable when it is tortuous as it lies directly lateral to the tonsil (Fig. B8.9).

Adenoiditis

Inflammation of the pharyngeal tonsils (adenoids) is called *adenoiditis*. This condition can obstruct the passage of air from the nasal cavities through the choanae into the nasopharynx, making mouth breathing necessary. Infection from the enlarged pharyngeal tonsils may also spread to the tubal tonsils, causing swelling and closure of the pharyngotympanic tubes. Impairment of hearing may result from nasal obstruction and blockage of the pharyngotympanic tubes. Infection spreading from the nasopharynx to the middle ear causes *otitis media* (middle ear infection), which may produce temporary or permanent hearing loss.

Foreign Bodies in the Laryngopharynx

Foreign bodies entering the pharynx may become lodged in the piriform fossae. If the object (e.g., a chicken bone) is sharp, it may pierce the mucous membrane and injure the internal laryngeal nerve. The superior laryngeal nerve and its internal laryngeal branch are also vulnerable to injury if the instrument used to remove the foreign body accidentally pierces the mucous membrane. Injury to these nerves may result in anesthesia of the laryngeal mucous membrane as far inferiorly as the vocal folds. Young children swallow various objects, most of which reach the stomach and subsequently pass through the alimentary tract without difficulty. In some cases, the foreign body stops at the inferior end of the laryngopharynx, its narrowest part. A medical image such as a radiograph or a CT scan, will reveal the presence of a radiopaque foreign body. Foreign bodies in the pharynx are often removed under direct vision through a pharyngoscope.

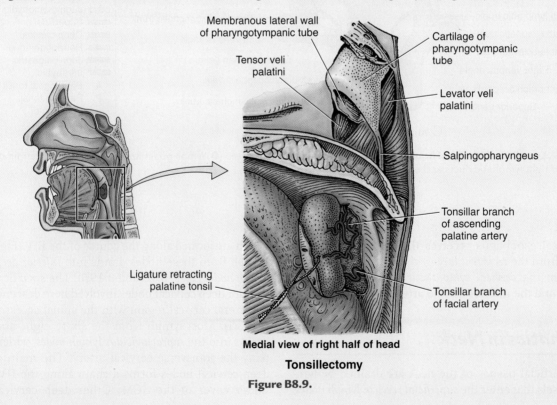

Membranous lateral wall of pharyngotympanic tube

Tensor veli palatini

Cartilage of pharyngotympanic tube

Levator veli palatini

Salpingopharyngeus

Tonsillar branch of ascending palatine artery

Ligature retracting palatine tonsil

Tonsillar branch of facial artery

Medial view of right half of head

Tonsillectomy

Figure B8.9.

Zones of Penetrating Trauma

Three zones are common clinical guides to the seriousness of neck trauma (Fig. B8.10). The zones give physicians an understanding of structures that are at risk with penetrating neck injuries.

- **Zone 1** includes the root of neck extending from the clavicles and manubrium to the inferior border of the cricoid cartilage. Structures at risk are the cervical pleurae, apices of lungs, thyroid and parathyroid glands, trachea, esophagus, common carotid arteries, jugular veins, and the cervical region of the vertebral column.
- **Zone II** extends from the cricoid cartilage to the angles of the mandible. Structures at risk are the superior poles of the thyroid gland, thyroid and cricoid cartilages, larynx, laryngopharynx, carotid arteries, jugular veins, esophagus, and cervical region of the vertebral column.
- **Zone III** occurs superiorly from the angles of the mandible. Structures at risk are the salivary glands, oral and nasal cavities, oropharynx, and nasopharynx.

Injuries in zones I and III obstruct the airway and have the greatest risk for **morbidity** (complications after surgical procedures and other treatments) and **mortality** (a fatal outcome) because injured structures are difficult to visualize and repair and vascular damage is difficult to control. Injuries in zone II are most common; however, morbidity and mortality are lower because physicians can control vascular damage by direct pressure and surgeons can visualize and treat injured structures more easily than they can in zones I and III.

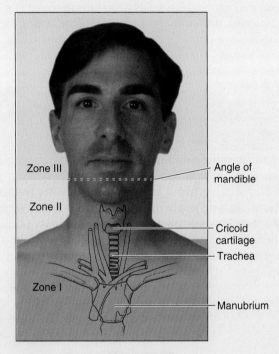

Figure B8.10.

---

include the prelaryngeal, pretracheal, paratracheal, and retropharyngeal nodes (Fig. 8.10). Efferent lymphatic vessels from the deep cervical nodes join to form the **jugular lymphatic trunks,** which usually join the thoracic duct on the left side. On the right side, the vessels enter the junction of the internal jugular and subclavian veins (*right venous angle*) directly or via a short right lymphatic duct.

The *thoracic duct* passes through the superior thoracic aperture along the left border of the esophagus. It arches laterally in the root of the neck, posterior to the carotid sheath and anterior to the sympathetic trunk and vertebral and subclavian arteries (Fig. 8.7*A*). The thoracic duct enters the left brachiocephalic vein at the junction of the subclavian and IJVs (*left venous angle*) (Fig. 8.19*C*). The thoracic duct drains lymph from the entire body, except the right side of the head and neck, the right upper limb, and the right side of the thorax, which drain through the *right lymphatic duct*. The right jugular, subclavian, and bronchomediastinal lymphatic trunks unite to form this duct, which enters the right venous angle. Often, however, these lymphatic trunks enter the venous system independently in the region of the right venous angle.

Radical Neck Dissections

Radical neck dissections are performed when cancer invades the lymphatics. During the procedure, the deep cervical lymph nodes and the tissues around them are removed as completely as possible. Although major arteries, the brachial plexus, CN X, and the phrenic nerve are preserved, most cutaneous branches of the cervical plexus are removed. The aim of the dissection is to remove all tissue that contains lymph nodes in one piece. The deep cervical lymph nodes, particularly those located along the transverse cervical artery, may be involved in the spread of cancer from the thorax and abdomen. Because their enlargement may give the first clue to cancer in these regions, they are often referred to as the *cervical sentinel lymph nodes*.

Medical Imaging of Neck

Radiographic examinations of the cervical vertebral column include anteroposterior (AP), lateral, and oblique projections. Lateral projections are common for evaluating severe neck injuries (Fig. 8.20). When a fracture is suspected, the lateral projection is examined before the person is moved for other projections. Observe the anterior and posterior margins of the vertebral bodies. Any deviation from the smooth curvature of these margins suggests a fracture and tearing of the associated ligaments. Observe that the intervertebral (IV) disc spaces are wider anteriorly than posteriorly. This difference exists because the IV discs are wedge

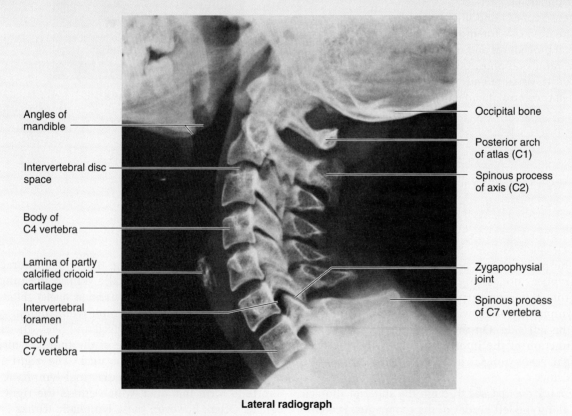

Angles of mandible

Intervertebral disc space

Body of C4 vertebra

Lamina of partly calcified cricoid cartilage

Intervertebral foramen

Body of C7 vertebra

Occipital bone

Posterior arch of atlas (C1)

Spinous process of axis (C2)

Zygapophysial joint

Spinous process of C7 vertebra

Lateral radiograph

Figure 8.20. Cervical region of vertebral column.

shaped. As the discs degenerate, the vertical height of the disc spaces decreases.

Transverse CT scans through the thyroid gland provide images of sections of the neck (Fig. 8.21A). They are oriented to show how a horizontal section of the person's neck appears to the physician standing at the foot of the bed. The superior edge of the CT image represents the anterior surface of the neck, and the right lateral edge of the image represents the left lateral surface. CT scans are used mainly as a diagnostic adjunct

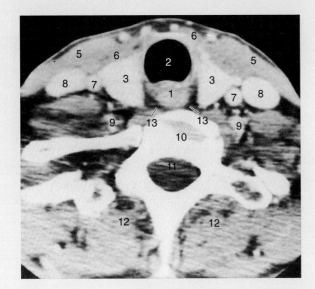

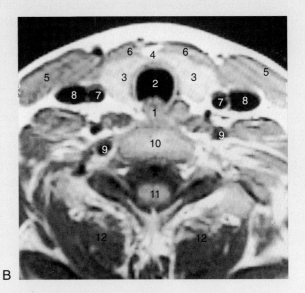

B

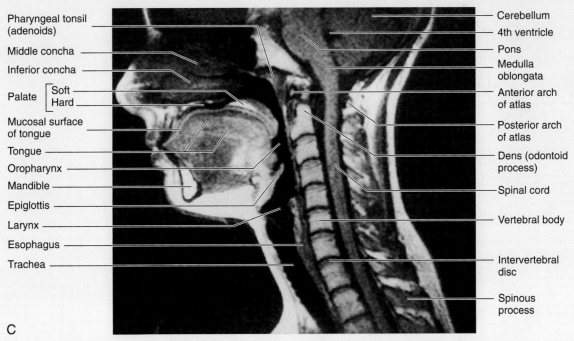

C

Figure 8.21. Scans of neck through thyroid gland. These transverse studies via CT (**A**) and MRI (**B**) reveal the structures of the neck. *1,* esophagus; *2,* trachea; *3,* lobes of thyroid gland; *4,* thyroid isthmus; *5,* SCM; *6,* sternohyoid; *7,* common carotid artery; *8,* IJV; *9,* vertebral artery; *10,* vertebral body; *11,* spinal cord in cerebrospinal fluid; *12,* deep muscles of the back; *13,* retropharyngeal space. (Courtesy of Dr. M. Keller, Assistant Professor of Medical Imaging, University of Toronto, Toronto, Ontario, Canada.) **C.** This median MRI study of the head and neck demonstrates that the air and food passages share the oropharynx. (Courtesy of Dr. W. Kucharczyk, Chair of Medical Imaging and Clinical Director, Tri-Hospital Resonance Centre, Toronto, Ontario, Canada.)

to conventional radiography. CT scans are superior to radiographs because they reveal radiodensity differences among and within soft tissues (e.g., in the thyroid gland).

MRI systems construct images of transverse, sagittal, and coronal sections of the neck and have the advantage of using no radiation (Fig. 8.21*B* & *C*). MRI studies of the neck are superior to CT studies for showing detail in soft tissues, but they provide little information about bones.

Ultrasonography is also a useful diagnostic imaging technique for studying soft tissues of the neck. Ultrasound provides images of many abnormal conditions non-invasively, at relatively low cost, and with minimal discomfort. Ultrasound is useful for distinguishing solid from cystic masses, for example, which may be difficult to determine during physical examination. Vascular imaging of arteries and veins of the neck is possible using intravascular ultrasonography (Fig. 8.22). The im-

ages are produced by placing the transducer within the blood vessel. Doppler ultrasound techniques help evaluate blood flow through a vessel (e.g., for detecting stenosis [narrowing] of a carotid artery). ●

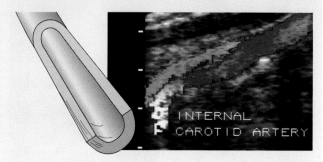

Figure 8.22. **Normal Doppler color flow study of internal carotid artery.**

Review of Cranial Nerves

The regional aspects of the cranial nerves are described in the preceding chapters, especially those for the head, neck, and thorax. This chapter summarizes the cranial nerves and the autonomic nervous system, using mainly figures and tables. Cranial nerve injuries, indicating the type or site of lesion and the abnormal findings, are also summarized.

Overview of Cranial Nerves

Cranial nerves, like spinal nerves, contain sensory or motor fibers or a combination of these fibers (Fig. 9.1). Cranial nerves innervate muscles or glands or carry impulses from sensory receptors. They are called cranial nerves because they emerge from foramina or fissures in the cranium and are covered by tubular sheaths derived from the cranial meninges. There are 12 pairs of cranial nerves, which are numbered I–XII, from rostral to caudal, according to their attachments to the brain (Fig. 9.2; Table 9.1). Their names reflect their general distribution or function.

Cranial nerves carry one or more of the following five main functional components (Fig. 9.1):

- Motor (efferent) fibers.
  1. *Motor fibers innervating voluntary (striated) muscle:*
     a. *Somatic motor* (general somatic efferent) axons innervate the striated muscles in the orbit, tongue, and external muscles of the neck (sternocleidomastoid and trapezius).
     b. *Branchial motor* (special visceral efferent) axons innervate striated muscle derived from the pharyngeal arches (face, palate, pharynx, and larynx).
  2. *Motor fibers involved in innervating involuntary (smooth) muscles or glands.* These include *visceral motor* (general visceral efferent) axons that constitute the cranial outflow of the parasympathetic division of the autonomic nervous system. The presynaptic (preganglionic) fibers that emerge from the brain synapse outside the central nervous system in a parasympathetic ganglion. The postsynaptic (postganglionic) fibers continue to innervate smooth muscles and glands.
- Sensory (afferent) fibers.
  3. *Fibers conveying sensation from the viscera.* These include visceral sensory (general visceral afferent) conveying information from the carotid body and sinus, pharynx, larynx, trachea, bronchi, lungs, heart, and gastrointestinal tract.
  4. *Fibers transmitting general sensation (e.g., touch, pressure, heat, cold, etc.) from the skin and mucous membranes.* These include *general sensory* (general somatic afferent) fibers mainly carried by CN V but also by CN VII, CN IX, and CN X.
  5. *Fibers transmitting unique sensations.* These include *special sensory* fibers conveying taste and smell (special visceral afferent fibers) and those serving the special senses of vision, hearing, and balance (special somatic afferent fibers).

The fibers of cranial nerves connect centrally to **cranial nerve nuclei,** groups of neurons in which sensory or afferent fibers terminate and from which motor or efferent fibers originate (Fig. 9.3). Except for CN 1 and CN II, which are extensions of the forebrain, the nuclei of the cranial nerves are located in the brainstem. Nuclei of similar functional components are generally aligned into functional columns in the brainstem.

Olfactory Nerve (CN I)

The **olfactory nerves** (CN I) convey the sense of smell. The cell bodies of the **olfactory receptor neurons** are located in the **olfactory organ** (the olfactory part of the nasal mucosa or olfactory area), in the roof of the nasal cavity, and along the nasal septum and medial wall of the superior nasal concha (Fig. 9.4). The central processes of the bipolar olfactory neurons are collected into bundles to form approximately 20 **olfactory nerves** on each side that collectively form the right or left olfactory nerve. The fibers pass through tiny foramina in the **cribriform plate** of the ethmoid bone, surrounded by sleeves of dura and arachnoid, and enter the **olfactory bulb** in the anterior cranial fossa (Fig. 9.4*B*). The olfactory nerve fibers synapse with **mitral cells** in the olfactory bulb. The axons of these cells form the **olfactory tract,** which conveys the impulses to the brain. The olfactory bulbs and tracts are technically anterior extensions of the forebrain.

Anosmia—Loss of Smell

Loss of olfactory fibers usually occurs with aging. The chief complaint of most people with anosmia is the loss or alteration of taste; however, clinical studies reveal that in all but a few people, the dysfunction is in the olfactory system (Sweazey, 2002). Transitory olfactory impairment occurs as a result of viral or allergic rhinitis, inflammation of the nasal mucous membrane.

Injury to the nasal mucosa, olfactory nerve fibers, olfactory bulbs or olfactory tracts may also impair smell. In severe head injuries, the olfactory bulbs may be torn away from the olfactory nerves, or some olfactory nerve fibers may be torn as they pass through a *fractured cribriform plate.* If all the nerve bundles on one side are torn, a complete loss of smell occurs on that side; consequently, anosmia may be a clue to a fracture of the cranial base and cerebrospinal fluid rhinorrhea (leakage of the fluid through the nose).

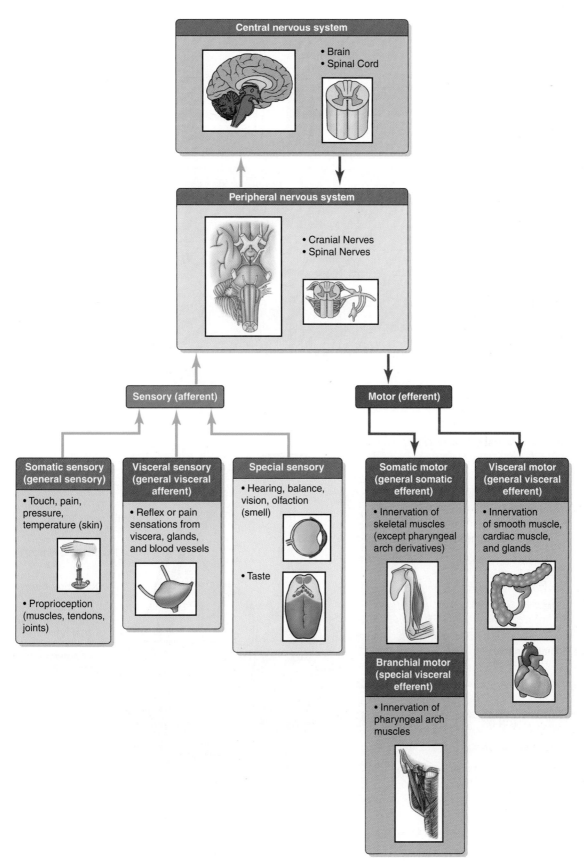

Figure 9.1. Overview of sensory and motor components of cranial and spinal nerves.

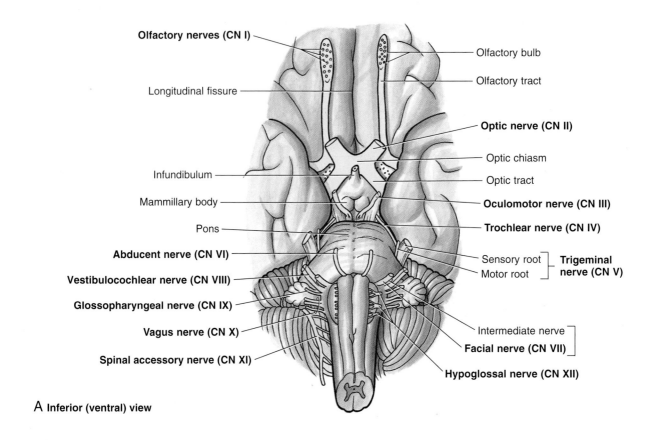

Olfactory nerves (CN I)

Olfactory bulb

Olfactory tract

Longitudinal fissure

Optic nerve (CN II)

Optic chiasm

Infundibulum

Optic tract

Mammillary body

Oculomotor nerve (CN III)

Pons

Trochlear nerve (CN IV)

Abducent nerve (CN VI)

Sensory root

Motor root

Trigeminal nerve (CN V)

Vestibulocochlear nerve (CN VIII)

Glossopharyngeal nerve (CN IX)

Vagus nerve (CN X)

Intermediate nerve

Facial nerve (CN VII)

Spinal accessory nerve (CN XI)

Hypoglossal nerve (CN XII)

A Inferior (ventral) view

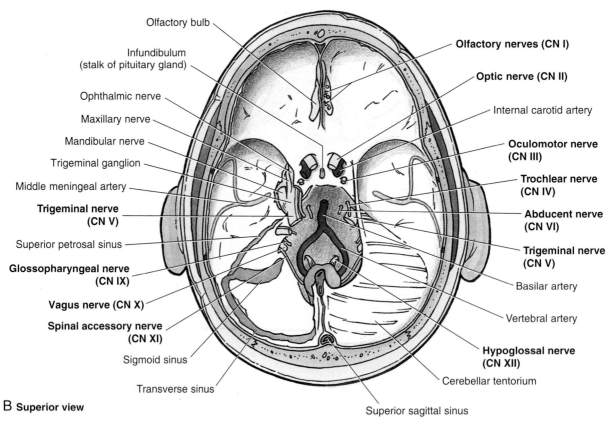

Olfactory bulb

Infundibulum (stalk of pituitary gland)

Olfactory nerves (CN I)

Optic nerve (CN II)

Ophthalmic nerve

Maxillary nerve

Internal carotid artery

Mandibular nerve

Oculomotor nerve (CN III)

Trigeminal ganglion

Trochlear nerve (CN IV)

Middle meningeal artery

Abducent nerve (CN VI)

Trigeminal nerve (CN V)

Trigeminal nerve (CN V)

Superior petrosal sinus

Glossopharyngeal nerve (CN IX)

Basilar artery

Vagus nerve (CN X)

Vertebral artery

Spinal accessory nerve (CN XI)

Hypoglossal nerve (CN XII)

Sigmoid sinus

Cerebellar tentorium

Transverse sinus

Superior sagittal sinus

B Superior view

Figure 9.2. Intracranial portions of cranial nerves. A. Superficial origins of the cranial nerves. **B.** Interior of the cranial base showing the proximal parts of the cranial nerves, dura mater, and blood vessels.

Table 9.1 Summary of Cranial Nerves

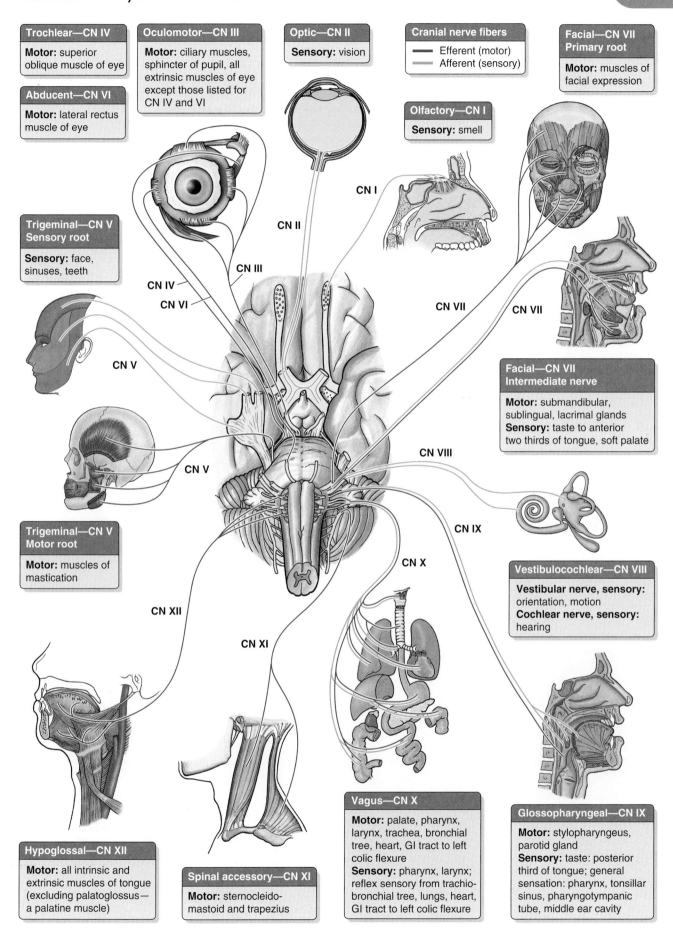

Trochlear—CN IV
Motor: superior oblique muscle of eye

Abducent—CN VI
Motor: lateral rectus muscle of eye

Oculomotor—CN III
Motor: ciliary muscles, sphincter of pupil, all extrinsic muscles of eye except those listed for CN IV and VI

Optic—CN II
Sensory: vision

Cranial nerve fibers
—— Efferent (motor)
—— Afferent (sensory)

Facial—CN VII Primary root
Motor: muscles of facial expression

Olfactory—CN I
Sensory: smell

Trigeminal—CN V Sensory root
Sensory: face, sinuses, teeth

Facial—CN VII Intermediate nerve
Motor: submandibular, sublingual, lacrimal glands
Sensory: taste to anterior two thirds of tongue, soft palate

Trigeminal—CN V Motor root
Motor: muscles of mastication

Vestibulocochlear—CN VIII
Vestibular nerve, sensory: orientation, motion
Cochlear nerve, sensory: hearing

Hypoglossal—CN XII
Motor: all intrinsic and extrinsic muscles of tongue (excluding palatoglossus—a palatine muscle)

Spinal accessory—CN XI
Motor: sternocleido-mastoid and trapezius

Vagus—CN X
Motor: palate, pharynx, larynx, trachea, bronchial tree, heart, GI tract to left colic flexure
Sensory: pharynx, larynx; reflex sensory from trachio-bronchial tree, lungs, heart, GI tract to left colic flexure

Glossopharyngeal—CN IX
Motor: stylopharyngeus, parotid gland
Sensory: taste: posterior third of tongue; general sensation: pharynx, tonsillar sinus, pharyngotympanic tube, middle ear cavity

(continued)

Table 9.1 Summary of Cranial Nerves (continued)

Nerve	Components	Location of Nerve Cell Bodies	Cranial Exit	Main Action(s)
Olfactory (CN I)	Special sensory	Olfactory epithelium (olfactory cells)	Foramina in cribriform plate of ethmoid bone	Smell from nasal mucosa of roof of each nasal cavity and superior sides of nasal septum and superior concha
Optic (CN II)	Special sensory	Retina (ganglion cells)	Optic canal	Vision from retina
Oculomotor (CN III)	Somatic motor	Midbrain	Superior orbital fissure	Motor to superior rectus, inferior rectus, medial rectus, inferior oblique, and levator palpebrae superioris muscles; raises superior eyelid; turns eyeball superiorly, inferiorly, and medially
	Visceral motor	Presynaptic: midbrain Postsynaptic: ciliary ganglion		Parasympathetic innervation to sphincter of pupil and ciliary muscle; constricts pupil and accommodates lens of eye
Trochlear (CN IV)	Somatic motor	Midbrain		Motor to superior oblique to assist in turning eye inferolaterally (or inferiorly when adducted)
Trigeminal (CN V)				
Ophthalmic (CN V_1)	General sensory	Trigeminal ganglion	Superior orbital fissure	Sensation from cornea, skin of forehead, scalp, eyelids, nose, and mucosa of nasal cavity and paranasal sinuses
Maxillary (CN V_2)	General sensory	Trigeminal ganglion	Foramen rotundum	Sensation from skin of face over maxilla, including upper lip, maxillary teeth, mucosa of nose, maxillary sinuses, and palate
Mandibular (CN V_3)	General sensory	Trigeminal ganglion	Foramen ovale	Sensation from skin over mandible, including lower lip, side of head, mandibular teeth, temporomandibular joint, mucosa of mouth, and anterior two thirds of tongue
	Branchial motor	Pons		Motor to muscles of mastication, mylohyoid, anterior belly of digastric, tensor veli palatini, and tensor tympani
Abducent (CN VI)	Somatic motor	Pons	Superior orbital fissure	Motor to lateral rectus to turn eye laterally
Facial (CN VII)	Branchial motor	Pons	Internal acoustic meatus; facial canal; stylomastoid foramen	Motor to muscles of facial expression and scalp; also supplies stapedius of middle ear, stylohyoid, and posterior belly of digastric
	Special sensory	Geniculate ganglion		Taste from anterior two thirds of tongue and palate
	Visceral motor	Presynaptic: pons Postsynaptic: pterygopalatine ganglion; submandibular ganglion		Parasympathetic innervation to submandibular and sublingual salivary glands, lacrimal gland, and glands of nose and palate
Vestibulocochlear (CN VIII)				
Vestibular	Special sensory	Vestibular ganglion	Internal acoustic meatus	Vestibular sensation from semicircular ducts, utricle, and saccule related to position and movement of head
Cochlear	Special sensory	Spiral ganglion		Hearing from spiral organ
Glossopharyngeal (CN IX)	Branchial motor	Medulla	Jugular foramen	Motor to stylopharyngeus to assist with swallowing
	Visceral motor	Presynaptic: medulla Postsynaptic: otic ganglion		Parasympathetic innervation to parotid gland
	Visceral sensory	Superior ganglion		Visceral sensation from parotid gland, carotid body and sinus, pharynx, and middle ear
	Special sensory	Inferior ganglion		Taste from posterior third of tongue
	General sensory	Inferior ganglion		Cutaneous sensation from external ear

Table 9.1 Summary of Cranial Nerves *(continued)*

Nerve	Components	Location of Nerve Cell Bodies	Cranial Exit	Main Action(s)
Vagus (CN X)	Branchial motor	Medulla	Jugular foramen	Motor to constrictor muscles of pharynx (except stylopharyngeus), intrinsic muscles of larynx, muscles of palate (except tensor veli palatini), and striated muscle in superior two thirds of esophagus
	Visceral motor	Presynaptic: medulla Postsynaptic: neurons in, on, or near viscera		Parasympathetic innervation to smooth muscle of trachea, bronchi, digestive tract, and cardiac muscle of heart
	Visceral sensory	Superior ganglion		Visceral sensation from base of tongue, pharynx, larynx, trachea, bronchi, heart, esophagus, stomach, and intestine
	Special sensory	Inferior ganglion		Taste from epiglottis and palate
	General sensory	Superior ganglion		Sensation from auricle, external acoustic meatus, and dura mater of posterior cranial fossa
Spinal accessory (CN XI)	Somatic motor	Spinal cord		Motor to sternocleidomastoid and trapezius
Hypoglossal (CN XII)	Somatic motor	Medulla	Hypoglossal canal	Motor to intrinsic and extrinsic muscles of tongue (except palatoglossus)

Optic Nerve (CN II)

The **optic nerve** (CN II) conveys visual information. The optic nerves are paired, anterior extensions of the forebrain (diencephalon) and are, therefore, CNS fiber tracts formed by axons of *retinal ganglion cells.* CN II is surrounded by extensions of the cranial meninges and subarachnoid space, which is filled with cerebrospinal fluid (CSF). CN II begins where the unmyelinated axons of the retinal ganglion cells pierce the sclera and become myelinated, deep to the **optic disc.** The nerve passes posteromedially in the orbit, exiting through the **optic canal** to enter the middle cranial fossa, where it forms the **optic chiasm** (L. *chiasma opticum*) (Fig. 9.5). Here, fibers from the nasal (medial) half of each retina decussate in the chiasm and join uncrossed fibers from the temporal (lateral) half of the retina to form the **optic tract.** The partial crossing of optic nerve fibers in the chiasm is a requirement for binocular vision, allowing depth-of-field perception (three-dimensional vision). Thus fibers from the right halves of both retinas form the right optic tract, and those from the left halves form the left optic tract. The decussation of nerve fibers in the chiasm results in the right optic tract conveying impulses from the left visual field and vice versa. The **visual field** is what is seen by a person with both eyes wide open and looking straight ahead. Most fibers in the optic tracts terminate in the **lateral geniculate bodies** of the thalamus. From these nuclei, axons are relayed to the visual cortices of the occipital lobes of the brain.

Oculomotor Nerve (CN III)

The **oculomotor nerve** (CN III) provides the following (Fig. 9.6):

- Motor innervation to four of the six extraocular muscles (*superior, medial,* and *inferior rectus* and *inferior oblique*) and to the elevator of the superior eyelid (L. *levator palpebrae superioris*).
- Proprioceptive innervation to the above muscles.
- Parasympathetic innervation through the ciliary ganglion to the smooth muscle of the sphincter pupillae, which causes constriction of the pupil and ciliary body to produce accommodation (allowing the lens to become more rounded) for near vision.

CN III is the chief motor nerve to the ocular and extraocular muscles. It emerges from the midbrain, pierces the dura, and runs through the roof and lateral wall of the *cavernous sinus.* CN III leaves the cranial cavity and enters the orbit through the *superior orbital fissure.* Within this fissure, CN III divides into a **superior division,** which supplies the superior rectus and levator palpebrae superioris and an **inferior division,** which supplies the inferior and medial rectus and inferior oblique. The inferior division also carries presynaptic parasympathetic (visceral efferent) fibers to the **ciliary ganglion,** where they synapse (Table 9.3). Postsynaptic fibers from this ganglion pass to the eyeball in the *short ciliary nerves* to innervate the ciliary body and the sphincter pupillae.

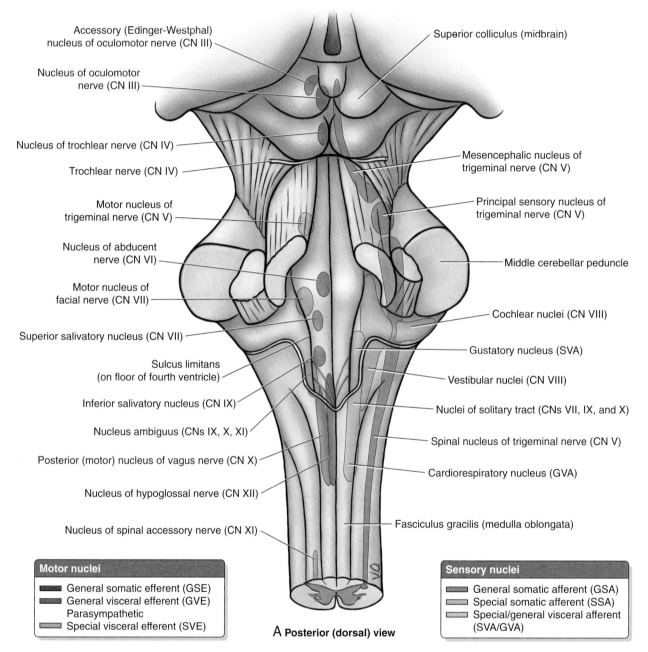

Accessory (Edinger-Westphal) nucleus of oculomotor nerve (CN III)

Nucleus of oculomotor nerve (CN III)

Nucleus of trochlear nerve (CN IV)

Trochlear nerve (CN IV)

Motor nucleus of trigeminal nerve (CN V)

Nucleus of abducent nerve (CN VI)

Motor nucleus of facial nerve (CN VII)

Superior salivatory nucleus (CN VII)

Sulcus limitans (on floor of fourth ventricle)

Inferior salivatory nucleus (CN IX)

Nucleus ambiguus (CNs IX, X, XI)

Posterior (motor) nucleus of vagus nerve (CN X)

Nucleus of hypoglossal nerve (CN XII)

Nucleus of spinal accessory nerve (CN XI)

Superior colliculus (midbrain)

Mesencephalic nucleus of trigeminal nerve (CN V)

Principal sensory nucleus of trigeminal nerve (CN V)

Middle cerebellar peduncle

Cochlear nuclei (CN VIII)

Gustatory nucleus (SVA)

Vestibular nuclei (CN VIII)

Nuclei of solitary tract (CNs VII, IX, and X)

Spinal nucleus of trigeminal nerve (CN V)

Cardiorespiratory nucleus (GVA)

Fasciculus gracilis (medulla oblongata)

Motor nuclei
- General somatic efferent (GSE)
- General visceral efferent (GVE) Parasympathetic
- Special visceral efferent (SVE)

Sensory nuclei
- General somatic afferent (GSA)
- Special somatic afferent (SSA)
- Special/general visceral afferent (SVA/GVA)

A **Posterior (dorsal) view**

Figure 9.3. Cranial nerve nuclei. The fibers of the cranial nerves are connected to nuclei (groups of nerve cell bodies in the CNS), in which afferent (sensory) fibers terminate and from which efferent (motor) fibers originate. The motor nuclei are shown on the left side of the brainstem and the sensory nuclei on the right side. The sensory and motor nuclei are all paired—that is, located in both the right and left sides of the brainstem.

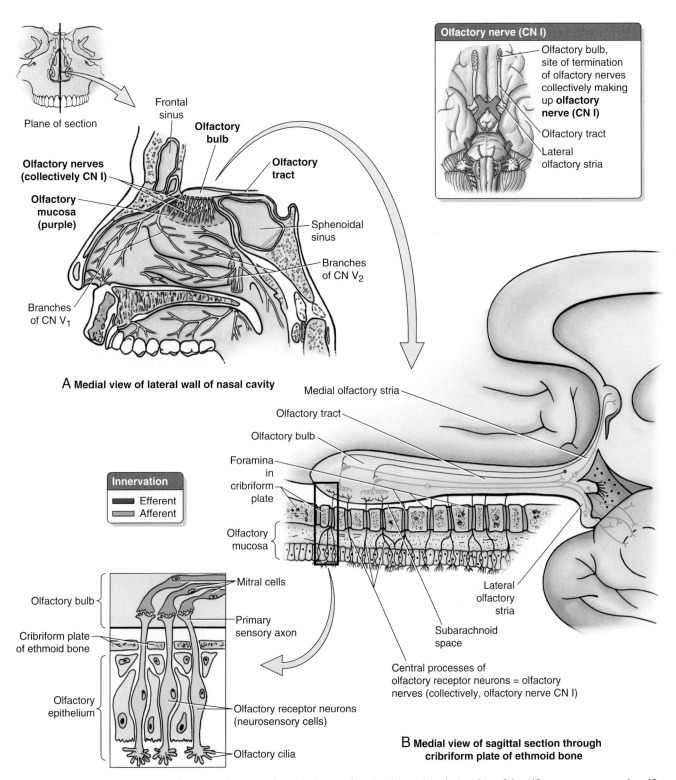

Plane of section

Frontal sinus

Olfactory bulb

Olfactory tract

Olfactory nerves (collectively CN I)

Olfactory mucosa (purple)

Branches of CN V₁

Sphenoidal sinus

Branches of CN V₂

A Medial view of lateral wall of nasal cavity

Olfactory nerve (CN I)

Olfactory bulb, site of termination of olfactory nerves collectively making up **olfactory nerve (CN I)**

Olfactory tract

Lateral olfactory stria

Medial olfactory stria

Olfactory tract

Olfactory bulb

Foramina in cribriform plate

Olfactory mucosa

Innervation

Efferent

Afferent

Lateral olfactory stria

Subarachnoid space

Central processes of olfactory receptor neurons = olfactory nerves (collectively, olfactory nerve CN I)

Olfactory bulb

Mitral cells

Cribriform plate of ethmoid bone

Primary sensory axon

Olfactory epithelium

Olfactory receptor neurons (neurosensory cells)

Olfactory cilia

B Medial view of sagittal section through cribriform plate of ethmoid bone

Figure 9.4. Olfactory system. A. This sagittal section through the nasal cavity shows the relationship of the olfactory mucosa to the olfactory bulb. **B.** The bodies of the olfactory receptor neurons are in the olfactory epithelium. These bundles of axons are collectively called the olfactory nerve (CN I).

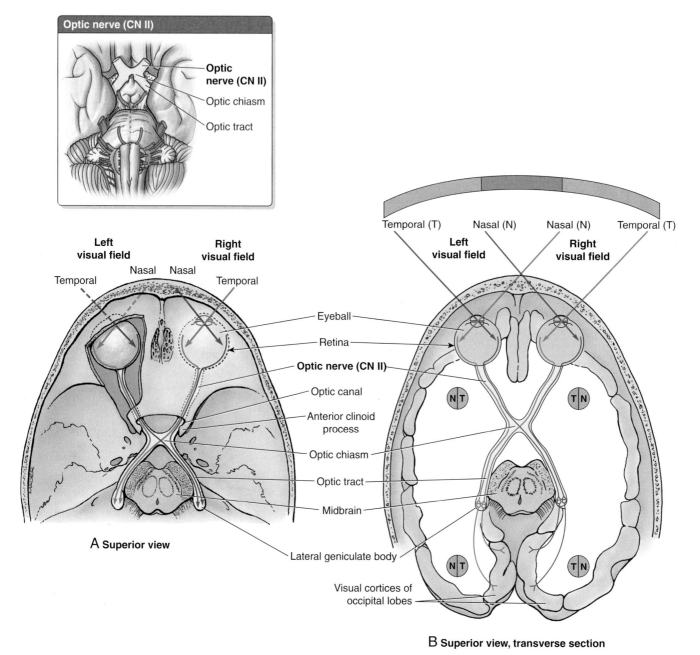

Optic nerve (CN II)

Optic
nerve (CN II)
Optic chiasm
Optic tract

**Left
visual field**

**Right
visual field**

Temporal
Nasal
Nasal
Temporal

Eyeball
Retina
Optic nerve (CN II)
Optic canal
Anterior clinoid
process
Optic chiasm
Optic tract
Midbrain
Lateral geniculate body

A **Superior view**

Temporal (T)
Nasal (N)
Nasal (N)
Temporal (T)

**Left
visual field**

**Right
visual field**

Visual cortices of
occipital lobes

B **Superior view, transverse section**

Figure 9.5. Visual system. The origin and course of the visual pathway are shown.

Demyelinating Diseases and the Optic Nerve

Because the optic nerves are actually CNS tracts, the myelin sheath that surrounds the fibers from the point at which they penetrate the sclera is formed by oligodendro-cytes (glial cells) rather than by neurolemma (Schwann cells). Consequently, the optic nerves are susceptible to the effects of demyelinating diseases of the CNS, such as multiple sclerosis (MS).

Visual Field Defects

Visual field defects result from lesions that affect different parts of the visual pathway (Fig. B9.1).

The type of defect depends on where the pathway is interrupted:

- *Complete section of right optic nerve* results in blindness (*black,* in Fig. B9.1) in the temporal (*T*) and nasal (*N*) visual fields of the right eye.
- *Complete section of optic chiasm* reduces peripheral vision, resulting in *bitemporal hemianopsia,* the loss of vision of one half of the visual field of both eyes.
- *Complete section of right optic tract* eliminates vision from the left temporal and right nasal visual fields. A lesion of the right or left optic tract causes a contralateral *homonymous hemianopsia,* indicating that the visual loss is in similar fields. This defect is the most common form of visual field loss and is often observed in patients with strokes.

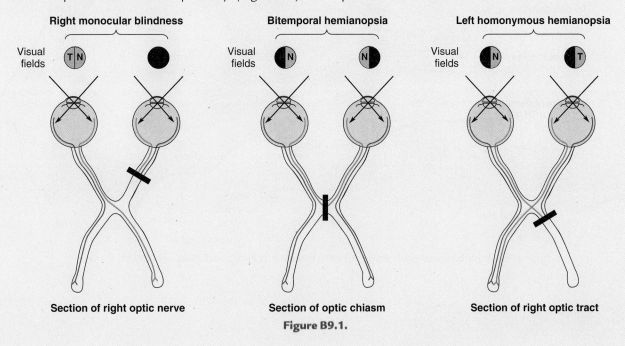

Right monocular blindness — Section of right optic nerve

Bitemporal hemianopsia — Section of optic chiasm

Left homonymous hemianopsia — Section of right optic tract

Figure B9.1.

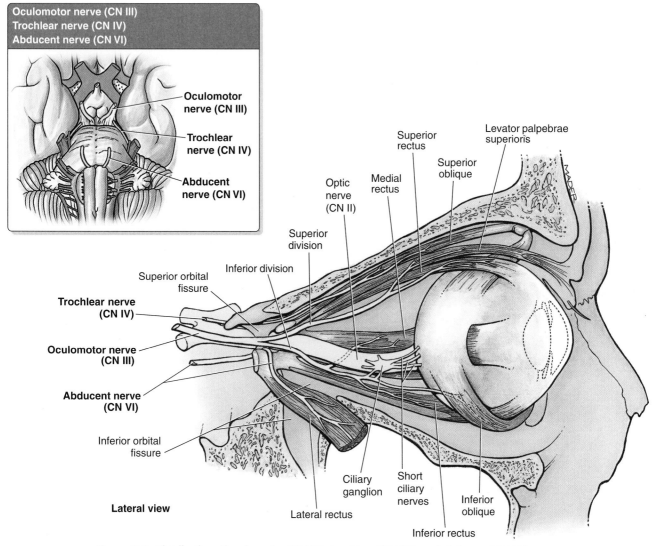

Figure 9.6. Distribution of oculomotor (CN III), trochlear (CN IV), and abducent (CN VI) nerves.

Oculomotor Palsy

Characteristic signs of a complete lesion of CN III are (Fig. B9.2)

- Ptosis (drooping) of the superior eyelid, caused by paralysis of the levator palpebrae superioris.
- Eyeball (pupil) abducted and directed slightly inferiorly (down and out) because of unopposed actions of the lateral rectus and superior oblique.
- No pupillary (light) reflex (constriction of the pupil in response to bright light) in the affected eye.

- Dilation of pupil, resulting from the interruption of parasympathetic fibers to the sphincter of the pupillae, leaving the dilator pupillae unopposed.
- No accommodation of the lens (adjustment to increase convexity for near vision) because of paralysis of the ciliary muscle.

An aneurysm of a posterior cerebral or superior cerebellar artery may exert pressure on CN III as it passes between these vessels. Because CN III lies in the lateral wall of the cavernous sinus, injuries, infections, or tumors may also affect this nerve. The effects depend on severity.

Compression of Oculomotor Nerve

Rapidly increasing intracranial pressure (e.g., resulting from an extradural hematoma) often compresses CN III against the petrous part of the temporal bone. Because autonomic fibers in CN III are superficial, they are affected first. As a result, the pupil dilates progressively on the injured side and there is ipsilateral slowness of the pupillary response to light.

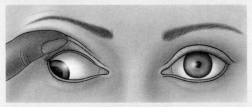

Figure B9.2.

Trochlear Nerve (CN IV)

The **trochlear nerve** (CN IV) provides motor and proprioceptive innervation to one extraocular muscle (**superior oblique**). The trochlear nerve is the smallest cranial nerve; it emerges from the posterior surface of the midbrain and passes anteriorly around the brainstem (Fig. 9.2). CN IV pierces the dura mater at the margin of the cerebellar tentorium (L. *tentorium cerebelli*) and passes anteriorly in the lateral wall of the cavernous sinus. The nerve continues past the sinus to course through the superior orbital fissure into the orbit, where it supplies the superior oblique (Fig. 9.6).

Trigeminal Nerve (CN V)

The **trigeminal nerve** (CN V) emerges from the lateral aspect of the pons by a large sensory root and a small motor root (Fig. 9.2A). CN V is the principal general sensory nerve for the head (face, teeth, mouth, nasal cavity, and dura of the cranial cavity) (Fig. 9.7). The **sensory root of CN V** is composed mainly of the central processes of neurons in the **trigeminal ganglion** (Fig. 9.2B). The peripheral processes of the ganglionic neurons form three nerves or divisions: **ophthalmic nerve** (CN V_1), **maxillary nerve** (CN V_2), and sensory component of the **mandibular nerve** (CN V_3). For a summary of CN V, see Figure 9.7 and Table 9.2. The fibers of the **motor root of CN V** are distributed exclusively via the mandibular nerve (CN V_3) to the muscles of mastication, mylohyoid, anterior belly of the digastric, tensor veli palatini, and tensor tympani.

Injury to the Trochlear Nerve

CN IV is rarely paralyzed alone. The nerve may be torn in severe head injuries because of its long intracranial course. Damage to CN IV nerve or its nucleus impair the ability to turn the affected eyeball inferomedially. The characteristic sign of trochlear nerve injury is *diplopia* (double vision) when looking down (e.g., when going down stairs). Diplopia occurs because the superior oblique normally assists the inferior rectus in depressing the pupil (directing the gaze downward) and is the only muscle to do so when the pupil is adducted. In addition, because the superior oblique is the primary muscle producing intorsion of the eyeball, the primary muscle producing extorsion (the inferior oblique) is unopposed when the superior oblique is paralyzed. Thus the direction of gaze and rotation of the eyeball about its anteroposterior axis is different for the two eyes, especially when looking downward and medially. The person can compensate for the diplopia by inclining the head anteriorly and laterally to the side of the normal eye.

Injury to the Trigeminal Nerve

CN V may be injured by trauma, tumors, aneurysms, or meningeal infections. Injury to CN V causes

- Paralysis of the muscles of mastication with deviation of the mandible toward the side of the lesion.
- Loss of the ability to appreciate soft tactile, thermal, or painful sensations in the face.
- Loss of the corneal reflex (blinking in response to the cornea being touched) and the sneezing reflex.

Trigeminal neuralgia (tic douloureux), the principal disease affecting the sensory root of CN V, produces excruciating, episodic pain that is usually restricted in the areas supplied by the maxillary and/or mandibular divisions of CN V.

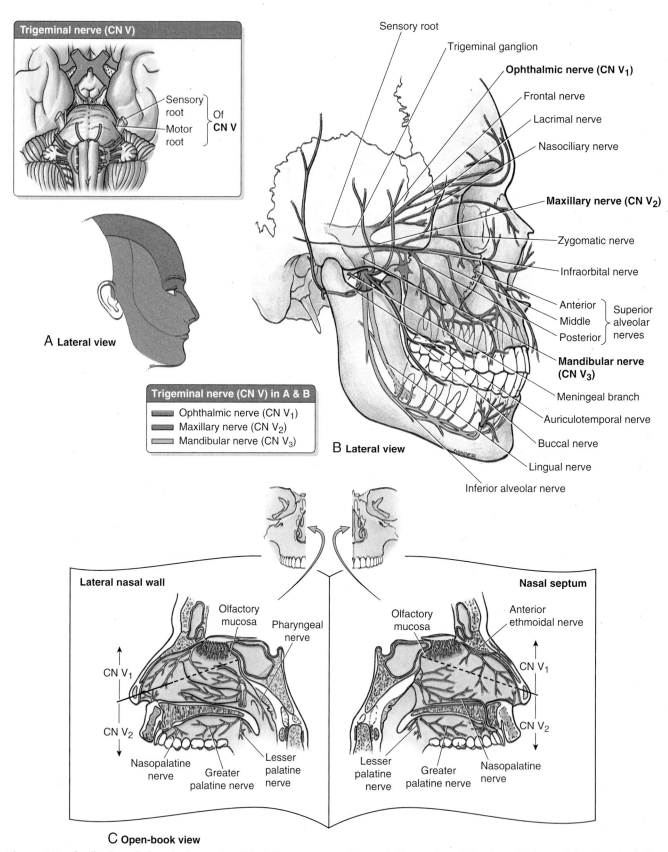

Figure 9.7. Distribution of trigeminal nerve (CN V). A. The cutaneous (sensory) distribution of the three divisions of the trigeminal nerve is shown. **B.** The branches of the ophthalmic, maxillary, and mandibular divisions are identified. **C.** This view shows CN V_1 and CN V_2 innervation of the lateral wall and septum of the nasal cavity and palate.

Table 9.2 Summary of the Divisions of the Trigeminal Nerve (CN V)

Divisions/Distributions	Branches
Ophthalmic nerve (CN V$_1$) Sensory only Passes through superior orbital fissure Supplies cornea, upper conjunctiva, mucosa of anterosuperior nasal cavity, frontal and ethmoidal sinuses, anterior and supratentorial dura mater, skin of dorsum of external nose, superior eyelid, forehead, and scalp	Tentorial nerve (a meningeal branch) Lacrimal nerve 　Communicating branch from zygomatic nerve Frontal nerve 　Supraorbital nerve 　Supratrochlear nerve Nasociliary nerve 　Sensory root of ciliary ganglion 　Short ciliary nerves 　Long ciliary nerves 　Infratrochlear nerves 　Anterior and posterior ethmoidal nerves
Maxillary nerve (CN V$_2$) Sensory only Passes through foramen rotundum Supplies dura mater of anterior part of middle cranial fossa; conjunctiva of inferior eyelid; mucosa of posteroinferior nasal cavity, maxillary sinus, palate and anterior part of superior oral vestibule; maxillary teeth; and skin of lateral external nose, linferior eyelid, anterior cheek, and upper lip	Meningeal branch Zygomatic nerve 　Zygomaticofacial branch 　Zygomaticotemporal branch 　Communicating branch to lacrimal nerve Ganglionic branches to (sensory root of) pterygopalatine ganglion Posterior superior alveolar branches 　Infraorbital nerve 　Anterior and middle superior alveolar branches 　Superior labial branches 　Inferior palpebral branches 　External nasal branches Greater palatine nerves 　Posterior inferior lateral nasal nerves Lesser palatine nerves Posterior superior lateral nasal branches Nasopalatine nerve Pharyngeal nerve
Mandibular nerve (CN V$_3$) Sensory and motor Passes through the foramen ovale Supplies sensory innervation to mucosa of anterior two thirds of tongue, floor of mouth, and posterior and anterior inferior oral vestibule; mandibular teeth; and skin of lower lip, buccal, parotid, and temporal regions of face; and external ear (auricle, upper external auditory meatus, and tympanic membrane)	General sensory branches 　Meningeal branch (nervus spinosum) 　Buccal nerve 　Auriculotemporal nerve Lingual nerve Inferior alveolar nerve 　Nerve to mylohyoid 　Inferior dental plexus 　Mental nerve Branchiomotor branches 　Masseter 　Temporal 　Medial and lateral pterygoids 　Mylohyoid 　Anterior belly of digastric 　Tensor tympani

Abducent Nerve (CN VI)

The **abducent nerve** (CN VI) provides motor and proprioceptive information to one extraocular muscle (**lateral rectus**). The abducent nerve emerges from the brainstem between the pons and the medulla and traverses the pontine cistern of the subarachnoid space, straddling the basilar artery (Fig. 9.2). It then pierces the dura and runs the longest intradural course within the cranial cavity of all the cranial nerves. During its intradural course, it bends sharply over the crest of the petrous part of the temporal bone and then courses through the cavernous sinus, surrounded by venous blood in the same manner as the internal carotid artery, which it parallels

Injury to the Abducent Nerve

Because CN VI has a long intracranial course, it is often stretched when intracranial pressure rises, partly because of the sharp bend it makes over the crest of the petrous part of the temporal bone after entering the dura. A space-occupying lesion such as a brain tumor may compress CN VI, causing paralysis of the lateral rectus muscle. Complete paralysis of CN VI causes medial deviation of the affected eye—that is, it is fully adducted owing to the unopposed action of the medial rectus, leaving the person unable to abduct the eye (Fig. B9.3). *Diplopia* is present in all ranges of movement of the eyeball, except on gazing to the side opposite the lesion.

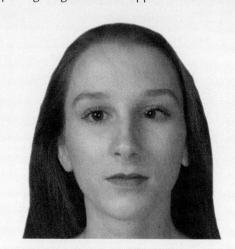

Abducent nerve injury
Figure B9.3.

in the sinus. CN VI then enters the orbit through the superior orbital fissure and runs anteriorly to supply the **lateral rectus**, which abducts the eye (Fig. 9.6).

Facial Nerve (CN VII)

The **facial nerve** (CN VII) emerges from the junction of the pons and medulla as two divisions: the motor root and the intermediate nerve (L. *nervus intermedius*) (Fig. 9.2*A*). The larger **motor root** (facial nerve proper) innervates the muscles of facial expression, and the smaller **intermediate nerve** carries taste, parasympathetic, and somatic sensory fibers (Fig. 9.8). During its course, CN VII traverses the posterior cranial fossa, internal acoustic meatus, facial canal, stylomastoid foramen of the temporal bone, and parotid gland. After traversing the internal acoustic meatus, the nerve proceeds a short distance anteriorly within the temporal bone and then turns abruptly posteriorly to course along the medial wall of the tympanic cavity. The sharp bend is the **geniculum of the facial nerve,** the site of the **geniculate ganglion** (sensory ganglion of CN VII). Within the facial canal, CN VII gives rise to the greater petrosal nerve, the nerve to the stapedius, and the chorda tympani nerve. After running the longest intraosseous course of any cranial nerve, CN VII emerges from the cranium via the *stylomastoid foramen;* gives off the posterior auricular branch; enters the parotid gland; and forms the **parotid plexus,** which gives rise to the following five terminal motor branches: temporal, zygomatic, buccal, marginal mandibular, and cervical.

Branchial Motor

As the nerve of the 2nd pharyngeal arch, the facial nerve supplies the striated muscle derived from its mesoderm, mainly the muscles of facial expression and auricular muscles. It also supplies the posterior bellies of the digastric, stylohyoid, and stapedius muscles.

Parasympathetic (Visceral Motor)

The parasympathetic distribution of the facial nerve is detailed in Figure 9.9. CN VII provides presynaptic parasympathetic fibers to the **pterygopalatine ganglion** for innervation of the lacrimal, nasal, pharyngeal, and palatine glands and to the **submandibular ganglion** for innervation of the sublingual and submandibular salivary glands. The main features of parasympathetic ganglia associated with the facial nerve and other cranial nerves are summarized in Table 9.3. Parasympathetic fibers synapse in these ganglia, whereas sympathetic and other fibers pass through them.

General Sensory

Some fibers from the **geniculate ganglion** supply a small area of skin close to the external acoustic meatus (Fig. 9.8).

Taste (Special Sensory)

Fibers carried by the chorda tympani join the **lingual nerve** to convey taste sensation from the anterior two thirds of the tongue and soft palate.

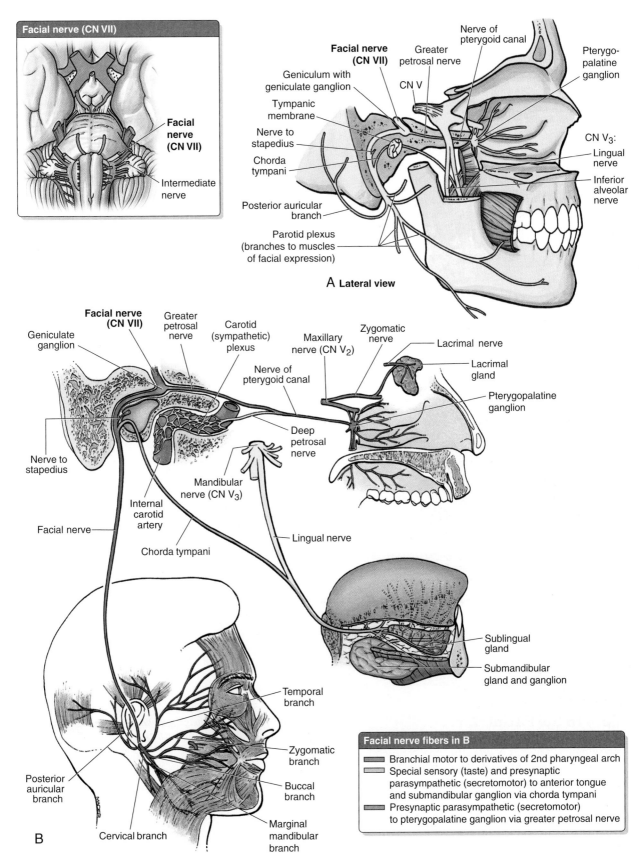

Figure 9.8. Distribution of facial nerve (CN VII). A. The facial nerve in situ demonstrates its intraosseous course and branches. **B.** The regional distribution of the facial nerve fibers is shown.

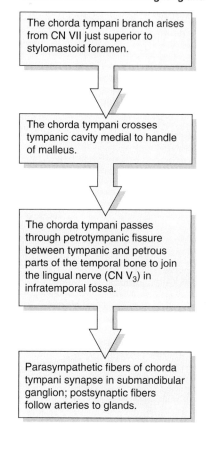

A. Parasympathetic (visceral motor) to lacrimal gland

> Greater petrosal nerve arises from CN VII at geniculate ganglion and emerges from superior surface of petrous part of temporal bone to enter middle cranial fossa.

> Greater petrosal nerve joins deep petrosal nerve (sympathetic) at foramen lacerum to form nerve of pterygoid canal.

> Nerve of pterygoid canal travels through pterygoid canal and enters pterygopalatine fossa.

> Parasympathetic fibers from nerve of pterygoid canal in pterygopalatine fossa synapse in pterygopalatine ganglion.

> Postsynaptic parasympathetic fibers from this ganglion innervate lacrimal gland via zygomatic branch of CN V₂ and lacrimal nerve (branch of CN V₁).

B. Parasympathetic (visceral motor) to submandibular and sublingual glands

> The chorda tympani branch arises from CN VII just superior to stylomastoid foramen.

> The chorda tympani crosses tympanic cavity medial to handle of malleus.

> The chorda tympani passes through petrotympanic fissure between tympanic and petrous parts of the temporal bone to join the lingual nerve (CN V₃) in infratemporal fossa.

> Parasympathetic fibers of chorda tympani synapse in submandibular ganglion; postsynaptic fibers follow arteries to glands.

Figure 9.9. Parasympathetic innervation involving facial nerve (CN VII).

Injury to the Facial Nerve

Among motor nerves, *CN VII* is the most frequently paralyzed of all the cranial nerves. Depending on the part of the nerve involved, injury to CN VII may cause paralysis of facial muscles without loss of taste on the anterior two thirds of the tongue or altered secretion of the lacrimal and salivary glands.

A *lesion of CN VII near its origin* or near the geniculate ganglion is accompanied by loss of motor, gustatory (taste), and autonomic functions. The motor paralysis of facial muscles involves upper and lower parts of the face on the ipsilateral (same) side.

A *central lesion of CN VII* (lesion of the CNS) results in paralysis of muscles of the inferior face on the contralateral side. However, forehead wrinkling is not visibly

Table 9.3 Summary of the Cranial Parasympathetic Ganglia

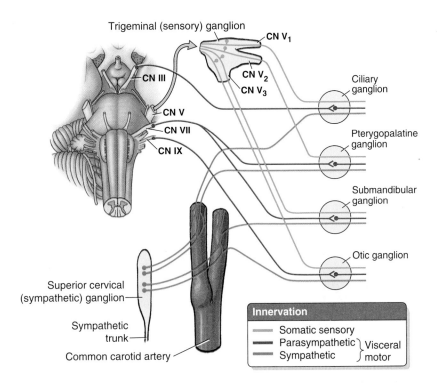

Ganglion	Location	Parasympathetic Root	Sympathetic Root	Main Distribution
Ciliary	Between optic nerve and lateral rectus, close to apex of orbit	Inferior branch of oculomotor nerve (CN III)	Branches from internal carotid plexus in cavernous sinus	Parasympathetic postsynaptic fibers from ciliary ganglion pass to ciliary muscle and sphincter pupillae of iris; sympathetic postganglionic fibers from superior cervical ganglion pass to dilator pupillae and blood vessels of eye
Pterygopalatine	In pterygopalatine fossa, where it is suspended by ganglionic branches of maxillary nerve (sensory roots of pterygopalatine ganglion); just anterior to opening of pterygoid canal and inferior to CN V_2	Greater petrosal nerve from facial nerve (CN VII) via nerve of pterygoid canal	Deep petrosal nerve, a branch of internal carotid plexus that is a continuation of postsynaptic fibers of cervical sympathetic trunk; fibers from superior cervical ganglion pass through pterygopalatine ganglion and enter branches of CN V_2	Parasympathetic postganglionic (secretomotor) fibers from pterygopalatine ganglion innervate lacrimal gland via zygomatic branch of CN V_2; sympathetic postsynaptic fibers from superior cervical ganglion accompany branches of pterygopalatine nerve that are distributed to blood vessels of nasal cavity, palate, and superior parts of pharynx
Otic	Between tensor veli palatini and mandibular nerve (CN V_3); lies inferior to foramen ovale of sphenoid bone	Tympanic nerve from glossopharyngeal nerve (CN IX); from tympanic plexus tympanic nerve continues as lesser petrosal nerve	Fibers from superior cervical ganglion come from plexus on middle meningeal artery	Parasympathetic postsynaptic fibers from otic ganglion are distributed to parotid gland via auriculotemporal nerve (branch of CN V_3); sympathetic postsynaptic fibers from superior cervical ganglion pass to parotid gland and supply its blood vessels
Submandibular	Suspended from lingual nerve by two ganglionic branches (sensory roots); lies on surface of hyoglossus muscle inferior to submandibular duct	Parasympathetic fibers join facial nerve (CN VII) and leave it in its chorda tympani branch, which unites with lingual nerve	Sympathetic fibers from superior cervical ganglion via plexus on facial artery	Parasympathetic postsynaptic (secretomotor) fibers from submandibular ganglion are distributed to sublingual and submandibular glands; sympathetic fibers supply sublingual and submandibular glands and appear to be secretomotor

impaired because it is innervated bilaterally. Lesions between the geniculate ganglion and the origin of the chorda tympani produce the same effects as that resulting from injury near the ganglion except that lacrimal secretion is not affected. Because it passes through the facial canal, CN VII is vulnerable to compression when a viral infection produces inflammation of the nerve (viral neuritis) and swelling of the nerve just before it emerges from the stylomastoid foramen.

Bell palsy is a unilateral facial paralysis of sudden onset resulting from a lesion of CN VII. This syndrome is illustrated and discussed in Chapter 7

Vestibulocochlear Nerve (CN VIII)

The **vestibulocochlear nerve** (CN VIII) is a special sensory (special somatic afferent) nerve of hearing and equilibrium. The vestibulocochlear nerve emerges from the junction of the pons and medulla and enters the *internal acoustic meatus* (Fig. 9.2*A*). Here, it separates into the vestibular and cochlear nerves (Fig. 9.10).

- The **vestibular nerve** is concerned with equilibrium. It is composed of the central processes of bipolar neurons in the **vestibular ganglion**; the peripheral processes of the neurons extend to the **maculae** of the utricle and saccule (sensitive to the linear acceleration relative to the position of the head) and to the **ampullae** of semicircular ducts (sensitive to rotational acceleration).
- The **cochlear nerve** is concerned with hearing. It is composed of the central processes of bipolar neurons in the **spiral ganglion**; the peripheral processes of the neurons extend to the spiral organ.

Injuries of the Vestibulocochlear Nerve

Although the vestibular and cochlear nerves are essentially independent, peripheral lesions often produce concurrent clinical effects because of their close relationship. Hence lesions of CN VIII may cause *tinnitus* (ringing or buzzing of the ears), *vertigo* (dizziness, loss of balance), and impairment or loss

of hearing. Central lesions may involve either the cochlear or vestibular divisions of CN VII.

Deafness

There are two kinds of deafness: conductive deafness, involving the external or middle ear (e.g., otitis media, inflammation in the middle ear) and sensorineural deafness, which results from disease in the cochlea or in the pathway from the cochlea to the brain.

Glossopharyngeal Nerve (CN IX)

The **glossopharyngeal nerve** (CN IX) emerges from the lateral aspect of the medulla and passes anterolaterally to leave the cranium through the *jugular foramen*. At this foramen are **superior** and **inferior ganglia**, which contain the cell bodies for the afferent (sensory) components of the nerve (Fig. 9.11). CN IX follows the stylopharyngeus, the only muscle the nerve supplies, and passes between the superior and the middle constrictor muscles of the pharynx to reach the oropharynx and tongue. It contributes sensory fibers to the *pharyngeal plexus* of nerves. The glossopharyngeal nerve is afferent from the tongue and pharynx (hence its name) and efferent to the stylopharyngeus and parotid gland.

Branchial Motor

Motor fibers pass to the one muscle, the stylopharyngeus, derived from the 3rd pharyngeal arch.

Parasympathetic (Visceral Motor)

Following a circuitous route initially involving the tympanic nerve, presynaptic parasympathetic fibers are provided to the otic ganglion for innervation of the parotid gland (Fig. 9.12; Table 9.3).

Visceral Sensory

The sensory branches of CN IX are as follows (Fig. 9.11):

- The *tympanic nerve.*
- The *carotid sinus nerve* to the carotid sinus, a baro–(presso) receptor sensitive to changes in blood pressure, and the carotid body, a chemoreceptor sensitive to blood gas (oxygen and carbon dioxide) levels.

The *pharyngeal, tonsillar,* and *lingual nerves* to the mucosa of the oropharynx and isthmus of the fauces (*L.* throat),

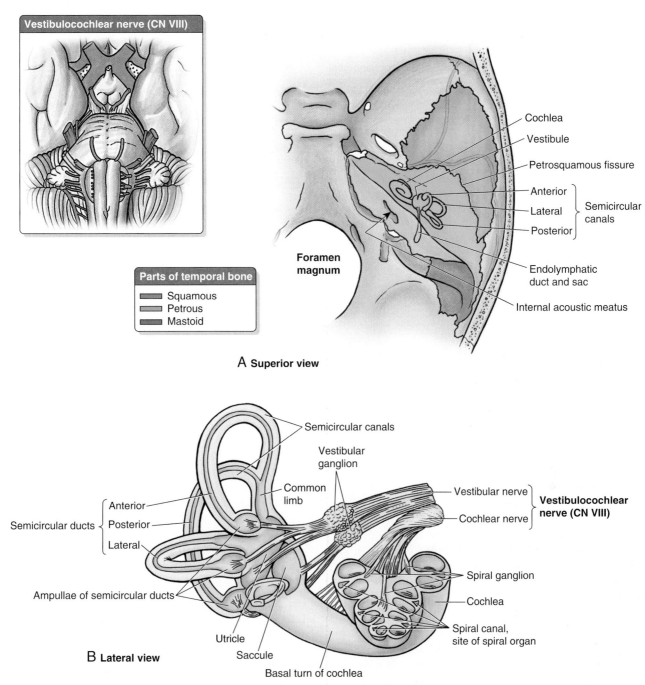

Figure 9.10. Distribution of vestibulocochlear nerve (CN VIII). A. The internal surface of the cranial base shows the location of the bony labyrinth of the internal ear within the temporal bone and the internal acoustic meatus for CN VIII. **B.** This view of the bony and membranous labyrinths shows innervation of the cochlea by the cochlear nerve of CN VIII and innervation of the vestibular apparatus by the vestibular nerve of CN VIII.

including the palatine tonsil, soft palate, and posterior third of the tongue. Stimuli determined to be unusual or unpleasant here may evoke the gag reflex or even vomiting.

Taste (Special Sensory)

Taste fibers are conveyed from the posterior third of the tongue to the sensory ganglia.

Vagus Nerve (CN X)

The **vagus nerve** (CN X) is

- Sensory from the inferior pharynx, larynx, and thoracic and abdominal organs.
- Sense of taste from the root of the tongue and the taste buds on the epiglottis.

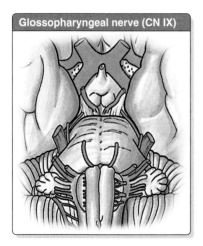

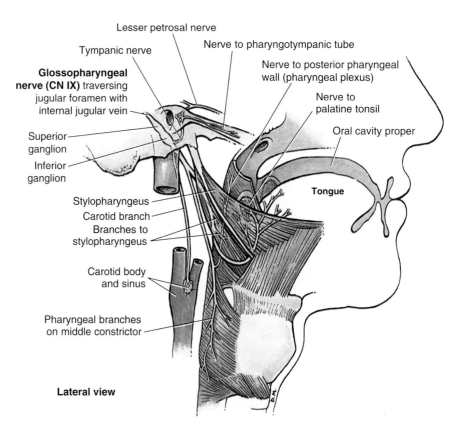

Glossopharyngeal nerve (CN IX)

Lesser petrosal nerve

Tympanic nerve

Nerve to pharyngotympanic tube

Glossopharyngeal nerve (CN IX) traversing jugular foramen with internal jugular vein

Nerve to posterior pharyngeal wall (pharyngeal plexus)

Nerve to palatine tonsil

Oral cavity proper

Superior ganglion

Inferior ganglion

Tongue

Stylopharyngeus

Carotid branch

Branches to stylopharyngeus

Carotid body and sinus

Pharyngeal branches on middle constrictor

Lateral view

Figure 9.11. Distribution of glossopharyngeal nerve (CN IX).

Lesions of the Glossopharyngeal Nerve

Isolated lesions of CN IX or its nuclei are uncommon and are not associated with perceptible disability. Taste is absent on the posterior third of the tongue, and the gag reflex is absent on the side of the lesion. Ipsilateral weakness may produce a noticeable change in swallowing. Injuries of CN IX resulting from infection or tumors are usually accompanied by signs of involvement of adjacent nerves. Because CN IX, CN X, and CN XI pass through the jugular foramen, tumors in this region produce multiple cranial nerve palsies—the *jugular foramen syndrome.*

- Motor to the soft palate, pharynx, intrinsic laryngeal muscles (phonation), and a nominal extrinsic tongue muscle, the palatoglossus, which is actually a palatine muscle based on its derivation and innervation.
- Proprioceptive to the above muscles.
- Parasympathetic to thoracic and abdominal viscera.

The vagus nerve arises by a series of rootlets from the lateral aspect of the medulla that merge and leave the cranium through the jugular foramen positioned between CN IX and CN XI (Fig. 9.13). What was formerly called "the cranial root of the accessory nerve" is actually a part of CN X. CN X has a **superior ganglion** in the jugular foramen that is mainly concerned with the general sensory component of the nerve. Inferior to the foramen is an **inferior ganglion** (nodose ganglion) concerned with the visceral sensory components of the nerve. In the region of the superior ganglion are connections to CN IX and the superior cervical (sympathetic) ganglion. CN X continues inferiorly in the carotid sheath to the root of the neck, supplying branches to the palate, pharynx, and larynx (Fig. 9.14; Table 9.4).

The course CN X in the thorax differs on the two sides. CN X supplies branches to the heart, bronchi, and lungs. The vagi join the *esophageal plexus* surrounding the

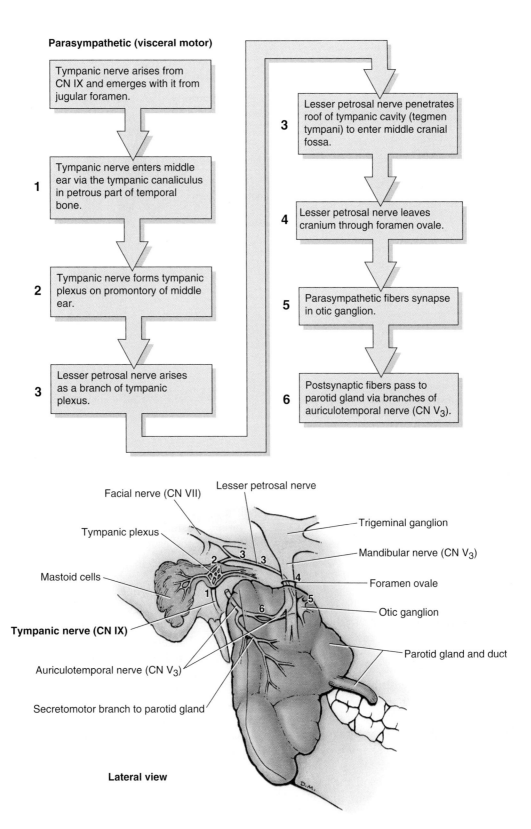

Parasympathetic (visceral motor)

Tympanic nerve arises from CN IX and emerges with it from jugular foramen.

1 Tympanic nerve enters middle ear via the tympanic canaliculus in petrous part of temporal bone.

2 Tympanic nerve forms tympanic plexus on promontory of middle ear.

3 Lesser petrosal nerve arises as a branch of tympanic plexus.

3 Lesser petrosal nerve penetrates roof of tympanic cavity (tegmen tympani) to enter middle cranial fossa.

4 Lesser petrosal nerve leaves cranium through foramen ovale.

5 Parasympathetic fibers synapse in otic ganglion.

6 Postsynaptic fibers pass to parotid gland via branches of auriculotemporal nerve (CN V₃).

Facial nerve (CN VII)
Lesser petrosal nerve
Tympanic plexus
Trigeminal ganglion
Mandibular nerve (CN V₃)
Mastoid cells
Foramen ovale
Otic ganglion
Tympanic nerve (CN IX)
Parotid gland and duct
Auriculotemporal nerve (CN V₃)
Secretomotor branch to parotid gland

Lateral view

Figure 9.12. Parasympathetic innervation involving glossopharyngeal nerve (CN IX).

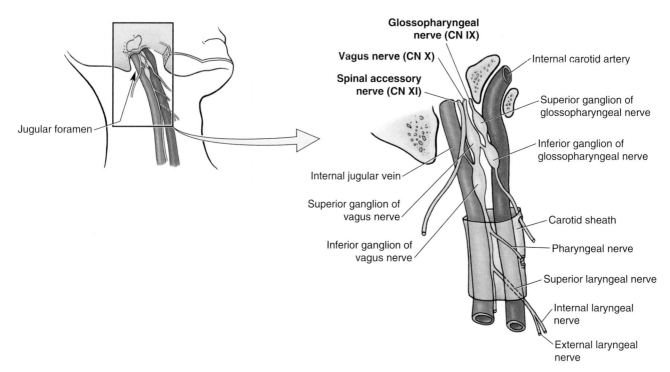

Figure 9.13. Relationship of structures traversing jugular foramen. CN IX, CN X, and CN XI are in numerical order, anterior to the internal jugular vein.

Lesions of the Vagus Nerve

Isolated lesions of CN X are uncommon. Injury to the pharyngeal branches of CN X results in *dysphagia* (difficulty in swallowing). Lesions of the superior laryngeal nerve produce anesthesia of the superior part of the larynx and paralysis of the cricothyroid muscle. The voice is weak and tires easily. Injury of a recurrent laryngeal nerve may be caused by aneurysms of the arch of the aorta and may occur during neck operations. Injury of the recurrent laryngeal nerve causes *hoarseness* and *dysphonia* (difficulty in speaking) because of paralysis of the vocal folds (cords). Paralysis of both recurrent laryngeal nerves causes *aphonia* (loss of voice) and *inspiratory stridor* (a harsh, high pitched respiratory sound). Because of its longer course, lesions of the left recurrent laryngeal nerve are more common than those of the right. Proximal lesions of CN X also affect the pharyngeal and superior laryngeal nerves, causing difficulty in swallowing and speaking.

esophagus, which is formed by branches of the vagi and sympathetic trunks. This plexus follows the esophagus through the diaphragm into the abdomen, where the **anterior** and **posterior vagal trunks** break up into branches that innervate the esophagus, stomach, and intestinal tract as far as the left colic flexure (Fig. 9.14).

Spinal Accessory Nerve (CN XI)

The spinal accessory nerve (CN XI) is motor to the sternocleidomastoid (SCM) and trapezius muscles (Fig. 9.15). The traditional "cranial root" of CN XI is actually a part of CN X. CN XI emerges as a series of rootlets from the first five or six cervical segments of the spinal cord (Lachman et al., 2002). It joins CN X temporarily as they pass through the jugular foramen, separating again as they exit (Fig. 9.11). CN XI descends along the internal carotid artery, penetrates and innervates the SCM, and emerges from the muscle near the middle of its posterior border. It crosses the posterior cervical region and passes deep to the superior border of the trapezius to innervate it. Branches of the cervical plexus conveying sensory fibers from spinal nerves C2–C4 join the spinal accessory nerve in the posterior cervical region, providing these muscles with pain and proprioceptive fibers.

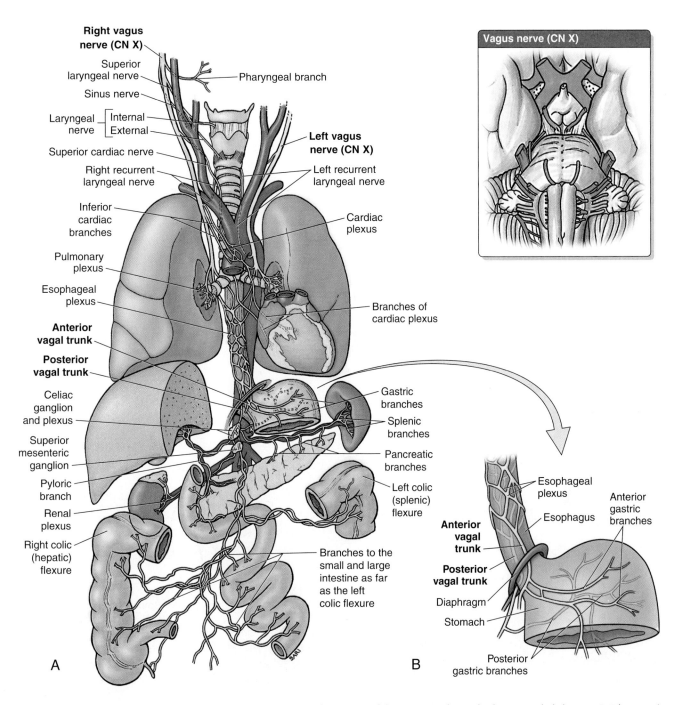

Figure 9.14. Distribution of vagus nerves (CN X). A. Observe the course of the nerves in the neck, thorax, and abdomen. **B.** The anterior and posterior vagal trunks are shown.

Table 9.4 Summary of Vagus Nerve (CN X)

Divisions (Parts)	Branches
Cranial Vagi arise by a series of rootlets from medulla (includes traditional cranial root of CN XI)	Meningeal branch to dura mater (sensory; actually fibers of C2 spinal ganglion neurons that hitch a ride with vagus nerve) Auricular branch
Cervical Exit cranium/enter neck through jugular foramen; right and left vagus nerves enter carotid sheaths and continue to root of neck	Pharyngeal branches to pharyngeal plexus (motor) Cervical cardiac branches (parasympathetic, visceral afferent) Superior laryngeal nerve (mixed), internal (sensory) and external (motor) branches Right recurrent laryngeal nerve (mixed)
Thoracic Vagi enter thorax through superior thoracic aperture; left vagus contributes to anterior esophageal plexus; right vagus to posterior plexus; form anterior and posterior trunks	Left recurrent laryngeal nerve (mixed; all distal branches convey parasympathetic and visceral afferent fibers for reflex stimuli) Thoracic cardiac branches Pulmonary branches Esophageal plexus
Abdominal Anterior and posterior vagal trunks enter abdomen through esophageal hiatus in diaphragm; distribute asymmetrically	Esophageal branches Gastric branches Hepatic branches Celiac branches (from posterior trunk) Pyloric branch (from anterior trunk) Renal branches Intestinal branches (to left colic flexure)

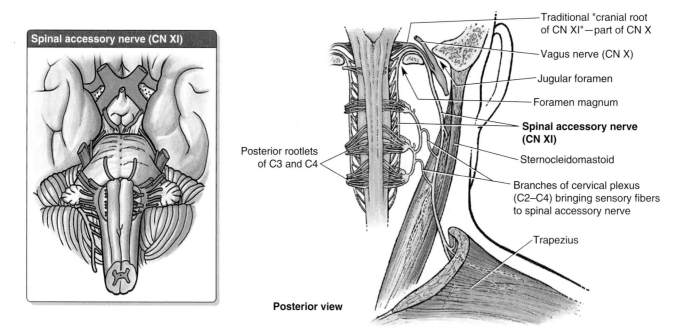

Figure 9.15. Distribution of spinal accessory nerve (CN XI).

Hypoglossal Nerve (CN XII)

The **hypoglossal nerve** (CN XII) is motor to intrinsic and extrinsic muscles of the tongue (styloglossus, hyoglossus, genioglossus). The hypoglossal nerve arises as a purely motor nerve by several rootlets from the medulla and leaves the cranium through the *hypoglossal canal* (Fig. 9.2A). After exiting the cranial cavity, the nerve is joined by a branch or branches of the cervical plexus (Fig. 9.16), conveying general somatic motor fibers from C1 and C2 spinal nerves and general somatic sensory fibers from the spinal ganglion of C2. These spinal nerve fibers "hitch a ride" with CN XII to reach the hyoid muscles, with some of the sensory fibers passing retrograde along it to reach the dura mater of the posterior cranial fossa. CN XII passes inferiorly medial to the angle of the mandible and then curves anteriorly to enter the tongue.

CN XII ends in many branches that supply all the extrinsic muscles of the tongue, except the palatoglossus

Injury to the Spinal Accessory Nerve

Because of its nearly subcutaneous passage through the posterior cervical region, CN XI is susceptible to injury during surgical procedures such as lymph node biopsy, cannulation of the internal jugular vein, and carotid endarterectomy. Lesions of CN XI produce weakness and atrophy of the trapezius and impairment of rotary movements of the neck and chin to the opposite side as a result of weakness of the SCM. Weakness of shrugging movements of the shoulder is the result of weakness of the trapezius.

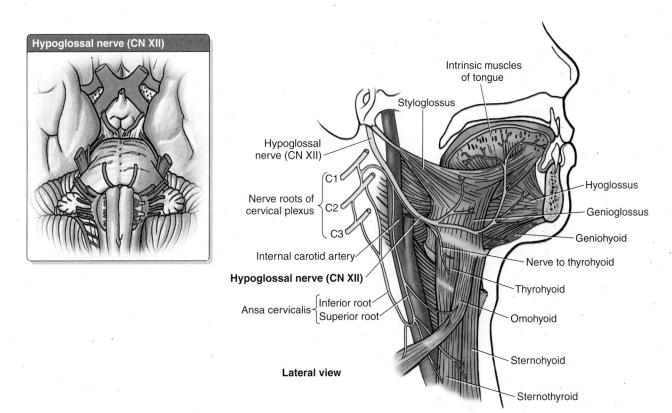

Figure 9.16. Distribution of hypoglossal nerve (CN XII).

Injury to the Hypoglossal Nerve

Injury to CN XII paralyzes the ipsilateral half of the tongue. After some time, the tongue atrophies, making it appear shrunken and wrinkled. When the tongue is protruded, its apex deviates toward the paralyzed side because of the unopposed action of the genioglossus muscle on the normal side of the tongue.

(which is actually a palatine muscle). CN XII has the following branches:

- A **meningeal branch** returns to the cranium through the hypoglossal canal and innervates the dura mater on the floor and posterior wall of the posterior cranial fossa. The nerve fibers conveyed are from the sensory spinal ganglion of spinal nerve C2, not from CN XII.
- The **superior root of the ansa cervicalis** branches from CN XII to supply the infrahyoid muscles (sternohyoid, sternothyroid, and omohyoid). This branch actually conveys only fibers from the cervical plexus (loop between the anterior rami of C1 and C2) that joined the nerve outside the cranial cavity. Some fibers reach the thyrohyoid muscle.
- Terminal **lingual branches** supply the styloglossus, hyoglossus, genioglossus, and intrinsic muscles of the tongue.

Figure Credits

All sources are published by Lippincott Williams & Wilkins, unless otherwise indicated.

Introduction

i.7: Moore KL, Dalley AF. *Clinically Oriented Anatomy,* 5th ed., 2006, i.15.

i.12*E* & *F:* Moore KL, Dalley AF. *Clinically Oriented Anatomy,* 5th ed., 2006, i.23.

i.16*B:* Based on Moore KL, Dalley AF. *Clinically Oriented Anatomy,* 5th ed., 2006, i.28A.

i.*22:* Moore KL, Dalley AF. *Clinically Oriented Anatomy,* 5th ed., 2006, I.38.

i.24: Moore KL, Dalley AF. *Clinically Oriented Anatomy,* 5th ed., 2006, i.40.

i.25: Moore KL, Dalley AF. *Clinically Oriented Anatomy,* 5th ed., 2006, i.41.

i.29*B:* Wicke L. *Atlas of Radiologic Anatomy,* 6th English ed., Ed. and Trans. AN Taylor, 1998. [Originally published, Wicke L. *Roentgen-Anatomie Normalbefunde,* 5th ed. Munich: Urban & Schwarzenberg, 1995.]

i.29*C:* Courtesy of E. Becker, University of Toronto, Canada.

i.30*B:* Courtesy of AM Arenson, University of Toronto, Canada.

i.30*C:* Wicke L. *Atlas of Radiologic Anatomy,* 6th English ed, Ed. and Trans. AN Taylor, 1998. [Originally published, Wicke L. *Roentgen-Anatomie Normalbefunde,* 5th ed. Munich: Urban & Schwarzenberg, 1995.]

i.31*A:* Moore KL. *Clinically Oriented Anatomy,* 3rd ed., 1992, 1.30.

i.31*B:* Dean D, Herbener TE. *Cross-Sectional Human Anatomy,* 2000.

i.32: Posner MI, Raichle M. *Images of Mind.* New York: Scientific American Library, 1994.

Bi.1: Willis MC. *Medical Terminology: The Language of Health Care,* 1995.

Bi.2: *Roche Lexicon Medizin,* 4th ed. Munich: Urban and Schwarzenberg, 1998.

Chapter 1

1.6*D* & *E:* Moore KL, Dalley AF. *Clinically Oriented Anatomy,* 5th ed., 2006,1.9*D* & *E.*

1.16: Courtesy of DE Sanders, University of Toronto, Canada.

1.17*A–C:* Moore KL, Dalley AF. *Clinically Oriented Anatomy,* 5th ed., 2006, 1.28*B, C,* & *D.*

1.19: Moore KL, Dalley AF. *Clinically Oriented Anatomy,* 5th ed., 2006, 1.30.

1.20*A* & *B:* Based on Moore KL, Dalley AF. *Clinically Oriented Anatomy,* 5th ed., 2006, 1.62 and 1.64.

1.22*A:* Moore KL, Dalley AF. *Clinically Oriented Anatomy,* 5th ed., 2006, 1.38.

1.23: Moore KL, Dalley AF. *Clinically Oriented Anatomy,* 5th ed., 2006, 1.36.

1.24*A–F:* Moore KL, Dalley AF. *Clinically Oriented Anatomy,* 5th ed., 2006, 1.39.

1.25*A* & *B:* Moore KL, Dalley AF. *Clinically Oriented Anatomy,* 5th ed., 2006, 1.40.

1.26*A:* Courtesy of MA Haider, University of Toronto, Canada.

1.26*B:* Moore KL, Dalley AF. *Clinically Oriented Anatomy,* 5th ed., 2006, 1.67*A* & *B.*

1.32*A* & *B:* Agur AMR, Dalley AF. *Grant's Atlas of Anatomy,* 11th ed., 2005, 1.45*A* & *B.*

1.33*A* & *B:* Agur AMR, Dalley AF. *Grant's Atlas of Anatomy,* 11th ed., 2005, 1.46*A* & *B.*

1.37*A:* Moore KL, Dalley AF. *Clinically Oriented Anatomy,* 5th ed., 2006, 1.58*A* & *B*(2).

1.39*A* & key: Agur AMR, Dalley AF. *Grant's Atlas of Anatomy,* 11th ed., 2005, 1.72

1.43: Moore KL, Dalley AF. *Clinically Oriented Anatomy,* 5th ed., 2006, 1.62.

1.44: Dean D, Herbener TE. *Cross-Sectional Human Anatomy,* 2000, 2.7.

1.45*A–C:* Agur AMR, Dalley AF. *Grant's Atlas of Anatomy,* 11th ed., 2005, 1.47; photos courtesy of I. Morrow, University of Manitoba, Canada.

1.46*A–F:* Photos from Madden ME. *Introduction to Sectional Anatomy,* 2001, 2.37*B,* 2.38*B,* 2.39*B,* 2.40*B,* 2.42*B,* and 2.43*B.*

SA1.1*A–C:* Moore KL, Dalley AF. *Clinically Oriented Anatomy,* 5th ed., 2006, SA1.3.

SA1.2: Moore KL, Dalley AF. *Clinically Oriented Anatomy,* 5th ed., 2006, SA1.6.

SA1.5: Moore KL, Dalley AF. *Clinically Oriented Anatomy,* 5th ed., 2006, SA1.7.

Table 1.5: Moore KL, Dalley AF. *Clinically Oriented Anatomy,* 5th ed., 2006, 1.35*D.*

B1.1*A* & *B:* Moore KL, Dalley AF. *Clinically Oriented Anatomy,* 5th ed., 2006, B1.2.

B1.2: Moore KL, Dalley AF. *Clinically Oriented Anatomy,* 5th ed., 2006, B1.5.

B1.4: Moore KL, Dalley AF. *Clinically Oriented Anatomy,* 5th ed., 2006, B1.3.

B1.5: Moore KL, Dalley AF. *Clinically Oriented Anatomy,* 5th ed., 2006, B1.4.

B1.9: Moore KL, Dalley AF. *Clinically Oriented Anatomy,* 5th ed., 2006, 1.34B.

B1.10: Moore KL, Dalley AF. *Clinically Oriented Anatomy,* 5th ed., 2006, B1.15.

B1.11: Moore KL, Dalley AF. *Clinically Oriented Anatomy,* 5th ed., 2006, B1.20B.

Chapter 2

2.8*B:* Moore KL, Dalley AF. *Clinically Oriented Anatomy,* 5th ed., 2006, 2.15.

2.9: Agur AMR. *Grant's Atlas of Anatomy,* 9th ed., 1991, 2.27.

2.15*C,* right: Courtesy of EL Landsdown, University of Toronto, Canada.

2.22: Moore KL, Dalley AF. *Clinically Oriented Anatomy,* 5th ed., 2006, 2.22.

2.23*C:* Courtesy of GB Haber, University of Toronto, Canada.

2.26: Moore KL, Dalley AF. *Clinically Oriented Anatomy,* 5th ed., 2006, 2.50.

2.27*A:* Agur AMR, Dalley AF. *Grant's Atlas of Anatomy,* 11th ed., 2005, 2.53.

2.27*B–E:* Agur AMR, Dalley AF. *Grant's Atlas of Anatomy,* 11th ed., 2005, 2.53.

2.28: Moore KL, Dalley AF. *Clinically Oriented Anatomy,* 5th ed., 2006, 2.54.

2.29*A:* Moore KL, Dalley AF. *Clinically Oriented Anatomy,* 5th ed., 2006, 2.53*A.*

2.29*C:* Courtesy of GB Haber, University of Toronto, Canada.

2.32: Agur AMR. *Grant's Atlas of Anatomy,* 9th ed., 1991, 2.108.

2.36*A* & *B:* Moore KL, Dalley AF. *Clinically Oriented Anatomy,* 5th ed., 2006, 2.65 and 2.68.

2.37: Moore KL, Dalley AF. *Clinically Oriented Anatomy,* 5th ed., 2006, 2.12.

2.38: Moore KL, Dalley AF. *Clinically Oriented Anatomy,* 5th ed., 2006, 2.69.

2.35: Agur AMR, Dalley AF. *Grant's Atlas of Anatomy,* 11th ed., 2005, 2.66*D.*

2.46*A–C:* Courtesy of MA Haider, University of Toronto, Canada.

2.46*D–E:* Courtesy of MA Haider, University of Toronto, Canada.

2.47: Courtesy of Tom White, Department of Radiology, The Health Sciences Center, University of Tennessee, Memphis.

2.48: Courtesy of AM Arenson, University of Toronto, Canada.

2.49*A:* Courtesy of M Asch, University of Toronto, Canada.

2.49*B:* Dean D, Herbener TE. *Cross-Sectional Human Anatomy,* 2000.

2.49*C:* Courtesy of CS Ho, University of Toronto, Canada.

SA2.1*A:* LWW Surface anatomy photo collection.

SA2.2: LWW Surface anatomy photo collection.

SA2.4: LWW Surface anatomy photo collection.

B2.2: Moore KL, Dalley AF. *Clinically Oriented Anatomy,* 5th ed., 2006, B2.1.

B2.3*A–E:* Moore KL, Dalley AF. *Clinically Oriented Anatomy,* 5th ed., 2006, 2.13 and 2.14.

B2.4: Moore KL, Dalley AF. *Clinically Oriented Anatomy,* 5th ed., 2006, B2.4*A* & *C.*

B2.5: Moore KL, Dalley AF. *Clinically Oriented Anatomy,* 5th ed., 2006, 2.3*D.*

B2.6*A–E:* Moore KL, Dalley AF. *Clinically Oriented Anatomy,* 5th ed., 2006, B2.14.

B2.7: *Roche Lexicon Medzin,* 4th ed. Munich: Urban & Schwarzenberg, 1998.

B2.8*C: Roche Lexicon Medzin,* 3rd ed. Munich: Urban & Schwarzenberg, 1993.

Chapter 3

3.1: Moore KL, Dalley AF. *Clinically Oriented Anatomy,* 5th ed., 2006, 3.1.

3.2: Moore KL, Dalley AF. *Clinically Oriented Anatomy,* 5th ed., 2006, 3.2.

3.4*A* & *B:* Moore KL, Dalley AF. *Clinically Oriented Anatomy,* 5th ed., 2006, 4.27 and 4.28.

3.4*C:* Moore KL, Dalley AF. *Clinically Oriented Anatomy,* 5th ed., 2006, 3.4*C.*

3.6: Moore KL, Dalley AF. *Clinically Oriented Anatomy,* 5th ed., 2006, 3.10*B.*

3.12: Moore KL, Dalley AF. *Clinically Oriented Anatomy,* 5th ed., 2006, 3.19.

3.14*B:* Courtesy of AM Arenson, University of Toronto, Canada.

3.20*B* & *D:* Courtesy of AM Arenson, University of Toronto, Canada.

3.23: Moore KL, Dalley AF. *Clinically Oriented Anatomy,* 5th ed., 2006, 3.36.

3.26: Moore KL, Dalley AF. *Clinically Oriented Anatomy,* 5th ed., 2006, 3.41*B* & *C.*

3.27*A* & *B:* Agur AMR. *Grant's Atlas of Anatomy,* 9th ed., 1991, 3.60*B* & *C.*

3.32*A* & *B:* Moore KL, Dalley AF. *Clinically Oriented Anatomy,* 5th ed., 2006, 3.47 & 3.51.

3.34*B:* Moore KL, Dalley AF. *Clinically Oriented Anatomy,* 5th ed., 2006, 3.56.

3.35*A–E:* Courtesy of MA Haider, University of Toronto, Canada.

3.36*A–D:* Courtesy of MA Haider, University of Toronto, Canada.

Table 3.1*A* & *B:* Moore KL, Dalley AF. *Clinically Oriented Anatomy,* 5th ed., 2006, Table 3.1.

Table 3.3: Moore KL, Dalley AF. *Clinically Oriented Anatomy,* 5th ed., 2006, Table 3.3.

B3.1: Moore KL, Dalley AF. *Clinically Oriented Anatomy,* 5th ed., 2006, B3.24*B.*

B3.2: Moore KL, Dalley AF. *Clinically Oriented Anatomy,* 5th ed., 2006, B3.7.

B3.3: Moore KL, Dalley AF. *Clinically Oriented Anatomy,* 5th ed., 2006, B3.9.

B3.4*A:* Moore KL, Dalley AF. *Clinically Oriented Anatomy,* 5th ed., 2006, B3.14*B.*

B3.5: Moore KL, Dalley AF. *Clinically Oriented Anatomy,* 5th ed., 2006, B3.18.

B3.6: Photo courtesy of RE Bristow, Johns Hopkins School of Medicine, Baltimore, MD.

B3.7: Moore KL, Dalley AF. *Clinically Oriented Anatomy,* 5th ed., 2006, B3.25.

B3.8: Moore KL, Dalley AF. *Clinically Oriented Anatomy,* 5th ed., 2006, B3.26*A.*

B3.9: Moore KL, Dalley AF. *Clinically Oriented Anatomy,* 5th ed., 2006, B3.26*B.*

B3.10: Moore KL, Dalley AF. *Clinically Oriented Anatomy,* 5th ed., 2006, B3.29.

Chapter 4

4.2*A–D:* Based on Moore KL, Dalley AF. *Clinically Oriented Anatomy,* 5th ed., 2006, 4.2.

4.3*D–F:* Based on Moore KL, Dalley AF. *Clinically Oriented Anatomy,* 5th ed., 2006, 4.9*B–D.*

4.14*C–E:* Based on Olson TR. *Student Atlas of Anatomy,* 1998.

4.15*D* & *E:* Based on Moore KL, Dalley AF. *Clinically Oriented Anatomy,* 5th ed., 2006, Table 4.7.

4.17*B:* Agur AMR, Dalley AF. *Grant's Atlas of Anatomy,* 11th ed., 2005.

4.18*A* & *B:* Agur AMR, Dalley AF. *Grant's Atlas of Anatomy,* 11th ed., 2005, 4.52*C.*

4.18*C:* Moore KL, Dalley AF. *Clinically Oriented Anatomy,* 5th ed., 2006, 4.39.

SA4.1*A–C:* LWW Surface anatomy photo collection.

SA4.2: LWW Surface anatomy photo collection.

Table 4.1*A* & *B:* Based on Agur AMR, Dalley AF. *Grant's Atlas of Anatomy,* 11th ed., 2005.

Table 4.1*C* & *D:* Agur AMR. *Grant's Atlas of Anatomy,* 9th ed., 1991, p. 211.

Table 4.2*A–C:* Agur AMR, Dalley AF. *Grant's Atlas of Anatomy,* 11th ed., 2005.

Table 4.3*A–D:* Moore KL, Dalley AF. *Clinically Oriented Anatomy,* 5th ed., 2006, Table 4.3.

Table 4.4*A–D:* Moore KL, Dalley AF. *Clinically Oriented Anatomy,* 5th ed., 2006, 4.5*A, C,* & *D.*

Table 4.7*A–D:* Moore KL, Dalley AF. *Clinically Oriented Anatomy,* 5th ed., 2006, Table 4.8*A–D.*

Table 4.8*A–E:* Moore KL, Dalley AF. *Clinically Oriented Anatomy,* 5th ed., 2006, Table 4.9*A–E.*

Table 4.9*A–D:* Moore KL, Dalley AF. *Clinically Oriented Anatomy,* 5th ed., 2006, Table 4.11.

Table 4.10: Moore KL, Dalley AF. *Clinically Oriented Anatomy,* 5th ed., 2006, Table 4.12.

B4.1: Moore KL, Dalley AF. *Clinically Oriented Anatomy,* 5th ed., 2006, B4.16*A–E.*

B4.2: Moore KL, Dalley AF. *Clinically Oriented Anatomy,* 5th ed., 2006, B4.1.

B4.3*A–C:* Moore KL, Dalley AF. *Clinically Oriented Anatomy,* 5th ed., 2006, B4.14, B4.15, B4.3.

B4.4*A* & *B:* Moore KL, Dalley AF. *Clinically Oriented Anatomy,* 5th ed., 2006, B4.10*A–C.*

B4.5*A* & *B:* Based on Moore KL, Dalley AF. *Clinically Oriented Anatomy,* 5th ed., 2006, B4.6.

Chapter 5

5.1*B:* Moore KL, Dalley AF. *Clinically Oriented Anatomy,* 5th ed., 2006, 5.14 and 5.3.

5.3*A–C:* Moore KL, Dalley AF. *Clinically Oriented Anatomy,* 5th ed., 2006, 5.6*A* & *B.*

5.7*A* & *B:* Moore KL, Dalley AF. *Clinically Oriented Anatomy,* 5th ed., 2006, 5.10*C* & *D.*

5.8*B:* Agur AMR, Dalley AF. *Grant's Atlas of Anatomy,* 11th ed., 2005, 5.6.

5.10*A:* LWW Anatomy Photo Collection.

5.10*G:* Moore KL, Dalley AF. *Clinically Oriented Anatomy,* 5th ed., 2006, Table 5.3.

5.11*C:* Moore KL, Dalley AF. *Clinically Oriented Anatomy,* 5th ed., 2006, Table 5.4.

5.12*B:* Moore KL, Dalley AF. *Clinically Oriented Anatomy,* 5th ed., 2006, 5.20*A.*

5.15*A* & *B:* LWW Anatomy Photo Collection.

5.15*D* & *E:* Moore KL, Dalley AF. *Clinically Oriented Anatomy,* 5th ed., 2006, Table 5.6*A* & *B.*

5.16*A:* LWW Anatomy Photo Collection.

5.16*B:* Moore KL, Dalley AF. *Clinically Oriented Anatomy,* 5th ed., 2006, Table 5.7*A.*

5.19*A* & *B:* LWW Anatomy Photo Collection.

5.21*B:* Moore KL, Dalley AF. *Clinically Oriented Anatomy,* 5th ed., 2006, SA5.3*C.*

5.21*C:* LWW Anatomy Photo Collection.

5.22*B:* LWW Anatomy Photo Collection.

5.23*A:* LWW Anatomy Photo Collection.

5.26: Moore KL, Dalley AF. *Clinically Oriented Anatomy,* 5th ed., 2006, 5.43*C.*

5.27*D:* Moore KL, Dalley AF. *Clinically Oriented Anatomy,* 5th ed., 2006, 5.14-II*B.*

5.28*A:* Moore KL, Dalley AF. *Clinically Oriented Anatomy,* 5th ed., 2006, 5.50*A.*

5.28*B:* Agur AMR, Dalley AF. *Grant's Atlas of Anatomy,* 11th ed., 2005, 5.32*A.*

5.29*C:* Moore KL, Dalley AF. *Clinically Oriented Anatomy,* 5th ed., 2006, 5.52*B.*

5.34*B:* Agur AMR, Dalley AF. *Grant's Atlas of Anatomy,* 11th ed., 2005, 5.50*B.*

5.36: Clay JH, Pounds DM. *Basic Clinical Massage Therapy,* 2002, Plate 10-1.

5.40: Moore KL, Dalley AF. *Clinically Oriented Anatomy,* 5th ed., 2006, 5.70*A.*

5.41*A* & *B:* Courtesy of P. Bobechko, University of Toronto, Canada.

5.43: Courtesy of D. Salonen, University of Toronto, Canada.

5.42: Wicke L. *Atlas of Radiologic Anatomy,* 6th English ed. Ed. and Trans. AN Taylor, 1998. [Originally published, Wicke L. *Roentgen-Anatomie Normalbefunde,* 5th ed. Munich: Urban & Schwarzenberg, 1995.]

SA5.1*A:* Moore KL, Dalley AF. *Clinically Oriented Anatomy,* 5th ed., 2006, SA5.1*A.*

SA5.1*B* & *C:* Moore KL, Dalley AF. *Clinically Oriented Anatomy,* 5th ed., 2006, SA 5.1*C* & *D.*

Table 5.8*A* & *B:* Moore KL, Dalley AF. *Clinically Oriented Anatomy,* 5th ed., 2006, Table 5.11.

T5.9*A* & *B:* Moore KL, Dalley AF. *Clinically Oriented Anatomy,* 5th ed., 2006, Table 5.12.

Table 5.13: Moore KL, Dalley AF. *Clinically Oriented Anatomy,* 5th ed., 2006, Table 5.15.

Table 5.15: Moore KL, Dalley AF. *Clinically Oriented Anatomy,* 5th ed., 2006, Table 5.2.

Table 5.20: Clay JH, Pounds DM. *Basic Clinical Massage Therapy,* 2002: Plate 10-1.

B5.1*A–C:* Moore KL, Dalley AF. *Clinically Oriented Anatomy,* 5th ed., 2006, B5.3.

B5.6: Moore KL, Dalley AF. *Clinically Oriented Anatomy,* 5th ed., 2006, B5.23.

B5.7*A–C:* Moore KL, Dalley AF. *Clinically Oriented Anatomy,* 5th ed., 2006, B5.25.

B5.8*D–E:* Moore KL, Dalley AF. *Clinically Oriented Anatomy,* 5th ed., 2006, B5.28.

B5.10*A:* Moore KL, Dalley AF. *Clinically Oriented Anatomy,* 5th ed., 2006, B5.34*A.*

Chapter 6

6.1: Moore KL, Dalley AF. *Clinically Oriented Anatomy,* 5th ed., 2006, 6.1.

6.7: Adapted from Moore KL, Dalley AF. *Clinically Oriented Anatomy,* 5th ed., 2006, 6.10*A.*

6.11: Moore KL, Dalley AF. *Clinically Oriented Anatomy,* 5th ed., 2006, 6.24*A.*

6.13: Moore KL, Dalley AF. *Clinically Oriented Anatomy,* 5th ed., 2006, 6.27*C.*

6.32*A:* Courtesy of EL Landsdown, University of Toronto, Canada.

6.33*A:* Courtesy of E Becker, University of Toronto, Canada.

6.37*A:* Courtesy of J. Heslin, University of Toronto, Canada.

6.37*B:* Courtesy of D. Armstrong, University of Toronto, Canada.

6.38*A* & *B:* Dean D, Herbener TE. *Cross-Sectional Human Anatomy,* 2000: Plate 7-8.

6.39: Courtesy of W. Kucharczyk, University of Toronto, Canada.

SA6.1*A:* Moore KL, Dalley AF. *Clinically Oriented Anatomy,* 5th ed., 2006, SA6.1.

SA6.3*A* & *B:* Moore KL, Dalley AF. *Clinically Oriented Anatomy,* 5th ed., 2006, SA6.8 and SA6.9.

SA6.4*A:* Moore KL, Dalley AF. *Clinically Oriented Anatomy,* 5th ed., 2006, 6.13.

SA6.4*C* & *D:* Moore KL, Dalley AF. *Clinically Oriented Anatomy,* 5th ed., 2006, SA6.16 and SA6.17.

SA6.4*B:* Moore KL, Dalley AF. *Clinically Oriented Anatomy,* 5th ed., 2006, SA6.15.

Table 6.1: Adapted from Moore KL, Dalley AF. *Clinically Oriented Anatomy,* 5th ed., 2006, Table 6.1.

Table 6.3: Adapted from Moore KL, Dalley AF. *Clinically Oriented Anatomy,* 5th ed., 2006, Table 6.2.

Table 6.4: Adapted from Moore KL, Dalley AF. *Clinically Oriented Anatomy,* 5th ed., 2006, Table 6.4.

Table 6.6: Adapted from Moore KL, Dalley AF. *Clinically Oriented Anatomy,* 5th ed., 2006, Table 6.6*A* & *B.*

Table 6.9: Moore KL, Dalley AF. *Clinically Oriented Anatomy,* 5th ed., 2006, Table 6.10.

Table 6.10: Moore KL, Dalley AF. *Clinically Oriented Anatomy,* 5th ed., 2006, Table 6.9.

Table 6.11: Moore KL, Dalley AF. *Clinically Oriented Anatomy,* 5th ed., 2006, Table 6.11.

Table 6.12: Moore KL, Dalley AF. *Clinically Oriented Anatomy,* 5th ed., 2006, Table 6.12.

Table 6.15: Photo courtesy of W. Kucharczyk, University of Toronto, Canada.

B6.4: Moore KL, Dalley AF. *Clinically Oriented Anatomy,* 5th ed., 2006, B6.4.

B6.5: Rowland LP. *Merritt's Textbook of Neurology,* 9th ed., 1995.

B6.7: Anderson MK, Hall SJ, Martin M. *Foundations of Athletic Training,* 3rd ed., 1995.

B6.8: Moore KL, Dalley AF. *Clinically Oriented Anatomy,* 5th ed., 2006, B6.15.

B6.11*A* & *B*: Moore KL, Dalley AF. *Clinically Oriented Anatomy,* 5th ed., 2006, B6.19*A* and B6.21.

B6.14*A* & *B*: Moore KL, Dalley AF. *Clinically Oriented Anatomy,* 5th ed., 2006, B6.29*E* & *F*.

B6.17: Moore KL, Dalley AF. *Clinically Oriented Anatomy,* 5th ed., 2006, B6.33.

B6.18: Moore KL, Dalley AF. *Clinically Oriented Anatomy,* 5th ed., 2006, B6.36.

Chapter 7

7.8: Agur AMR, Dalley AF. *Grant's Atlas of Anatomy,* 11th ed., 2005, 7.26*B, C,* & *F*.

7.15*A* & *B*: LWW Surface Anatomy Photo Collection.

7.16*A:* Courtesy of W. Kucharczyk, University of Toronto, Canada;

7.16*B*: Agur AMR, Dalley AF. *Grant's Atlas of Anatomy,* 11th ed., 2005, 7.39*C*.

7.16*C:* Moore KL, Dalley AF. *Clinically Oriented Anatomy,* 5th ed., 2006, 7.23*A*.

7.17*A* & *B*: LWW Surface Anatomy Photo Collection.

7.22*A* & *B*: Moore KL, Dalley AF. *Clinically Oriented Anatomy,* 5th ed., 2006, 7.40.

7.22*C*: Agur AMR, Dalley AF. *Grant's Atlas of Anatomy,* 11th ed., 2005, 7.44*F*.

7.25*A* & *B*: Agur AMR, Dalley AF. *Grant's Atlas of Anatomy,* 11th ed., 2005, 7.48*A* and 7.49*A*.

7.28: Moore KL, Dalley AF. *Clinically Oriented Anatomy,* 5th ed., 2006, 7.45.

7.36*A:* Moore KL, Dalley AF. *Clinically Oriented Anatomy,* 5th ed., 2006, 7.60.

7.39*C:* Agur AMR, Dalley AF. *Grant's Atlas of Anatomy,* 11th ed., 2005, Table 9.7.

7.40*C:* Courtesy of D. Armstrong, University of Toronto, Canada.

7.41*A:* LWW Surface Anatomy Photo Collection.

7.42*A* & *B:* Moore KL, Dalley AF. *Clinically Oriented Anatomy,* 5th ed., 2006, 7.73*A* & *B;* photo courtesy of Welch Allen, Inc., Skaneateles, NY.

7.48*A* & *B:* Courtesy of E. Becker, University of Toronto, Canada.

7.48*C:* Courtesy of D. Armstrong, University of Toronto, Canada.

7.50*A:* Photo courtesy of W. Kucharcyzk, University of Toronto, Canada.

7.50*B:* Photo courtesy of D. Armstrong, University of Toronto, Canada.

Table 7.2*A–C:* Moore KL, Dalley AF. *Clinically Oriented Anatomy,* 5th ed., 2006, 7.3.

Table 7.4: Moore KL, Dalley AF. *Clinically Oriented Anatomy,* 5th ed., 2006, Table 7.5.

Table 7.5: Moore KL, Dalley AF. *Clinically Oriented Anatomy,* 5th ed., 2006, Table 7.6.

Table 7.6: Moore KL, Dalley AF. *Clinically Oriented Anatomy,* 5th ed., 2006, Table 7.8.

Table 7.7: Agur AMR, Dalley AF. *Grant's Atlas of Anatomy,* 11th ed., 2005, Table 7.6.

B7.3: Courtesy of Dr. Gerald S. Smyser, Altru Health System, Grand Forks, ND.

B7.4: Moore KL, Dalley AF. *Clinically Oriented Anatomy,* 5th ed., 2006, B7.15.

B7.6: Moore KL, Dalley AF. *Clinically Oriented Anatomy,* 5th ed., 2006, B7.21.

B7.8*A:* Welch Allen Inc, Skaneateles Falls, NY.

B7.8*B: Roche Lexikon Medzin,* 3rd ed. Auflage, Munich, Germany: Urban & Schwarzenberg, 1998.

Chapter 8

8.1*A–C:* Based on Moore KL, Dalley AF. *Clinically Oriented Anatomy,* 5th ed., 2006, 8.3.

8.2*A–C:* Based on Moore KL, Dalley AF. *Clinically Oriented Anatomy,* 5th ed., 2006, 8.4.

8.3: Based on Moore KL, Dalley AF. *Clinically Oriented Anatomy,* 5th ed., 2006, 8.10.

8.5*C:* Based on Moore KL, Dalley AF. *Clinically Oriented Anatomy,* 5th ed., 2006, 8.18.

8.7*C:* Based on Moore KL, Dalley AF. *Clinically Oriented Anatomy,* 5th ed., 2006, 8.9.

8.10*B:* Based on Moore KL, Dalley AF. *Clinically Oriented Anatomy,* 5th ed., 2006, 8.41*C*.

8.16*A–C:* Biebgott B. *The Anatomical Basis of Dentistry.* Philadelphia: Saunders, 1982, 9.22.

8.19*A* & *B:* Based on Moore KL, Dalley AF. *Clinically Oriented Anatomy,* 5th ed., 2006, 8.41*A* & *B*.

8.21*A:* Courtesy of M. Keller, University of Toronto, Canada.

8.21*B* & *C:* Courtesy of W. Kucharczyk, University of Toronto, Canada.

8.22: Courtesy of Acuson Corp, Mt View, CA.

SA8.1*A–E:* Moore KL, Dalley AF. *Clinically Oriented Anatomy,* 5th ed., 2006, SA8.1*A–D* & *F*.

SA8.2: LWW Surface Anatomy Photo Collection.

Table 8.1A: LWW Surface Anatomy Photo Collection.

Table 8.2*C:* Moore KL, Dalley AF. *Clinically Oriented Anatomy,* 5th ed., 2006, p. 1052.

Table 8.3*A–D:* Moore KL, Dalley AF. *Clinically Oriented Anatomy,* 5th ed., 2006, Table 8.3*A–D*.

Table 8.5: Moore KL, Dalley AF. *Clinically Oriented Anatomy,* 5th ed., 2006, Table 8.5.

B8.4: Moore KL, Dalley AF. *Clinically Oriented Anatomy,* 5th ed., 2006, B8.4.

B8.5: Based on Moore KL, Dalley AF. *Clinically Oriented Anatomy,* 5th ed., 2006, B8.7.

B8.6: Rohen JW, Yokochi C, Lutjen-Drecoll E, Romrell LJ. *Color Atlas of Anatomy: A Photographic Study of the Human Body,* 5th ed., 2002.

B8.7: Moore KL, Dalley AF. *Clinically Oriented Anatomy,* 5th ed., 2006, B8.11.

Chapter 9

9.3: Based on Agur AMR, Dalley AF. *Grant's Atlas of Anatomy,* 11th ed., 2005, 9.3*A* & *B.*

9.5*A:* Based on Agur AMR, Dalley AF. *Grant's Atlas of Anatomy,* 11th ed., 2005, 9.4*A.*

9.5*B:* Based on Agur AMR, Dalley AF. *Grant's Atlas of Anatomy,* 11th ed., 2005, p. 801.

9.7: Based on Moore KL, Dalley AF. *Clinically Oriented Anatomy,* 5th ed., 2006, 9.6.

9.10: Based on Moore KL, Dalley AF. *Clinically Oriented Anatomy,* 5th ed., 2006, 9.8*A* & *B.*

9.13: Based on Moore KL, Dalley AF. *Clinically Oriented Anatomy,* 5th ed., 2006, 9.11.

9.16: Based on Moore KL, Dalley AF. *Clinically Oriented Anatomy,* 5th ed., 2006, 9.15.

Table 9.1: Based on Moore KL, Dalley AF. *Clinically Oriented Anatomy,* 5th ed., 2006, Table 9.1.

References and Suggested Readings

Agur AMR, Dalley AF. *Grant's Atlas of Anatomy,* 11th ed. Baltimore: Lippincott Williams & Wilkins, 2005.

Brust JCM. Coma. *In* Rowland LP (ed), *Merritt's Textbook of Neurology,* 10th ed. Baltimore: Lippincott Williams & Wilkins, 2000.

Callen PW. *Ultrasonography in Obstetrics and Gynecology,* 4th ed. Philadelphia: WB Saunders, 2000.

Cormack DH. *Essential Histology,* 2nd ed. Baltimore: Lippincott Williams & Wilkins, 2001.

Cotran RS, Kumar V, Collins T. *Robbin's Pathologic Basis of Disease,* 6th ed. Philadelphia: WB Saunders, 1999.

Dean DX, Herbener TE. *Cross-Sectional Human Anatomy.* Baltimore: Lippincott Williams & Wilkins, 2002.

Foerster O. The dermatomes in man. Brain 56:1, 1933.

Gartner LP, Hiatt JL. *Color Textbook of Histology,* 2nd ed. Philadelphia: WB Saunders, 2001.

Hardy SGP, Nafrel JP. *Viscerosensory pathways. In* Haines DE (ed). *Fundamental Neuroscience,* 2nd ed. New York: Churchill Livingstone, 2002.

Haines DE. *Neuroanatomy: An Atlas of Structures, Sections, and Systems,* 6th ed. Baltimore: Lippincott Williams & Wilkins, 2004.

Haines DE (ed). *Fundamental Neuroscience,* 2nd ed. New York: Churchill Livingstone, 2002.

Hutchins JB, Naftel JP, Ard MD. The cell biology of neurons and glia. *In* Haines DE (ed). *Fundamental Neuroscience,* 2nd ed. New York: Churchill Livingstone, 2002.

Keegan JJ, Garrett FD. The segmental distribution of the cutaneous nerves in the limbs of man. *Anat Rec* 102:409, 1948.

Lachman N, Acland RD, Rosse C. Anatomical evidence for the absence of a morphologically distinct cranial root of the accessory nerve in man. *Clin Anat* 15:4, 2002.

Mihailoff GA, Haines DE. Motor system II: Corticofugal systems and the control of movement. *In* Haines DE (ed). *Fundamental Neuroscience,* 2nd ed New York: Churchill Livingstone, 2002.

Moore KL, Dalley AF. *Clinically Oriented Anatomy,* 5th ed. Baltimore: Lippincott Williams & Wilkins, 2006.

Moore KL, Persaud TVN. *The Developing Human: Clinically Oriented Embryology,* 7th ed. Philadelphia: WB Saunders, 2003.

Moore KL, Persuad TVN, Shiota K. *Color Atlas of Clinical Embryology,* 2nd ed. Philadelphia: WB Saunders, 2002.

Myers RP, Cahill DR, Devine, RM, King BF. Anatomy of radical prostatectomy as defined by magnetic resonance imaging. *J Urol* 159:2148, 1998a.

Myers RP, King BF, Cahill DR. Deep perineal "space" as defined by magnetic resonance imaging. *Clin Anat* 11:132, 1998b.

Oelrich TM. The urethral sphincter in the male. *Am J Anat* 158:229, 1980.

Oelrich TM. The striated urogenital sphincter muscle in the female. *Anat Rec* 205:223, 1983.

Ross MH, Kaye G, Pawlina W. *Histology. A Text and Atlas,* 5th ed. Baltimore: Lippincott Williams & Wilkins, 2006.

Rowland LP (ed). *Merritt's Neurology,* 11th ed. Baltimore: Lippincott Williams & Wilkins, 2005.

Salter RB. *Textbook of Disorders and Injuries of the Musculoskeletal System,* 3rd ed. Baltimore: Lippincott Williams & Wilkins, 1999.

Swartz MH. *Textbook of Physical Diagnosis, History and Examination,* 4th ed. Philadelphia: WB Saunders, 2002.

Sweazy RD. Olfaction and taste. *In* Haines DE (ed). *Fundamental Neuroscience,* 2nd ed. New York: Churchill Livingstone, 2002.

Tank PW. *Grant's Dissector,* 13th ed. Baltimore: Lippincott Williams & Wilkins, 2005.

Torrent-Guasp F, Buckburg GD, Clemente C, Cox JL, Coghlan HC, Gharib M. The structure and function of the helical heart and its buttress wrapping. I. The normal macroscopic structure of the heart. *Semin Thoracic Cardiovasc Surg* 13:301–319, 2001.

Wendell-Smith C. Muscles and fasciae of the pelvis. *In* Williams PL et al. (eds). *Gray's Anatomy. The Anatomical Basis of Medicine and Surgery,* 38th ed. New York: Churchill Livingstone, 1995.

Wilson-Pauwels L, Akesson EJ, Stuart PA, Spacey SO. *Cranial Nerves in Health and Disease.* Hamilton, ON, Canada: Decker, 2002.

Wilson-Pauwels L, Stuart PA, Akesson EJ. *Autonomic Nerves-Basic Science. Clinical Aspects, Case Studies.* Hamilton, ON, Canada: Decker, 1997.

Index

Page numbers in *italics* denote figures; those followed by t denote tables.